PRAISE FOR A WOMAN'S DECISION

"A timely book that should be read by every woman."

—*The Los Angeles Times*

"This remarkable and informative book...will help women deal with the fear and reality of breast cancer by enabling them to become informed participants in the treatment planning process."

—*Charles M. Balch, MD*

"My doctor gave this book to me, and I read it cover to cover. It was enormously helpful in sorting through my options and understanding the choices that lay before me."

—*J. Pane*

When my sister was diagnosed with breast cancer, I went to the library and researched every book and article I could find on the topic. *A Woman's Decision* was a godsend. It provided information that helped me and my sister understand our risks and sort through our options. Thank you.

—*A. Hansen*

I had a bilateral mastectomy with TRAM flap reconstruction in May. The decisions I had to make were agonizing. This book was the best I found on the subject, and I read and reread the case histories that were closest to my own situation. The information proved to be accurate and gave me a realistic expectation of the process and the results. I recommend this book to anyone undergoing breast surgery, with or without reconstruction, as it covers a wide array of decisions that other women have made.

—*T. Scully*

My plastic surgeon gave me this book to read. It was the best book on breast cancer I've found, and I've built up quite a library lately. It aided me in my treatment decisions as well as my reconstruction choice. It also explained my pathology report better than any of my doctors did. A great book for any breast cancer patient or her family.

—*J. West*

There are many, many books out there dealing with breast cancer and treatment, but this was the only one I could find that really helps a woman decide what course to take if she thinks she wants to have reconstructive surgery. I found it so helpful I recommended it to my doctor. Making a decision to have reconstructive surgery is hard enough, but then you have to decide what type you would like to have, what your choices are depending on your type of cancer and treatment and when to have the surgery. Especially helpful are the black and white photos of the results of each type of operation as well as touching and honest real-life descriptions of experiences by women who have had these types of surgeries. Having actually gone through a mastectomy with simultaneous "TRAM flap" reconstruction, I can attest to the accuracy of both the medical information and the emotional descriptions contained in the book.

—*K. McDonnell*

I thoroughly enjoyed this book! The personal stories of those who have been through breast reconstruction were especially interesting. Each subject discussed their type of reconstruction, why they chose that particular type, their surgery (pain, recovery, and results) and how breast surgery and reconstruction affected their relationships with their mate and family. The rest of the book is filled with so much valuable information on reconstruction procedures and various aspects of breast cancer. I would heartily recommend this book to anyone who is wrestling with the decision to have reconstruction. Even those who are already reconstructed will enjoy this book. They will learn more about the surgical procedures and can compare their experiences with those in the personal stories. Definitely a five-star book!

—*Amazon reviewer*

A *Woman's* DECISION

Breast Care, Treatment, & Reconstruction

A Woman's DECISION

Breast Care, Treatment, & Reconstruction

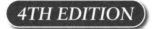

Karen Berger
John Bostwick III, MD
Glyn Jones, MD

Quality Medical Publishing, Inc.

ST. LOUIS, MISSOURI
2011

EDITING   Suzanne Wakefield
PRODUCTION   Carolyn Garrison Reich
COMPOSITION   Carol Hollett
COVER DESIGN   David Berger
MEDICAL ILLUSTRATION   Amanda Yarberry Behr, Brenda L. Bunch

Quality Medical Publishing, Inc.
2248 Welsch Industrial Court
St. Louis, Missouri 63146
Telephone: 1-314-878-7808
Website: http://www.qmp.com

Library of Congress Cataloging-in-Publication Data

Berger, Karen.
  A woman's decision : breast care, treatment & reconstruction / by Karen Berger,
John Bostwick III, Glyn Jones. -- 4th ed.
      p. ; cm.
  Includes bibliographical references and index.
  ISBN 978-1-57626-230-6 (pbk.)
  1. Breast--Cancer--Surgery. 2. Breast--Care and hygiene. 3. Mammaplasty.
4. Breast--Cancer--Psychological aspects. I. Bostwick, John. II. Jones,
Glyn E. (Glyn Evan), 1954- III. Title.
  [DNLM: 1. Mammaplasty. 2. Breast Neoplasms--surgery. 3. Breast
Neoplasms--therapy. WP 910]
  RD667.5.B47 2011
  616.99′449059--dc22
                                                           2010039446
QM/SB/SB   10   9   8   7   6   5   4   3   2   1

To My Family

My dear husband, Phil,
whose love and encouragement sustain and inspire me.

And my wonderful children, David, Andrew, and Michelle,
who fill me with pride at their many accomplishments
and joy at their humanity.

My family has been an unwavering source of love,
laughter, and support.

K.B.

With love and appreciation to my mother, Mary Jones,
who should be astonished but isn't.

G.J.

NOTE: THE GENDER PROBLEM

In writing this book, we were confronted with the dilemma of which gender pronouns to use to refer to the physicians, surgeons, and plastic surgeons we discussed. Because all of the patients in this book are female and are referred to as she, we decided to avoid confusion by using the male pronoun for all the doctors in this book.

A SPECIAL NOTE TO OUR READERS

This edition has taken more than 10 years to complete, because John Bostwick III, my co-author and friend, passed away during its preparation. The world and breast cancer patients everywhere have felt his loss. John Bostwick was a wonderful person and an amazing surgeon who popularized the art of breast reconstruction. He recognized the importance of this transformative surgery for women who wanted to be whole again, and he led the way in refining reconstructive techniques so that women could feel good about themselves after cancer surgery. John was a gentle, sensitive man who truly cared about and empathized with his breast cancer patients. Although he had written a landmark book for surgeons that was world renowned, he still regarded *A Woman's Decision* as one of his most valued contributions, because he saw every day how much it helped women to cope with breast cancer diagnosis, treatment, and rehabilitation.

It was difficult for me to work on this new edition without John's input. If it had not been for the wonderful and heartfelt letters and phone calls that I received from women, physicians, and breast centers who relied on this book, I might never have completed it. They let me know how important this book was to them and how it had affected their lives or the lives of their patients. Their requests for an updated version could not be denied. So here we are again with a new edition. You will note that I have retained John Bostwick's name as an author on the cover and title page in deference to his special wisdom and expertise that still pervade these pages.

In John's absence, I have asked a number of specialists to assist me in updating current data and in providing information on the latest advances. This outstanding team of world-class experts has worked closely with me to produce this new edition. They, and the many other friends and colleagues who have provided support and helped to make this book possible, are cited in the acknowledgments that follow.

Karen Berger

ACKNOWLEDGMENTS

A book progresses through many stages and numerous revisions during its evolution. Initially the authors struggle in isolation while committing their thoughts to paper. Transforming their rough manuscript into a published book, however, requires the assistance of others. This book was no exception. Although this is a fourth edition, the writing process was as intense as if it were a new creation. All aspects of the book were carefully reexamined, a new chapter added, and most chapters rewritten to incorporate the latest information in a field that has become increasingly complex and dynamic.

Enormous progress has been made in breast cancer diagnosis and therapy, and it was important to include these advances in this new edition. For a time, the book seemed to be a moving target that shifted its direction at every turn. Each day brought news of dramatic new developments and promising new genetic therapies to shrink tumors, disrupt cell growth, and interfere with cell signals. These amazing discoveries led to chronic last-minute changes with no end in sight. Ultimately, as all authors must, we relinquished the manuscript, ever hopeful that it was as current as the publishing process allows. Most likely, we would still be revising the manuscript had it not been for the assistance of numerous experts who contributed their time and knowledge to help finalize this writing project. We were fortunate to have the advice of medical experts, skilled editors, sensitive friends and family, and business associates. With their guidance and encouragement, we brought the book to a conclusion. Therefore there are many people to acknowledge and to thank for their contributions and their participation.

First among them is Glyn Jones, MD. You will note that he is now listed on the cover and title page as a co-author.

Glyn Jones, MD
Professor of Surgery (Plastic), Department of Surgery,
University of Illinois College of Medicine, Peoria, Illinois

Glyn Jones is a talented plastic surgeon who trained with John Bostwick and was his colleague at Emory University in Atlanta. Glyn is an outstanding surgeon who possesses superb patient communication skills. It has been a pleasure to work with him on this edition. His input and expertise have added tremendously to the value of this endeavor. He has also helped to coordinate the patient interviews and carefully critiqued and updated all of the chapters to ensure that the latest information on breast reconstruction was included. He also added new case examples of surgical results and worked with our artists to include additional drawings to illustrate some of the reconstructive techniques that have been added. It is an honor and a pleasure to include him as a co-author.

In addition to Dr. Jones, a number of experts have contributed important information to this edition. They are listed and acknowledged below:

Catherine M. Appleton, MD
Assistant Professor, Breast Imaging Section, Mallinckrodt Institute of Radiology, Washington University School of Medicine, St. Louis, Missouri

Barbara S. Monsees, MD
Ronald and Hanna Evens Professor, Mallinckrodt Institute of Radiology, Washington University School of Medicine, St. Louis, Missouri

Catherine Appleton, MD, and Barbara Monsees, MD, are respected radiologists who wrote the chapter on breast imaging. This chapter provides critical information about breast screening and imaging options; it also helps women interpret current screening guidelines. Dr. Monsees is a valued friend and a noted radiologist, who has been a contributor to each edition of the book. She is a knowledgeable and insightful individual who brings significant experience, both personal and professional, to this topic. She helped to recruit new contributors, including Dr. Appleton. She and Dr. Appleton carefully reviewed the chapter and provided helpful additions and updates.

John M. Bedwinek, MD
Clinical Professor, Department of Radiation Oncology, St. Louis University, St. Louis; Director, Department of Radiation Oncology, Missouri Cancer Care, Lake St. Louis, Missouri

John Bedwinek, MD, is a radiation oncologist whose expertise is matched only by his skill as an educator and a communicator. Dr. Bedwinek contributed to previous editions as well. His information on breast conservation and irradiation provides our readers with the facts they need to make informed decisions about treatment options.

Dan W. Luedke, MD
President and Founder, Missouri Cancer Care, PC; Medical Director, Cancer Program, St. Joseph Health Center, St. Charles, Missouri

Dan Luedke, MD, a medical oncologist, is a new contributor to this edition. He has taken the complex subjects of chemotherapy and hormonal therapy and made them accessible and understandable for all women. That is a challenging task that he accomplished with great skill.

Julie A. Margenthaler, MD, FACS
Associate Professor of Surgery, Department of Surgery, Washington University School of Medicine, St. Louis, Missouri

Julie Margenthaler, MD, a surgical oncologist, is also a new contributor to this edition. She carefully reviewed the chapters on breast lumps and breast cancer treatment options—providing important updates and revisions.

Peter C. Neligan, MD
Professor, Division of Plastic Surgery, University of Washington, Seattle, Washington

Peter C. Neligan, MD, is a plastic surgeon, an educator, and a skilled microsurgeon. He reviewed the chapter on surgical options, updated information on microsurgical technique, and added a new section on perforator flaps.

Charles M. Balch, MD
Professor of Surgery, Oncology, and Dermatology; Deputy Director for Clinical Trials and Outcomes Research; Director, Johns Hopkins Clinical Research Network, Institute for Clinical and Translational Research, Johns Hopkins Medical Institutions, Baltimore, Maryland

Charles Balch, MD, is a renowned oncologic surgeon and a leading authority on breast cancer and melanoma; he is the editor-in-chief of *Annals of Surgical Oncology*, past president of the Society of Surgical Oncology, an educator, and a friend. Dr. Balch wrote the foreword for the previous edition, and we are fortunate to have him as a reviewer and contributor for this edition. He has carefully reviewed the chapters on breast conditions and breast cancer therapy, adding new information on current therapies, updating statistics, and providing us with the benefit of his vast experience.

Jennifer Ivanovich, MS
Genetic Counselor and Research Instructor, Department of Surgery, Washington University School of Medicine, St. Louis, Missouri

Jennifer Ivanovich, genetics counselor par excellence, has written a valuable new chapter that puts the topic of familial breast cancer and breast cancer risk into perspective as I have never seen it presented before. Her explanation of what a genetic counselor does is incredibly helpful to all women who are faced with a breast cancer diagnosis and with a family history of breast cancer.

Additionally, I would also like to thank the contributors from previous editions, some retired and some still practicing, whose material has been retained, revised, and updated. These professionals include Kenneth J. Arnold, MD; Benjamin A. Borowsky, MD; Roger S. Foster, Jr., MD; Mary Ellen Hawf, RN, OCN; Jacob Klein, MD; Lynne A. McCain, BSN, RN; John S. Meyer, MD; and William C. Wood, MD. Recognition is also due to Mimi Greenberg, PhD, who allowed us to reprint excerpts on the patient's responsibilities from her book, *Invisible Scars*.

The contributions from these experts have resulted in a comprehensive update on current breast cancer therapy and breast reconstruction technique that is unavailable elsewhere in a single book for the general public.

I would be remiss without mentioning two plastic surgeons who critiqued the book and added their insightful suggestions and comments:

Thomas J. Francel, MD, FACS
Associate Clinical Professor, Department of Surgery, St. Louis University; Chief of Plastic Surgery, Department of Surgery, St. John's Mercy Medical Center, St. Louis, Missouri

Thomas Francel, MD, is a respected plastic surgeon in St. Louis, Missouri. He critically reviewed the book, filling the margins with notes as he commented on information that should be added or revised. His suggestions were instrumental in shaping our writing. He also helped recruit patients to interview.

Albert Losken, MD, FACS
Associate Professor of Surgery, Department of Surgery, Division of Plastic and Reconstructive Surgery, Emory University, Atlanta, Georgia

Albert Losken, MD, a talented plastic surgeon at Emory University in Atlanta, Georgia, is an expert in oncoplastic surgery; he offered numerous suggestions for updating and expanding the book. His input has been invaluable.

This manuscript would never have been completed had it not been for the efforts of the outstanding team at Quality Medical Publishing. Michelle Berger, a woman of many talents, provided ongoing assistance throughout every phase of book development. She critically read the interviews and provided insightful comments and editing suggestions. She also led the effort to compile the comprehensive appendices, working tirelessly contacting different agencies and support organizations to check the accuracy of our data.

Amy Debrecht reviewed the manuscripts, offered invaluable comments, and processed them for turnover. She also read the interviews and provided important feedback. Taira Keele transcribed the interviews, often with tears in her eyes as she listened to the touching stories that unfolded. Taira, Julie Dill, and Olivia Ayes played a key role in compiling the appendices, glossary, and bibliography. They searched the literature and the Internet to provide us with the latest information on new developments and to ensure that all references were current. I was truly overwhelmed when they proudly presented me with five legal boxes packed full of possible references to include.

The editing skills of Suzanne Wakefield were very helpful; she polished our prose and offered critical suggestions for reworking the manuscript. I am grateful for the care she lavished on our book. Amanda Behr and Brenda Bunch created and revised the beautiful new drawings for this book, adding to those originally provided by William Winn. Additional assistance came from Carol Hollett, who skillfully prepared the layouts for the book and worked and reworked them until they were just right. Carolyn Reich deftly managed and coordinated this publishing project, checking and reviewing the pages and helping to ensure a quality publication. She arranged for the book's scheduling, production, and publication in record time. Carolyn's expert management made all of the difference. Andrew Berger provided the enthusiastic marketing and sales support so necessary for any publishing project, and Julie Dill managed the social media promotion. Brett Stone, Keith Roberts, Becky Sweeney, Sandy Hanley, and other staff members of Quality Medical Publishing also provided support and expertise throughout this endeavor.

They say that a book is often judged by its cover. If that is true, this new edition will receive high marks. It is graced by the beautiful artwork of Colleen Randall, a gifted artist and my beloved friend and sister-in-law. The design of the cover was created by David Berger, who used his considerable skill as a graphic designer to determine the ideal color scheme and look for the book.

My friends, relatives, and associates were an ongoing source of support during the preparation of this book. Jeff Friedman, my wonderful brother and a much-published poet in his own right, wrote the back cover copy and provided needed encouragement during the writing process. I am in awe of his ability with words. My husband, Phil, was always understanding of the late nights spent working and reworking chapters; I couldn't have completed this without his moral support, morning coffees, and faith in my abilities. My friends have been incredibly supportive. They are amazing individuals who willingly give of themselves to help others. Harriet Kopolow, Ann Smith Carr, Pat Simons, Vicki Friedman, Susan Goldberg, Kathleen Arink, Steven Stout, Diane Feldman, Dr. Joel Feldman, Johnna Hart Matthews, Anitra Sheen, and Marjorie Jackson have always been there to provide help or needed encouragement. Dr. Jessica Lewis was one of the reasons the book was written; it meant a great deal to know that she believed in the project and in the authors.

Finally, I would like to acknowledge the great debt of gratitude owed to the many individuals whose voices are heard throughout these pages. Over the years, thousands of women have taken the time to respond to our surveys, providing detailed answers to our questions and providing us with letters, phone calls, and a general outpouring of advice. Their words not only inspired us but also taught us how to improve this edition to better meet the needs of breast cancer patients.

Particular thanks are reserved for the women and men whose stories are recorded here. Much of the tone and focus of this book was derived from the emotion-packed interviews I conducted with the women and men who allowed me to record their feelings about, and relive their experiences with, breast cancer and reconstruction. Even though the names and personal details of these individuals have been changed to protect their privacy, their feelings and experiences reflect their real-life encounters with breast cancer and breast reconstruction.

Karen Berger

CONTENTS

Appendices

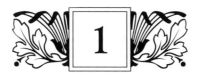

OUR PURPOSE IN WRITING

Today women diagnosed with breast cancer have more and better options for treatment, preservation, and reconstruction of the breast. No longer is the choice reduced to saving a life or saving a breast. Now the choices are more promising, but they are also more complex. Current diagnostic methods and medical and surgical therapies allow women to make their own decisions based on available information about the effectiveness of treatment, risk factors, and possibilities for breast preservation and restoration. In this context, access to reliable, balanced information becomes increasingly important. This new edition is written to fill that need. Our purpose is to provide our readers with the latest information and to assist them in understanding and evaluating the many factors that will influence a decision that will profoundly affect their lives.

Options now available to women include local therapy that focuses on optimal cancer removal with simultaneous breast preservation or reconstruction and systemic therapy using new chemotherapy and hormonal therapy regimens. Breast-conserving surgery with irradiation has become a widely accepted and increasingly appealing option for most women with early breast cancer. It offers excellent cancer treatment with survival rates equivalent to those for mastectomy. Furthermore, new oncoplastic procedures are now used to reconstruct deformities associated with breast-conserving surgery. Mastectomy operations have also been modified and improved. Many women who require or choose mastectomy can now have skin-sparing procedures for breast removal, followed by immediate breast reconstruction.

Women and their families are far better educated about their health than they were a mere 11 years ago. Vast resources are readily available to them. Logging on to the Internet can yield a wealth of information on a wide variety of topics. Breast cancer and breast reconstruction are covered in abundant detail. In fact, the array of available materials can be overwhelming. The challenge lies in sorting through the data to glean the information that is pertinent, meaningful, and appropriate. Our goal is to give women and their loved ones an overview of current health issues, new developments, and approaches to breast cancer diagnosis, treatment, and rehabilitation. Armed with this information, they can take control of their health, their lives, and their destinies.

This fourth edition reflects the transformation in breast cancer therapy. When we wrote the first edition 26 years ago, our primary emphasis was on mastectomy and breast reconstruction. At that time total breast removal was the most effective therapy for local treatment of breast cancer, and we wanted to let women know that breast restoration was available to them. The second and third editions were written as breast-conserving surgery was gaining more advocates and had become a viable and often preferable option for women with early breast cancer. This edition represents the changing face of breast cancer diagnosis and treatment and the exciting new developments on the horizon.

This book describes the diverse choices that are increasingly available to women. It includes tips on routine breast self-examination; guidelines for mammography, including a discussion of current controversies about screening guidelines; descriptions of commonly occurring breast problems; risk factors for breast cancer; and updates on hormone replacement therapy. Recent research developments and therapeutic approaches to breast cancer are fully explored, as is new information on breast cancer genetics. Image-guided biopsy techniques, sentinel node biopsy, breast-conserving surgery and irradiation, oncoplastic surgery, skin-sparing and nipple-sparing mastectomies, and promising drug therapies for breast cancer prevention are among the many topics that now share the spotlight with breast reconstruction.

Even so, breast reconstruction remains a major focus, and this edition continues to offer a comprehensive yet understandable account of this topic for women who wish to explore this option. All aspects of breast reconstruction are covered: Why do women seek breast restoration? Who is a candidate? What is the correct timing for this surgery? What is the best method for breast reconstruction? What defects can be reconstructed? What are the least invasive methods for breast reconstruction? What are the risks and benefits associated with the different types of breast reconstruction? What are the facts about breast implants? Answers to these frequently asked questions and many others are combined with personal accounts of women who have had their breasts restored. Pain, recuperation, and expense are issues of primary concern to any woman contemplating elective surgery, and these have been dealt with in detail, as have the special problems encountered when dealing with insurance carriers. We itemize the costs, risks, and benefits and describe and illustrate the different reconstructive techniques available. We try to present all sides of this topic from an unbiased perspective. Clearly, breast reconstruction is not for every woman. Many will not wish to undergo further surgery, pain, or expense. But for those who are interested, we provide a source of current, reliable information to enable them to make an educated decision.

This is not intended to be a medical text. We are speaking as professionals, but the scope of our book extends far beyond statistical analysis or scientific explanations of tumor behavior. Rather, we address the concerns of women confronting their fears of breast malignancy and monitoring their breasts. We believe that women with breast problems need to take a commonsense approach in dealing with physicians and the treatments they prescribe. We try to provide a personal yet medically accurate account.

Readers will find these pages liberally sprinkled with medical terms. Care has been taken to define these words, not to eliminate them. We are not proponents of medical jargon—just realists who respect the intelligence of our readers. Despite doctors' best efforts to give their patients understandable explanations, it is only natural for them to rely heavily on the communication tools they routinely use. For a woman to feel fully in control, she must familiarize herself with this terminology if she is not to be frustrated in her efforts to learn more about her condition and to communicate more fully with her physicians. We strongly believe that it is important for women to understand the language they will encounter during the treatment process.

Because breast cancer touches so many people's lives, the audience for this book is a broad one. Since the first edition was published in 1984, more than 2 million women have developed breast cancer in the United States alone. Now the alarming news is that it will strike one out of eight women during her lifetime. For the female author of this book, these statistics have come home. She notes with each passing year that breast cancer is an intimate reality for more and more relatives and friends. She feels that she is writing this book for herself, to answer all of those questions that have always worried and haunted her. The physician contributors see the need for such a book to help answer patient questions. Over the years they have seen significantly greater numbers of women in search of breast cancer treatment and breast reconstruction; alarmingly, many of these women are in their thirties and forties, far younger than the patient population they were treating a mere 15 years ago. We wish to reach women all over the world who have had mastectomies or lumpectomies as well as the more than 192,000 women each year who develop breast cancer in this country. We want these women to know about the options for breast cancer treatment and breast reconstruction and to understand that a diagnosis of breast cancer does not necessarily equate with permanent breast loss or disfigurement.

This book is also directed at women who are disease free. If they know that lumpectomy and irradiation and breast reconstruction are available, they might be less prone to procrastinate about seeking medical attention for suspected breast problems. Early detection remains the key to survival. Women need to understand the critical importance of mammography, breast self-examination, and physician examination.

We are also writing for men, not because they will suffer from breast cancer (the incidence of breast cancer among men is 1% that of women), but because they will know, love, work with, and live among women who have had this experience. Perhaps this knowledge will sensitize them to the psychological and physical concerns that this disease generates.

Much of the information in this book is drawn from more than 26 years of research, over 5000 questionnaires, hundreds of letters and comments received from our readers, and numerous interviews with men and women. We principally surveyed women who had lumpectomies and mastectomies for breast cancer and asked them to relate their feelings about and experiences with this disease, their methods for coping, as well as their subsequent therapy and rehabilitation. We asked women to supply us with questions they wanted answered and issues they would like to see addressed.

We continue to be amazed by the enthusiastic response we have received to our questionnaires. One only has to page through the typed and handwritten pages of these surveys to see that the women who have responded have invested considerable time pondering our questions and thoughtfully answering them. They have painstakingly recorded their thoughts on the backs of pages, typed extra sheets, written letters and personal notes, and attached articles and reading lists that they thought would assist us. They even emailed their responses and articles to us and suggested online resources that we should check out. Especially gratifying for us were communications received from women who had read the first three editions of this book; they graciously described the book's impact on their lives and provided suggestions for revision.

These women's responses prompted us to make critical changes in the tone and direction of the book. Because of them, we have carefully reexamined all of the information in existing chapters, adding, rewriting, and amplifying as we went along and significantly updating this material. We have also updated the Appendix to include current information on support services, patient education resources, comprehensive cancer centers, and online resources, and have expanded the Glossary so that it reflects the latest terminology, research, therapies, and surgical techniques.

Since our last literary excursion, many new developments have occurred in breast cancer research and therapy. Despite the numerous books and articles on the general health issues related to breast disease, our surveys indicate that many women remain woefully ignorant of them. Therefore we have interwoven basic information on these subjects throughout. Of particular interest are expanded sections on new tests and therapies for diagnosing and treating breast cancer, sentinel node biopsy, methods for breast cancer staging, updated criteria for choosing lumpectomy with irradiation, information about oncoplastic techniques for reconstructing lumpectomy defects, and the latest chemotherapy and hormonal therapy regimens. In addition, we have greatly expanded the discussion of breast cancer genetics and the breast cancer genes (*BRCA1* and *BRCA2*), with a new chapter devoted to this topic and a new section on the role of the genetic counselor in advising women about their risks. We have also placed greater emphasis on the social, psychological, and wellness issues confronting breast cancer patients. Consequently, the chapter on breast cancer and its effect on relationships has been expanded to include more input from men and single women and greater attention to the practical realities of daily life. In our surveys and interviews we probe the strategies others have used to help them cope with dating, sex, communication, making new acquaintances, and building lasting relationships. Their solutions are surprising, creative, and always inspiring.

Finally, we have totally updated the chapters on breast reconstruction to incorporate the numerous advances that have taken place in the past 11 years and to respond to women's questions about breast restoration. All of the currently available reconstructive techniques, from the simplest to the most complex, are described in detail and accompanied by numerous photographs and drawings of the procedures and the anticipated results, as our readers requested. We have also expanded the chapter on frequently asked questions about breast reconstruction, incorporating information about currently available implants and expanders and adding details on perforator flaps and on fat grafting. In view of the mounting demand for and trend toward more immediate breast reconstructions, this topic has been explored in depth. We have also added information on oncoplastic reconstruction after lumpectomy and partial mastectomy, and perforator flap procedures, such as the DIEP flap.

The concluding chapter of the book has always been cited by our readers as being particularly helpful to them in understanding the possibilities and limitations of breast reconstruction. It captures conversations with breast reconstruction patients throughout the country. In this edition five new interviews have been added to reflect the latest reconstructive techniques and to capture special reconstructive scenarios for women who have been diagnosed with breast cancer genes and have opted for preventive mastectomy or those who have had particular risk factors that have complicated their recoveries. These women poignantly explain their motivations for seeking breast reconstruction. They candidly discuss such diverse issues as dating and sex after breast cancer, postsurgical depression, and the doctor/patient relationship. All of these women share the details of their surgery as well as their intense feelings about it and about the breast cancer experience. To assist the reader in differentiating among these interviews, we have included a short index at the beginning of this chapter that lists each woman's name, age, and type of reconstructive surgery.

Breast cancer is a complex and terrifying disease. It attacks a woman's self-confidence, her physical being, and her very life. It affects friends, family, and acquaintances alike. It does not discriminate. Wealth, power, and privilege offer no protection against its assault. Knowledge, however, is the common defense that unites all women. It is the secret to overcoming fear and regaining control. Early detection is still the key to long-term survival.

It is our hope that this book will educate women about the full spectrum of options available for dealing with breast cancer, thereby empowering them with the strength and understanding required to confront this life-threatening disease. Many exciting developments are taking place in breast cancer research and therapy that offer new hope for improved quality of life and for a potential cure. Equipped with this knowledge, women will be able to more effectively influence their own destinies and play an active role in their own health care.

BREAST ANATOMY AND PHYSIOLOGY

How much do most women really know about their breasts? Most likely, very little. Unless they develop breast problems, they usually are not motivated to learn about the inner structure of this intimate female body part. Yet women need to be more familiar with the normal anatomy and physiology (function) of their breasts if they are going to be able to recognize the earliest and most treatable signs of breast cancer. With this knowledge, they will not be so frightened every time they notice a breast change. This chapter provides that information in a simple, straightforward manner. It offers women a baseline for evaluating their own health care requirements. Additionally, it provides assistance for women interested in performing breast self-examination, a crucial routine for proper breast surveillance.

The breast is a mound of glandular, fatty, and fibrous tissue located over the pectoralis muscles of the chest wall and attached to these muscles by fibrous strands (*Cooper's ligaments*). The breast itself has no muscle tissue, which is why exercises (often vigorously engaged in by teenagers intent on enlarging their breasts) will not build up the breasts. A layer of fat surrounds the breast glands and extends throughout the breast. This fatty tissue gives the breast a soft consistency and gentle, flowing contour. The actual breast is composed of fat, glands (with the capacity for milk production when stimulated by special hormones), blood vessels, milk ducts to transfer the milk from the glands to the nipples, and sensory nerves that give feeling to the breast. These nerves extend upward from the muscle layer through the breast and are highly sensitive, especially in the nipple and areola region, which accounts for the sexual responsiveness of some women's breasts.

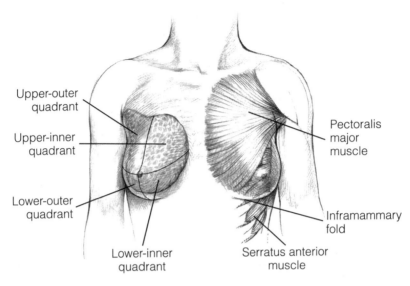

Upper-outer quadrant

Upper-inner quadrant

Lower-outer quadrant

Lower-inner quadrant

Pectoralis major muscle

Inframammary fold

Serratus anterior muscle

Because the breast is made up of tissues with different textures, it may not have a smooth surface and often feels lumpy. This irregularity is especially noticeable if a woman is thin and has little breast fat to soften the contours; it becomes less obvious after menopause, when the cyclic changes and endocrine stimulation of the breast cease and the glandular tissue softens. Estrogen supplements after menopause can cause continued lumpiness. The breast glands drain into a collecting system of ducts that go to the base of the nipple. The ducts then extend through the nipple and open on its outer surface. In addition to serving as a channel for milk, these ducts are often the source of breast problems. Experts now believe that most breast cancer begins in the lining of the ducts and sometimes the milk glands. Benign fibrocystic changes also originate in these ducts.

The ducts end in the nipple, which projects from the surface of the breast; these ducts are a conduit for the milk secreted by the glands and suckled by a baby during breast-feeding. There is considerable variation in women's nipples. In some, the nipple is constantly erect; in others it only becomes erect when stimulated by cold, physical contact, or sexual activity. Still other women have inverted nipples. Surrounding the nipple is a slightly raised circle of pigmented skin called the *areola*. The nipple and areola contain specialized muscle fibers that make the nipple erect and give the areola its firm texture. The areola also contains *Montgomery's glands*, which may appear as small, raised lumps on the surface of the areola. These glands lubricate the areola and are not symptoms of an abnormal condition.

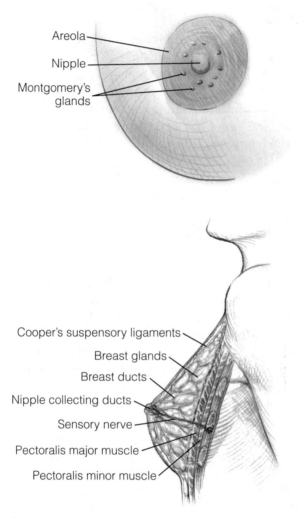

Areola

Nipple

Montgomery's
glands

Cooper's suspensory ligaments

Breast glands

Breast ducts

Nipple collecting ducts

Sensory nerve

Pectoralis major muscle

Pectoralis minor muscle

   Beneath the breast is a large muscle, the pectoralis major, which
assists in arm movement; the breast rests on this muscle. (Portions of
three other muscles are also found under the lower and outer portions
of the breast.) Originating on the chest wall, the pectoralis major extends from deep under the breast to attach on the upper arm. It also
helps form the axillary fold, created where the arm and chest wall
meet. The *axilla* (armpit) is the depression behind this fold. Removal

of the pectoralis major muscle, as was formerly done during a radical mastectomy (an operation rarely performed anymore), left a considerable deformity: the chest had a hollowed-out appearance under the collarbone, the skin was tight and drawn over the rib cage, and the axillary fold and axilla were missing.

A rich system of blood vessels supplies nutrients and hormones to the breast. Because blood flow is increased during the menstrual cycle, pregnancy, and sexual stimulation, the breasts become engorged.

Fluid exits the breast through the venous network of the bloodstream and the lymphatic channels. The lymphatics are small vessels that carry tissue fluid away from the breast, where it passes through a system of filters known as *lymph nodes*. As part of the body's immune system, the lymph nodes can enlarge in response to local infection or tumor. Trapped breast cancer cells multiplying in these lymph nodes also can cause them to swell. The two main lymph drainage areas are under the breastbone and in the axilla. Enlarged lymph nodes in the axilla usually can be felt.

In examining a woman's breasts, the physician first checks the appearance of the skin and nipple-areola for any changes such as dimpling, nipple inversion, or crusting. He then feels the glandular tissue of the breast to detect suspicious or unusual lumps or thickenings. Despite the beneficial value of mammograms (breast x-ray films), the physical breast examination is still the most common way of detecting breast masses. In addition, the physician examines the underarm to determine whether the lymph nodes are enlarged. When breast cancer spreads, it often can be detected first in the underarm. Thus in a patient who is being treated for breast cancer, some of these lymph nodes from the underarm are usually removed and examined by a pathologist to see whether the cancer has spread to them, and if so, to what extent. Removal of the lymph nodes can accentuate the depth or hollow appearance of the armpit.

Each woman's breasts are shaped differently. Individual breast appearance is influenced by the volume of a woman's breast tissue and fat, her age, a history of previous pregnancies and lactation, her heredity, the quality and elasticity of her breast skin, and the influence of breast hormones.

The breast is responsive to a complex interplay of hormones that causes the breast tissue to develop, enlarge, and produce milk. The three major hormones affecting the breast are estrogen, progesterone, and prolactin, which cause glandular tissue in both the breast and uterus to change during a woman's menstrual cycle. Because of reduced hormonal levels the breasts are less full for 1 to 2 weeks after menstrual flow; therefore it may be easier to detect breast lumps during this time. Reduction of hormonal levels is also responsible for the breast's return to its prepregnant state after a woman stops breast-feeding.

The cells lining the small lobular ducts of the breast change with each menstrual cycle. They grow under the influence of estrogen early in the cycle, and in the latter part they replicate their DNA and divide under the influence of progesterone and estrogen. This process continues through the onset of menstruation until, with declining levels of estrogen and progesterone, a number of cells equal to those that have been divided is destroyed. By this process the cells of the terminal lobular ducts are essentially replaced with each menstrual cycle in young women. This process of cell loss and renewal slows as a woman approaches menopause. After menopause, the terminal lobular ducts atrophy, cell renewal all but ceases, and the lobules atrophy unless supplemental hormones are given. The process of cell renewal in the breast lobules during the reproductive years is reminiscent of a similar process in the *endometrium* (lining of the uterus). It provides a continually fresh cell population ready to undergo growth and development in preparation for lactation during pregnancy. Proliferation and turnover of cells in the lobular breast ducts are particularly rapid in women below age 35, especially in the teens and twenties. Radiation exposure should be minimized during these younger years because the risk of inducing cancer is high when cells are proliferating.

Some women have a large amount of breast tissue and/or breast fat and thus have large breasts. Others have a small but normal amount of breast tissue with little breast fat and thus have small breasts. After weight loss, pregnancy, or menopause, many women experience a decrease in breast size and volume. If the skin does not have sufficient elasticity, the breasts may droop or sag. The size of a woman's breasts often influences whether the breasts will sag. The larger the breasts, the more likely they are to succumb to the constant force of gravity. This sagging appearance (ptosis) often accompanies the aging process, particularly if the breast size decreases.

Few women have completely balanced breasts; one side is often larger or smaller, higher or lower, or its shape is different from that of the other side. The underlying chest wall may also be asymmetrical. Breast asymmetry is normal, even though some women are not aware of it unless it is pointed out to them.

Breast shape and appearance change as a woman ages. In a young woman the breast skin is stretched and expanded by the developing breasts. The breast in an adolescent is usually hemispherical, rounded, and equally full in all areas. As a woman gets older, the top side of the breast tissue settles to a lower position, the skin stretches, and the shape of the breast changes. After menopause, with the decrease of hormonal activity, the composition of the breast changes: the amount of glandular tissue decreases and fat and ductal tissues become the pre-dominant components of the breast. Reduction in glandular volume can result in further looseness of the breast skin.

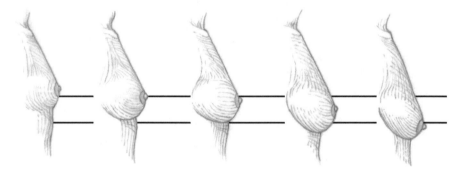

Skin quality influences breast shape. Although breast skin con-tains special elastic fibers, there is much natural and hereditary vari-ation in the amount of elasticity and thickness of each individual's breast skin. Some women have thicker skin, with considerable elas-ticity or stretch. They tend to have tighter and firmer breasts longer than women who have thinner skin with less elasticity. Women with very thin skin may even develop stretch marks, or striae. These marks are actual tears of the deeper layers of the thin skin and usually indicate a lack of elasticity.

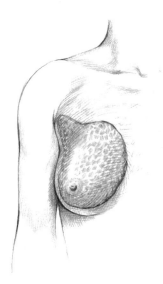

Few women realize the large area of their chest that is actually covered by breast tissue; it may extend from just below the collarbone to the level of the sixth rib and from the edge of the breastbone to the underarm area. A portion of the breast even reaches into the armpit region. The breast also has mobility on the chest wall because of loose fibrous (fascial) attachments to the underlying muscles. This breast motion is limited and the breasts are given support by special ligaments known as Cooper's ligaments. When a breast is removed, these ligaments, their fascial attachments and some lymph nodes from the armpit area are also removed. Thus the deformity created encompasses more than a missing breast, and for breast reconstruction to be successful, it must fill in or restore all of these areas.

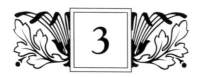

BREAST SELF-EXAMINATION

Breast self-examination (BSE) can save a woman's life. Many women are so fearful of finding a lump in their breast that they avoid checking their breasts. This neglect can prove to be foolishly dangerous; it may even allow cancer to go undetected and spread outside the local breast tissue, thus decreasing the chance for cure and long-term survival. Periodic breast examinations are important for early detection of breast cancer, which ranks second to lung cancer as the most frequent cause of cancer death in women. Statistics reveal that most breast cancers are first discovered by women themselves. If more women practiced routine BSE and became familiar with the normal feel of their breasts, the incidence of death from breast cancer could possibly be reduced by as much as 18%, because BSE-detected tumors usually are discovered when the tumor is in its early, more curable stages. In addition to checking her own breasts, a woman should have her gynecologist, internist, or family physician examine them at least once a year.

BSE is clearly an essential part of a woman's health care. It is easy to learn and perform, does not require a special setting, and can be incorporated into any woman's normal routine. BSE is basically a "familiarity exercise" that helps acquaint a woman with the look and feel of her breasts and their normal cyclic changes, making it easier for her to detect breast changes early, when treatment is most likely to be effective. If breast cancer is detected early, a less extensive operation may be needed.

Many women are puzzled by their breasts' natural lumpy texture and question their ability to find a small lump within this irregular breast tissue. Initially it may be difficult to differentiate abnormal from normal breast tissue. A woman may even want to ask her doctor to go through the procedure with her the first time. He can examine her breasts, tell her what he feels and why, and help her to understand what she is looking for. Eventually, with monthly inspection, she will feel more comfortable and knowledgeable about this process.

Some women have fibrocystic changes that give their breasts a lumpy texture and confound their attempts at BSE. These lumps frequently shrink and swell with the menstrual cycle. Women with fibrocystic breasts should identify the ordinary bumpy areas of their breasts so that they can monitor cyclic changes and thus discover any new, distinct lumps.

Ideally, BSE should be conducted once a month. If you are still menstruating, you should inspect your breasts approximately 7 to 10 days after the beginning of menstruation, when they are not swollen and tender. If you are no longer menstruating, you should still perform regular monthly examinations; the first day of each month is often an easy-to-remember schedule. Monthly BSE should also remain a part of your routine after mastectomy or lumpectomy or after breast reconstruction.

HOW TO PERFORM BSE

BSE consists of visual inspection and palpation (feeling).

Visual Inspection

To examine your breasts visually, stand in front of a mirror in a well-lighted room and carefully observe all sides of your breasts for unusual characteristics. Any differences in the size or shape of your breasts should be noted. You are looking for discharge from your nipples, sudden nipple inversion (if your nipples were previously erect), a skin rash, scaling, redness, puckering, or dimpling. Some women may notice that they have prominent veins in their breasts. This condition, in itself, is not cause for alarm if it is the normal state of a woman's breasts. Changes in the appearance of these veins are important. If you notice any of these variations in your breast appearance, you should immediately report them to your doctor.

To identify any changes in the shape of your breasts, observe yourself in three positions: (1) standing straight with your hands at your sides, (2) hands raised and clasped behind your head with hands pressed forward, and (3) hands pressed firmly on your hips with shoulders and elbows pulled forward. As you assume the last two positions, you should be able to feel your chest muscles tense. The outline of your breasts should have a smooth curve in all positions.

Visual Inspection

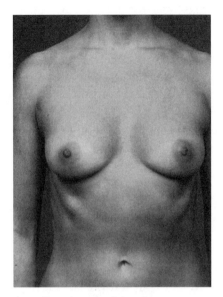

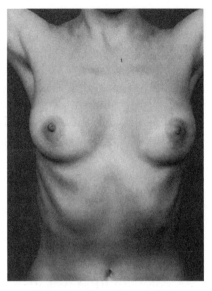

Stand up straight with your
hands at your sides.

Raise your hands and clasp
them behind your head with your
hands pressed forward.

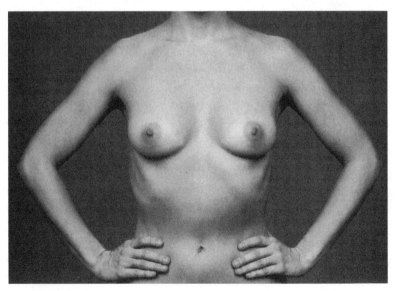

Press your hands firmly on your hips with your shoulders and
elbows pulled forward.

If you have had a mastectomy or lumpectomy or breast reconstruction, you must also observe the breast scar for any sign of new swelling, lumps, redness, or color change. Although redness may be caused by chafing from your undergarments or your prosthesis, it should be reported to your doctor.

Palpation (Feeling)

The most important part of the examination, feeling your breasts, can be done while you are standing up or lying down. There is no need to be embarrassed about feeling your breasts; this is a normal part of a woman's health care.

Many women prefer the privacy of the shower for this inspection. The soap and water make their skin feel slippery, and their fingers can glide smoothly over their breasts, making it easier for them to detect any textural changes underneath.

If you perform palpation while standing, begin the inspection by raising your left arm and using the flat, cushioned part of your fingers of your right hand (not the fingertips) to feel your left breast. Place your fingers at the outer edge of your breast and slowly press or compress the breast tissue gently down to the chest wall beneath.

Several patterns can be used for examining your breasts. With one, the strip pattern, you start at the top of your chest and palpate your breasts in a vertical pattern, carefully compressing the breast tissue, strip by strip, until all breast tissue has been inspected. With another pattern, you examine your breasts by moving your fingers in small circles around your breast, gradually working toward the nipple. Still another pattern approaches the breast as if it were a circle divided into wedges (sometimes referred to as the *wedge pattern*). You examine your breast wedge by wedge, working from the outer portion of your breast toward the nipple until the whole breast is examined. Which pattern you choose is not important. What is important is selecting one, using it consistently, and allowing yourself enough time for a thorough and deliberate examination. With all of these patterns, be sure to palpate the entire breast region as well as the areas above the breast and under the collarbone and the underarm, including the armpit. Sometimes lumps are discovered in this area. You are looking for any thickening, masses, swollen lymph nodes, or unusual lumps under the skin and especially a change from previous examinations. They might feel like firm, distinct bumps. Repeat this examination on your right side.

Palpation

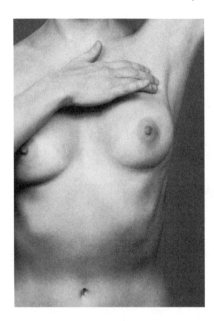

Place your fingers at the outer edge of your breast and slowly compress the breast tissue.

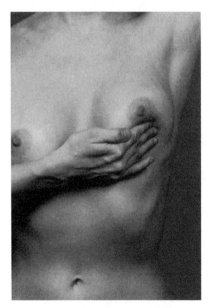

Move your fingers in small circles, working toward the nipple.

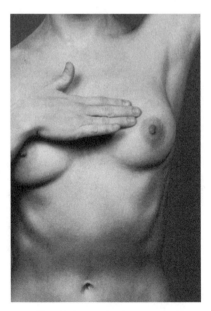

Check the entire breast and underarm, including the armpit.

Palpation Patterns

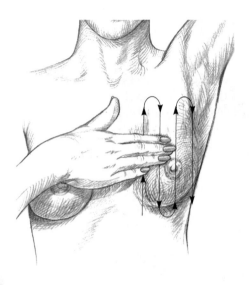

Vertical pattern

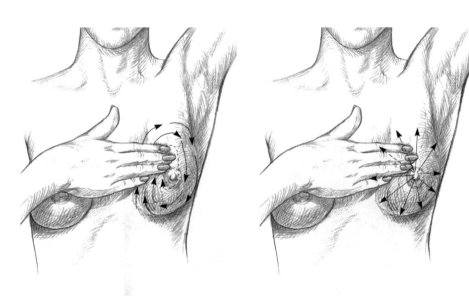

Circular pattern   Wedge pattern

If you have had a mastectomy, a lumpectomy, or breast recon-struction, you should feel your chest area, paying close attention to the scar and tissue surrounding it. Raise your arm on the unoperated side (or opposite side if you have had bilateral surgery), and using your opposite hand, place three or four fingers at the top of the scar. Press gently, using the circular motion described previously. Inspect the entire length of the scar. You are looking for lumps, bumps, hard spots, or thickenings. As with your breasts, familiarity with your scar will make it easier for you to recognize any changes and report them to your physician.

If you perform the inspection while lying down, lie flat on your back with your left arm over your head and a pillow or rolled towel under your left shoulder. This position flattens your breasts and makes

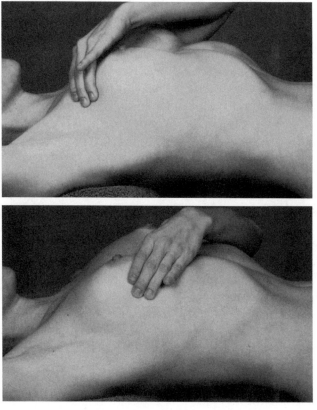

Breast self-examination while lying down

it easier for you to examine them. Use the same strip, circular, or wedge pattern described previously and repeat the procedure on your right breast.

Remember, most women's breasts have a bumpy texture, and the upper-outer portion is usually the lumpiest. The best way to discover abnormal breast lumps is to know what is normal for your breasts; then if a problem develops, you can spot it immediately. Essentially what you are looking for is persistent lumps that do not disappear or change size after menstrual cycles. These are dominant lumps that appear suddenly and persist. Abnormal breast lumps will vary in size, firmness, and sensitivity. They may be hard or irregular, with sharp edges. Still others appear as thickened areas with no distinct outlines. Some lumps are painful and tender. Pain and/or tenderness is not ordinarily a sign of breast cancer, however, and may simply indicate the development of a breast cyst. Sometimes natural underlying anatomic structures such as breast glands, the breastbone, or ribs can be mistaken for lumps. A firm ridge in the lower curve of each breast is normal. Don't worry about making a mistake. *Suspicious lumps should always be reported to your doctor. It never hurts to be wrong, but it can be fatal to ignore a cancer.*

Whether you perform BSE while standing up or lying down, the important point is to make the commitment to do a self-inspection each month. Any breast changes, unusual pain or tenderness, or lumps you discover should be investigated further by your doctor. Along with your monthly BSE, you should have regular checkups by your family physician, internist, or gynecologist. A breast examination should be a routine part of your yearly office visit. The American Cancer Society recommends the following guidelines for the detection of breast cancer in asymptomatic women:

- Women 20 years of age and older should perform monthly BSE.
- Women 20 to 39 years of age should have a physical examination every 3 years by a health care professional (such as a physician, physician assistant, nurse, or nurse practitioner).
- Women 40 years of age and older should have a physical examination of the breast every year by a health care professional.
- Women 40 years of age and older should have a yearly mammogram. (See Chapter 4 for more information on breast imaging guidelines.)

Most breast lumps are benign, but for those that are malignant, mammography, BSE, and physician surveillance will ensure early detection and a significantly higher cure rate.

MAMMOGRAPHY AND OTHER BREAST IMAGING METHODS FOR EARLY DETECTION AND DIAGNOSIS

Catherine M. Appleton, MD, and Barbara S. Monsees, MD

Screening mammography (x-ray examination of the breast) is a valuable and widely available tool for early detection of breast cancer that has been shown to reduce the death rate from breast cancer. Yet surprisingly, despite extensive media coverage about the value of screening mammography, many women still fail to take advantage of this lifesaving diagnostic tool. It is estimated that 40% of women between ages 40 and 49, 35% of women between ages 50 and 64, and 46% of women older than 65 have not had a mammogram in the past 2 years. Fear of finding that their worst suspicion is confirmed, apprehension that radiation exposure from mammography may cause the very breast cancer it seeks to detect, fear of possible breast loss from mastectomy, concerns about the costs of this test and lack of insurance, and lack of support by their physicians often deters women from having mammograms performed. These fears may prove to be a woman's worst enemy. Fortunately, today many of the barriers that have discouraged compliance with screening recommendations have now been addressed. The risk of the radiation delivered during mammography is so small that the benefits of detecting a possible tumor far outweigh the theoretical risk of developing breast cancer. Cost deterrents have also been greatly reduced through mandated insurance coverage in most states, Medicare coverage, and the availability of low-cost or free mammograms through a variety of programs.

Many well-documented studies have demonstrated that women who have routine screening for breast cancer with mammography have a lower death rate from breast cancer than those who do not. When properly performed and interpreted, mammography has the potential to detect most breast cancers; however, it is not a perfect test, and not all cancers will be detected before they are felt by the woman herself. Although about 5% to 10% of women may be recalled from a screening mammogram for additional imaging, most are told that they are fine, and that no further testing is needed until the next regular mammogram. About 1% to 2% of women who have a screening mammogram have an abnormality for which biopsy is recommended. Most of these biopsies (about 75%) yield benign results (that is, no cancer is found). Many of the cancers detected by screening mammograms are smaller, and thus they cannot be felt by the woman or her physician. Because they have been found while they are still small, most of these tumors have a better prognosis, may be more easily treated, and a large percentage may be treated with breast-conserving therapy and do not require mastectomy.

There are two basic approaches to using mammography to address breast problems: screening mammography and diagnostic mammography. Although they use the same type of technology, it is the target group of women, whether they are with or without signs or symptoms, that dictates whether a woman should receive a screening mammogram or a diagnostic mammogram.

SCREENING MAMMOGRAMS

Screening is the process of evaluating healthy people with no signs or symptoms to detect disease. The term *baseline* screening mammogram is often used to describe a woman's first mammogram. The baseline mammogram is used the same way that her subsequent mammograms are used: to determine whether she has a finding that could be breast cancer. Subsequent mammograms are usually compared with the prior examinations, and fewer women are usually recalled from a subsequent examination than from the baseline examination, because the comparison is helpful. The job of the interpreting radiologist is to find possible abnormalities that could be breast cancer. As mentioned previously, about 5% to10% of women may be recalled for further evaluation with additional mammographic images (a diagnostic mammogram), or ultrasound to determine the significance of the finding.

Most of these women will not require a biopsy, and of the few who will need a biopsy to determine the diagnosis, most will not have breast cancer. Although mammograms are extremely effective in finding most breast cancers, they cannot provide a definitive diagnosis; that can only be done by a biopsy (see Chapter 5).

Mammography is a highly sensitive method for detecting breast cancer, but it is not perfect. For this reason, a woman should not request a screening examination if she suspects that she has a breast lump or other signs or symptoms suggestive of breast cancer. A mammogram interpreted as normal in that circumstance may offer false assurance that breast cancer is not present. Therefore, if a lump or area of breast thickening is present, a woman should seek the advice of her personal physician and possibly a breast surgeon. When there is a suspected sign or symptom of breast cancer, a diagnostic mammogram is warranted for full evaluation. Furthermore, for the same reason, if a woman had a negative screening mammogram and then later feels a lump or finds a suspicious sign, she should see her physician and should not wait until her next regular mammogram appointment.

DIAGNOSTIC MAMMOGRAMS

A diagnostic mammogram is used to evaluate a woman in any of the following situations: when a lump or thickening has been felt, when a screening mammogram reveals a finding that requires further investigation, when she is being followed for a finding that is probably not cancer, and sometimes when she has a personal history of breast cancer.

Specially tailored views and/or ultrasound may be performed to better assess an area of abnormality found on either mammography or physical examination. Preferably, the diagnostic examination should be monitored by a radiologist so that any additional imaging can be performed at that same time; then the radiologist can determine whether a biopsy should be recommended based on the imaging findings.

The radiologist will evaluate the mammogram not only to determine whether a biopsy is needed, but also to identify other findings in different locations in the same or the opposite breast. The location, character, and extent of disease seen on mammography and ultrasound can often be helpful in determining whether a woman would be a good candidate for breast-conserving surgery if she does have cancer.

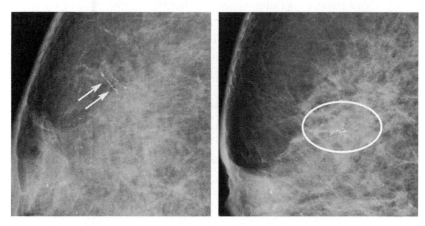

Diagnostic mammogram magnification images depict suspicious
microcalcifications. (These appear as small white dots
in branching patterns; see *arrows* and *circle.*)

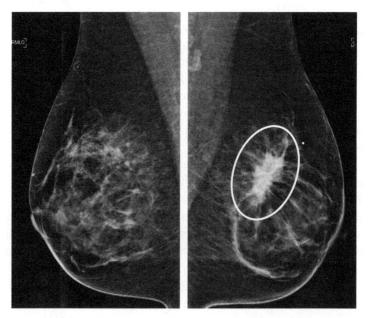

Mammogram of woman with a cancer in her left breast. Mediolateral views
(looking from the side) show an irregular spiculated mass *(circle).*

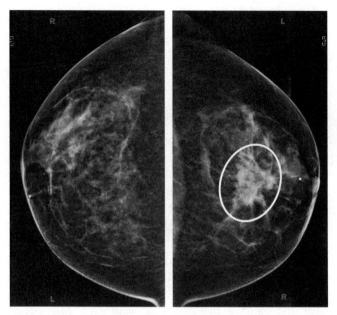

Mammogram of another patient with a cancer in the left breast: craniocaudal views (looking from above) show an irregular spiculated mass *(circle)*.

If a biopsy confirms a cancer, additional imaging such as a breast MRI may be recommended, because it may help to better document the extent of disease and is very useful for treatment planning and medical decision-making.

SCREENING RECOMMENDATIONS

When should a woman have her first mammogram, and how often should she have follow-up mammograms? Much media attention and public confusion have been generated over conflicting reports about the value of screening mammography. The most recent controversy erupted after the United States Preventive Services Task Force (USPSTF) issued recommendations that women in their forties consult with their health care providers regarding whether they want to be screened, and that women over 50 years of age be screened every other year rather than yearly. In addition, the USPSTF suggested that clinical breast examination and teaching breast self-examination were of little value, and that since there were no randomized trials that included older women, screening should stop at age 75.

Although the USPSTF agreed that mammography does save lives, it weighed the benefits and harms of the test for differing age groups and derived its recommendations based on conservative estimates of the benefits. It included data only from randomized, controlled trials and excluded other types of evidence that provide information suggesting that the death rate can be more substantially reduced than seen in the randomized trials. In addition, many professionals believe that the USPSTF overemphasized the potential *harms* from mammography screening. The harms that they considered included the necessity for patient recalls because of screening for additional workup, biopsy for findings that did not turn out to be cancer, and cancers for which the natural history is unknown, and may not have caused a problem for the woman if left untreated. *Surveys of women have shown that women are very accepting of these false-positive results (harms) and would rather deal with these than risk a breast cancer death that could be avoided.*

The recent discovery of specific genes that carry a very high risk of breast cancer for affected women is hopeful as well as frightening. If a woman has a family history suggestive of familial breast cancer, she should speak to her physician regarding supplemental screening with MRI (see the section on MRI, p. 40), genetic counseling, genetic testing, and risk reduction strategies (see Chapter 7, Breast Cancer Genetics, and Chapter 15, Prophylactic Mastectomy).

The American Cancer Society (ACS) has continually revised its guidelines through the years to conform to the best-known science in this field. Unlike the USPSTF, the ACS considers all the available evidence in making its screening recommendations. *The ACS recommends annual screening for women beginning at age 40 and continuing as long as the woman is in good health.*

AMERICAN CANCER SOCIETY RECOMMENDATIONS FOR EARLY BREAST CANCER DETECTION IN WOMEN WITHOUT BREAST SYMPTOMS

Women age 40 and older should have a mammogram every year and should continue to do so for as long as they are in good health.

- Current evidence supporting mammograms is even stronger than in the past. In particular, recent evidence has confirmed that mammograms offer substantial benefit for women in their forties. Women can feel confident about the benefits associated with regular mammograms for finding cancer early. However, mammograms also have limitations. A mammogram can miss some cancers, and it may lead to follow-up of findings that are not cancer.
- Women should be told about the benefits and limitations linked with yearly mammograms. But despite their limitations, mammograms are still a very effective and valuable tool for decreasing suffering and death from breast cancer.
- Mammograms should be continued regardless of a woman's age, as long as she does not have serious, chronic health problems such as congestive heart failure, end-stage renal disease, chronic obstructive pulmonary disease, and moderate to severe dementia. Age alone should not be the reason to stop having regular mammograms. Women with serious health problems or short life expectancies should discuss with their doctors whether to continue having mammograms.

Women in their twenties and thirties should have a clinical breast exam (CBE) as part of a periodic (regular) health exam by a health professional preferably every 3 years. Starting at age 40, women should have a CBE by a health professional every year.

- CBE is done along with mammograms and offers a chance for women and their doctors or nurses to discuss changes in their breasts, early detection testing, and factors in the woman's history that might make her more likely to have breast cancer.
- There may be some benefit in having the CBE shortly before the mammogram. The exam should include instruction for the purpose of getting more familiar with your own breasts. Women should also be given information about the benefits and limitations of CBE and breast self-examination (BSE). The chance of breast cancer occurring is very low for women in their 20s and gradually increases with age. Women should be told to promptly report any new breast symptoms to a health professional.

Data from *http://www.cancer.org.*

Continued

AMERICAN CANCER SOCIETY RECOMMENDATIONS
FOR EARLY BREAST CANCER DETECTION IN WOMEN
WITHOUT BREAST SYMPTOMS—cont'd

Breast self-examination (BSE) is an option for women starting in their twenties. Women should be told about the benefits and limitations of BSE. Women should report any breast changes to their health professional right away.

Women at high risk (greater than 20% lifetime risk) should have an MRI and a mammogram every year.

Women at moderately increased risk (15% to 20% lifetime risk) should talk with their doctors about the benefits and limitations of adding MRI screening to their yearly mammogram. Yearly MRI screening is not recommended for women whose lifetime risk of breast cancer is less than 15%.

If MRI is used, it should be in addition to, not instead of, a screening mammogram, because although an MRI is a more sensitive test (it's more likely to detect cancer than a mammogram), it may still miss some cancers that a mammogram would detect.

For most women at high risk, screening with MRI and mammograms should begin at age 30 and continue for as long as a woman is in good health. But because the evidence is limited regarding the best age at which to start screening, this decision should be based on shared decision-making between patients and their health care providers, taking into account personal circumstances and preferences.

Women at high risk include those who:
- Have a known *BRCA1* or *BRCA2* gene mutation
- Have a first-degree relative (parent, brother, sister, or child) with a *BRCA1* or *BRCA2* gene mutation and have not had genetic testing themselves
- Have a lifetime risk of breast cancer of 20% to 25% or greater, according to risk assessment tools that are based mainly on family history (see below)

Data from *http://www.cancer.org.*

- Had radiation therapy to the chest when they were between the ages of 10 and 30
- Have Li-Fraumeni syndrome, Cowden syndrome, or Bannayan-Riley-Ruvalcaba syndrome, or a first-degree relative has one of these syndromes

Women at moderately increased risk include those who:
- Have a lifetime risk of breast cancer of 15% to 20%, according to risk assessment tools that are based mainly on family history (see below)
- Have a personal history of breast cancer, ductal carcinoma in situ (DCIS), lobular carcinoma in situ (LCIS), atypical ductal hyperplasia (ADH), or atypical lobular hyperplasia (ALH)
- Have extremely dense breasts or unevenly dense breasts when viewed by mammograms

THE MAMMOGRAM EXAM

Mammographic units have compression plates to thin and flatten the breast to a uniform thickness. Adequate compression not only improves the quality of the breast images, but also lowers the x-ray dose to the breast. During a typical examination, two views are taken of each breast, one view of each at different angles. More than one view of each breast is necessary to unfold the overlapping breast tissue seen on the image. Larger breasts or fibrocystic breasts may require additional views or adjustments to include all the tissue or to adequately view dense tissue.

Some women complain of discomfort from the manipulation and compression necessary to pull the breast tissue away from the chest wall. However, this process takes only a few seconds for each exposure. The entire examination usually takes less than 5 minutes. Most women have minimal discomfort. Women who complain of breast tenderness should consider delaying the test until early in their monthly cycle (if they are still menstruating, right after their period) or a time when their breasts are less tender. Mammograms may also be delayed for a few weeks after a breast operation, because the breast compression may prove uncomfortable. As with any test or procedure, the ability to tolerate pain and discomfort varies among individuals. Most admit, however, that any pain associated with mammography is short lived, and the benefits far outweigh the momentary discomfort.

WHERE TO GET YOUR MAMMOGRAM

Many women wonder where to go to ensure they get a high-quality mammogram. Screening mammography may be performed in a breast diagnostic center, at a radiology office, at a physician's office, or on a mobile mammography unit. Federal law dictates that any mammography facility has to meet certain minimum standards delineated in the Mammography Quality Standards Act. All facilities should be certified by the Food and Drug Administration. Before making a decision about where to go, you should consult with your personal physician. If you have found a good facility, try to return there year after year; that strategy will make it easier to compare current with older films. If you switch facilities, try to bring your old films for comparison. If your mammogram is a digital examination, it is best to ask for a DICOM-compatible disk to transport the prior examination to the new facility. Asking the following questions may help you determine the quality of a facility.

How many mammograms are performed each day?

If 20 or more mammograms are performed per day, there is a higher likelihood that the technologist and radiologist will be experienced. For screening mammography, there is no need for the radiologist to be present at the time of the mammogram. However, if the mammogram is a diagnostic mammogram, the radiologist should be present so that the examination can be monitored while the woman is having the examination. In addition, ultrasound should be immediately available to expedite the workup and problem-solving.

Does the facility offer digital mammography?

Digital mammography has been shown to have advantages in women with dense breasts, and women under age 50. Most busy facilities have probably invested in this new technology. Currently, approximately one third of radiology facilities offer digital mammography. This has been changing as facilities buy new equipment. Film mammography is still an excellent exam for detecting breast cancer. Therefore it is most important to get a mammogram performed rather than delay in order to obtain a digital mammogram.

If the facility is using analog (nondigital) equipment, is the film processor expressly devoted to developing mammograms, or does it develop other x-ray films in the same processor?

Film processors used for chest or bone x-ray films are not likely to result in top-quality mammograms and are unacceptable.

Is the person who takes the mammograms a dedicated registered mammography technologist, or does he or she take other types of x-ray films as well?

The more experienced the technologist, the greater the likelihood that this professional will do a better job of breast positioning, and thus will obtain better-quality images.

Is the radiologist who reads the mammograms specially trained to do so?

The radiologist should be board certified and should have taken specific training courses in mammography. A radiologist who specializes in breast imaging is likely to be more experienced in interpreting the findings.

WHAT ARE THE COSTS?

Because of widespread recognition of the importance of breast-imaging examinations, many hospitals, clinics, and medical centers are offering low-cost screening mammograms, and many states require insurance carriers to cover the expenses of this test. Additionally, Medicare pays for annual mammograms. Insurance carriers and Medicare should reimburse for both screening and diagnostic mammography when indicated. If an ultrasound is warranted to evaluate a lump or an abnormal finding on the mammogram, it should be covered by the insurance company. If an image-guided biopsy or MRI is recommended, you or your provider should find out whether precertification is needed before these are performed.

To find the least expensive source for mammograms, a woman can compare prices. Many facilities participate in programs that underwrite the cost for low-income women.

MAMMOGRAPHY IN SPECIAL CIRCUMSTANCES

Augmentation Mammaplasty

Breast implants can affect the quality of the mammogram and the radiologist's ability to detect breast cancer. Because the implant, *whether silicone or saline*, is opaque to x-rays, any breast tissue underlying the implant cannot be seen on the images. If a woman is at higher risk for developing breast cancer because of her family history, she should discuss this matter with her plastic surgeon before undergoing augmentation.

Implant-displaced views (see p. 37, *bottom*) should be obtained to allow visualization of the breast that might otherwise be obscured by the implant. Implant-displaced views provide better visualization if the implant has been placed under rather than over the chest wall muscle, when a smaller implant has been used, and if the breast has remained soft. A woman should tell the facility at the time she schedules her mammogram, and again notify the technologist if she has breast implants before having a mammogram taken.

Reduction Mammaplasty

Women who have had breast reduction surgery should inform the radiologic technologist of this before a mammogram is taken. Although scarring from breast reduction is sometimes seen on the mammogram, it does not usually present a problem for radiographic interpretation. Unless an implant has been placed in the breast at the time of reduction, no special views are necessary.

If a woman is contemplating having reduction or augmentation mammaplasty, a preoperative mammogram should be obtained to screen for breast cancer if she is over the age of 30 to avoid missing a nonpalpable breast problem. This should be discussed with the plastic surgeon before the surgery.

After Mastectomy

A woman who has had a mastectomy for breast cancer needs routine surveillance of the opposite breast to screen for breast cancer. Mammography should be performed every year following the initial diagnosis, regardless of the patient's age. Women often ask if they need mammograms taken on the mastectomy side. Some facilities obtain special chest wall views to evaluate for recurrence in the skin or muscle of the chest wall. There is no evidence that such views can change the outcome by earlier detection of recurrences on the chest wall. However, if a woman or her physician can feel a nodule on the chest

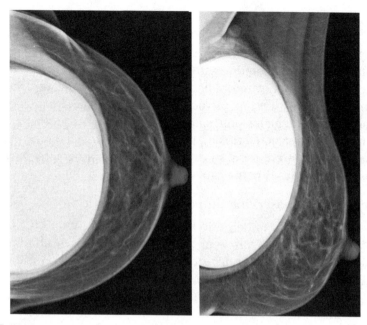

Full mammographic views of the left breast in a woman with subpectoral
silicone implants

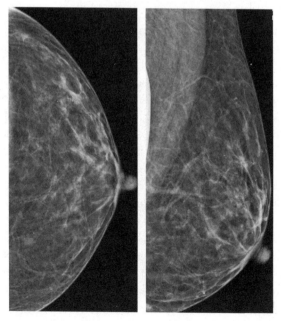

Special implant-displaced views of the left breast in the same woman with
subpectoral implants

wall, views of that area or ultrasound can be helpful in evaluation and may determine the need for a biopsy. If a woman has had a mastectomy and subsequent reconstruction, yearly mammography of the opposite breast is warranted to screen for breast cancer. However, as in the case of a woman who has had a mastectomy with reconstruction, mammography of the reconstructed breast is not necessary, because no breast tissue remains on the mastectomy side. If a problem develops in the reconstructed tissue, special views of the region can be obtained and are often useful in evaluation. Ultrasonography may also be used under these circumstances.

After Breast-Conserving Surgery and Irradiation

A woman who has undergone lumpectomy and radiation therapy must have meticulous follow-up mammograms. If a new abnormality (such as a mass or area of microcalcifications) is found on the mammogram or felt to be present on physical examination, then biopsy may be necessary to determine whether there is a recurrence in the treated breast.

OTHER IMAGING MODALITIES

Ultrasonography

Ultrasonography (ultrasound, sonogram) is an extremely useful adjunct to mammography. Its ability to differentiate a breast mass containing fluid (a cyst) from a solid mass (a benign or malignant tumor or other finding) offers distinct benefits. If a mammogram discloses the presence of a mass or finding in the breast that cannot be felt, an ultrasound is often performed. If the mass is a simple cyst containing fluid, then biopsy is not necessary. In most instances, however, unless the cyst is painful, aspiration is usually not warranted. However, if the cyst exhibits irregularities, aspiration or biopsy may be recommended.

There have been many advances in ultrasonography in recent years, and this technology may be useful in a variety of circumstances. The ultrasound characteristics of a palpable (one that can be felt) abnormality can often indicate whether a lesion is more likely to be benign or malignant. It can also be used to assess a patient with signs or symptoms of infection or a patient with breast implants to evaluate a lump or the integrity of the implants. However, as is true of mammography, this test is not tissue specific, and biopsy is often warranted

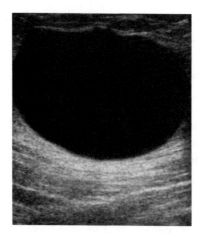 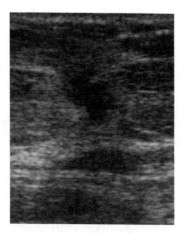

Ultrasound image of a large simple cyst

Ultrasound image of a tiny invasive ductal carcinoma

for a definite diagnosis. Often an ultrasound technologist may perform the actual scan, but the radiologist should be present in the department and available to participate in the ultrasound examination if needed.

Ultrasonography is extremely effective for providing guidance for diagnosis during breast biopsy. This has been a major advance for women. If an image-guided biopsy gives a definitive benign diagnosis, open surgical biopsy can be avoided. (See the section on image-guided biopsy in Chapter 5.)

More recently, ultrasound has been used to evaluate the lymph nodes. If an abnormal lymph node is detected in a woman newly diagnosed with breast cancer, ultrasonography can be used to guide the lymph node biopsy. (See the section on sentinel node biopsy, p. 44.)

Recent research has addressed the use of ultrasonography for breast cancer screening. Results have shown that although ultrasonography used in conjunction with mammography can result in the detection of more cancers, there are many more benign biopsies performed because of the use of ultrasound compared with the number that would be performed because of a finding detected by mammography. Furthermore, ultrasound screening has to be performed by an experienced radiologist and has not been validated for technologists or other nonexpert radiologists. In addition, if supplemental screening is to be performed for high-risk women, MRI is more sensitive than ultrasonography in detecting additional cancers, and *in such cases, the best combination of screening tests is mammography plus MRI, excluding ultrasonography unless something is detected.*

Breast MRI

Magnetic resonance imaging (MRI) is now frequently used as an adjunct to mammography. An MRI is performed with the patient lying face down on a moveable examination table with her breasts hanging free into cushioned openings; the unit itself is a special cylindrical magnet tube. The procedure takes approximately 20 to 30 minutes, and the patient must be able to remain still during the study. If the woman feels discomfort in the prone position, she should report this to the technologist before the exam begins so comfort adjustments can be made. For cancer detection, intravenous gadolinium, a contrast agent, is given through an IV catheter. If the exam is performed simply to evaluate breast implants (ruptured or not), no contrast agent is required. Some patients with claustrophobia may require medication, but overall the exam is painless and well tolerated by most. As with other MRI examinations, patient with pacemakers and other implantable metal devices cannot undergo the test.

It is recommended that the women who get an MRI do so at a facility that can do an MRI-guided breast biopsy if it is needed. Otherwise, the woman may have to have a second MRI for diagnosis at another facility before the biopsy can even be planned.

The American Cancer Society (ACS) recommends breast MRI for supplemental breast cancer screening in certain groups of high-risk women. (See the ACS recommendations, pp. 31-33.) MRI is not a replacement for mammography in this group of women; it should be used as a complement to clinical breast examination and mammography.

MRI is also often used to evaluate the extent of disease in a patient with newly diagnosed breast cancer to help in medical decision-making. In addition, MRI has been shown to detect cancers in the opposite breasts of newly diagnosed women about 3% of the time, even when mammographic findings are normal. The false-positive rate of MRI is higher than in mammography. This means that more women will have a finding that needs further investigation with other methods, such as ultrasound, and some women will need to undergo

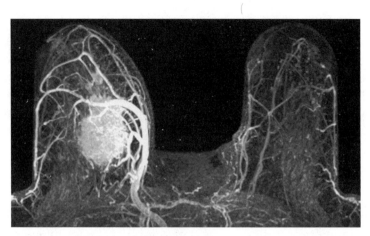

Contrast-enhanced MRI in a patient
with newly diagnosed cancer in her right breast

MRI-guided biopsy. Therefore it is important to discuss the exam with your doctor ahead of time, so you can understand the pros and cons of having such an examination.

MRI can also be used to monitor response to therapy in certain circumstances where the tumor is not yet removed from the breast. It may also be used in certain clinical trials of new chemotherapy drugs.

There are some special considerations for breast MRI. In premenopausal women, the exam should be performed between days 7 to 12 of the menstrual cycle (counting the first day of bleeding as day 1). Imaging in the latter half of the cycle can make the images more difficult to interpret. Because the study requires an intravenous contrast agent, which is excreted by the kidneys, a simple blood test should be performed before the exam to check kidney function.

OTHER LESS FREQUENTLY USED MODALITIES

Computed tomography (CT) is rarely useful in breast imaging but is under investigation for potential future use. Whole-body positron emission tomography (PET) may be used in newly diagnosed breast cancer patients or patients with recurrence, to look for the extent of disease in the whole body. It may also prove useful in estimating the response to systemic therapy such as chemotherapy or hormone therapy. Breast PET, scintimammography, and breast-specific gamma imaging are nuclear medicine techniques, some of which have received FDA approval and are being used clinically in practices across the United States. Unfortunately, although "safe," their utility and effectiveness in detection and diagnosis have not been well studied. They may or may not be covered by most insurance companies. More research is needed to evaluate the role of these technologies.

IMAGE-GUIDED BIOPSY

Image-guided biopsy represents one of the most exciting developments in breast biopsy and reflects the increasing use of minimally invasive surgery in different areas of the body. These image-guided biopsy techniques should now be the standard of care in practice. Open surgical biopsy as the first line for diagnosis should be discouraged and avoided, except in certain unusual circumstances. The imaging methods used include ultrasound, stereotaxis, and MRI guidance. These biopsy techniques remove small pieces of tissue or cells from the area of abnormality with a high degree of accuracy, through a tiny nick in the skin. Often a small metal marker is inserted in the region of the biopsy after the tissue has been taken. This is important, because it allows the radiologist and surgeon to know where the biopsy was performed and aids future procedure planning, if needed. If the biopsy yields a definitive benign diagnosis, open surgical biopsy may be avoided. If a definitive malignant diagnosis is made, then the woman can begin discussion with her surgeon regarding her treatment options before she has surgery.

The stereotactic unit is a variation of a mammogram unit in which two images are obtained at different angles. Identifying an imaged abnormality on both views allows a computer to calculate coordinates to accurately guide placement of a needle into a breast lesion. For small breast lesions that can be seen only on mammography, stereotactic biopsy is usually the method of guidance used.

Ultrasound is the most frequently used method of guidance; it is easier on the patient and more cost effective than stereotactic biopsy. If a lesion can be seen by both mammography and ultrasonography, biopsy is usually performed using ultrasonography. In addition, ultrasound of the axillary lymph nodes can often detect a suspicious node, even if it cannot be felt by the woman or her doctor. Performing an ultrasound-guided biopsy of such a node can often mean that a sentinel node biopsy can be avoided if the node is positive, saving the woman from unnecessary procedures.

If a lesion is seen by MRI only, and cannot be seen by ultrasonography or mammography, then an MRI-guided biopsy may be used for diagnosis. If an MRI-detected lesion can be seen by ultrasonography or mammography in retrospect, or with a "second look" with detailed imaging, then biopsy should be done by ultrasound or stereotactic guidance, since these are less costly methods of biopsy.

Sentinel Node Biopsy

Sentinel node biopsy is an excellent technique for lymph node evaluation. It is now the accepted standard of care for determining whether breast cancer has spread to the axillary (underarm) lymph nodes. The sentinel lymph node (the first draining node or nodes) is biopsied to determine whether the tumor has spread. Two different methods are used for localizing the sentinel node. One approach involves injecting blue dye in the region of the breast cancer and following the dye to the sentinel node. Alternatively, a radioisotope can be injected near a tumor to localize the lymph nodes using nuclear medicine cameras and handheld probes. Once identified, the sentinel node is removed and sent to the pathologist for evaluation. If it is negative for tumor, then other nodes do not need to be evaluated, because the sentinel node status is a good indicator of whether the tumor has spread. This biopsy technique has replaced complete axillary lymph node dissection in women with newly diagnosed breast cancer, thereby virtually eliminating some of the associated problems and complications (such as lymphedema) that have sometimes been associated with axillary lymph node dissection. (See Chapter 5 for more detailed information on sentinel node biopsy.) If the sentinel lymph node shows cancer, a complete axillary lymph node dissection will be required.

The growing incidence of breast cancer demands women's attention. Breast cancer currently accounts for 32% of new cancers and 19% of cancer deaths among women in the United States. Any test that can facilitate early detection and improve the chance of surviving this disease merits consideration. Mammography is such a test; in most cases it is capable of detecting breast cancer as early as 1 to 4 years before it can be felt on physical examination. However, as with most tests, mammography is not infallible and may fail to find about 20% of breast cancers, particularly in younger women, underscoring the complementary role of mammography and breast physical examination.

Ultrasonography is an extremely important tool in breast imaging. It is used for a wide variety of purposes, including evaluation of abnormalities found by mammography or clinical examination, image-guided biopsy of the breast and lymph nodes. Contrast-enhanced breast MRI is the most sensitive imaging test for cancer detection and evaluation of the extent of disease in the breast, but it is less specific than mammography, and thus its pros and cons need consideration before it is used.

BREAST LUMPS AND OTHER BREAST CONDITIONS

When a woman discovers a lump in her breast, she naturally fears that she has breast cancer. Fortunately, most breast masses are benign and are not related to breast cancer. Nevertheless, such a discovery can cause a woman and her family considerable anxiety. Although many women immediately equate breast pain with cancer, most tender lumps are benign (not malignant). Lumpy breasts, however, can be a problem and may make it more challenging for a woman or her doctor to detect new changes in her breast that may be a sign of an early breast cancer. Therefore it is extremely important to be aware of commonly occurring benign breast conditions to alleviate unwarranted fears, to understand when and how a biopsy should be performed, and to assist in early detection of a cancer if it does occur.

Although breast cancer occurs in women of all ages and the incidence among younger women has risen, one of the important factors in predicting whether an isolated breast lump is a cancer is the person's age. Less than 3% of breast cancers occur in women under the age of 35. Most breast cancers develop after menopause. When a woman in her thirties or forties finds a lump, it is more likely to be a simple fluid-filled cyst than a cancer. Less than one third of breast cancers occur in women under the age of 50. After menopause, benign breast conditions occur less frequently and the incidence of breast cancer rises; thus any lump is viewed with more concern.

BENIGN BREAST CONDITIONS
Fibroadenomas

When lumps are found in the breasts of teenagers and young adult women (without a strong family history of breast cancer), they are almost always benign. The most common benign breast lump found in this age group is a firm, rounded, rubbery tumor known as a *fibroadenoma*. Fibroadenomas are not related to and are not precursors of breast cancer. Surgical removal of these tumors is usually recommended.

Fibrocystic Breasts

It is normal for many women in their childbearing years to notice that their breasts swell and become painfully tender before their menstrual periods. Along with this swelling, the breasts often develop a lumpy texture that in some cases becomes a permanent breast characteristic. Although this lumpy condition reflects normal changes within the glandular tissue and milk ducts of the breast, it is often described as fibrocystic disease. Calling this condition a disease is inappropriate and unnecessarily frightening to women, since these physiologic changes occur in at least half of all North American women and are particularly common in women from age 20 to menopause. Because they occur during a time when a woman has a high level of female hormones, they are related to the response of the breast to those hormones. After menopause, fibrocystic activity usually subsides as a result of a woman's reduced hormonal levels. Women taking hormones after menopause may note a persistence of fibrocystic activity and breast fullness.

The symptoms of *fibrocystic change* frequently vary with a woman's monthly cycle and are often associated with breast tenderness or pain, which may be constant or may be accentuated when her breasts are swollen. Breast tenderness further increases a woman's anxiety that a tumor could be present, even though diffuse pain and tenderness are rarely manifestations of breast cancer. The soreness also can prevent a careful breast examination by the woman herself or by her physician.

Fibrocystic breasts usually feel lumpy because of cysts, irregularities, or thickened areas; some of these lumps are indistinguishable from tumors. These fibrocystic changes are not believed to be precancerous, but they may produce noticeable breast lumps that can be confused with cancer or even obscure the diagnosis of a small cancer. The newer image-guided needle biopsy techniques have further reduced the need for operations for fibrocystic disease.

Fibrocystic changes are usually managed without surgery if the doctor confirms that no other breast condition is present. Because it is a chronic condition, it may require surveillance over a long period by both the woman and her doctor, including regular breast self-examination, physician follow-up and examination, mammograms, ultrasound studies, aspiration of cysts, and biopsies of lumps that persist after aspiration.

Some experts believe that caffeine can accentuate the symptoms of fibrocystic breasts and recommend that women with this condition try to avoid caffeine-containing substances such as colas, coffees, teas, and chocolates. Some women notice a significant improvement in breast tenderness after abstinence from these foods, whereas others notice no change in their breasts. Vitamin E in a daily dosage of 800 IU (international units) is believed by some to lessen the symptoms of fibrocystic change in some women, although controlled studies have demonstrated no benefit from vitamin E. Diclofenac gel, a topical nonsteroidal anti-inflammatory medication similar to ibuprofen, was recently approved for symptomatic relief of breast pain secondary to fibrocystic change. It is safe and very effective for most women. In exceptionally severe cases, the doctor can prescribe danazol (Danocrine) or tamoxifen (Nolvadex) to control the pain and swelling. These drugs are indicated infrequently, however, because of their undesirable side effects, expense, and lack of efficacy.

Nipple Drainage

Nipple discharge is generally not caused by cancer. The only nipple discharges that are significant are those that are bloody and those that occur spontaneously without manipulating or squeezing the nipple. (It is normal to be able to express or squeeze a small amount of fluid from the nipples.) A discharge of blood or serum, however, can indicate the presence of cancer and should never be ignored. The doctor can take a sample of the nipple discharge by spreading a thin layer of fluid on a glass slide; it is then sent to the pathologist for examination under the microscope. Definitive diagnosis, however, can only be made by a biopsy of the involved duct.

Small, benign tumors within the nipple ducts (ductal papillomas) as well as fibrocystic changes or inflammation can be the source of drainage. Sometimes a localized infection within a duct can cause persistent drainage. Treatment occasionally involves removal of the source of the drainage within the ductal system. The doctor also may order some hormonal studies of the blood to identify other benign causes of nipple discharge.

Calcifications

Calcifications are deposits of calcium flecks in the breast that can only be detected by mammography. These deposits are common in the breasts of women over the age of 50 and in a smaller percentage of younger women. Calcifications are associated with benign or noncancerous conditions and most likely represent degenerative changes in a woman's breasts related to aging of the breast arteries, old injuries, inflammations, or common benign conditions such as fibrocystic changes. Calcifications may be large and coarse (macrocalcifications) or tiny (microcalcifications).

Sometimes minute particles of calcium are discovered on mammography. Although these microcalcifications can be an indication of precancerous changes or of breast cancer itself, this is not usually the case, and a woman should not panic if these are diagnosed. Microcalcifications are common in breast tissue, and most (more than 80%) are benign and are not markers of breast cancer.

A woman who has numerous scattered microcalcifications in both breasts is not likely to have cancer. Of more concern is a cluster of microcalcifications in one breast, especially if it is new; this may be the earliest finding indicating intraductal cancer. *Grouped or clustered microcalcifications are perhaps the most significant secondary sign of malignancy, frequently suggesting the presence of a breast cancer.* The probability of malignant disease increases with the degree of irregularity in the shapes of the microcalcifications as well as their size variations. Calcifications can also be noted after operations such as breast reduction and breast reconstruction. Most calcifications seen on mammography are benign.

Currently, mammography cannot accurately distinguish between some benign and malignant microcalcifications; therefore, in such cases, biopsy is needed for a definitive diagnosis and to rule out the possibility of breast cancer. A new density in the breast visible on two mammographic views should always be investigated or followed up with another mammogram in a short interval (3 to 4 months). If a questionable abnormality is discovered on a woman's first mammogram, the doctor may sometimes delay biopsy for several months and then order another mammogram to see if the findings are stable or have changed. Usually, however, unless the findings indicate a very low level of suspicion about possible malignancy, this abnormality needs to be positively identified by the pathologist after a biopsy.

If a woman is concerned about a lump in her breast, she should insist on appropriate and prompt evaluation that leads to a definitive diagnosis. Sometimes, particularly when the woman is young, this process may be complicated by several forces operating in divergent directions. Although breast cancer is rare in women under age 35, it does occur, even in women in their early twenties. This is especially true for women whose family members have developed breast cancer at an early age (premenopausal). Cancers in young women are generally faster growing than those in older women, and early diagnosis is critical. However, because a lump in a young woman's breast is usually not malignant, the physician may be less likely to suspect breast cancer. He may have referred other patients to surgeons, only to have further evaluations yield negative findings. Furthermore, some health maintenance plans penalize primary care physicians for excessive referrals to specialists. Mammography is less effective in detecting cancer in the breasts of young women than in older women. *A negative mammogram in such a case does not rule out cancer; in fact, it may be worrisome unless it actually reveals a benign condition.* Reevaluation of the mass at a different stage of the menstrual cycle and needle aspiration for fluid (a cyst) or to obtain cells for microscopic examination are appropriate measures. A breast ultrasound or MRI may be helpful in characterizing the nature of the mass if a biopsy is not performed. If a benign diagnosis is not established by these or other measures within 6 weeks, the patient should have a biopsy (minimally invasive, if possible).

DIAGNOSIS AND MANAGEMENT

Assuming that a breast problem is detected on a mammogram or that a woman finds a lump in her breast, what can she expect when she visits her doctor? The procedure varies, depending on her symptoms and her doctor's preferences. Some physicians will refer her to a breast-imaging specialist or a surgeon immediately, whereas others might prefer to examine her first. A medical history is always taken.

It is important to understand that referral to a breast surgeon or surgical oncologist does not necessarily mean that a biopsy will be done. Surgeons do not just operate; they are skilled in examining breast lumps, advising women about commonly occurring breast conditions and breast disease, and helping to detect and treat cancer at an early stage.

As a preliminary step, when a lump is first detected, the physician can use several noninvasive (nonsurgical) diagnostic tools. The doctor may suggest that the woman have diagnostic mammography or ultrasonography, in which sound waves are used to evaluate lumps. Ultrasonography is less specific and less dependable for detecting breast abnormalities than mammography and therefore is not as effective for screening. Unlike mammography, ultrasonography usually does not detect microcalcifications or identify very small cancers. However, it is particularly useful for distinguishing a simple cyst from a solid lump. It is also useful for examining younger women who have normally glandular breasts. The most frequently used and reliable nonoperative diagnostic test is mammography. Magnetic resonance imaging (MRI), a technique that does not use radiation, is increasingly being used in some diagnostic situations. (More detailed information on mammograms and other imaging modalities is provided in Chapter 4.)

Breast examination and mammography are complementary diagnostic tools. Mammography alone without breast examination is inadequate. Sometimes even obvious breast lumps will not show up on x-ray examination; this is more often the case when the woman is under 40 years of age and her breasts are relatively dense. A mammogram is a very valuable diagnostic tool, because it can indicate a breast abnormality at a very early stage before it can be felt and while it is still small and curable. However, it cannot positively identify a calcification or a mass as cancerous; this can only be done through a biopsy of the area for examination under a microscope. A biopsy is done after all appropriate imaging tests have been completed.

Needle Aspiration

When there is a palpable lump in the breast that feels like a cyst, it is usually drained (aspirated) with a thin needle. Occasionally the doctor may tell the patient to return to his office after her next menstrual cycle so that he can reexamine her breast before doing needle aspiration. Tissue that shrinks and then swells again before her next cycle could indicate a cyst or an area of fibrocystic change (both are benign and not related to cancer).

Needle aspiration is a method for determining whether a breast mass is cystic or solid. It is a simple and relatively painless procedure that can be done in the surgeon's office. A surgical biopsy may be avoided if the lump disappears after the fluid has been withdrawn from the suspected cyst. The doctor may want to send the fluid for analysis to a pathologist, especially if it is bloodstained. If no fluid is aspirated, the lump could be a fibroadenoma, a fibrocystic change, or a cancer. Most cysts are benign; breast cancer is usually a solid tumor.

If the fluid is bloody or if a mass cannot be aspirated, further investigation is warranted to rule out the possibility of breast cancer regardless of the findings on mammography. In these cases the surgeon removes the lump or samples a portion of the lump so that a specific diagnosis of the tissue can be made by a pathologist. This sampling is called a *biopsy* and can be performed by needle aspiration or surgery. Stereotactic or ultrasound-guided needle biopsy is usually the first approach when an abnormality is seen on the mammogram but cannot be felt. An open biopsy is reserved only for situations in which results are inconclusive or indeterminate.

Fine-Needle Aspiration Biopsy
JOHN S. MEYER, MD

Fine-needle aspiration biopsy (FNAB) is a method for making a definitive diagnosis of breast carcinoma without an incision or surgical procedure. This approach uses a narrow-gauge needle (similar to or smaller than the type employed to draw blood) that is attached to a syringe. The mass is localized (located) by touch, and the needle is introduced into it as the syringe plunger is drawn back to produce negative pressure, thereby drawing cells and fluid into the needle. Several repeat passes of the needle are necessary to obtain a satisfactory sample. A local anesthetic may be used during the procedure to prevent discomfort. From a few to more than 100,000 cells may be obtained in a drop or two of fluid. The cells are deposited on glass slides, stained, and examined microscopically. Interpretation is similar to that for Papanicolaou (Pap) smears. Malignant cells are recognized by their large abnormal nuclei (centers) and disorderly relationships to one another.

The results of aspiration biopsy can be available relatively quickly so that a decision on therapy can be reached before surgery. A number of studies have shown accuracy to be very high when cancer is diagnosed with FNAB; only about 1 in 1000 such diagnoses have been in error. Fibroadenoma (a benign tumor, discussed earlier in this chapter) may rarely be indistinguishable from carcinoma in needle aspiration biopsies, and premalignant changes accompanying fibrocystic breasts can at times be confusing to the cytopathologist. For the most part, however, a positive aspiration cytologic diagnosis of cancer can be considered equivalent to a diagnosis by surgical biopsy.

FNAB is not as accurate, however, when the results are negative, indicating that no cancer is present. There are several reasons for this diminished reliability. One is the possibility of missing the tumor with the needle. This risk increases as the tumor size becomes smaller. Another reason is that some breast carcinomas have small nuclei with minimal abnormalities, and these cells are difficult to distinguish from the cells of fibroadenomas or other benign conditions. Therefore cytopathologists err on the side of caution in diagnosing carcinoma and in certain cases may withhold diagnosis, recommending surgical biopsy for further clarification. If a suspicious lump persists after a negative needle biopsy, a surgical biopsy is necessary for definitive diagnosis.

FNAB may also be indicated when the physician is uncertain about the existence of a breast mass or a mammogram shows a focus of uncertain significance. In this situation the suspicious area can be examined by FNAB to help exclude the possibility of carcinoma. If the FNAB is positive, a diagnosis may be made at an early stage in the evolution of the disease.

Although FNAB is often sufficient for diagnosis of cancer, it is not sufficient for complete classification of the cancer type. The structural pattern of the cancer cannot be ascertained and the cancer cannot be graded by standard pathologic criteria. Estrogen and progesterone receptor assays can be done if several slides are specially prepared for this procedure, but often these assays are not possible from a simple FNAB procedure. Because of these limitations, the current recommendation is to perform a core-needle or a minimally invasive biopsy for definitive diagnosis.

Core-Needle Biopsy

Core-needle biopsy uses a cutting-type needle (somewhat larger than the needle used for FNAB) to remove a sample of the breast mass for microscopic examination. A core of tissue 1 mm in diameter ($\frac{1}{32}$ inch) and 1 to 2 cm ($\frac{3}{8}$ to $\frac{3}{4}$ inch) long is obtained with each pass of the needle. Often, it is necessary to take two or more core biopsies to be sure the sampling is representative of the whole mass. This quantity of tissue is sufficient for histologic grading, estrogen and progesterone receptor analysis, and assay for *HER-2/neu* and other molecular entities for genetic studies of the cancer cells (such as Oncotype DX or MammaPrint assays). The role of this type of needle biopsy is to make a reasonably definitive diagnosis without the need for an operation. With the assistance of image guidance, core-needle biopsy can be performed on even very small tumors.

Stereotactic and Ultrasound-Guided (Minimally Invasive) Biopsy

One biopsy method for suspicious areas that can be seen on mammograms but cannot be felt is called *minimally invasive* or *closed-needle biopsy*. This technique combines core-needle biopsy with three-dimensional computer imaging (stereotactic guidance) or with ultrasonography. It allows a needle to be introduced into a lesion that is ultrasonically or mammographically visible. (See Chapter 4 for additional information on minimally invasive biopsy.) This nonoperative or minimally invasive technique requires only a small incision and is performed with the patient under local anesthesia; recovery time is minimal. Both biopsy methods are used, depending on whether the abnormality is best seen by mammography or ultrasonography. These image-guided biopsy approaches are now considered the standard of care in lieu of open surgical biopsies.

Stereotactic-guided and ultrasound-guided core-needle biopsy techniques are sufficiently accurate for diagnosing small tumors less than $\frac{1}{2}$ inch in diameter. These tumors need not be palpable. By this means, the great majority of breast lesions, both benign and malignant, can be identified. If the lesion is benign, excisional surgery is unnecessary. If it is malignant, the surgeon can plan the definitive operation with full knowledge of the nature of the cancer. Multiple samples (4 to 20 cores) may be used to maximize the accuracy of this procedure. Some techniques remove larger amounts of breast tissue and may require stitches to close the incision.

When stereotactic guidance is used, computer-assisted mammography equipment maps the precise location of the lesion or suspicious area. Then the needle can be inserted through the skin and into the lesion, which is accurately pinpointed on the three-dimensional x-ray image. Either cells or tissue samples are removed and sent to the pathologist for evaluation. This technique, however, requires expensive specialized machinery and the skilled use of this equipment by a radiologist or surgeon to position the needle and collect the samples. Its advantages are a smaller incision and a shorter recovery period. New technology permits even smaller samples to be identified and removed with increasing accuracy.

As mentioned in the previous discussions on fine-needle and core-needle biopsy, false-negative results may occur, because the needle may miss the malignant lesion (that is why multiple samples are often suggested to improve accuracy) or may not yield sufficient tissue or cells for a diagnosis. However, this is uncommon in a core-needle biopsy, where pieces of tissue (rather than cells) are obtained. It is very important for the surgeon and/or radiologist to determine whether the pathology results of the core-needle specimen are in agreement with their level of suspicion on the imaging. This process is called determining *concordance*. If the pathologist's findings agree with the imaging appearance, the results are considered concordant. If the findings do not agree with the imaging appearance, the results are considered discordant, and additional biopsies are recommended. This technique is becoming more widely used and is available in most major cities and large teaching hospitals.

Surgical Biopsy
CHARLES M. BALCH, MD

A more specific and definitive procedure is known as an open *biopsy*. This method requires a small incision in the skin; the surgeon then directly identifies the lump and either removes the entire lump (excisional biopsy) or a representative sample (incisional biopsy). This open biopsy remains the gold standard method for obtaining a specific diagnosis of a breast lump or of a suspicious area that is discovered on mammography. It can be done with the use of a local anesthetic; however, most surgeons and patients prefer light general anesthesia supplemented by local anesthesia.

When calcifications or suspicious abnormalities are seen on a mammogram but are not palpable, an open biopsy is usually performed with preoperative needle localization. Needle localization is usually done by a breast radiologist with the use of local anesthesia. The clinician performing the needle localization may use a film image, stereotactic equipment, or ultrasound equipment to insert a small needle into the breast pointing toward the lesion. Then a wire with a hook on the end is passed through the needle and positioned so that it rests where the calcification, density, or suspicious area has been seen. The wire (and sometimes the needle) is left in the breast when the patient goes to the operating room to guide the general surgeon when he performs the open biopsy. After the incision is made for the biopsy, the surgeon follows the wire or needle and removes the area of tissue surrounding the wire and/or the area containing the dye. The tissue is then sent to the radiology department, where it is x-rayed to determine that the correct area has been removed. Once the accuracy is confirmed, the specimen is sent to pathology for evaluation. To be sure that all of the calcifications or suspicious areas have been removed, in some cases the patient may need a follow-up mammogram 3 to 6 months later.

When a surgical biopsy is recommended, the surgeon is concerned that the suspicious area or lump may be malignant. Plans must be made before the biopsy to consider the options for treatment so that if the lump proves cancerous, a definitive local procedure (lumpectomy) with clear surgical margins or mastectomy can be performed at the time of the open biopsy (a one-step procedure). Alternatively, the surgeon can remove the lump and delay treatment to allow the patient time to consider her options (a two-step procedure). In the latter situation, more breast tissue is removed with an increased potential for complications and deformity than when a one-step approach is used.

If her doctor recommends a surgical biopsy to clarify the diagnosis of a lump, a woman should ask questions about this procedure in advance so that she fully understands what is involved.

One-step procedures are usually done with the patient under general anesthesia after the biopsy. The woman remains on the operating table while the tissue specimen is sent to the pathologist for a frozen-section analysis. The pathologist places the specimen on a chuck (holder) and secures it in a microtome (slicer); it is frozen and then cut into thin slices of tissue, which are placed on glass slides, stained, and examined under the microscope. With this technique the pathologist is able to make an immediate determination as to whether the lump is benign or malignant. Although frozen-section examination is more expensive than routine histologic examination, this expense is more than justified by the large savings realized by avoiding the need for a second surgical procedure in the breast. Occasionally the pathologist cannot make a specific diagnosis based on these findings. If the report indicates that the lump is benign, the incision is closed and the woman is returned to the recovery room. If malignancy is diagnosed in the one-step approach, the doctor will proceed with the mastectomy or lumpectomy with lymph node removal during this one-step procedure.

The two-step procedure allows a woman with breast cancer time to investigate her options and make an informed decision. She may wish to obtain a second opinion and explore the different types of therapy available for treating her cancer and for possible breast reconstruction. In a two-step procedure, the biopsy and treatment are done at separate times. The biopsy usually can be done on an outpatient basis with a local anesthetic or by fine-needle aspiration or core-needle biopsy. The pathologist performs a "definitive histologic study," which takes longer but yields results that are easier to read than a frozen section. In addition to the standard staining techniques used for the definitive histologic study, other staining methods can be used to help make a correct diagnosis. Some methods employ immuno-histochemistry, which enables the detection of specific molecular entities. These can include estrogen and progesterone receptors and "oncogene" products (*HER-2/neu* [see Chapter 6] and epidermal growth factor receptor) and proteins specific for proliferative cells (such as Ki-67). The latter studies help to determine hormonal responsiveness, growth rate, and prognosis of cancer. A positive test result suggests that a patient may respond to treatment with Herceptin. This definitive histologic study takes about 24 hours. At its completion, the pathologist is able to make a final report.

A woman should also ask about the length and location of the biopsy scar. Often these scars are short and can be hidden around the outer edge of the areola, placed in inconspicuous areas, or planned to facilitate a future incision for lumpectomy or mastectomy and reconstruction. Usually such scars are nearly invisible once they have faded, but the final appearance depends on how the person heals.

A woman who detects a breast lump either during self-inspection or after a physician's examination should constantly keep in mind the most significant fact that countless women overlook: not all lumps are cancerous—80% of all breast lumps are benign. If a calcification or suspicious area is detected on a mammogram, she should not panic. Early detection and conclusive identification can ensure a better chance for cure if a cancer is present and can quickly alleviate a woman's needless fears if the breast condition is benign.

BREAST CANCER FACTS
AND TREATMENT OPTIONS

Breast cancer typically strikes healthy women in their prime years. Disbelief and shock are the natural responses of women faced with this shattering experience. Frequently they are as worried about the loss of a breast as about the presence of cancer. To them, "cancer" is a frightening word, a remote medical entity that strikes other people, whereas a breast is a personal and intimate body part, and its loss directly threatens them in many ways.

Breast cancer is the most common cancer occurring in U.S. women today. (The incidence of breast cancer in men is only 0.5%.) The American Cancer Society reports that one of every eight women in the United States will develop breast cancer in her lifetime, and it is the second most common cause of death from cancer for women in the United States. (Because of smoking, lung cancer, a much less treatable form of cancer, has become the most common cause of cancer death in women.) Today, for the first time we are seeing a reduction in breast cancer deaths as a result of the impact of early screening and adjunctive therapies. Hopefully this encouraging information will prompt more women to have regular checkups and to be vigilant with breast self-examination (BSE) and mammographic screening.

Breast cancer treatment now costs over $3.8 billion per year in the United States; that represents more than 1% of the total health care budget. This year alone, more than 192,000 U.S. women will develop breast cancer. For many of these women, attempts to treat their disease and save their lives will also result in partial or complete breast loss. Knowledge about cancer, its *prognosis* (projected outcome), and the options for therapy is necessary before they can make informed and enlightened decisions about their future.

THE NATURAL HISTORY OF BREAST CANCER

Breast cancer usually originates in the ducts of the mammary glands and is called *ductal carcinoma*. This is the most common type of breast cancer, occurring in 70% to 80% of all cases. In most other instances it originates in the mammary or milk glands (called breast lobules) and is called *lobular carcinoma*. These two types of breast cancer have somewhat different behavior.

A precursor type of breast cancer, *intraductal carcinoma* or *ductal carcinoma in situ* (DCIS), has been diagnosed with increasing frequency with more widespread use of mammography for screening. Recent reports indicate that 15% to 20% of all breast cancers currently being diagnosed are intraductal; these cancers are usually very small, often less than 1 cm (that is, less than ½-inch) in diameter, and may be too small to be felt. They usually are detected by mammography, thus underscoring the importance of this test for early detection. Intraductal cancers are not invasive and therefore do not spread, but if left untreated, may develop into invasive cancer with the potential capacity to spread. When intraductal cancers are found at this early stage, the prognosis for cure and long-term survival is excellent (approaching 100%). A special type of intraductal cancer, known as *Paget's disease* of the nipple, is characterized by a rash on the nipple associated with underlying cancer; this may be only intraductal cancer, or it may be intraductal and invasive ductal cancer.

Breast cancer does not appear overnight; in fact, it typically grows for years before reaching a detectable size. It is not precipitated by injury or a bump to the breast. Instead, it is thought to be a gradual process in which certain cells lining the ducts (the epithelial cells) change from normal cells showing an abnormal amount of growth (hyperplasia) to cells that are noticeably different from normal breast cells (atypical) but are not cancerous by definition. These atypical cells may eventually undergo further change and begin to regenerate themselves (autonomous growth), an uncontrolled growth that can extend through the cells lining the breast ducts. Thus breast cancer begins when a change in a breast duct cell gives that cell a growth advantage over other breast duct cells. The advantage may be a faster rate of cell division or a lower probability of cell death, or both.

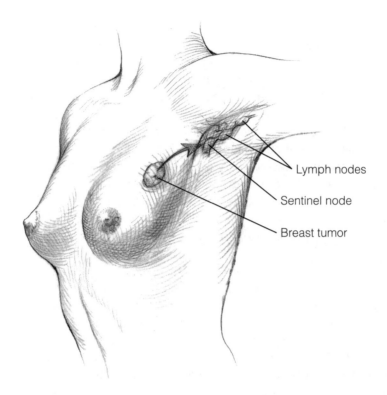

Lymph nodes

Sentinel node

Breast tumor

These cancerous cells initially grow inside the breast ducts (intraductal cancer) before they spread. If the cancer is discovered in the intraductal phase (or in situ), it has not yet spread outside the duct lining and potentially gained access to the surrounding lymphatic vessels, where it can then spread to other parts of the body. When the intraductal carcinoma cells break through the outer lining of the breast ducts, the cancer is described as *invasive*. Once the cancer cells become invasive, they can further invade into the lymph vessels of the breast and be transported to the lymph nodes in the armpit (axilla) or beneath the breastbone. Less commonly, the breast cancer cells can also invade the bloodstream and be carried directly to other parts of the body. When tumor cells are carried or spread outside the breast to other parts of the body and continue to grow, the process is known as *metastasis*. Current information indicates local growth factors that promote new blood vessel formation (*angiogenesis*) also facilitate the process of metastasis.

Because breast cancer develops from extremely small, microscopic cells, some experts believe that it often takes 4 to 10 years for the cancer to grow large enough to be felt as a mass or tumor. (Mammograms help identify breast cancers in their earliest stages, even years before they can be felt.) These tiny cancer cells have the potential to become invasive and spread to other parts of the body before the tumor can be felt, accounting for the high mortality from breast cancer and the serious and sometimes unpredictable nature of this disease. This invasive potential is also the reason it is so important to identify the patient at high risk so that through increased surveillance, breast cancer can be found in its earliest stages, before it has a chance to spread.

RESEARCH IN BREAST CANCER GENETICS

JOHN S. MEYER, MD

Research in breast cancer genetics offers hope for new treatments aimed at blocking the process that makes cells cancerous. Investigation of the mechanisms by which cells become cancerous has identified the existence of growth-regulating genes that are normally present in all cells. These genes appear to play an important role during the years of childhood growth and development but are normally dormant or relatively inactive once a person reaches adulthood. If these genes become activated, tumors can result. Because these genes play a role in producing cancers, they are called *oncogenes* (from the Greek root "onkos," meaning bump or tumor). Several of these oncogenes have been identified as factors causing breast cancer. The activity of some of these genes can now be measured in the clinical laboratory. For instance, breast carcinomas with overactivity of the *HER-2/neu* genes, or epidermal growth factor receptor (EGFR) genes, are known to have rapid growth rates and an increased capacity to metastasize.

Increased knowledge in this area has also led to a better understanding of how an inherited tendency toward breast carcinoma can be passed from one generation to another in certain families. Families in which more than one woman develops breast cancer are not uncommon, but in most instances probably do not represent inherited tendencies for breast cancer. The disease is sufficiently common to account for multiple instances in families by chance. The probability of an inherited mutation becomes higher when affected women of a given family are relatively young. The current challenge is to recognize women who carry a heritable breast cancer tendency. Two genes, BRCA1 (breast cancer 1) and BRCA2 (breast cancer 2), have been identified that, when changed or mutated, lead to an increased susceptibility to breast cancer. These two genes are thought to account for many instances of breast cancer caused by inherited genetic errors, but there are more genetic susceptibility genes yet to be discovered. (Human cells have 46 distinct chromosomes.) (See Chapter 7 for a detailed discussion of breast cancer genetics.)

More than 50 oncogenes have now been identified, and several of them are implicated in breast carcinoma, indicating that a breast duct cell can become cancerous by more than one pathway. Therefore it is not surprising that there are also different types of breast cancers and that these cancers vary in their growth rates and in their ability to invade and metastasize (grow in other parts of the body). Certain types have an excellent prognosis, even without chemotherapy or hormonal therapy, and others are more aggressive and have a poorer prognosis. Histologic assessment (microscopic analysis of cells and tissues) of breast cancer cell characteristics is helpful in determining whether the cancer might have spread. Molecular tests are used to identify *biomarkers*, characteristics of tumor cells that provide information on tumor behavior. These are used to predict the prognosis of a cancer and/or its responsiveness to particular treatments. Growth rate measurements are also helpful in prognosis. Cancers with high rates of growth are more likely to produce recurrences within a few years of treatment than those with slow growth rates. (These tests are discussed later in this chapter, p. 69, and in Chapter 7.)

RISK FACTORS

Some women are at higher risk of developing breast cancer than others. Age, family history, and previous breast cancer are three factors associated with high risk. (More information on risk factors is included in Chapter 7.)

Age

A woman's age strongly influences her risk of developing cancer. The largest number of breast cancers are detected in postmenopausal women between the ages of 50 and 70 years. A third of the cases occur in patients under the age of 50 and 25% in women over 65. As our population ages, however, a larger proportion of breast cancer cases will occur in women over 65. Any individual woman's risk is slightly higher with each year of age.

During the past 15 years, however, the breast cancer rate among women age 25 to 44 has increased, as it has in women of all ages. Our surveys and interviews confirm these findings. Many of the women we canvassed during the last 11 years were in their thirties and early forties with no previous family history of breast cancer. This increase in young women with breast cancer excludes the statistical increase resulting from better detection through mammography. Experts cite various reasons for the rise. Some point to late childbearing, fat in the diet, toxins in the environment, or some other unknown cause. Whatever the cause, it is crucially important that breast lumps in young women be thoroughly evaluated to rule out the possibility of cancer. This disease does occur in young women, and if a suspicious lump persists, a biopsy should be performed to obtain a definitive diagnosis.

Family History

Having first-degree maternal relatives (mothers and sisters) who developed breast cancer increases a woman's risk by two or three times, with a lifetime risk of about 20%. Your father's family's cancer history is of equal importance to that of your mother's. Too often, a woman's paternal family history of breast cancer is mistakenly discounted as insignificant. Since we inherit our genes from both parents, a woman may inherit a gene responsible for hereditary cancer from her father.

If a family member developed breast cancer before age 50, the risk is somewhat greater (30%). If the cancer was bilateral, the risk may approach 50%. Some women with these family histories have genetically identifiable heritable risk of breast cancer, such as women who have tested positive for *BRCA1* or *BRCA2* mutations. Other families simply have random occurrences of multiple sporadic cancers. Increasingly, laboratory testing can define which of these two situations accounts for a particular woman's family history.

Previous Breast Cancer

When breast cancer occurs in one breast, the cumulative risk of a cancer in the other breast is about 14% for women younger than 50 years of age with a first cancer. It is less, approximately 4%, for women older than 50. If the first was lobular carcinoma or if lobular carcinoma in situ was present, some experts once thought the risk of a second invasive breast cancer was somewhat greater. However, more recent studies have not confirmed that there is a higher risk after lobular cancers than after ductal cancers. The risk of a second breast cancer is greater if the first cancer is diagnosed before age 50.

Additional Risk Factors

The following factors also influence a woman's risk of developing breast cancer:

- History of breast cancer in a maternal or paternal grandmother, the father's sister, or the mother's sister.
- Excessive exposure to radiation in the breast area, particularly before age 20. Currently used diagnostic x-ray examinations (even cumulatively) do not reach these levels. Women who underwent radiation therapy of the chest for previous malignancies such as Hodgkin's disease are included in this at-risk group.
- Early menarche (beginning of menstruation).
- Birth of first baby after age 30.
- Never having borne children (*nulliparity*).
- Late menopause.
- Obesity.
- Socioeconomic status: women of higher socioeconomic status have a higher risk than poorer women do.
- History of some types of fibrocystic change.
- Alcohol consumption: Studies demonstrate a link between alcoholic consumption even in moderate amounts and a woman's risk of breast cancer. This may be related to the fact that alcohol raises the level of estrogen in the bloodstream of women. Many experts recommend limited or no consumption. Although alcohol is an established risk factor for breast cancer, results of a recent study published in the *Journal of the National Cancer Institute* in 2010 suggest that alcohol primarily increases the risk of lobular and hormone receptor–positive breast cancer. (Ductal carcinomas account for roughly 70% of invasive breast cancers in the United States while lobular carcinomas account for 15% to 20% of invasive cancers.)
- Race: Although the incidence of breast cancer is a little lower for black women than for white women, once they get the disease, women of African American heritage do not fare nearly as well. In fact, their survival rate dropped by 14% in the 1980s, whereas the survival rate for white women actually increased

during the same period. This may be attributed in part to socioeconomic status, education, and access to mammography and physician examination to ensure early detection, but there may be other factors as well, perhaps dietary.

- Environmental factors: At this time no conclusive findings have linked environmental factors to an increased risk of breast cancer. However, there seem to be geographic "hot spots" for breast cancer, or areas in the United States where there is a higher incidence of breast cancer than one would ordinarily suspect. For example, the high incidence of breast cancer on Long Island has been widely reported. Breast cancer rates are also lower in warmer climates, perhaps related to sun exposure.

Diet and Nutrition

Although no clear link has been found between a high-fat diet and breast cancer, the National Academy of Sciences and many experts recommend reducing total fat intake from 40% of calories (average U.S. consumption) to 30% to try to reduce serious health problems. Generally, low-fat diets are recommended to prevent excess body fat, which is widely thought to be the primary culprit in heart disease. This applies particularly to saturated fats found in many cooking oils, butter, and animal fats, not to the monounsaturated or polyunsaturated fats found in olive and canola oils. In the case of breast cancer, a low-fat diet is recommended, because estrogen accumulates in body fat. Conversion of steroid hormones to estrogen occurs in fat through action of the enzyme aromatase. Because estrogen has been found to be a "promoter" of breast cancer, it is believed that reducing body fat might prevent an overload of estrogen in the body and therefore a reduced risk of breast cancer.

A recent study published in the *American Journal of Clinical Nutrition* concluded that postmenopausal women who consume a traditional Mediterranean diet—one that is rich in fish, olive oil, vegetables, whole grains, nuts, and legumes and lower in red meat and dairy—may have a decreased risk of breast cancer. This study followed 15,000 Greek women for 10 years and showed that premenopausal women with greater adherence to the diet had a 22% reduced risk of breast cancer.

Exercise

Women who exercise regularly, whether they are premenopausal or postmenopausal, have a decreased incidence of breast disease. The benefits of exercise are of particular importance for postmenopausal women, because for them weight gain and obesity are associated with an increased incidence of breast cancer. A regular exercise regimen can help to avoid weight gain and the risks associated with it.

Estrogen Supplements and Hormone Replacement Therapy

For decades, women have used hormone replacement therapy (HRT) (either estrogen or estrogen combined with progestin) to ease the symptoms of menopause. Several large studies have investigated possible links between hormone replacement therapy and breast cancer. Results from the Women's Health Initiative, a large, randomized trial of women receiving either continuous combined HRT or a *placebo* (an inactive substance used for comparison) showed that daily use of combined HRT increases a woman's chance of developing breast cancer by about 5% to 6% with each year of use. If 10,000 women took combined HRT for a year, this would add up to about eight more cases of breast cancer per year than if they had not taken HRT. In this study, the longer HRT was used, the more the risk increased. Women who took combined HRT also had a higher risk of having breast cancer detected at a more advanced stage and were more likely to have breast changes seen on mammograms. Most of the increased risk of breast cancer from combined HRT is thought to be caused by progestin. Women who have had a total hysterectomy should take estrogen replacement therapy (ERT) instead of combined HRT. These women do not need progestin to protect against uterine cancer and are increasing their risk by taking combined HRT. The Women's Health Initiative also looked at women who had had hysterectomies. Those who were taking only estrogens did not appear to have an increased risk of breast cancer.

HRT risks apply only to current and recent users. A woman's breast cancer risk is thought to decrease after she stops HRT and returns to the same risk level as that of the general population within 3 years of stopping.*

Although it is now well established that menopausal hormone therapy with estrogen plus progestin increases the risk of breast cancer, new investigations are ongoing to determine which subgroups of women are at greatest risk. A recent study of menopausal hormone

---

*Information from American Cancer Society: Menopausal Hormone Replacement Therapy and Cancer Risk, 2009.

therapy and risk of breast cancer reported that risk may vary by body weight and the type of hormone therapy. These results were published in the journal *Cancer Epidemiology, Biomarkers, and Prevention*. In this study, the increased risk of breast cancer among users of hormone therapy was most apparent among thinner women. Use of hormone therapy increases the risk of cancers that were estrogen receptor–positive and progesterone receptor–positive.

BREAST CANCER STAGES

Once breast cancer has been diagnosed, the stage of the breast cancer is determined to assist your physicians in making treatment decisions. Physicians classify the localization and spread of cancer in terms of stages. A basic element of staging is classifying the cancer as *invasive*, meaning it has the potential to metastasize (grow in other parts of the body), or *noninvasive*. A noninvasive breast cancer (such as DCIS) is classified as stage 0. Invasive breast cancers are graded from stage I to stage IV, and both treatment and prognosis are directly related to the stage of the cancer when it was detected. Unquestionably, it is best to discover the breast cancer before it becomes stage I (that is, in its preinvasive form) and before it has spread beyond the breast ducts. Breast cancer in this preinvasive form is known as *in situ* cancer (in situ means that the cancer is "in its original place" and has not spread), and if a woman's breast tissue is removed at this stage, invasive cancer can be prevented. If no treatment is undertaken, up to 40% of these women may develop a more serious invasive cancer.

Staging is determined by the size of the tumor, its grade of differentiation, whether there is local extension to the chest wall or skin, the number and location of lymph nodes involved, and whether there are metastases to other areas of the body. To provide a more precise and standardized approach to staging, the TNM system was developed: *T* stands for tumor size, *N* stands for nodal spread, and *M* stands for distant metastases. The TNM staging system ranks patients as having stage group TIS (tumor in situ, or noninvasive cancer) or stages 0 through IV, with stage IV indicating known distant metastases. Although there are various staging methods, the system devised by the American Joint Commission on Cancer Staging is now considered the standard method. (See Appendix E for details of this classification system.)

PROGNOSIS OF CANCER

CHARLES M. BALCH, MD

The prognosis, or projected outcome, for a woman with breast cancer is related to the extent or spread of the disease at the time of diagnosis. Most experts agree that survival is directly related to the size of the tumor at the time of diagnosis. Women with small cancers (less than 1 cm, or less than ½-inch in diameter) have a better long-term survival rate, while those with large tumors with direct extension to the chest wall or with skin involvement have a significantly worse prognosis. Other features of the primary breast cancer are also important in classifying their risk of spreading.

The lymph nodes removed during axillary staging are also important predictors of the course of the disease and outcome for the patient. The number of lymph nodes in each armpit (axillary) area varies. The *sentinel lymph nodes* (the first draining node or nodes in the axilla) lying between the muscles and below the axillary vein are removed by the surgeon during surgery and are examined by the pathologist to determine whether the breast cancer has spread to this area. The pathologist checks each of these lymph nodes carefully under the microscope. Usually the pathologist can determine whether there are breast cancer cells in the lymph node within 10 to 15 minutes after receiving the specimen (a "frozen section exam"). If no tumor is detected, no further surgical removal of lymph glands is required. However, if there is evidence of tumor spread to the sentinel lymph node, other surrounding lymph nodes might also contain cancer spread, and the surgeon will perform a partial axillary lymph node dissection. The total number of lymph glands containing cancer is a vital part of staging and treatment planning. If any axillary nodes are involved, chemotherapy usually is recommended in an attempt to improve the patient's chances of survival.

After pathologic identification of the tumor type, other microscopic studies of the cells can be conducted to determine whether they are likely to be aggressive. Additional information can be obtained by examining the tumor to determine histologic type. For instance, some cancers are of special histologic types, such as tubular carcinomas and papillary carcinomas, that have a more favorable prognosis. Cell differentiation is also an indicator. Cancer cells that closely resemble normal mature breast cells are considered well differentiated and are associated with a better prognosis than poorly differentiated cancer cells that are less normal, or *atypical*, in appearance and have a less favorable prognosis, because they are thought to be more aggressive. The prognosis is also less promising when tumor *necrosis* (areas of dead cells) is identified or when there is evidence of tumor invasion through the blood vessels or lymphatic vessels.

The microscopic appearance of the cancer is especially valuable in node-negative breast cancer (cancer that has not spread to the lymph nodes). Measurement of how many cells are dividing (the Ki67 index) and the degree of cell division (nuclear grade) are reliable indicators of risk of cancer recurrence in most pathology laboratories and are used as standard measures of risk. The most aggressive cancers tend to have many cells dividing at the same time because of rapid growth. Less-aggressive cancers tend to have very few cells dividing. Pathologists usually grade on a scale of 1 to 3 or 4 (a measurement of how aggressive the cancer is), with the lower number being the best.

In addition to the microscopic description of the tumor and lymph nodes, a panel of tests may be used to better estimate a woman's risk of recurrent breast cancer.

BIOMARKERS

A major thrust of breast cancer research seeks new markers (biomarkers) that can predict a patient's prognosis and, in some cases, predict the outcome after specific therapy. Increasingly, physicians are using advanced molecular tests to identify characteristics of tumor cells that provide information on tumor behavior. There are a number of biomarkers to choose from, but scientists are still trying to determine which ones are the best for making these predictions. Biomarkers can be divided into three different groups: those that predict the prognosis of a particular cancer, those that predict whether a cancer will respond to a particular treatment, and those that predict both prognosis and treatment responsiveness.

Estrogen and Progesterone Hormone Receptors

Measurement of the estrogen and progesterone hormone receptors on the tumor cells is probably the most common biomarker analysis performed today; this is helpful in predicting prognosis and response to hormonal therapy. If laboratory evaluation shows the breast mass to be cancerous, hormone receptor tests will be run to determine whether proteins called *receptors* are present. Estrogen and progesterone are female hormones that can affect breast cancer cell growth. When breast cancer cells have higher levels of receptors for these hormones (estrogen-receptor positive, or ER+), that often indicates that the tumor is slower growing, and the prognosis is somewhat better. It also suggests that this patient's tumor will probably respond favorably to hormonal manipulation. Generally, postmenopausal women are more likely to be ER-positive, whereas premenopausal women are less likely to be ER-positive. Hormone receptor tests help your doctors determine whether cancer cells might be destroyed or slowed by administering antiestrogen or other antihormones.

Growth Rate Measurements

Growth rate measurements are also helpful in determining prognosis. Cancers with high rates of growth are considered more aggressive and more likely to produce recurrences within a few years of treatment than those with slow growth rates. Scientists have identified growth factors that are important in the transformation of normal breast cells to those with atypical features that then progress to actual cancer cells. With such unlikely names as S-phase, ploidy, *HER-2/neu* oncogene, epidermal growth factor receptor, and cathepsin-D, these markers can tell physicians how the malignant cells are growing and how likely the cancer is to spread or recur. For example, measurement of the genetic material (DNA) in tumor cells enables the physician to determine the growth rate of cells (S-phase fraction) and whether or not the tumor cells contain normal or abnormal quantities of DNA (ploidy). Other potential markers are related to the genes in cells that influence cell behavior (the oncogenes mentioned earlier). In particular, scientists are studying the *HER-2/neu* oncogene and its protein products to predict the response to certain types of chemotherapy. Epidermal growth factor receptors, nm23 and p53, are among the many other biomarkers that have now been identified and more are being detected on a regular basis. (See p. 99 in this chapter for a detailed discussion of *Her-2/neu* and other biomarkers.)

When all of these factors are assessed together, physicians are able to construct a fuller picture of the tumor, its prognosis, and its projected behavior. Then therapy can be tailored to the patient's particular circumstance, and reasoned decisions can be made about the need for adjunctive hormonal therapy or chemotherapy.

Gene Expression Panels

Researchers are also looking at patterns of a number of genes at the same time (gene expression profiling) to help predict whether an early stage breast cancer is likely to recur after treatment. These tests can be helpful to your doctors when deciding whether more treatment, such as chemotherapy, might be useful. Although there are several reported grouped gene tests, only two are available commercially: Oncotype DX® and MammaPrint®.

Oncotype DX

The Oncotype DX test evaluates a set of 21 genes from fresh tumor samples to determine a recurrence score of 0 to 100. Results are classified as low, intermediate, or high risk for recurrence within 10 years after diagnosis. This test is useful for determining whether adjuvant chemotherapy might be helpful in women with early stage breast cancers (stage I or II) who are ER positive, with no lymph node involvement. Recent data have shown that this test may also be useful for women with positive lymph nodes. (See p. 107 for more information on this test.)

MammaPrint

The MammaPrint test looks at the activity of 70 different genes to determine whether the cancer is low risk or high risk. It is used to predict how likely it is that some early stage (stage I or II) breast cancers will recur in a distant part of the body after initial treatment. It can be used for either estrogen positive or estrogen negative tumors. To perform this test, the tumor must be collected and stored in a specific way. Therefore the decision to perform the test must be made before surgery.

The Benefits of Testing

The Oncotype DX test has been recommended by both the American Society of Clinical Oncology (ASCO) and the National Cancer Center Network (NCCN), which publishes cancer treatment guidelines, as a means of predicting the risk for women with newly diagnosed ER-positive, node-negative breast cancer.

The benefit of both Oncotype DX and MammaPrint tests is that treatment can be customized to the specific risks and needs of each individual in determining the best treatment plan. Although these tests cannot predict with certainty whether any woman will have a recurrence, they are useful along with other factors in helping doctors and their patients determine whether additional therapy might be helpful. Currently, these tests are used primarily for women with very small ER-positive tumors who are node negative and who otherwise may be considered too low a risk to warrant receiving prophylactic chemotherapy or targeted therapy and can be treated with hormone therapy alone. These tests are generally covered by health insurance, but it is always wise to check with your carrier to be certain. The role of these and other new tests is still being evaluated, but promising advances are being made in understanding the nature of changes in cells that make them cancerous.

Despite the increasing ability of scientists to tailor risk estimates, most women with a breast cancer greater than 1 cm in diameter will benefit from treatment with chemotherapeutic or anti-estrogen drugs to lower the risk of local and distant tumor recurrence.

Breast cancer remains a threat because of its unpredictable growth and potential to invade and spread to other parts of the body before the tumor can be detected. Death from breast cancer and virtually all symptoms result from the spread to other organs of the body, such as the liver, lungs, bone, or brain. Research continues to seek the answer to why cancers invade and metastasize. Early detection is critical today, but an understanding of the basic nature of cancer will allow innovative treatments to prevent invasion or spread.

Even though cancer statistics can be quite frightening and information on oncogenes, DNA, and cell growth factors is intimidating, it is important to remember that progress is being made. Recent American Cancer Society data suggest an improved 5-year breast cancer survival rate for whites and blacks alike. This is exciting news and underscores the importance of early detection combined with the effectiveness of local and systemic therapy in influencing survival rates as well as improving the length and quality of life. The use of chemotherapy and/or hormonal therapy as part of the patient's initial treatment for breast cancer represents a significant advance in the care of cancer patients and is one method for improving the prospects of women at high risk by preventing further spread or recurrence of their breast cancer.

PERSONALIZED THERAPY

As our understanding of genetic differences among individuals increases, physicians are also learning how to use this information to tailor drug treatments and dosages to each patient. When you take a drug, your body metabolizes it and converts it to different molecules using enzymes. Some of these molecules are responsible for the benefits of the drug. The body's drug-processing enzymes are present in different amounts in different individuals. The targets for the drugs also vary from person to person. These differences in enzymes and the targets they bind to can affect the safety and effectiveness of drugs. This is particularly true for anti-tumor drugs that have low margins of safety and are given in relatively high doses. For example, with tamoxifen, women who are poor metabolizers get the least benefit from this drug, whereas rapid metabolizers respond the best. Personalized therapy is based on studies intended to help physicians choose drug treatments for individual patients that are tailored to their specific genetic characteristics.

LOCAL THERAPY: SURGERY AND RADIATION

Surgery with or without radiation therapy has always been considered the primary local treatment for breast cancer and the best means of eliminating cancer in the breast and in the adjacent lymph nodes. This is still the case, but the means for achieving this goal has changed dramatically over the years. Whereas cancer surgery once sought to remove as much tissue as possible to eradicate all local traces of malignancy and all possibilities for local recurrence, today the same goal can be accomplished with less-extensive surgery and without loss of the entire breast. Thus breast-conserving surgery (lumpectomy or partial mastectomy) followed by radiation therapy is an appealing option for many women whose cancers are detected early and are confined to a specific area of the breast.

Large, randomized studies and experience with outcomes have taught surgeons that less-radical surgery can provide equivalent survival for most women without the deformity previously associated with these operations. Mastectomies have also undergone transformation as new skin-sparing techniques have been introduced that, combined with immediate reconstruction, offer many women a viable and aesthetic alternative when a complete mastectomy is necessary or is chosen by the patient. The good news is that women's breast cancer treatment options are expanding; today they can realistically expect less-extensive surgery that does not compromise treatment or survival, yet produces excellent cosmetic results. Women can now have the most appropriate treatment for their breast cancer and still have a breast, either through lumpectomy and radiation therapy or skin-sparing mastectomy and immediate reconstruction.

What follows is a discussion of local surgical therapies, with and without radiation therapy, that are used for breast cancer treatment. Although surgery of the breast and sentinel node or axillary node dissection are commonly performed as a single procedure, in the interest of clarity, our discussion will treat these topics separately. We will start with an explanation of the regional lymph nodes, including sentinel node and axillary node dissection. Then we will explore the range of surgical treatments, from breast-conserving surgery and irradiation to the various mastectomies with and without immediate breast reconstruction. The role of adjunctive radiation therapy as a supplement to surgery will conclude our discussion of local therapy.

REGIONAL LYMPH NODES

JOHN M. BEDWINEK, MD, and ROGER S. FOSTER, JR., MD

When breast cancer becomes invasive, it can spread to the regional lymph nodes. The nodes most commonly involved with metastases are the axillary (armpit) lymph nodes. Less commonly, cancer may spread to the internal mammary lymph nodes just behind the ribs near the sternum (breast bone) or to the supraclavicular lymph nodes (above and below the collarbone).

Surgical removal of regional lymph nodes in breast cancer patients serves two purposes: (1) diagnosis (or staging) and (2) treatment by removing nodes containing cells that could proliferate. At the present time, for patients with an invasive breast cancer, the number of nodes containing cancer is the single most important prognostic indicator as to the probability of having microscopic cancers elsewhere in the body (*micrometastases*); these can then be treated to prevent a recurrence.

When the lymph nodes in the axilla are not involved by metastasis, the chance that the tumor will spread to other parts of the body in the future is decreased. When there are metastases to one or more lymph nodes, the risk for microscopic spread elsewhere in the body becomes higher. The greater the number of involved nodes, the greater the risk. The lymph nodes provide further information about the spread or extent of the cancer so that the course of the tumor can be predicted. This information on the involvement of the lymph nodes plus information on the size and character of the tumor are used in making therapeutic decisions. Knowing whether these nodes contain cancer helps the medical oncologist decide whether to recommend systemic therapy (chemotherapy and/or hormone therapy) and, if so, what kind of systemic therapy.

Radiation therapy can also be used to treat the regional nodes if they are not enlarged. The effectiveness of radiation therapy is roughly equivalent to surgical removal of the nodes. Radiation therapy of the axillary nodes may be indicated when it is judged that no useful additional information will be gained by pathologic examination of the lymph nodes. Radiation therapy is also used when it is felt that there is a high risk for spread to the lymph nodes over the collarbone (*supraclavicular nodes*) or behind the breastbone (*internal mammary lymph nodes*). There are fewer adverse effects when lymph nodes in these areas are treated by radiation rather than surgery. Radiation to the axilla combined with complete surgical axillary node removal should be avoided if possible because of the increased possibility of swelling (*lymphedema*) of the area. (The lymphatic vessels of the arm also drain through the axilla.)

Lymphatic Mapping and Sentinel Node Biopsy
CHARLES M. BALCH, MD

The most common drainage pathway for lymphatic vessels from all portions of the breast is the axillary lymph nodes. Even if the axillary lymph nodes are normal on physical examination or needle biopsy, there is still a 15% to 20% chance that cancer cells exist in the lymph nodes. Since there is a predictable drainage pattern through the lymphatics of the breast, it is possible for the surgeon to use a blue dye or a radioisotope (or both) to identify the *sentinel* lymph node in the armpit (the first node that would harbor breast cancer cells). Therefore a sentinel node biopsy, in which only the first draining node or nodes are removed through a small incision, is generally considered the standard approach to determine possible tumor spread. When no tumor is found in the sentinel node or nodes, it is unlikely that other axillary nodes will contain breast cancer cells, and no further surgery is necessary. Thus axillary node dissection can be eliminated as a staging procedure for the vast majority of women with a sentinel node that is negative for the spread of cancer.

A study recently published in the *Journal of Clinical Oncology* concluded that among early-stage breast cancer patients without evidence of cancer in their sentinel lymph node, sentinel lymph node biopsy alone is as effective as more extensive lymph node surgery. In another study presented at the 2010 American Society of Clinical Oncology meeting, researchers reported that women with early breast cancer and no evidence of cancer in the sentinel lymph node who did not require additional lymph node removal report fewer side effects to the arm and breast than women who undergo additional lymph node removal.

Axillary Node Dissection

When there is pathologic evidence of breast cancer spread to the axillary lymph nodes, either by needle biopsy or sentinel node biopsy, the standard surgical procedure for evaluating these nodes is called an *axillary node dissection*. This is a partial removal of the lymph nodes, not a complete, or radical, dissection, as was used in the past. With this procedure, the surgeon removes the lymph nodes lying below the axillary vein and those between the major back muscle that attaches to the arm (latissimus dorsi) and the major chest wall muscles beneath the breast (pectoralis major and minor muscles). Axillary dissection to remove these lymph nodes can be performed in conjunction with a standard mastectomy, with a skin-sparing mastectomy and breast reconstruction, or with breast-conserving surgery when a partial mastectomy or lumpectomy is performed. Surgeons may refer to these axillary dissections as "removal of level I and level II axillary lymph nodes." Ten or more lymph nodes are usually found by the pathologist in the excised tissue after this type of surgery.

BREAST-CONSERVING SURGERY AND IRRADIATION
JOHN M. BEDWINEK, MD

Lumpectomy

Breast-conserving surgery and irradiation is an option for primary treatment of breast cancer that has become widely accepted and today can be considered one of the standard treatment approaches for stage I and II breast cancers. As its name implies, the chief advantage of this treatment approach in comparison with mastectomy is that a woman's natural breast is preserved. The surgeon removes only the cancerous lump, along with a small margin of normal breast tissue. This procedure is referred to as a *lumpectomy* or *partial mastectomy*. When a lumpectomy is performed, it is important that the surgical margins are "negative." A pathologist examines the removed breast tissue under the microscope to judge whether or not the cancer cells come up to the edges of removed tissue. If the cancer cells border the edge of the removed tissue, then the margins are said to be "positive," and there is a high risk that a significant amount of cancer is left behind in the patient's breast. In this circumstance, it is usually necessary to go back and remove more of the surrounding breast tissue or revert to a total mastectomy if there is extensive involvement at the margin. On the other hand, if the cancer cells do not border the edge of the removed breast tissue, then the margins are said to be "negative," and the risk of a significant amount of cancer left behind in the breast is low. In addition to removing the lump, the surgeon also performs a sentinel lymph node sampling (see earlier discussion).

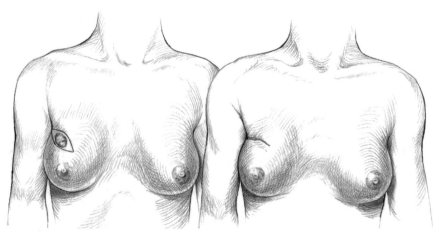

Lumpectomy

Breast Irradiation

After a lumpectomy, residual cancer cells remain in the breast in about 30% of woman. For this reason, the entire breast is treated with radiation to kill these residual cancer cells. Chemotherapy and hormone therapy can reduce the number of these residual cells, but not to the same extent as radiation. The 10-year breast recurrence rate with lumpectomy and chemotherapy (no radiation) is about 25% to 30% but drops to 5% to 10% with the addition of radiation.

The radiation therapy course consists of a single daily treatment 5 days a week for a total of 25 to 35 treatments (5 to 6 weeks of therapy). A total radiation dose of approximately 5000 centiGrays is delivered to the entire breast (centiGray, abbreviated cGy, is a unit of radiation dosage). Before starting radiation, a CT scan of the breast area is performed. This may take 30 to 45 minutes. The radiation oncologist uses this CT information to plan the treatment. The goal is to deliver a homogeneous dose to the breast tissue while sparing the heart and lungs. With today's modern computer-generated treatment techniques, this can almost always be accomplished. Following the planning day, subsequent radiation treatments should last only 10 to 15 minutes. Most women continue to work and lead normal lives during their radiation therapy.

After irradiation of the entire breast is completed, an additional radiation dose of approximately 1000 to 2000 cGy is usually applied only to the site from which the tumor was removed. This additional dose to the tumor site, referred to as the *boost,* is given to ensure that all residual cancer in that area is eradicated. The rationale for this boost is that the number of residual cancer cells at the excision site is greater than the number of cancer cells elsewhere in the breast.

The radiation used in breast-conserving treatment does not cause hair loss, nausea, or any significant loss of energy, although about 30% of patients do experience some day's-end fatigue that usually does not occur until about the fourth or fifth week of treatment. The radiation also causes a temporary reddening of the breast skin, similar to a moderate sunburn. This reddening usually occurs 3 to 4 weeks after radiation therapy is started and usually disappears by 2 weeks after completion of therapy. In about 10% of cases, slight thickening of the skin and the breast occurs because of increased fluid in the skin (edema). This skin edema, if it occurs, results from inflammation from the radiation combined with the axillary node surgery, which severs the small lymph vessels through which breast fluid normally escapes. In 18 to 24 months these vessels regenerate, and the edema usually disappears. Breast irradiation can result in late-term and potentially irreversible adverse effects after 5 years or more, consisting of breast contraction, skin thickening, and pain in the breast.

Investigators at Harvard University Medical School tried to determine whether there are certain women for whom irradiation after lumpectomy might not be necessary. They selected women with small tumors that were less than 1 cm in diameter and very slow growing and treated these women with lumpectomy without irradiation. Unfortunately, many of them developed a recurrence in the breast. The investigators concluded that even women with small, slow-growing tumors need breast irradiation after lumpectomy.

Who Is a Candidate for Breast-Conserving Therapy?

In 1983, when the first edition of this book was being prepared, breast-conserving surgery followed by irradiation was controversial, and many surgeons questioned whether it was as safe as mastectomy. Today, at the writing of the fourth edition of this book, breast-conserving surgery followed by irradiation has become a standard of treatment for many women with stage I and II breast cancers. The long-term results of the randomized trials mentioned above continue to show that it is just as effective as mastectomy with respect to survival rates. For example, results of the recent National Surgical Adjuvant Breast Project (NSABP) Trial of Induction Chemotherapy indicate that tumor size is no longer a limiting factor. If a tumor is too large to be completely excised with a reasonable cosmetic result, *induction chemotherapy* (preoperative chemotherapy) may first be used to shrink the tumor to a size that can be treated by breast-conserving therapy. This trial indicates that survival at 10 years is identical. These results now give women with breast cancer a choice between two treatments with equivalent survival rates. Nevertheless, there are very few medical reasons for not doing breast-conserving surgery and irradiation and these are listed on the following pages.

Medical Reasons for Not Doing Breast-Conserving Surgery and Irradiation

Pregnancy Radiation should not be delivered to the breast during pregnancy because of the potential for exposing the fetus to radiation. Even though the scattered radiation to the fetus is extremely low, fetal tissues are many times more susceptible to radiation than adult tissues are. Small amounts of radiation to a developing embryo can cause congenital malformations, and small amounts to a fetus can increase the risk of cancer or leukemia. However, if a pregnant woman with breast cancer wants to preserve her breast, she can have lumpectomy and node sampling during the pregnancy and can even have chemotherapy if she is in her third trimester. She can then have breast irradiation immediately after delivery of her child. Thus pregnancy is not an absolute contraindication to breast conservation.

Prior radiation therapy to the involved breast Women who have had radiation treatment of all or part of a breast for a prior malignancy (such as Hodgkin's disease) should not have breast-conserving surgery and irradiation for a cancer of that breast. The radiation that a given volume of tissue receives is additive, and the amount of radiation used for breast-conserving surgery plus irradiation, when added to the previous radiation dosage, may exceed the radiation tolerance of the breast tissue and thereby cause damage, such as severe scarring or ulceration.

The presence of collagen-vascular disease The three main rheumatologic disorders, referred to as *collagen-vascular diseases,* are rheumatoid arthritis, lupus, and scleroderma. Women with scleroderma or lupus that involves the skin should have mastectomy, since radiation in the presence of these disorders can increase the risk of severe scarring of the breast. Women with rheumatoid arthritis and most other forms of lupus, however, can be safely treated with breast-conserving surgery and radiation.

Extensive intraductal component in which excision with negative margins would create a significant surgical deformity Occasionally an invasive breast cancer will be accompanied by a large amount of intraductal cancer. This intraductal portion, if it comprises more than 25% of the entire cancer and if it extends beyond the main cancer, is said to be extensive. The name applied to this situation is *extensive intraductal component* (EIC). Investigators at Harvard showed that invasive cancer with EIC has a very high rate of recurrence if the margins are positive. For this reason, if the pathologist notes that EIC is present and the margins are positive, the surgeon must excise more breast tissue to achieve negative margins. If excising more breast tissue will create a significant surgical defect, the patient should strongly consider mastectomy and subsequent reconstruction instead of breast-conserving surgery and irradiation. In this situation, preoperative chemotherapy is usually not helpful in reducing the size of the intraductal component, and mastectomy should be recommended.

Two cancers in the same breast Although this is a rare occurrence, occasionally a woman will have two separate cancers in one breast. If all of the following conditions are met, then the women can safely have breast-conserving therapy: (1) both of the cancers are within the same quadrant and can be removed through a single incision, (2) there is not an extensive intraductal component (see above), and (3) the excision margins are negative. If one or more of these conditions cannot be met, then the patient is better treated with mastectomy, since the risk of recurrence in the breast after tumor excision and irradiation in this circumstance can be as high as 40%.

Diffuse malignant microcalcifications seen on mammogram One of the ways a mammogram can detect a very early cancer is by showing tiny flecks of calcium. These tiny flecks are referred to as *microcalcifications*. If there are microcalcifications that have been proven by biopsy to be malignant, and if these microcalcifications extend throughout a large area of the breast, this means that there are small amounts of cancer (usually intraductal cancer) extending widely throughout the breast. Under these circumstances the risk of recurrence following lumpectomy and irradiation is extremely high, even if all the microcalcifications can be removed. It is recommended that these women have mastectomy.

Having a BRCA1 or BRCA2 mutation (see Chapter 7) Having one of these genetic mutations is not an absolute contraindication to having breast-conserving surgery; however, women with one of these mutations who are treated with breast conservation have approximately a 40% chance of having a second cancer in the treated breast and about the same risk of getting a new cancer in the opposite breast. For this reason, many of these women opt for bilateral mastectomies and reconstruction. For women who do not choose bilateral mastectomy, breast-conserving surgery followed by radiation is still an option, but risk-lowering measures such as oophorectomy (removal of the ovaries) or administration of tamoxifen should be considered. Women with one of the BRCA gene mutations who do not undergo bilateral mastectomies should have their annual mammogram supplemented with breast MRI. This is the one instance in which a screening MRI may be useful.

Large locally advanced tumors or inflammatory breast cancer Most radiation oncologists agree that patients with more aggressive or advanced cancers are not good candidates for breast-conservation therapy. The standard treatment for stage III cancers is usually neoadjuvant chemotherapy, followed by mastectomy and postoperative radiation.

Nonmedical Reasons for Not Performing Breast-Conserving Surgery and Irradiation

In addition to the medical reasons for not performing breast-conserving surgery and irradiation, there may be nonmedical reasons for choosing mastectomy instead of breast conservation.

Lack of a strong desire for breast preservation Some women will say, "You're telling me that all I have to do to save my breast is to come in for a 15-minute radiation treatment once a day for 33 treatments? I'd come in for 100 treatments to save my breast!" Other women, however, might say, "You mean I have to come in every day, 5 days a week, for 6 weeks? I don't have time for that kind of foolishness. I'd rather have my breast off and get it over and done with!" Every woman is different, and these two responses probably reflect opposite ends of the spectrum. However, it is clear that not every woman has a strong desire for breast preservation. There are some women who don't mind having one breast and don't mind wearing a prosthesis every day. For these women, mastectomy is the better option, since it is quicker in that radiation treatments are usually not necessary.

Inability to get to and from a radiation center on a daily basis For some women, daily radiation treatments can be a real hardship because of logistical problems or a physical disability. A logistical problem might be lack of transportation or living a long distance from the radiation oncology center. An example of physical disability would be severe arthritis, making it difficult, and even painful, to travel on a daily basis. Some patients with kyphoscoliosis (the humpback that is caused by osteoporosis) find it very painful to lie on a hard table (which is necessary during radiation treatments). For all of the above reasons, mastectomy may be a kinder and easier option than breast-conserving surgery and irradiation. However, there is now an option that allows breast conservation for women who have difficulty getting to and from a radiation oncology center or who find it uncomfortable to lie on a table. That option is *partial breast irradiation* (PBI) (discussed below).

Fear of radiation Some women have heard horror stories about radiation or remember a relative who "got burnt up by that cobalt." These fears, while they may not be based on facts, are very real for the patient and difficult to dispel. Such women may be better off psychologically if they are treated by mastectomy so that radiation can be avoided.

Fear of the cancer-producing breast Some women view the affected breast as a cancer-forming organ and will experience continued anxiety unless they are rid of it. Obviously, for these women mastectomy is the treatment of choice. Anxiety can influence a woman's choice, as in the case of the breast imager who chose mastectomy and reconstruction over lumpectomy because she didn't want to have to worry about her breasts in light of the breast disease she was seeing on a daily basis.

•   •   •

There are few medical reasons today for not doing breast-conserving surgery and irradiation, but physicians (surgeons and radiation oncologists) should be able to recognize these reasons when they exist. They should also realize that there are valid nonmedical reasons that may be just as important, if not more important, than medical reasons.

PARTIAL BREAST IRRADIATION

Partial breast irradiation is a relatively new procedure that, like standard breast conservation, involves lumpectomy and irradiation; however, in partial breast irradiation, only the portion of the breast that surrounds the lumpectomy site is irradiated. The theory is that most of the residual cancer after lumpectomy is in the breast tissue immediately adjacent to the lumpectomy cavity, and if only this area is irradiated, there will be very few recurrences elsewhere in the breast. In other words, whole-breast irradiation may not be necessary. The

5-year data on PBI are encouraging in that the breast cancer recurrence rate seems to be no different than it is for standard whole-breast irradiation. Whether with longer follow-up there will be more breast recurrences for PBI in the unirradiated portions of the breast remains to be seen. Remember that we have more than 25 years of experience with standard breast irradiation compared with only 5 years with PBI.

An advantage of PBI is that it can be accomplished in 1 week instead of the standard 5 to 6 weeks. Why does treating only the tissue around the lumpectomy cavity make this possible? The amount of tissue damage and scarring following irradiation is related, not just to the total dose of radiation, but even more so to the amount of radiation given in each radiation session, sometimes referred to as the *daily fraction*. This is the reason that most radiation treatment today is given in multiple small daily fractions. Breaking the total dose up into many small fractions decreases the effect of the radiation on normal tissue. Thus late tissue scarring and damage are much less than they would be for fewer but larger fractions. However, if the volume of scar tissue that forms is small, then it may not be clinically significant. In partial breast irradiation, only a small volume of tissue is irradiated, compared with whole-breast irradiation; therefore large fractions can be given without worrying about the scar tissue that these large doses may cause. This allows fewer daily fractions and hence a much shorter overall treatment time.

Radiation oncologists have learned that the overall treatment time can be made even shorter if the patient receives two fractions in 1 day; this can be done if the fractions are separated by at least 6 hours, the time interval required for normal cells to repair radiation damage. We do not really need to wait a full day between fractions—6 hours is sufficient.

Radiation oncologists have determined what dose per fraction will make two large fractions per day for 5 days (a total of 10 fractions) be roughly equivalent to standard radiation (28 to 30 much smaller once-daily fractions) in their tumor-killing effect. These large fractions do cause more damage to the normal breast tissue; however, as noted above, if the volume of tissue receiving these large fraction sizes is kept small, the scarring that results from this additional damage is not clinically noticeable.

There are three forms of partial breast irradiation:

1. *Interstitial irradiation:* In this technique, hollow needles are inserted around the excision cavity. These needles are then replaced by hollow catheters, which are left in place for 1 week. Highly radioactive material is inserted into the needles for a short time twice daily for 5 days (10 fractions). This type of PBI is not used very frequently.

2. *MammoSite:* In this type of PBI, a balloon surrounding a catheter is placed into the excision (lumpectomy) cavity, either at the time of excision or a few days later, using ultrasound guidance to identify the cavity. The balloon and catheter are left in place for a week, and a highly radioactive source is inserted into the catheter to the central portion of the balloon twice a day for 5 days (10 fractions). The term MammoSite is the manufacturer's trade name for the balloon-catheter device. There are now balloon-catheter devices that are not from the MammoSite manufacturer, but the procedure is still referred to as MammoSite.

3. *Three-dimensional conformal PBI:* In this type of PBI, the radiation is delivered to the tissue surrounding the excision cavity by using multiple shaped radiation beams. This form of PBI is similar to standard breast irradiation in that external beam irradiation is used, but it differs in two important ways: (1) the high dose area is limited only to the excision cavity and immediate surrounding tissue, and (2) the dose is given in 10 large fractions administered twice daily for days (just like the interstitial irradiation and the MammoSite techniques.)

ONCOPLASTIC SURGERY

GLYN JONES, MD

Oncoplastic operations combine cancer therapy with aesthetic reconstruction. These procedures are performed in conjunction with breast-conserving surgery when removal of an appropriate amount of breast tissue to provide adequate margins for surgical clearance during lumpectomy may result in significant loss of breast volume and even a breast deformity. This is particularly true in a woman with small breasts or someone with a large tumor, regardless of her initial breast size. The deformity caused by surgery is further affected by the addition of radiation therapy and the long-term effects of radiation, which can result in fibrosis, firmness, and shrinkage of the breast over time. If the breast starts out deformed after a lumpectomy, it appearance will usually get worse over the next 5 to 10 years after radiation therapy, resulting in breasts that do not match. This can be frustrating and embarrassing for the woman who was seeking to preserve her breast, and it can also be an inconvenience, making it difficult for her to find a bra that fits.

Another issue that is not often understood by women requesting lumpectomy is that the larger the breast, the more difficult it is for the radiation oncologist to deliver adequate therapy to the entire breast to achieve treatment goals in breast conservation. It is easier to irradiate a smaller breast effectively, and smaller breasts tolerate radiation better than large breasts do, with less firmness and distortion in the long term.

If the breast is large, an oncoplastic breast reduction can be performed at the time of lumpectomy, thereby making radiation treatment easier to administer. This also allows the surgeon to rearrange the remaining breast tissue to prevent or minimize any defect or deformity associated with the lumpectomy. Standard breast reduction techniques are used, resulting in smaller, more uplifted breasts. This approach has the added benefit of reducing the symptoms associated with large breasts, such as neck pain and rashes; it also improves the breast shape and may provide some psychological reassurance to women who are already worried about the impact cancer treatment will have on their appearance.

If there is concern about the adequacy of the initial lumpectomy tumor margins, the lumpectomy can be performed, results obtained, and once it is certain that the margins are clear of cancer, the breast reduction can then be performed. This secondary procedure is usually done a week after the lumpectomy.

If the patient has a small breast and a large lumpectomy is planned, the defect that is created can be filled with a latissimus dorsi muscle flap that is brought from the back through the underarm to the front of the chest, where it is placed in the lumpectomy defect. This approach uses the woman's own natural tissues; the muscle is soft and warm and is easily visible on mammograms, allowing for accurate follow-up after surgery.

TYPES OF MASTECTOMY

The primary types of mastectomy performed today are modified radical mastectomy, total or simple mastectomy, skin-sparing mastectomy, and, less frequently, nipple-sparing mastectomy for preventive mastectomy.

Modified Radical Mastectomy

Today, modified radical mastectomy with sentinel node dissection is the method for *total breast removal* chosen by most surgeons for operable breast cancer. It has been shown that this operation is effective for local control of the breast tumor. Women who want to avoid permanent breast loss can have immediate breast reconstruction performed during the same operation or delayed reconstruction performed as a separate operation at a later date.

With a modified radical mastectomy, the surgeon removes the breast, nipple-areola, and sentinel node(s) in the axilla. The largest chest wall muscle, the pectoralis major, remains intact. This muscle is located in the front of the chest and helps to support the breasts; preservation of this muscle greatly reduces the deformity resulting from a mastectomy.

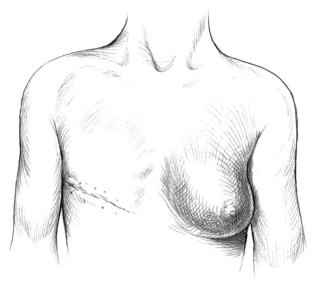

Modified radical mastectomy

After a modified radical mastectomy, the chest wall will not have a hollowed-out appearance, and the ribs will still be covered by muscle and therefore will not seem overly prominent. The loss of the breast and nipple will result in chest flatness. A scar will extend horizontally or diagonally across the chest. In addition, the area of the mastectomy is usually numb because the nerves that supply sensation to the chest and breast were threaded through the breast tissue, which is now gone. The inside of the upper arm can also be numb, because the nerves to this area that go through the axillary region may have been removed with the node dissection. Many surgeons can now spare these nerves and reduce the numbness of the inner upper arm area. After the mastectomy, the armpit is usually deeper and harder to shave, and many women notice less perspiration on that side than on the other normal side. Because the operation extends beneath the upper arm into the axilla, a woman may experience temporary pain after the operation when she moves her arm. The cancer surgeon usually will recommend postoperative exercises to ensure the return of full use and function of the arm. Some women also report experiencing a phenomenon called *phantom pain* in the area of the missing nipple or breast. They may feel throbbing, tingling, numbness, or stabbing pains. These sensations are probably caused by the nerve endings that were cut during surgery and that regrow incompletely after the operation. Exercise and pain medication might alleviate this discomfort.

Total or Simple Mastectomy

A total mastectomy or simple mastectomy may be done without removing the lymph nodes. It is very much the same operation as the breast removal portion of the modified radical mastectomy; all or nearly all of the breast tissue is removed. Depending on the extent of the tumor in the breast and on whether the patient is to have immediate breast reconstruction, variable amounts of skin are removed. When no reconstruction is planned, the surgeon usually removes a relatively large amount of skin.

Skin-Sparing Mastectomy

WILLIAM C. WOOD, MD

For patients who are to have mastectomy with immediate reconstruction, a skin-sparing mastectomy may be considered. This approach is only appropriate for individuals who have *no tumor involvement of the skin area to be saved.* For women requiring mastectomy who are appropriate candidates for this skin-sparing approach, this operation provides the best cosmetic result. With this procedure, only the nipple and areola are excised as well as the overlying skin in those areas. If necessary, the incision extends to the side of the nipple and areola in a horizontal or vertical line approximately ½ to 1 inch to allow all of the breast and the lower axillary nodes to be removed. During the immediate breast reconstruction the skin envelope is refilled to provide a symmetrical breast appearance that is very similar to the premastectomy appearance. The appearance and symmetry are enhanced by preservation or re-creation of the anatomic landmarks of the breast, such as the inframammary fold, the lateral breast line, and the cleavage line.

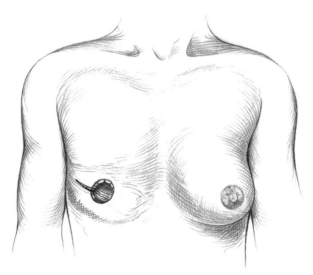

Skin-sparing mastectomy

Nipple-Sparing Mastectomy

In some situations a nipple-sparing mastectomy can be performed in which all of the skin, including the nipple, is preserved. This type of mastectomy is appropriate for preventive procedures, but its application is still the subject of debate when the mastectomy is performed for cancer excision.

IMMEDIATE BREAST RECONSTRUCTION
WILLIAM C. WOOD, MD

Many surgeons who recommend a mastectomy for women with breast cancer also inform them of the option of breast reconstruction to rebuild their breasts and fill in the defects left from their cancer surgery. Immediate breast reconstruction has become the preferred timing option for women undergoing mastectomy, and they are choosing it with increasing frequency because it combines a safe and effective treatment for breast cancer with immediate breast restoration. Immediate breast reconstruction often permits a skin-sparing mastectomy to be performed (if there is no tumor involvement in the skin), which requires less skin removal and sensory nerve division and produces shorter scars. By removing the breast and replacing the volume immediately, the skin that is not excised as a part of the cancer operation can then be used for the reconstruction. If the mastectomy is performed separately, more breast skin must be removed initially to create a smooth skin surface over the chest wall and to avoid leaving redundant folds of breast skin that would thicken and toughen over time. Later, when breast reconstruction is performed, the missing breast skin must be replaced either by transferring new skin from another part of the body on a muscle-skin (*musculocutaneous or myocutaneous*) flap or by stretching the skin at the mastectomy site (tissue expansion) to make it expand to the desired size.

With this approach, the cancer surgeon and plastic surgeon must closely coordinate their efforts and work as a team, since the mastectomy and the breast reconstruction are done during one operation, which means the patient will have to undergo anesthesia only once. Since there is only one initial procedure, a woman will not have to wear a breast prosthesis or experience breast loss. The nipple-areola is usually reconstructed later, and any other adjustments are performed to enhance symmetry and appearance. Most women prefer this approach, because they don't have to face a mastectomy deformity. Depending on the reconstructive procedure chosen, the patient may need a blood transfusion.

In the past some expressed concern that breast reconstruction, particularly when done immediately, would make it difficult to examine the chest wall for recurrent disease. This has not proved to be the case. In most instances there is no contraindication to immediate reconstruction for patients with stage I or II breast cancer. However, women with stage III breast cancer (locally advanced) must have a combination of surgery, chemotherapy, and chest wall radiation therapy. Therefore, for these patients it may be prudent to complete all therapy before pursuing breast reconstruction. Although patients with stage III breast cancer can safely have reconstructive surgery, some oncologists suggest that these very high-risk patients wait 1 to 2 years before proceeding with further surgery. An alternative approach is initial chemotherapy (neoadjuvant or induction) to shrink the tumor, followed by a mastectomy, immediate breast reconstruction, and follow-up radiation therapy. Cancer treatment should be the first priority, and any complication of reconstruction that would delay therapy should be avoided. For the majority of women facing mastectomy, however, immediate reconstruction is a welcome option that permits them to receive optimal treatment of their breast cancer without the trauma of breast loss.

POSTOPERATIVE IRRADIATION

JOHN M. BEDWINEK, MD, and WILLIAM C. WOOD, MD

The term *postoperative irradiation* is used to indicate radiation treatment that is delivered to the chest wall and regional lymph nodes (those in the axilla and those beneath and over the collarbone) after a total or modified radical mastectomy in patients who, for one of the reasons noted previously, are not good candidates for breast conservation. Not all patients who have mastectomy require postoperative radiation. It is indicated when there is a high risk (25% risk or greater) that microscopic cancer cells will remain in the local area (chest wall and/or regional lymph nodes) after mastectomy. This level of risk occurs when the breast tumor is greater than 5 cm (about 2 inches) in maximum diameter, when 4 or more of the nodes removed form the axilla contain cancer, and/or when there is invasion of the skin or underlying muscle by cancer. Approximately 25% to 35% of patients with these tumor characteristics will develop a recurrence of cancer on the chest wall or in the regional lymph nodes if radiation is not given to these areas after mastectomy. Most patients for whom postoperative radiation is indicated will also be receiving adjuvant chemotherapy. Usually all of the chemotherapy is given before starting the radiation.

In 1990, two articles, one from Denmark and another from British Columbia, were published that suggested that postoperative radiation improved the survival (cure rate) in women not just with high risk features (four or more positive nodes, large tumors and skin involvement) but also for those women with only one to three positive lymph nodes. For this reason many radiation oncologists advocate radiation after mastectomy, not just for women with high risk features but for all women with any number of positive lymph nodes. However, not all radiation oncologists agree with this policy. They argue that the mastectomy performed in the British Columbia and Danish studies did not have as thorough an axillary dissection as is usually done in this country and therefore the survival advantage seen with post operative radiation may not be as great.

SYSTEMIC THERAPY: CHEMOTHERAPY, HORMONAL THERAPY, AND GENETIC THERAPY

Surgery and radiation therapy are used for local cancer removal in the breast and axilla, whereas chemotherapy, hormonal therapy, and genetic therapy are intended to interfere with the growth and spread of cancer to other parts of the body. As such, these therapies are often referred to as *adjunctive*, because they supplement the effectiveness of surgery.

When a woman learns that she requires additional therapy after her surgery and/or possible radiation treatment, this is often devastating news. The last thing she wants to deal with is another assault on her body with potentially toxic drugs. However, chemotherapy and hormonal therapy are essential, lifesaving treatments and integral to current breast cancer treatment regimens. Their long-term benefits should not be overlooked because of side effects that will pass relatively quickly, are often not as debilitating as might be feared, and are not permanent. A woman owes it to herself to seriously weigh the life-sustaining value of these therapies. Even though surgery will greatly reduce the risk of cancer spread, particularly if the cancer is detected in its earliest stages (in situ cancer), some risk still remains. Despite the increasing ability to tailor risk estimates, any woman with a breast cancer over 1 cm in diameter will probably benefit from treatment with chemotherapeutic or antiestrogen (hormonal) drugs to lower her risk of tumor recurrence. If microscopic cancer cells are found in the lymph nodes or if the tumor has other unfavorable prognostic signs, we know that cancer has a higher chance of being in other parts of the body. That is where systemic therapy takes over. Chemotherapy and hormonal therapy drugs travel through the bloodstream to attack cancer in distant sites, thereby significantly reducing the risk of recurrence by as much as one half and profoundly affecting the life span of women with breast cancer. Chemotherapy can also play a role preoperatively (neoadjuvant or induction chemotherapy) when used to shrink the tumor before surgery, often permitting a less extensive surgical procedure to be performed. Monoclonal antibodies and anti-angiogenesis drugs that shrink tumors and prevent growth of tumors that have spread also hold promise.

CHEMOTHERAPY

DAN W. LUEDKE, MD

Chemotherapy often conjures visions of nausea, vomiting, diarrhea, and hair loss in the minds of breast cancer patients and their families. The mythology of most families contains an "Aunt Sarah" who was diagnosed with breast cancer and suffered horribly from the treatment. Such may have been the case years ago, but that is not the case today. Fortunately, we have come a long way in treating breast cancer and reducing the side effects of therapy.

What Is Chemotherapy?

Chemotherapy is treatment involving chemical agents to destroy cancer cells. It is a systemic therapy given by vein, mouth or injection and traveling throughout the body to kill cancer cells and prevent recurrence of disease.

Who Are Candidates for Chemotherapy?

Candidates for chemotherapy include patients with invasive breast cancer who are at high risk for recurrence and are not candidates for hormonal therapy or those who have failed or been intolerant of hormonal therapy in the past. Patients with metastatic disease may also be candidates for chemotherapy, particularly those who are not candidates for hormonal therapy. In deciding who is a candidate for chemotherapy, the physician must consider whether the patient is healthy enough to tolerate the toxicities related to chemotherapy and the comorbid conditions the patient has. For example, if a patient has an underlying heart condition, she should not undergo chemotherapy with a drug that has cardiac toxicity.

How Is Chemotherapy Administered and What Is the Usual Course of Treatment?

Most chemotherapy drugs are given by intravenous injection, but capecitabine, and on occasion cyclophosphamide and methotrexate, are given orally. These routes of administration provide access to the bloodstream and hence are called *systemic;* that is, they go all over the body. Other routes of administration are usually reserved for special situations. One example is the injection of methotrexate directly into the spinal fluid when cancer has spread to the meninges (the covering over the brain and spinal cord). Most chemotherapy drugs can be given on an outpatient basis.

The course of chemotherapy depends on the drugs given and the characteristics of the drug. Treatments are usually scheduled in cycles to allow the patient to recover from side effects. A cycle typically lasts 3 or 4 weeks, with drugs given on the first day only, or once each week. Patients with metastatic disease are usually treated until no progression of disease is found. For adjuvant treatment, chemotherapy is given for a prescribed period of time and then discontinued. Toxicities may also necessitate discontinuation of treatment. A patient may also choose to discontinue treatment altogether.

Timing for Chemotherapy

The timing of chemotherapy depends on the situation and treatment the patient will be getting. A patient needs to be adequately healed from surgery before starting chemotherapy, because the treatments may delay wound healing. For a patient with metastatic cancer, treatment should begin as soon as disease progression is confirmed and eligibility is ensured.

Chemotherapy Drugs

The first family of chemotherapy drugs used for widespread metastatic breast cancer were called *alkylating agents*. These drugs penetrate the nucleus of the cell and bind together strands of DNA, disrupting cell proliferation. The best known of these drugs, cyclophosphamide (Cytoxan), is still the backbone of many chemotherapy regimens for breast cancer. Newer alkylating agents include the platinum derivatives, cisplatin (Platinol) and carboplatin (Paraplatin); these appear active in selected situations.

Subsequent chemotherapy drug development focused on killing the dividing (proliferating) cancer cell. Drugs found to be most useful in killing breast cancer cells included the fluorinated pyrimidine fluorouracil (5-FU) and the folate antagonist methotrexate. Another class of agents, the anthracyclines, including doxorubicin (Adriamycin) and epirubicin (Ellence), showed benefit in metastatic breast cancer, as did a growing list of FDA-approved drugs such as the taxanes, which act to stabilize cell microtubules that are crucial to cell division. Other taxanes that received FDA approval include paclitaxel (Taxol/Abraxane) and docetaxel (Taxotere). A historical footnote is that the taxanes were initially derived from the yew tree, which is found in the old-growth forests of the western United States. A brief media-fueled controversy arose over possible depletion of the yew and the old-growth forest environment in order to obtain drugs to treat breast cancer. This quickly became a moot point when the drugs were able to be synthesized in a laboratory, sparing the yew tree.

Today the search continues for the perfect drug to kill the proliferating breast cancer cell. FDA approval has been given to a relative of fluorouracil, gemcitabine (Gemzar); a prefluorouracil; capecitabine (Xeloda); and a vinca alkaloid, vinorelbine (Navelbine); this class of drugs also interferes with microtubules. This class also includes vincristine, which is no longer in common use for breast cancer. The most recent addition to the FDA-approved list of drugs directed toward killing proliferating breast cancer cells is ixabepilone (Ixempra). This is the first of a new class of agents, the epothilones, which also work on microtubules. It is primarily used in refractory breast cancer.

Adjuvant Chemotherapy

Adjunctive chemotherapy represents an exciting advance in breast cancer therapy. Although chemotherapy originally focused on management of widespread metastatic disease, adjunctive applications are used to prevent breast cancer recurrence or spread. This approach to chemotherapy was ushered in by a bright and daring group of Italian researchers who gave a combination of three drugs, cyclophosphamide, methotrexate, and fluorouracil (CMF) to women with breast cancer. The daring aspect of this treatment was that it was given to women who had undergone breast cancer surgery and radiation therapy and who had no evidence of cancer. They conducted a careful randomized trial: all women enrolled in the trial had disease clinically confined to the breast and axillary lymph nodes. All had appropriate breast surgery and, if indicated, radiation therapy. Then, by a flip of the coin, half of the women received CMF and the other half received no additional therapy. All were carefully followed. As expected, some of the women developed metastatic disease over the course of follow-up. But the exciting result was that many more women who had received CMF were alive and cured of their cancer compared with those who did not. Similar trials using different drugs have been conducted in the United States, spearheaded by superb trials by the National Surgical Adjuvant Breast Project (NSABP) Trial of Induction Chemotherapy, which confirmed the benefits of adjuvant chemotherapy. The era of adjuvant chemotherapy had arrived.

If metastatic breast cancer can be treated when it is so early in its growth that it cannot be seen on imaging studies such as CT, MRI, bone scan, or even PET scan (this is called *micrometastatic disease*), then there is a chance of killing all of the cancerous cells before they can develop resistant mutants. This concept has been extended to the preoperative setting. For patients with large primary tumors, these can be reduced in size by neoadjuvant chemotherapy. There is no difference in survival rates, whether adjuvant chemotherapy is given before or after surgery, but selected women may require less extensive surgery if they are first treated with chemotherapy, and a better cosmetic effect can be achieved. By selecting combinations of the most active single-agent chemotherapy drugs, we have improved the results of adjuvant therapy. Some of these combinations include the previously mentioned cyclophosphamide/methotrexate/fluorouracil. Please note that medical oncologists are addicted to eponyms and hence this combination is CMF. To achieve memorable acronyms, they also mix generic with brand names, as with cyclophosphamide/Adriamycin (CA) and cyclophosphamide/Taxotere (CT). Other effective combinations include cyclophosphamide/epirubicin/fluorouracil (FEC), Taxotere/Adriamycin/cyclophosphamide (TAC); and fluorouracil/Adriamycin/cyclophosphamide (FAC). Recently some of these combinations have been sequenced with a taxane with some additional success in high-risk patients. These include FEC for three cycles, followed by Taxol and CA, followed by Taxol or Taxotere. These regimens are usually given as *pulse doses,* with each drug given only on the first day of a 3-week cycle. This allows recovery from toxicity, which principally consists of lowered blood cell counts.

Efforts have been made to accelerate the doses of these combinations, including high-dose chemotherapy and autologous stem cell transplantation. This had proven benefit in the treatment of relapse lymphoma and was extended to the treatment of breast cancer patients. Patients at very high risk of recurrence had bone marrow (stem cells) harvested. High-dose chemotherapy was then given. The dose was so high that it destroyed the patients' bone marrow in an effort to destroy all of the microscopic cancer cells. The harvested stem cells were then reinfused in the patient to allow bone marrow recovery. However, results have been very disappointing, and this is no longer a standard therapy.

There are many ongoing therapeutic trials attempting to find more effective and less toxic chemotherapy combinations. The selection of one or another combination depends on the patient, her risk

COMMONLY USED CHEMOTHERAPY DRUGS

Anthra-cyclines	Taxanes	Alkylating Agents	Anti-metabolites	Epo-thilones	Vinca Alkaloids
Doxo-rubicin (Adria-mycin)	Paclitaxel (Taxol) Docetaxel (Taxotere) Paclitaxel (Abraxene)	Cyclophos-phamide (Cytoxan) Carboplatin (Paraplatin)	Fluorouracil (5-FU, Adrucil) Metho-trexate (Amethop-terin)	Ixa-bepilone (Ixempra)	Vinorelbine (Navelbine) Vincristine (Oncovin)
Epi-rubicin (Ellence)			Gemcitabine (Gemzar)		
			Capecitabine (Xoleda)		

of relapse, and existing medical problems that may be worsened by the side effects of one or the other drug in combination. The treatments are improving, but have not yet been perfected.

Treating Metastatic Breast Cancer

As mentioned earlier, the initial use of all of the *cytotoxic* (toxic to cells) drugs in the treatment of breast cancer was in the context of metastatic disease; that is, disease that had spread from the breast to other parts of the body. What quickly became apparent was that no matter which of these agents was given or in what sequence they were given, cancer cells ultimately became resistant, and the patient succumbed. So late in the sixth decade of the last century, investigators began using chemotherapeutic drugs in combination After all, in America, if one is good, two is better, and three has to be great. To some extent this is true with combination chemotherapy. The response rate (the number of patients in a study who demonstrate a meaningful reduction in the size of the measured cancer metastases) and the complete response (complete disappearance of the measured metastases) are greater with combination chemotherapy than with the sequential use of single agents. However, the toxicity is greater, and there is yet to be convincing evidence that combination chemotherapy prolongs survival. So when chemotherapy is used to treat metastatic breast cancer, doctors usually use a single drug until it proves ineffective, then move on to another drug, and then another. However, there are times when combination chemotherapy is used, such as when it is important to obtain a fast response or on occasion when there is relatively low–volume metastatic disease and we are attempting possible cure. Treating metastatic breast cancer with chemotherapy can produce excellent responses with prolonged survival and improved quality of life; but a cure is frustratingly elusive.

The answer lies within the very enemy we are trying to destroy. Breast cancer is composed of mutated normal breast ductal and lobule cells. Breast cancers probably arise from a single mutant cell, which gives rise to a clone of the same mutant cell. However, one of the characteristics of the cancer cell is that it is genetically unstable and will tend to develop further mutations. These mutations can, and all too frequently do, include drug resistance. The more cancer cells that are present, the greater the chance that a mutational event will occur. A mass of cancer cells the size of the tip of a finger contains approximately 1 billion cells. With metastatic disease, cells have already slipped into the bloodstream and lymphatic system and have spread throughout the body, giving rise to additional clones of cells numbering in the many tens of billions to even a trillion cells. Drug-resistant mutations are inevitable and ultimately lead to the death of the patient.

Beyond TNM Staging

Investigators gathering data on many thousands of women with breast cancer discovered that they could select women at the time of their initial breast surgery who, if followed over time, would very likely develop widespread metastatic disease. They could also select those who would not. This process is called *staging*. Currently the American Joint Commission on Cancer Staging (AJCCS) system is used, which is the TNM system in which *T* represents the size and local invasion of the primary tumor, *N* represents the number and extent of regional lymph node involvement, and M represents the presence or absence of detectable metastatic disease. (See Appendix E for more on this classification.) Please note that the primary tumor T and the lymph node involvement N are described in excruciating detail as we try desperately to sort out who will and will not have micrometastatic disease so that those who need it can be treated with systemic therapy and those who do not need it can be spared the treatment. On the other hand, M is either 1 (present) or 0 (absent), acknowledging that once cancer can be detected beyond the regional lymph nodes, the patient cannot be definitively cured. Since the primary purpose of the staging system is to predict who can and cannot be cured, going beyond M1 carries little value for the TNM system. Yet knowing more about M is crucial in defining appropriate therapy for the woman with metastatic disease.

It became apparent early on that there were characteristics of a woman's breast cancer that went beyond the size and number of lymph nodes involved that determined the probability of microscopic metastases. Breast cancers were mined microscopically to get more information, and such things as grade (how much the cancer looks like the corresponding normal tissue), the percentage of cells that can be seen in cell division *(mitotic index)*, and whether cancer cells can be seen in the blood vessels or lymphatic tissue contained within the cancer *(lymphovascular invasion)* were found to be of value in describing prognosis. However, scientists had to dig deeper into the cell than the microscope would allow to discover information crucial to prognosis and, as it turns out, for more effective therapy as well.

Think of a cell as being like a communications satellite. It has little prongs and projections on it that allow communication with the rest of the body. Earlier, we discussed the crucial need for the body to exert control over the individual cell for the body to function in an organized fashion. The same command and control function is exerted over every cell of our body, including the lobular and ductal cells of the breast. Unlike bone marrow, little reproductive activity is going on in breast cells until pregnancy and subsequent lactation occur. But those cells need to be controlled at all times. How that control is exerted and lost appears to be the key to understanding how cancer of the breast occurs.

Normal breast cells have a similar knobby appearance to them. Those "knobs" are called *receptors*. Receptors are proteins that, like any other protein, are the products of genes. The genes are located on chromosomes in the nucleus of the cell. The genes are composed of DNA sequences that tell the cell how to properly make each protein, and the body tells the genes when to do it. For example, if a woman becomes pregnant, the breast cells must divide and grow. The ovary increases production of estrogen and progesterone, among other molecules, to effect that growth. Some molecules bind (attach themselves) to receptors on the surface of the cell. This activates the receptor which in turn triggers one or more protein pathways within the cell that carry the message (also called a signal) to divide and grow. Other pathways lead to milk production in the lobule cell and even pathways that lead to programmed cell death (*apoptosis*). Each of the proteins along a pathway transmits the message to the next. Each may also amplify that signal or may be part of a second or third pathway and will send that signal down another one or more of those pathways.

HER2-Positive Breast Cancer

Let's return to ductal or lobular cells of the breast. Like other normal cells, they have on their surface a family of receptors called *epidermal growth factor receptors* (EGFRs). The second family member has received a variety of names but now is most often called *HER2*. It is a protein and therefore is a product of a gene located on one of our chromosomes. *HER2* has two "domains": one portion of the molecule sits on the surface of the cell and receives signals; the other portion lies within the cell beneath the cell membrane and transmits the signal to the molecular pathways within the cell. (Think of a party hostess who gets a word from the dictionary and then passes it on to the first guest at the table, and so on.) HER2 plays a crucial role in growth regulation of the cell. Certain molecular signals (including epidermal growth factor) will cause activation of pathways leading to cell growth and division via the HER2 receptor.

All goes well as long as the gene coding for HER2 makes the correct number of receptors necessary to regulate growth and that HER2 is properly constructed so it may be faithful in its reception and transmission of incoming signals. However, about 12% to 14% of women with breast cancer have an abnormal HER2 within their breast cancer cells. Now, it is crucial to remember that the abnormal HER2 is found in the cancer cells, not in the germ cell line (sperm and egg). That is, the mistake is part of the cancer transformation process and is not inherited (very different from the breast cancer genes, BRCA1 and BRCA2). HER2 is abnormal in structure so that it does not properly receive signals, and it is abnormal in number; that is, there are many more in the membrane of the cancer cell than in a normal cell. Oncologists call this cancer HER2-positive, which is shorthand for abnormal and overexpressed. The result of this defect is a cancer cell deaf to the outside world and wildly replicating. The HER2-positive cancer is also characterized by a high incidence of metastatic disease relative to its size and other previously described microscopic prognostic factors.

HER2 status has added a new, important prognostic indicator in breast cancer. It also ushers in a new era of understanding of what makes a good cell go bad. What is more important, because the HER2-positive cancer cell has a crucial error unique to that cell, it becomes an attractive target for cancer cell specific therapy. So far there are two drugs licensed by the FDA that are specific for HER2-positive cancer. One is an antibody specifically targeting the extracellular domain; that is, the portion of HER2 on the surface of the cell. It is called trastuzumab (Herceptin). The other is a small molecule, lapatinib (Tykerb), which crosses the membrane into the cell, where it interrupts the signal transmitted by the inner domain of HER2. This prevents HER2 from exerting its effects. Herceptin is given intravenously and is used as an adjuvant treatment with combination chemotherapy for women with high-risk HER2-positive breast cancer. In this context, Herceptin has reduced the recurrence of breast cancer by 50%, a truly remarkable achievement. Side effects include chills, fever, and allergic reactions while being given. There is also possible heart damage, which requires regular but infrequent monitoring of the heart's ejection fraction during the course of therapy. But for most women it is extremely well tolerated.

Herceptin is also very effective in combination with either hormonal therapy or chemotherapy for the treatment of metastatic breast cancer. It has increased both the frequency and duration of response. Lapatinib is generally reserved for women with metastatic *HER2*-positive breast cancer that is resistant to Herceptin. It is more toxic, particularly related to its gastrointestinal side effects, including diarrhea and nausea. It does have the advantage of being available in pill form.

Beyond *HER2*

Recognition of the presence of receptors on the surface of the cell and their role in cell regulation has ushered in a new area of research that has taken us into the circuitry that lies beneath the cell surface. Here key molecules along various *signal transduction* pathways relay the messages vital to cell growth and function. Just as mutations within the gene that codes for *HER2* can result in cancerous growth; so too mutations within the genes that code for key proteins along the various signal transduction pathways can cause "downstream" modifications of the signal, with disastrous results. Other mutations are of little consequence to the cell. It is very difficult, theoretically, to figure out what is important and what is not. Much research has been and will be devoted to signal transduction blind alleys that do not lead to better prognostication or more effective therapies. But that is the nature of research—trial and error. Currently candidate pathways and molecules are being studied in breast cancer and other cancers for targeting, including EGFR1, M-Tor, and K-RAS. It is too early to tell whether any of these molecules along the various signaling pathways will be important targets in breast cancer. But that makes research all the more important.

HORMONAL THERAPY

Another crucial prognostic marker in breast cancer was based on the early observation that most breast cancers occur in women; therefore there must be a role for estrogen in the development of breast cancer. This led to the discovery of the estrogen-receptor protein (ER) and the similar progesterone-receptor protein (PR). The presence of the estrogen receptor in the breast cancer cell confers a more indolent growth rate and an improved overall prognosis. The science behind ER and estrogen is similar in concept to that of *HER2*. However, estrogen is a steroid molecule and therefore can move into the cell without a membrane receptor. However, estrogen alone cannot activate pathways leading to cell proliferation. It first has to bind to the estrogen receptor protein within the cell nucleus. The ER-estrogen complex is vital to activation of cell proliferation and even survival pathways of a cell that is ER positive. Those cells without ER do not need estrogen for survival or proliferation. For example, most *HER2*-positive cells lack ER and thrive with or without estrogen. However, depriving an ER-positive breast cancer cell of estrogen may slow or shut down proliferation, and, depending on how dependent the cell is on estrogen, this could result in cell death.

Women who have ovarian function (that is, premenopausal women) produce a tremendous amount of ovarian estrogen by direct synthesis. Postmenopausal women, on the other hand, produce small amounts of estrogen within fat tissue and the adrenal glands. They can only produce estrogen from a precursor molecule, *estrone*. Conversion of estrone to estrogen requires the presence of an enzyme, *aromatase*. Without aromatase, there is no estrogen production.

The presence of the estrogen receptor protein is a good prognostic indicator. What is even more important, the bonding of estrogen and its receptor has become a target along a signaling pathway that is crucial for cancer cell growth. Targeting that receptor-estrogen complex has become the cornerstone of hormonal therapy for breast cancer. In women with metastatic cancer, hormonal therapy has improved response rates and extended survival, and in some cases responses have lasted for many years. In addition, if a woman responds to one class of drugs that alters her hormonal environment, she has an excellent chance of responding to a second or even a third different class of agent. For most women with metastatic breast cancer who are ER positive, hormonal therapy is the treatment of choice, because it offers the best chance of response with the least amount of toxicity. However, for women with metastatic ER-positive breast cancer, hormonal therapy will not be curative, and the cancer will become independent of the hormonal signaling pathway. For these women with cancer that is resistant to hormone therapy, treatment with chemotherapy becomes the best option, which in turn can lead to additional responses and prolongation of survival similar to what one sees with women who have ER-negative breast cancer at diagnosis.

For women with ER-positive breast cancer who have disease clinically confined to the breast, with or without axillary lymph node involvement, hormonal therapy can play a major role in adjuvant treatment. For many postmenopausal women, particularly those who do not have lymph node involvement, hormonal therapy may be the only adjuvant treatment necessary. This can be true for a small, select population of premenopausal women as well. Moreover, hormonal therapy in a high-risk ER-positive patient can have an additive benefit when used in conjunction with chemotherapy. In this setting, chemotherapy is given first, followed by hormonal therapy. Why? Proliferating cancer cells are more sensitive to chemotherapy drugs. Hormonal therapy will inhibit growth of the cancer cells. Slowing cancer cell growth would decrease the effectiveness of such drugs and allow the cancer cell more time to recover from chemotherapy-induced damage.

Toxicity associated with hormonal therapy is, to some extent, dependent on the individual drug. However, all have in common side effects that one would expect from estrogen deprivation; that is, menopausal symptoms, including hot flashes, weight gain, vaginal dryness, and loss of libido.

Postmenopausal ER-Positive Breast Cancer

Two classes of agents provide the bulk of hormonal therapy for treating postmenopausal ER-positive breast cancer. The first are selective estrogen-receptor modifiers (SERMs); these drugs include tamoxifen (Nolvadex), toremifene (Fareston) and raloxifene (Evista). The majority of the world's data on the effectiveness of hormonal therapy for breast cancer has been with tamoxifen. These drugs bind tightly to the estrogen-receptor protein, preventing estrogen access to the molecule. They are called *receptor modifiers* because they alter the receptor. For some tissue (breast cancer, vaginal tissue) they are antiestrogenic, because they deprive the tissue of estrogen. For some tissue such as bone (and for tamoxifen, the endometrium of the uterus) the SERM-receptor complex has an estrogenic effect and will actually promote bone health. In the case of tamoxifen, it will cause proliferation of the endometrium and with that, an increased risk of endometrial cancer. The SERMs as a class increase the risk of blood clots as well, particularly in elderly individuals.

The other class of agents is the aromatase inhibitors/inactivators (AI), which prevent aromatase from converting estrone to estrogen. They include anastrozole (Arimidex), letrozole (Femara), and exemestane (Aromasin). In randomized trials comparing these agents with tamoxifen given as an adjuvant treatment and to patients with metastatic cancer, they appear to have a modestly better efficacy of about 2% to 3%. They are associated with fewer hot flashes, but perhaps more of the other menopausal symptoms. There is little in terms of increased problems with blood clots, and no increased risk of endometrial cancer. They can cause joint pain and swelling, which can be unacceptable in some cases. Since they totally shut down estrogen production in a postmenopausal woman, there is increased risk of osteoporosis. SERMs can be sequenced in a patient with metastatic cancer; that is, the patient can receive tamoxifen until there is a relapse, and then an AI is given. A considerable amount of research is ongoing to determine how best to sequence the SERMs with the AIs as an adjuvant treatment and how long to give them.

Additional agents are licensed by the FDA for the treatment of patients with postmenopausal breast cancer. One class is the estrogen receptor downregulators; they act by blocking and effectively eliminating the estrogen receptor. Only one is available in the United States: fulvestrant (Faslodex). It is primarily used in patients with metastatic cancer after there has been disease progression on SERMs and AIs. The adverse effects are similar to those with the other estrogen-depriving drugs.

Premenopausal ER-Positive Breast Cancer

ER-positive premenopausal breast cancer provides a different hormonal environment and with it a different approach. The direct synthesis of estrogen by the ovaries negates any possible benefit from the aromatase inhibitors. Indeed, if one is to use an AI in this patient population, one must first castrate the patient. This can be done by surgically removing the ovaries, irradiating them, or by shutting down estrogen production (medical castration). This can be done by using luteinizing hormone–releasing hormone (LH-RH) agonists. Specific agents include leuprolide (Lupron) and goserelin (Zoladex). For metastatic premenopausal breast cancer, the hormone treatment of choice is tamoxifen. This will produce pronounced menopausal symptoms. When relapse occurs, castration by one means or another followed by an AI is appropriate. This further deepens the menopause but less drastically than castration and an AI up front. In premenopausal adjuvant therapy, the only FDA-approved hormonal treatment is tamoxifen. Because it forms a tighter bond to the receptor than does estrogen, the concentration of estrogen in the body has little effect on the efficacy of tamoxifen. Research is ongoing to determine whether there is greater efficacy in adjuvant treatment using castration and an AI compared with treatment with tamoxifen. For a premenopausal woman who is thrust into an immediate and deep menopause with castration and an AI, the menopausal symptoms can be horrific. Until data prove otherwise, this is not the standard premenopausal adjuvant therapy.

DRUGS THAT ALTER HORMONE METABOLISM

Progestational Agent	Aromatase Inhibitor (Inactivator)	SERMs	Estrogen Downregulators	GNRH Agonist	Targeted Therapy
Megestrol (Megace)	Anastrozole (Arimidex)	Tamoxifen (Nolvadex)	Fulvestrant (Faslodex)	Goserelin (Zoladex)	Trastuzumab (Herceptin)
	Letrozole (Femara)	Toremifene (Fareston)			Lapatinib (Tykerb)
	Exemestane (Aromasin)	Raloxifene (Evista)			

TREATING THE MICROENVIRONMENT

An area of growing interest is the microenvironment of the cancer cell. We know, for example, that colonies of cancer cells cannot grow in the human body much larger than the size of the head of a pin without having a blood supply. The relatively recent discovery that *angiogenesis* (making of blood vessels) is crucial to cancer growth has produced a new class of compounds designed to interfere with that process. This occurs through an antibody that is directed against *vascular endothelial growth factor* (VEGF), which is a small molecule produced by normal as well as cancer cells, including breast cancer cells. It is part of that complex signaling pathway system of the cell discussed earlier. However, this molecule has its major effect outside the cancer cell itself, because it stimulates new blood vessel formation. Additional drugs are being studied that are multi-targeting agents. These agents inhibit a number of molecules that are crucial in cancer cell signaling. Some of these also target angiogenesis. Whether they will find use in breast cancer remains to be seen. So-called *metronomic therapy* is another attempt at inhibiting angiogenesis. This regimen consists of low-dose daily cyclophosphamide and weekly low-dose methotrexate treatments, with both drugs given orally. This has met with limited success.

WHO NEEDS WHAT?
Predicting What Treatments Will Provide the Most Benefit

What should be apparent by now is the complexity inherent in determining whether a woman with an invasive breast cancer is or is not harboring micrometastatic disease and what should be done for that specific patient to reduce the risk of recurrence. The new term for this is *personalized medicine*. Information can be gathered by the TNM staging system, by characteristics of the cancer seen under the microscope, and by molecular markers. Indeed, the science is growing so rapidly that by the time of this book's publication, new developments will have been added.

This discussion is not meant to be exhaustive, but rather a primer to provide a foundation of knowledge to understand what is now known and to build on that foundation with information as it becomes available to us in the future. But we have to use the information currently available to us to predict metastatic disease and what we might do to reduce that risk. Medical oncologists do this every day with their patients, with online tools such as Adjuvant Online (*www.adjuvantonline.com*), which has a database of thousands of women with their prognostic indicators and the results of follow-up only (that is, they received no systemic therapy after definitive treatment of their primary breast cancers and regional lymph nodes). Their rate of relapse and resulting death is then compared with data on women with similar prognostic indicators who have been treated with either hormonal manipulation and/or chemotherapy. Adjuvant Online has its limitations because of the relatively low number and level of sophistication of the prognostic factors on which risk and risk reduction are based. It also has a time horizon of 10 years, meaning it provides information about the chances of relapse or death, the benefits of therapy, and the risk of death from other causes at 10 years from diagnosis only. These data then tend to be less useful for an elderly or a younger patient with serious medical problems.

The newest approaches to prognostication are based on what an array of identified "cancer genes" are expressing. Investigators take a sample of a patient's cancerous tissue and look at a series of genes that in breast cancer seem to carry prognostic importance (among them, genes coding for ER-positive and *HER2*). The pattern of expression of this collection of genes then gives a more accurate forecast of relapse and the benefits of various therapies. The only one currently in widespread use is Oncotype DX (see p. 70). The recommendation for use of this 21-gene array by the American Society of Clinical Oncology (ASCO) and the National Cancer Center Network (NCCN) is limited to premenopausal women who have ER-positive tumors and no lymph node metastases. This field is expanding rapidly, and it is to be hoped that it will provide us with more accurate information and on a larger group of breast cancer patients.

The bottom line for the patient becomes what is the estimated risk of metastatic disease in the future, how much can we lower that risk, and what cost in toxicity does that risk reduction bring with it? The final answer must lie with the individual patient.

TACKLING TOXICITY

Considering that all of these drugs work to destroy the proliferating cancer cell, it would seem reasonable that the list of adverse effects would include damage to the normal cells of our body that are dividing. To a greater or lesser degree, all these drugs can produce a lowering of the red blood cell, white blood cell, and platelet counts, because the bone marrow, which makes these cells, is like a factory churning them out 24 hours a day. The same is true for hair follicles, as our hair continuously grows. Many of the drugs produce hair loss (*alopecia*) which is reversible. Those that interfere with microtubules and those derived from heavy metals can produce damage to the nerves (*peripheral neuropathy*). This typically causes numbness and tingling in the fingertips and toes. Many of the drugs can also produce mouth sores (stomatitis), a rash, and diarrhea as the cells that line our digestive tracts and cover the surface of our bodies proliferate as well. And, of course, the drugs can cause nausea and vomiting. The mechanism for this is not stomach irritation but rather stimulation of the emetic centers in the brain. There are also side effects that are specific to the agent or class of drugs. For instance, the anthracyclines can cause heart damage, and cyclophosphamide can cause bladder irritation. Because most of the side effects of all of these agents are dose related (the higher the dose, the greater the chance that the side effect will occur and the more severe it will be), adjusting the dose or the schedule of the drug (how much and how frequently the drug is given) can reduce the toxicity or possible severity of the adverse effect.

Until the last two decades of the twentieth century, little research was devoted to supportive care of the cancer patient. Billions of dollars were spent in efforts to find curative treatments, but a relative pittance was spent to make the treatments tolerable. But then a trickle of articles were published on supportive care, which soon became a tsunami. Much of the impetus for such research came from advocacy groups and private foundations. *Yes, you do make a difference.* Today oncologists have become much more aggressive in treating chemotherapy-induced toxicity. This is because patients have made us more aware of their suffering, and better medications are available to control that suffering.

I would encourage a breast cancer patient to take an active role in tackling toxicity. Much of chemotherapy-related toxicity is either subjective or is experienced at home, away from the doctor's office. We will know the patient has had vomiting or diarrhea only if she tells us. It is important to share that information with the doctor and to be an active partner in treatment and prevention.

Perhaps the most dreaded of toxicities are chemotherapy-induced nausea and vomiting (CINV). Until recently physicians were poorly equipped to prevent CINV, because it was not well understood and effective medications were not available to treat it. There were the old standby medications such as the phenothiazines; this family of drugs includes chlorpromazine (Thorazine) and prochlorperazine (Compazine). Another agent of some benefit is metochlorpropamide (Reglan). These agents are still used today in an ancillary role or with chemotherapy drugs that cause minimal nausea. However, none of these has the specificity necessary to treat CINV.

Advances in brain research opened the door to specific treatment. There are centers within the brain that receive messages that tell us to vomit (think of it as signal transduction that is going on in the brain). Seeing something truly revolting can produce instant nausea and vomiting. Messages are sent from our eyes to the brain and then to an emetic center, and vomiting occurs. Based on this growing understanding of brain chemistry, there appear to be three types of CINV.

The first type is immediate and occurs within the first 24 hours after treatment. This nausea is triggered by the drug's stimulating a vomiting center in the brain. That center of the brain is inhibited by a family of drugs called *type three 5-hydroxytryptamine ($_5HT_3$) antago-*

nists. The first generation of these antagonists consists of granisetron (Kytril/Sancuso), ondansetron (Zofran), and dolasetron (Anzemet). All are of equal effectiveness and can be given intravenously or orally. When given with the steroid drug dexamethasone (Decadron) before chemotherapy, they are very effective in controlling immediate nausea. They are metabolized rapidly. However, repeat dosing does not appear to improve results. Granisetron also comes in a longer-acting patch; the drug is absorbed through the skin (Sancuso). A second-generation $_5HT_3$ antagonist is now available called palonosetron (Aloxi). This drug is more potent and is metabolized more slowly. In some studies it has been shown to be more effective than first-generation $_5HT_3$ inhibitors. It too is more effective when used with dexamethasone. It also helps to control the second type of nausea, delayed nausea, which comes on more than 24 hours after chemotherapy is administered. A new class of agents called *neurokinin-1* (NK-1) *inhibitors* acts on different receptors in the brain that appear to be responsible for delayed nausea. Two of these drugs are currently available, an oral agent, aprepitant (Emend), and its intravenous counterpart, fosaprepitant. Together with dexamethasone and a $_5HIAA$ inhibitor, this drug has dramatically reduced CINV, both immediate and delayed.

The third type of nausea and vomiting is anticipatory. This occurs before chemotherapy when a patient has had poorly controlled CINV with previous cycles of chemotherapy. The Russian psychologist Pavlov showed that he could condition dogs to salivate with the ringing of a bell if he repetitively rang the bell when he gave the dogs meat. This was conditioned or anticipatory salivating. Humans are a lot brighter than dogs: it usually takes but one bad experience with CINV to "condition" us to have anticipatory nausea and vomiting. Anticipatory nausea is best treated by prevention. Controlling nausea with the first cycle of chemotherapy is the key to preventing further anticipatory nausea. When it does occur, anticipatory nausea is difficult to control and requires the addition of sedation, hypnosis, or other forms of psychotherapy.

Chemotherapy drugs have also been graded in the frequency of nausea and vomiting they induce. The scale goes from minimal (less than a 10% chance) to high (greater than a 90% chance). This grading also reflects, to some extent, the severity of the *emetogenic* (vomit producing) effect as well. This grading allows selection of the appropriate "cocktail" for a given regimen of chemotherapy. One thought would be to give everything to everybody before the first cycle of any chemotherapy regimen to prevent CINV. However, this "shotgun" approach is to be avoided, because antiemetic drugs have their own side effects, which can in some cases make the cure worse than the disease.

Constipation and diarrhea are troubling chemotherapy toxicities. The principal task of the colon is water resorption. Waste, in the form of a fecal slurry from the small bowel, is ushered into the cecum, which is the antechamber of the colon. As the stool courses through the colon, water is absorbed until a formed stool is eliminated through the rectum. Anything that speeds up transit through the colon or damages the colon's ability to absorb water will cause diarrhea; conversely, that which slows transit will cause constipation. Chemotherapy drugs can cause all of the above. Diarrhea is most frequently treated with drugs that reduce bowel motility; these include over-the-counter loperamide (Imodium) and the prescription drug diphenoxylate/atropine (Lomotil). A long-acting form of somatostatin (Octreotide) can be used to reduce secretory diarrhea that results from bowel injury. Probiotics such as *Lactobacillus* can help to restore healthy colon flora. Prolonged diarrhea can be life threatening primarily as a result of dehydration. The patient must take in more fluids than the diarrhea coming out. If that is not possible, intravenous fluids must be given. The major mistake made by patients is to think that the water they drink is "just running right through me." It is not. Much of it is absorbed in the stomach and small bowel. You cannot stop diarrhea by not drinking fluids. Attempting this fool's errand can result in severe dehydration with resulting low blood pressure, possible kidney damage, and even shock and death. Severe diarrhea warrants a call to the doctor. Constipation can usually be treated with over-the-counter drugs. A bowel regimen should be discussed with your physician.

The most common dose-limiting adverse effect of chemotherapy is bone marrow suppression. The bone marrow is a factory that continually produces red blood cells (RBCs) to carry oxygen to our tissues and carbon dioxide back to our lungs; white blood cells (WBCs) to fight infection; and platelets to initiate blood clot formation. When chemotherapy is given, the bone marrow may be promptly damaged, yet the damage is not appreciated for perhaps a few days to a week or more. That is because the cells in the bone marrow that are damaged are not scheduled to make their appearance in our bloodstream and carry out their duties until then. Calculating doses of chemotherapy is not an exacting science. In addition, it is not desirable to start chemotherapy at a very low dose and scale upward, since that may encourage cancer cell resistance. Consequently, overdosing the bone marrow is not uncommon as oncologists try to tread a fine line between too much and too little. For chemotherapy regimens that have a high probability of causing low WBCs, there are several agents available to stimulate rapid bone marrow recovery. They include filgrastim (Neupogen), longer-acting pegfilgrastim (Neulasta), and sargamostatin (Leukine). They are usually given beginning the day after chemotherapy to prevent or shorten the period of *neutropenia* (low WBC count). This reduces the risk of infection.

Chemotherapy-induced anemia has become a contentious topic. Two agents that can stimulate RBC production include epoetin alfa (Epogen and Procrit) and darbepoetinalfa (Aranesp). These agents can prevent or treat anemia caused by chemotherapy and reduce some of the associated fatigue and malaise. However, there are data to suggest they may also stimulate breast cancer cell growth. The use of these agents to treat breast cancer is to be discouraged.

Chemotherapy-induced *thrombocytopenia* (a decrease in blood platelets) remains a vexing problem. Currently there are no effective agents licensed by the FDA to treat or prevent this toxicity. At present, dose reduction is the best preventive therapy, because thrombocytopenia is a dose-related toxicity.

One recently recognized toxicity that is under investigation is *cognitive dysfunction;* that is, impairment of memory and reduced concentration. This syndrome, coined "chemobrain" by patients, is a phenomenon described by some patients receiving chemotherapy. It is poorly understood and is variable in severity. Patients may experience trouble with immediate memory, have trouble finding words, or difficulty concentrating. It appears to be different from depression and is usually reversible over time.

• • •

I have not attempted to be encyclopedic in this discussion of chemotherapy toxicity. There are many more drug-related toxicities, most of which are drug or drug family specific. I would recommend that the breast cancer patient bring at least one relative or friend to the visit with the medical oncologist when he or she discusses the potential benefits and toxicities of therapy. Prepare questions that you want answered before the visit. Listen carefully and take notes. Be certain the physician has a complete list of your prescriptions and over-the-counter medications; we know that more than 60% of our patients take herbal medications; provide a list of those as well. Potentially dangerous drug-drug and drug-herbal interactions can be avoided if all medications are known. Finally, your medical history provides critical information for the choice of chemotherapy regimens, whether provided as adjuvant treatment or for metastatic cancer. No single chemotherapy regimen is best for everyone. For example, if you have a history of heart failure (weak heart), you are probably not a good candidate for doxorubicin (Adriamycin), but excellent regimens exist that do not contain that drug. But if you do not tell your oncologist, he will not know to choose the appropriate one for you. Finally, it is all about *you*, the patient with breast cancer. It is not about the doctor or his nurse or your family. *You* need to feel comfortable with the chemotherapy you are going to receive, who will administer it, and where it will be administered.

FOLLOW-UP SURVEILLANCE AFTER BREAST CANCER TREATMENT
WILLIAM C. WOOD, MD

After completion of primary treatment of breast cancer, patients are routinely placed under follow-up surveillance to detect and treat any recurrence of the first cancer or to discover any new breast cancer in the opposite breast at the earliest possible stage. As mentioned previously, women who develop breast cancer have an increased risk of cancer in the other breast. For women over 50, this risk is about 4% for their remaining years; for those under 50, it is about 14%. Although the risk is not as great as many women imagine, careful evaluation is essential. It is vital that a cancer in the opposite breast be detected as early as possible to increase the likelihood of cure, as is the case with a primary tumor.

Detecting a new breast tumor in the opposite breast is accomplished by a familiar triad: monthly breast self-examination of the opposite breast, clinical examination by a physician or nurse practitioner every 6 to 12 months, and annual mammography. This combination provides the greatest assurance of early diagnosis. More frequent examinations have not been shown to be beneficial.

Surveillance for evidence of recurrence of the initial breast cancer is also a collaborative effort by the patient, her surgeon, medical or radiation oncologist, and primary physician. The goal of self-examination of the chest wall or reconstructed breast (or the irradiated breast, if breast-conserving therapy was performed), like examination of the normal breast, is to detect an area that feels different to the examining fingers or looks different in the mirror. Lumps, thickenings, or areas of different color can all be normal, but they should be checked by a woman's surgeon as soon as they are detected. Any new lump or swollen lymph gland that is discovered may arouse anxiety. If it persists for several weeks, the surgeon should check it to make a diagnosis and confirm whether there is reason for concern.

Initially, follow-up consists of a brief history and physical examination performed every 4 to 6 months. Physical examination focuses on parts of the body that are common sites for the spread of breast cancer. In time, this interval can be increased and a woman can return to her normal "whole person care" examination by her internal medicine physician, gynecologist, or family doctor.

The follow-up pattern of testing and its frequency are determined by a woman's physicians. Blood tests are used to screen for liver, bone, or bone marrow involvement. Chest x-ray films can screen for asymptomatic lung metastases, and mammograms can be used to detect recurrences and screen for second (new) cancers of the breast. The great majority of recurrent cancers and second breast cancers are detected by self-examination, by physical examination, or by mammography. Unless specific symptoms are present, there is little evidence to support the use of additional laboratory studies such as chemistry studies, blood tumor markers, and even bone scans that are inconvenient for the patient, costly, and do not appear to improve survival rates. The value of these follow-up studies remains controversial. The American Society of Clinical Oncology (ASCO) has written a position paper discouraging the *routine* practice of follow-up laboratory studies, since these do not change outcome (survival). On the other hand, any new symptom (such as an ache or a pain) or a new finding (a mass or lump) discovered on physical examination is a clear indication for specific studies. Because tumors that are faster growing recur sooner, whereas more slowly growing tumors recur later, the interval between follow-up examinations can be increased over a period of years, but at no time should these examinations be discontinued.

Routine mammography of the reconstructed breast is not needed if a complete mastectomy has been done. Monthly self-examination of the rebuilt breast has proved the best method for detecting a recurrence. There is no evidence that reconstruction causes any significant delay in detecting the rare cases of recurrent disease behind or beneath the reconstructed breast.

CLINICAL TRIALS: THEIR ROLE IN ASSESSING BREAST CANCER TREATMENT OPTIONS

DAN W. LUEDKE, MD

Before new treatments for breast cancer are accepted by the medical community for use on patients, they need to be compared with alternative treatments in carefully conducted scientific studies. The clinical trial represents an excellent method for comparing and assessing different treatment approaches to breast cancer management. In these clinical trials, groups of doctors and their patients agree to participate in studies in which the cancer treatment alternatives that these patients will ultimately receive may be decided by randomization, meaning that neither the patient nor her doctor chooses between the alternative treatments; instead, the treatments are chosen arbitrarily to avoid bias. Randomized studies are particularly important when the differences between treatments being compared are likely to be either small or nonexistent.

Most breast cancer clinical trials require cooperation from physicians in many different medical centers. Numerous experts contribute to the design of each trial, thus providing "multiple second opinions." The National Cancer Institute reviews each trial design and commonly covers the expenses incurred in collecting the scientific data. In addition, each participating medical center has its own human investigation review committee that must approve the trial before it can begin at a medical center.

Clinical trials in breast cancer have now involved many thousands of women whose medical data have been carefully collected to answer a variety of questions about breast cancer. Out of these trials has come an understanding that *breast cancer is not one disease but many different diseases, or perhaps a disease with many variations.* Increasingly, appropriate treatment requires understanding these many variations of breast cancer.

Clinical research has provided us with new and better treatments for breast cancer; at no time has the potential for such research and the clinical studies associated with it been better. Since World War II, tight controls have been instituted to ensure that the potential benefits and hazards of therapy have been thoroughly explained to the patient and written informed consent has been obtained. For a new cancer drug to be marketed in the United States, it must go through a rigorous process, including preclinical trials (before it can be given to humans) with animals to establish toxicities and some estimate of dose. It must also be shown to have an anti-tumor effect in one or another of the many models of human cancer there are. An example is the growth of human cancer cells in a growth medium on a sterile petri dish. A new drug may kill these cells at promising low concentrations. Once these criteria have been met, the new drug is ready for testing in humans.

There are three phases of drug testing before FDA approval. Phase I provides toxicity information. Cancer patients who have exhausted all reasonable alternative drug therapies are the first humans to receive the new drug. It is first given in very low doses; then in a series of patients, dose escalation occurs until toxicity is produced. Phase I trials are completed when a dose and schedule (how frequently it is given) have been selected.

Phase II trials consist of testing for efficacy and better delineation of toxicity. Patients with advanced cancers who have had extensive prior treatments are enrolled in these trials. Groups of patients with different cancers are tested, including patients with breast cancer. If the drug shows real promise of benefitting breast cancer patients, it proceeds to phase III trials to see where it might fit into the therapeutic options for breast cancer. If the drug appears to produce an exceptionally good response, it may be given temporary FDA approval before proceeding to the next phase.

Phase III breast cancer trials are conducted on women with metastatic disease who have had a limited number of chemotherapy regimens or who may not have been previously treated. They are randomized; that is, women who volunteer for the trial are divided into two (or sometimes more) treatment groups by a "flip of the coin." (Today, of course, this is done through a computer-generated randomization.) One group will receive a regimen containing the new drug, and the other group will receive a regimen without the new drug. If it is a "blinded study," then neither the patient nor the physician knows whether the patient is receiving the study drug or not. The two groups are then followed for response to therapy, toxicity, and other factors. If the regimen with the new drug is proved superior to the regimen without, it becomes a new standard of therapy.

Similar randomized trials can be conducted in the adjuvant setting to test different surgical procedures, different kinds of medical devices, or different treatments with radiation therapy. The randomized trial has become the gold standard for clinical cancer research.

Unfortunately, less than 5% of patients eligible for clinical trials actually participate. There is a desperate need for volunteers to help in the quest for new and better treatments for tomorrow. However, doing so is a personal decision.

By participating in clinical trials, physicians are able to keep current with the most recent developments in cancer treatment, and patients can expect to receive either the best recognized treatment or a new treatment that a consensus of experts believes may represent an advance. In addition, information gained from the treatment will influence the future care of others. (Search for a list of clinical trials at the National Cancer Institute website at *www.cancer.gov/clinical trials.*)

The feelings of attachment a woman has about her breasts are profound and should not be lightly dismissed by the physician treating her. These feelings will influence a woman's decision to seek help initially and eventually will help determine the therapy she selects. Once the surprise of being stricken by a dreaded disease has passed, a woman desires and deserves honest information about her disease, her prognosis, and her options for treatment. In addition, she needs a physician who is sensitive to her psychological and aesthetic requirements. The physician who treats a woman with breast cancer must consider the effect of therapy, not only on ultimate survival and rehabilitation, but also on enhanced quality of life. Optimal patient care extends beyond medical management of the disease itself.

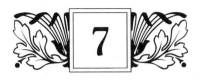

BREAST CANCER GENETICS: WHAT YOU NEED TO KNOW

Jennifer Ivanovich, MS

In the past 20 years, critical discoveries regarding the genetic basis of cancer have been incorporated in the medical care of women diagnosed with breast cancer. As part of your own research about breast cancer, you will read about "breast cancer genes." Some of this information relates to the genetic makeup of a breast tumor, or *tumor genetics*. For example, the number of copies of the *Her-2/neu* gene found in a breast tumor can be determined, and this information is used in planning the treatment for that specific tumor. The focus of this chapter, however, is on our *inherited genetic makeup* and specifically, hereditary cancer. Identification of an inherited gene abnormality is used to plan the medical care of a woman diagnosed with breast cancer and is essential for selecting the most appropriate medical follow-up for her children and extended family.

WHAT ARE THE GENETIC CLASSIFICATIONS OF BREAST CANCER?

From a genetic point of view, breast cancer is classified into three broad categories: sporadic, familial, and hereditary. These classifications reflect the inherited genetic contribution to the development of breast cancer.

The majority of women with breast cancer have *sporadic* cancer; that is, breast cancer that develops from the transformation of a single breast cell with no inherited genetic contribution. Women with sporadic disease tend to have a *very limited* family history of breast cancer and are most likely to be older at the time of diagnosis.

In contrast, one third of all breast cancer has some inherited genetic involvement. The *familial* classification refers to families with a *modest* breast cancer risk resulting from the inheritance of either a single gene abnormality (mutation) or multiple genes acting in concert. Families with familial disease tend to have a modest family history of cancer. To date, more than 10 genes linked to a modest or low risk have been identified. These genes are more common than genes that carry a high cancer risk and account for a larger fraction of all breast cancers. Most of the "breast cancer genes" discovered within the past 5 years confer a modest or low breast cancer risk.

Hereditary breast cancer results from the inheritance of a single gene mutation and is associated with a *high* breast cancer risk. Families with hereditary cancer tend to have a strong family history of cancer. Although the media have focused on the *BRCA1* and *BRCA2* genes, currently there are six genes known to be associated with a high breast cancer risk. Each gene is responsible for a distinct hereditary cancer predisposition syndrome. It is important to understand that a person does not inherit cancer. Rather, a person inherits a gene abnormality that renders the gene unable to function properly. As a consequence, that individual has a predisposition or higher likelihood of developing certain types of cancers. Inheriting a gene mutation does not mean a woman will develop cancer, but it does mean she has a high chance for certain types of cancers to develop in her lifetime. Women and their families with a high cancer risk may benefit for early screening or prophylactic (preventive) medical and surgical options. The vast majority of genes responsible for hereditary breast cancer have yet to be discovered, and this fact is critical when considering the evaluation and genetic testing of a family with a strong family history of cancer.

The medical care team uses data known about a given cancer syndrome to direct a woman's and her family's medical care. A diagnosis of hereditary cancer must first be made to incorporate these valuable data in her treatment plan.

HOW DO WE IDENTIFY FAMILIES WITH HEREDITARY CANCER?

The first and primary step in determining whether a family has hereditary breast cancer is to assess the family cancer history. A diagnosis of hereditary cancer is not made, or refuted, based on a single family member's diagnosis. (A review of how to document your family cancer history can be found in Chapter 8.)

Most hereditary cancer syndromes follow a dominant pattern of inheritance. Genetics professionals will assess the family history for features consistent with this pattern of inheritance. Some of these features include:

- Multiple affected family members who are closely related to one another
- Multiple generations affected with cancer
- Different cancer types that may be associated with one another as part of a hereditary cancer syndrome
- Bilateral breast cancer (in both breasts) or bilateral cancer in paired organs (for example, breasts, kidneys, and ovaries)
- Young age at diagnosis

You may benefit from a genetics evaluation if your family has at least one of these features. A genetic counselor will indicate the likelihood that your family has hereditary cancer based on the family cancer history. It is important to remember that *hereditary cancer is rare*. Most women diagnosed with breast cancer do not have a personal or family cancer history consistent with hereditary cancer.

For women diagnosed at a young age (less than 40 years), the possibility of hereditary cancer should always be considered, regardless of their family cancer history. There are two primary reasons for this consideration:

1. Young age at diagnosis is a feature of hereditary cancer. Studies have shown that compared with older women, young women are much more likely to have an underlying gene mutation that contributes to the development of their breast cancer.

2. A young woman's family may be "young" and consequently difficult to evaluate. Consider a 22-year-old woman diagnosed with breast cancer. Her parents are 40 and 41 years of age. Her parents are the oldest of their siblings. This is a "young" family, and the family cancer history may not have "expressed itself" yet. In essence, a negative family history in a young woman may be deceptive; thus the lack of a positive family history should not exclude the evaluation of hereditary cancer in a young woman diagnosed with breast cancer.

HOW IS A HEREDITARY CANCER SYNDROME INHERITED IN A FAMILY?

Most hereditary cancer syndromes follow a dominant pattern of inheritance. Each person has two copies of every gene found in each cell of the body. One copy is inherited from your mother and one copy from your father. A person with a hereditary cancer syndrome has a mutation or abnormal alteration in one copy of a specific gene. The presence of only one mutation is sufficient to cause a high risk of cancer.

Hereditary cancer does not skip a generation. A person with a gene mutation may not develop cancer, but he or she may pass on the gene mutation to a child. Each child has a 50% chance to inherit the mutation and an equally likely 50% chance *not* to inherit the mutation. A person who does not carry a gene mutation cannot pass it on. In essence, you cannot pass on what you do not have.

Your father's family cancer history is of equal importance to your mother's. Too often, a woman's paternal family history of breast cancer is mistakenly discounted as insignificant. Because we inherit our genes from both parents, a woman may inherit a gene responsible for hereditary cancer from her father.

The risks of developing certain types of cancers may vary based on which gene has a mutation, but also based on a person's sex. For example, a man with a gene mutation may have a low risk of developing breast cancer, whereas his female family member, with the same gene mutation, has a high risk.

If your family appears to have hereditary cancer, the next questions are: *What specific cancer syndrome does your family have?* and *How can you use information about the specific cancer syndrome in your medical decision-making?*

WHAT ARE THE KNOWN HEREDITARY BREAST CANCER SYNDROMES?

Several hereditary cancer syndromes associated with a high breast cancer risk have been described. The specific cancer syndrome considered for a family is based on the family cancer history. If your family has a history of breast and ovarian cancer, the hereditary breast cancer 1 *(BRCA1)* or hereditary breast cancer 2 *(BRCA2)* syndromes may be considered. If your family has a history of breast cancer, leukemia, and sarcoma, the Li-Fraumeni syndrome may be considered. Your medical care team will use information known about a given cancer syndrome to make treatment and follow-up recommendations for you and your family. A list of the hereditary cancer syndromes associated with a high breast cancer risk, the causative genes, the cancer risks, and some of the medical recommendations made for affected families are presented in the table below and on the next page.

HEREDITARY CANCER SYNDROMES ASSOCIATED WITH HIGH BREAST CANCER RISK

Syndrome (Gene)	Associated Cancers	Medical Recommendations*
Hereditary breast cancer 1 syndrome (BRCA1)	**High risk** Breast and ovarian cancer **Increased risk** Prostate and pancreatic cancer	**Female family members** • Mammography and breast MRI screening beginning by 25-35 years and repeated annually • Consideration of prophylactic mastectomy or prophylactic tamoxifen • Transvaginal ultrasound and CA-125 testing for ovarian cancer beginning by 25-35 years of age and repeated annually • Consideration of prophylactic oophorectomy (removal of ovaries)
Hereditary breast cancer 2 syndrome (BRCA2)	**High risk** Breast and ovarian cancer **Increased risk** Prostate, pancreatic, melanoma (including ocular melanoma), male breast cancer, gastric cancer (stomach)	**Female family members** • Mammography and breast MRI screening beginning by 25-35 years and repeated annually • Consideration of prophylactic mastectomy or prophylactic tamoxifen • Transvaginal ultrasound and CA-125 testing beginning by 25-35 years of age and repeated annually • Consideration of prophylactic oophorectomy (removal of ovaries) **All family members** • Annual clinical examinations of the skin

*See GeneReviews at *www.genetests.org* for more extensive information. The medical recommendations listed in this table are from cancer genetics experts. Because there are limited studies available to confirm the most appropriate screening guidelines for families with hereditary cancer, your medical care team may modify these recommendations based on your personal and family cancer history.

Continued

HEREDITARY CANCER SYNDROMES ASSOCIATED WITH HIGH BREAST CANCER RISK—cont'd

Syndrome (Gene)	Associated Cancers	Medical Recommendations*
Li-Fraumeni syndrome (Tp53)	**High risk** Breast cancer, sarcoma (primary bone cancer), leukemia (diagnosed in childhood), and other types of childhood tumors **Increased risk** Melanoma, colon, pancreatic, and brain cancer	**Screening for children, performed annually** • Physical examination • Complete blood cell count (CBC) • Abdominal ultrasound examination • Consider additional organ-targeted surveillance based on family cancer history **Screening for adults, performed annually** • Physical examination with skin examination • Complete blood cell count (CBC) • Women only: breast MRI and mammogram screening starting by 25 years of age • Consider additional organ-targeted surveillance based on family cancer history
Peutz-Jeghers syndrome (STK11)	**High risk** Breast cancer **Increased risk** Colon and small bowel polyps and cancer; gastric, ovarian, pancreatic, cervical, and testicular tumors	**Screening for children beginning by 10 years of age** • Upper gastrointestinal endoscopy screening • For boys: testicular examination during physical exam **Screening for adults** • Women only: mammogram and breast MRI starting by 25 years; pelvic ultrasound by 20 years of age • Pancreatic cancer screening beginning by 30 years of age
Hereditary diffuse gastric cancer syndrome (*e-cadherin*)	**High risk** Lobular breast cancer and diffuse gastric cancer (stomach cancer) **Increased risk** Colon cancer	• Upper gastrointestinal endoscopy screening performed annually • Consideration of prophylactic gastrectomy (removal of stomach) for individuals with mutation • Women only: mammogram and breast MRI starting by 25 years and performed annually
Cowden syndrome (PTEN)	**High risk** Benign and cancerous tumors of breast **Increased risk** Benign and cancerous tumors of thyroid and uterus	• Women only: mammogram and breast MRI starting by 30-35 years and performed annually • Consider uterine cancer screening with ultrasound and uterine biopsy by 35-40 years of age • Consider baseline thyroid ultrasound at 18 years and annual thyroid examination

HOW IS INFORMATION ABOUT A HEREDITARY CANCER SYNDROME USED IN A WOMAN'S CARE?

Currently, health care providers use information about a hereditary cancer syndrome to make screening recommendations, to offer approaches to avoid or prevent cancer from developing, and to identify family members with a high cancer risk. Research is underway to incorporate information regarding a woman's gene mutation into planning her chemotherapy.

Women with breast cancer and their at-risk female family members may benefit from earlier and more extensive breast health screening. Mammography and breast MRI screening are often recommended to begin by 25 years of age for women with a high breast cancer risk. The rationale for early screening is based on the observation that individuals with a gene mutation may develop cancer at a young age. Additional types of screening, such as MRI, are used because the cancer risk among women with a mutation is much higher than the average likelihood of developing breast cancer. Screening for cancers other than breast cancer may also be recommended. For example, it is recommended that women with an *e-cadherin* gene mutation undergo upper gastrointestinal endoscopic screening because of their high risk for developing gastric (stomach) cancer.

Individuals may also consider prophylactic medical or surgical options as a means to reduce their cancer risk. The word *prophylactic* refers to a procedure or medicine used before a disease develops. A woman with a *BRCA1* gene mutation may consider having her ovaries removed to reduce her chance to develop ovarian cancer. A woman with a *BRCA2* gene mutation may take tamoxifen to reduce the chance for breast cancer to develop. How much a woman's cancer risk is reduced depends on the option chosen. Prophylactic mastectomy reduces a woman's chance of developing breast cancer by more than 90%. Prophylactic administration of tamoxifen reduces a woman's chance of developing breast cancer by 50%. It is important to understand, however, that an option that is best for one woman may be different from one that is right for another woman with the same cancer risk.

Preliminary but exciting clinical trials that target a specific gene's biologic pathway are being tested. These protocols may target only the cancer cells, leaving normal tissue alone. Although these trials are in very preliminary stages, they provide the first glimpse of how knowledge of inherited gene mutations can be used to tailor a woman's chemotherapy.

HOW CAN WE TEST FOR HEREDITARY CANCER?

The primary step in determining whether a woman has hereditary cancer is to evaluate her family cancer history. Genetic testing is performed to identify the specific gene mutation responsible for the family's cancer syndrome. For most families with hereditary cancer, the underlying gene mutation will not be identified using the currently available genetic testing.

For genetic testing, a gene is assessed for the presence or absence of a mutation. A mutation is an abnormal alteration that ultimately disrupts normal gene function. As a result of this dysfunction, individuals with a mutation in a "cancer gene" have an increased cancer risk. Genetic testing is typically performed on one or two genes at a time, using a sample of blood or saliva. Which gene is tested is based on the specific cancer syndrome that is suspected. As technology improves, analysis of multiple, if not hundreds, of genes using one blood sample can be performed in the future.

It is recommended that genetic testing only be performed after evaluation of the family cancer history and following a thorough discussion of the possible test results and a review of how this testing may be useful in a woman's immediate and long-term medical care. By recommending genetic testing, the health care provider suspects the possibility of hereditary cancer. Because hereditary cancer extends well beyond the treatment of a single tumor, special attention should be paid to evaluation and testing for hereditary cancer.

Every medical test or screening procedure has its limitations. Consider the fact that not all breast cancers can be detected using mammography, and that additional tests, such as ultrasound or MRI, are needed to visualize some tumors. Genetic testing also has its limitations. No single type of analysis can detect all mutations. Two studies have recently shown that 10% of *BRCA1* and *BRCA2* gene mutations are not detected by gene sequencing, a common technique used to detect gene mutations. If you have had negative *BRCA1* or *BRCA2* gene testing, ask your genetic counselor about the additional analyses that can now be performed on these two genes. You may have a mutation in the *BRCA1* or *BRCA2* gene that is not detectable using gene sequencing. No matter how the mutation is detected, a mutation is associated with a high breast cancer risk.

Genetic testing is most informative when first performed in a ·
family member who has been diagnosed with cancer. In essence, testing should begin with a person most likely to have a gene mutation.
When testing is not performed for an affected family member first, it
is critical that the test results be interpreted cautiously. If genetic testing is performed for a woman who has not been diagnosed with breast
cancer and a gene mutation has not been identified in her family, a
negative test result may give false reassurance.

The results of medical testing or screening are often interpreted
as either *good* or *bad*. No tumor was detected on the MRI scan and
this result is interpreted as *good*. For genetic testing we need to shift
how the results are interpreted. Genetic testing results should be
viewed as either *informative* (I have gained new information to aid in
my medical decision-making) or *noninformative* (I did not gain any
new information).

Let's consider the three possible test results for a woman who has
genetic testing of a "cancer gene." For this discussion, we make the
following assumptions:
- She has a personal history of breast cancer.
- She is the first person in the family to be tested.
- She has a strong family cancer history suggestive of hereditary
  cancer.

1. **Positive**—a gene mutation is identified. This mutation is the basis for the cancer predisposition in her family. This testing is *informative*, because the woman has gained new information that is
   useful in planning her treatment and the medical care of her family. Identification of a mutation provides her with an explanation
   as to why her breast cancer developed. Once a mutation is identified, family members may then choose to pursue genetic testing.
   Their testing is much cheaper, because only targeted analysis of
   the specific mutation is necessary.

2. **Negative**—no mutation is identified in the specific gene analyzed
   using defined techniques. A negative test result is considered *noninformative*, because this woman has not gained any new information to aid in her medical decision-making. When interpreting
   this test result, the genetic counselor will review the techniques
   used and will determine whether further analyses of the same gene
   are indicated. For some women, analysis of additional genes may
   be appropriate. It is important to note that a negative test result
   for the woman described in our example does not eliminate her
   personal or family cancer history. A negative result did not pro-

vide her with information about why her breast cancer developed or why her family has a strong cancer history. Unaffected family members should not pursue genetic testing until a mutation is identified for an affected family member. For most women with hereditary breast cancer, the currently available genetic testing will be noninformative.

3. **Variant, clinical significance unknown**—a variation in the gene sequence is identified, but there are insufficient data to declare whether the variation disrupts the normal gene functioning. The laboratory will need to collect additional data from multiple (if not hundreds) of families to determine the significance, if any, of the variant. This data collection process may take several years. This test result is also considered *noninformative* and cannot be used in planning a woman's care. Family members should not pursue genetic testing, because the interpretation or meaning of the gene variant is unknown.

CAUTION: Do not misinterpret this test result as a positive test result. Further data are needed to clarify this test result, and until these data become available, this result should not be used in your medical planning. When these data become available, the laboratory will reclassify your test result as either *positive* or *negative*. The health care provider who ordered this testing will be notified. If your genetic testing identified a variant of unknown clinical significance, contact your medical care team annually to learn whether your testing has been reclassified.

Genetic testing cannot provide all of the practical information that would be useful in planning your medical care. Genetic testing cannot determine:

- Whether cancer is currently present in the body
- Whether there is a 100% certainty that an individual will develop cancer
- If a cancer is to develop in a person's lifetime, when that cancer will begin

It is evident that genetic testing is not a simple blood test. The results are complex and should always be interpreted cautiously.

DNA STORAGE

DNA storage is a clinical service in which a sample of blood is taken, the DNA or genetic material is removed, and it is stored in a freezer for testing at a later date. DNA storage is an important clinical option for women with advanced breast cancer who have either had negative results to genetic testing or who do not wish to pursue genetic testing. By storing a sample of DNA, the woman makes this "genetic history" available to her children. *Remember, genetic testing is always most informative when it is first performed in an affected family member.* Her DNA sample can be accessed and tested in the future as new "cancer genes" are identified. The woman who stores her DNA designates which family member may access the sample for testing. DNA storage generally costs $100 to $150 for approximately 10 years of storage. Talk with a genetic counselor about this important clinical option.

TWO FAMILIES WITH HEREDITARY CANCER

Consider the following two families for a practical demonstration of the potential benefits and limitations of genetic testing.

Family 1

Jeanne is a young woman who was diagnosed with lobular breast cancer at 34 years of age. See the pedigree for family 1 below.

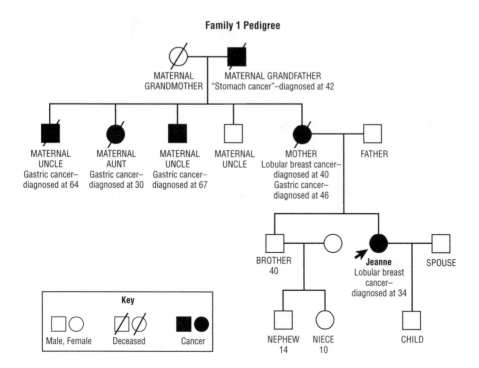

Family 1 Pedigree

MATERNAL GRANDMOTHER

MATERNAL GRANDFATHER
"Stomach cancer"–diagnosed at 42

MATERNAL UNCLE
Gastric cancer–diagnosed at 64

MATERNAL AUNT
Gastric cancer–diagnosed at 30

MATERNAL UNCLE
Gastric cancer–diagnosed at 67

MATERNAL UNCLE

MOTHER
Lobular breast cancer–diagnosed at 40
Gastric cancer–diagnosed at 46

FATHER

BROTHER
40

Jeanne
Lobular breast cancer–diagnosed at 34

SPOUSE

Key

Male, Female   Deceased   Cancer

NEPHEW
14

NIECE
10

CHILD

Jeanne's physician ordered *BRCA1* and *BRCA2* gene testing based *only* on her young age at diagnosis. Her test results are negative, with no mutation or variant or unknown clinical significance identified in the *BRCA1* or BRCA2 gene.

Is this the correct genetic test to order?

Answer: No. Jeanne's family cancer history reveals a striking family history of diffuse gastric cancer, a cancer of the stomach. Jeanne's personal and family cancer history are diagnostic for the hereditary diffuse gastric cancer (HDGC) syndrome, caused by *e-cadherin* gene mutations (see p. 122). The *BRCA1* and *BRCA2* genes are causative for the hereditary breast cancer 1 *(BRCA1)* and hereditary breast cancer 2 *(BRCA2)* syndromes, not the HDGC syndrome. Jeanne's physician did not consider her family history and ultimately did not identify the correct hereditary cancer syndrome in her family.

The hereditary diffuse gastric cancer syndrome is associated with a 40% lifetime chance of developing lobular breast cancer and an 80% lifetime risk of developing diffuse gastric cancer. The term *diffuse* refers to how the cancer grows; flat, rather than forming a distinct, round mass. Lobular breast cancer may also grow flat, making it more difficult to detect.

Genetic testing of the *e-cadherin* gene is available. If Jeanne has an *e-cadherin* gene mutation, it would give her family powerful information to aid in their medical care. Genetic testing would be used to determine who in the family has inherited the gene mutation and has a high risk of developing gastric and lobular breast cancer. These individuals may benefit from more extensive breast health and gastrointestinal screening or prophylactic surgical options to reduce their cancer risks.

Jeanne's family could not take advantage of this information because the family cancer history was not taken into consideration when her initial genetic testing was ordered. For women with breast cancer, it is important to know your family cancer history, communicate this information to your medical care team, and ask what impact your family cancer history may have on your medical care team's recommendations for you.

Family 2

Barbara is a 39-year-old woman who was recently diagnosed with a stage III ductal carcinoma. See the pedigree for family 2 below.

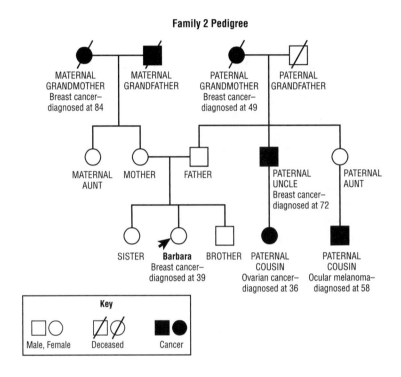

Family 2 Pedigree

She has a paternal family cancer history that is diagnostic for hereditary cancer, including multiple affected generations, multiple affected family members (including a male relative with breast cancer), and young age at diagnosis. *BRCA1* and *BRCA2* gene testing was ordered for Barbara. The test results were negative; that is, no mutation or variant of unknown clinical significance was identified.

Is this the correct genetic test to order?

Answer: Yes. The pattern of the cancers in the family is most consistent with either the hereditary breast cancer 1(*BRCA1*) or hereditary breast cancer 2 (*BRCA2*) syndromes. Women with one of these two syndromes have a 70% to 80% lifetime risk of developing breast cancer and a 20% to 40% chance of developing ovarian cancer. Male breast cancer is rare; any man with breast cancer should be referred for genetic assessment, because a large percentage of men diagnosed with breast cancer have either the *BRCA1* or *BRCA2* hereditary cancer syndrome. Ocular melanoma is another rare type of cancer and is known to be associated with the hereditary breast cancer 2 *(BRCA2)* syndrome.

Barbara's negative test result does not exclude or eliminate the possibility of hereditary cancer in this family. The negative test result only informs Barbara that she and her family do not have a *BRCA1* or *BRCA2* gene mutation that is detectable by gene sequencing.

Can additional genetic testing be performed for Barbara?

Answer: Yes. Additional testing of the *BRCA1* and *BRCA2* genes can now be performed. This additional analysis is used to detect gene deletions and rearrangements. These types of mutations cannot be detected using gene sequencing, the technique that was used for Barbara's initial genetic testing. Additional analysis of the *BRCA1* and *BRCA2* genes is warranted for Barbara. A gene mutation is associated with a high breast cancer risk, no matter how the mutation is detected.

ADVICE TO WOMEN WHO HAVE BEEN DIAGNOSED WITH BREAST CANCER

A woman diagnosed with breast cancer is faced with complex medical decisions, having received overwhelming amounts of information with multiple statistics to decipher. It is important to recognize that genetics is only one piece of this complex puzzle we know as breast cancer. *You need to document your family cancer history.* Even if you have a limited family cancer history, this information is becoming increasingly more useful in planning your medical care and the care of your children. *Ask questions.* Seek the counsel of a genetics professional about your family cancer history and the utility of any available genetic testing. Make certain all of your questions are answered in a way that reflects your personal decision-making approach. *Stay informed.* Maintain annual contact with your genetic counselor. As new advances in cancer genetics research are made, you may incorporate this new knowledge into your medical follow-up. A woman cannot change or take responsibility for her personal or family cancer history; she can only respond to it. The best response is an informed response.

THE BREAST CANCER TEAM

We live in an age of specialization. Nowhere is this phenomenon more obvious than in the field of medicine, where a single individual is no longer capable of staying current with all of the latest scientific data. Thus, when a woman has a breast problem, she may consult with several experts before she can decide on the appropriate course of action. Most likely she will begin by visiting her primary care physician, who is familiar with her medical history and whom she has grown to trust for advice about her health care. This doctor may be her gynecologist, family practitioner, or internist, and he is the person she will first see for diagnosis of her problem and treatment advice. This doctor will refer her to other specialists if he feels that they can contribute to the diagnosis or treatment of her suspected problem. When her doctor sends her to another specialist, he is playing an important coordinating role by using his knowledge and taking advantage of recent developments in medicine to help her get the best specialty care possible.

A woman's needs, of course, will vary with her individual situation. Sometimes her breast problem will be diagnosed as fibrocystic changes by her primary care physician, and he will monitor her breasts with regular checkups and mammograms. These mammograms will be interpreted by the diagnostic radiologist. A diagnostic radiologist who specializes in breast diseases is a *breast imager*. If a lump or another suspicious area is discovered on physical examination or on a mammogram and warrants further investigation, possibly a biopsy (image-guided or surgical), she may be referred to either a breast imager, who will perform an image-guided biopsy, or a surgeon (either a cancer surgeon or breast surgeon) for further examination and evaluation.

If a biopsy is performed, a pathologist now becomes involved in the woman's health care. He analyzes the biopsy specimen and reports whether a cancer has been found, and if so, what kind it is, and biomarkers that influence prognosis and treatment. If no cancer is found, the pathologist reports on whether the biopsy revealed something that indicates the woman is at high risk for developing breast cancer.

Although the pathologist has no direct contact with a woman diagnosed with breast cancer or even with a woman whose biopsied lump proves benign, his report has a great influence on what happens to each of these women in the future. If the pathologist's report indicates cancer, the woman is referred to members of the breast management team; this includes the surgeon, the medical oncologist, and the radiation oncologist who help to explain her treatment options and to devise the best course of therapy for her individual situation. If reconstructive surgery is a consideration, she also meets with the plastic surgeon. In the course of these consultations, she may also be referred to the genetic counselor to assess her risk status.

The thought of facing more than one doctor is often frightening, because we don't understand what each of these specialists does, who will coordinate care, and what questions to ask so they can help us. To clear up some of the confusion surrounding these specialists, we have asked experts we know and respect in each of the previously mentioned fields to write descriptions of what they do, how they interact, and how they can help you. The descriptions are organized according to the roles these medical professionals play in a woman's health care and the stage at which she might consult with each expert. Therefore the gynecologist and internist are included under the heading "Primary Care: Diagnosis, Management, and Referral," and the diagnostic radiologist, surgeon, pathologist, genetic counselor, radiation oncologist, medical oncologist, plastic surgeon, and nurse are listed under "The Breast Management Team: Diagnosis, Treatment, and Rehabilitation."

The genetic counselor's role is new to this edition of the book. Today many women with a breast cancer diagnosis, a high-risk status, or a previous breast cancer are referred to a genetic counselor for assessment of their risk status. This professional plays a key role in counseling women about their options.

The nurse's role is also included in the discussion of the breast management team. When a woman has a breast problem, she is usually referred directly to a physician. Nurses, however, are active in all phases of the woman's breast care and play a valuable part in patient education, therapy, and rehabilitation. Therefore we have asked two nursing experts we know and admire, an oncology nurse and a plastic surgery nurse, to describe what they do and how they can assist you during this difficult time.

The final member of the team is the woman herself. As one of our readers reminded us, "A woman has an important role to play in this team effort. She needs to maintain a positive attitude, keep informed, and take responsibility for maintaining good basic health habits with attention to nutrition and exercise. In other words, the woman does not passively submit to treatments imposed by her doctors and other team members; rather, she is an active participant in her own treatment and recovery." We couldn't agree more. It is in a woman's best interest to play an active role in her own health care and to become an integral part of this team effort that contributes so significantly to her ultimate health and survival. The first step in this effort is learning what these health professionals do and how they can help you.

All of the physicians listed are board-certified members of their specialties. We feel that it is important for a woman to choose a physician who has met this standard. All physicians can practice medicine after medical school or residency, but board certification indicates that they have completed an approved training program and, after an initial period of clinical practice, have passed an examination that certifies that they meet the criteria for practice in the specialty.

PRIMARY CARE: DIAGNOSIS, MANAGEMENT, AND REFERRAL

A yearly visit to the obstetrician-gynecologist or internist is routine for many women. If they develop a breast problem, they look to one of these doctors for advice and help.

The Obstetrician-Gynecologist's Role in a Woman's Breast Care
JACOB KLEIN, MD

Specializing in the care of women and their reproductive organs, the obstetrician-gynecologist is in reality the primary care physician for most women and frequently is the only doctor that they see on a regular, ongoing basis. During a woman's annual or semiannual visits to her gynecologist, he performs physical examinations that include a breast examination, pelvic examination, and Papanicolaou (Pap) smear, which is a screening test for cervical cancer.

In the absence of breast disease, the gynecologist is usually the physician who orders breast-screening tests. It is his responsibility to be knowledgeable about the types of tests available, their advantages and disadvantages, and the frequency with which these examinations should be made. The newest developments in the area of breast screening must be part of every gynecologist's fund of knowledge.

The gynecologist is frequently the person most responsible for educating his patients about their bodies. This education includes information about the normal structure and function of their reproductive organs and what happens when these organs malfunction. In addition, the gynecologist stresses the value of regular gynecologic examinations and the importance of breast self-examination for early detection of breast cancer.

It is vital for the gynecologist to educate patients about the need for regular, monthly breast self-examination as well as the best timing for these inspections. Because a woman's hormonal cycle has a profound influence on her breast tissue, she needs to understand these cyclic changes so that she knows when to examine her breasts. Women have numerous reasons for not performing this test, including fear of discovering a mass, ignorance of inspection techniques or the importance of early diagnosis, and lack of awareness of the prevalence of breast cancer. The gynecologist must be sensitive to a woman's concerns and aware of her reasons for procrastinating about initiating this health routine. With these reasons in mind, he should take responsibility for actually teaching his patients the appropriate techniques for breast self-inspection and then monitor a woman's performance to make sure that her inspections are adequate and to help her gain confidence in her ability to successfully practice self-examination. He also can assure her that she will gain proficiency with this inspection if she makes it a monthly routine.

When a woman discovers a questionable breast mass, the gynecologist is usually the first physician she contacts. The relationship that exists between a woman and her gynecologist is a unique and particularly trusting one. It allows the physician to deal with the physical and psychological aspects of a woman's breast disease. Therefore a gynecologist must sensitively respond to the patient's breast problem from a total perspective, realizing that the discovery of a breast mass provokes unparalleled fear and anxiety in most women. The stress caused by the discovery of a breast lump must be dealt with as well as the treatment for the actual breast problem.

The process leading to definitive treatment of a suspected breast problem is initiated by the gynecologist after a routine breast examination. His findings will either reassure him that a disease state does not exist or prompt him to evaluate the breast mass further. The gynecologist will direct this evaluation by arranging for breast cyst aspiration, mammograms, or referral to a surgeon who is familiar with and sensitive to the issues involved with treating breast diseases. The patient will rely on her gynecologist for direction in her health care and will expect him to provide her with an explanation of the course of events that will likely follow. Once evaluation of her breast problem is complete and definitive treatment planned, a woman frequently needs to be reassured by her gynecologist that the other specialist's approach is medically sound. At this time the gynecologist plays an important role as a reliable source of information. He will continue the relationship with the patient concomitant with the care being provided to her by the members of the breast management team.

Prevention of breast disease and referral for treatment of pathologic breast conditions when they do occur are an integral part of routine gynecologic care and should be expected and demanded by every patient.

The Internist's Role in a Woman's Breast Care
BENJAMIN A. BOROWSKY, MD

In current medical practice the internist is the specialist responsible for the comprehensive medical care of his patients and the monitoring of their ongoing health care needs. His involvement in the treatment of a woman with a breast problem or breast cancer is continuous, beginning before the disease is detected and continuing after treatment is complete.

As part of health maintenance counseling, the internist will advise women on the need for self-examination and physician examination, appropriate use of mammograms, and effects of various drugs and hormones on her breasts, and the need for genetic counseling when there is a family history or a potential increased risk of breast cancer. As more data become available on the influence of diet and environment on the incidence of breast cancer, he will discuss this information with her as well. In short, the internist's first duty is to educate the patient about practices that will prevent cancer when possible and lead to prompt detection if it does occur.

Once a breast mass has been discovered, the internist's first effort is to confirm its presence by examination. He must then choose from several options. If he feels certain that there is no indication of malignancy, he may decide not to proceed further. Repeat examination at a more suitable time in the menstrual cycle may be needed. In some cases the use of mammography is helpful. If he is uncertain about the diagnosis, he may wish to refer the patient to a surgeon for another opinion.

In selecting a breast surgeon for patient referral, the internist is guided by more than the surgeon's technical knowledge and skills; he must also consider how the individual woman will relate to a particular surgeon. Each person differs in the extent she wants to be informed about the many surgical options now available. Some women (and their families) wish to play an active role in planning treatment, whereas others prefer not to have to make a choice. It is important for the internist, who usually knows the patient best, to consider her preferences in recommending a surgeon. It is also his responsibility to advise the surgeon as to the woman's feelings. The surgeon and his colleagues in the breast management team will usually provide the technical information regarding the woman's local and adjunctive treatment options, but the internist can help her and her family understand these options and can offer his advice when a treatment choice is to be made.

During and immediately after surgery and adjunctive therapy the internist or the medical oncologist manages any other coexisting conditions a patient may have. He also will participate in decisions regarding postoperative x-ray treatment or chemotherapy.

After the initial therapy is complete, follow-up is a coordinated effort between the breast management team and the internist. The internist is often responsible for long-term follow-up and appropriate examinations to screen for signs of recurrent cancer. He also tailors his management of subsequent complaints based on the effect treatment may have on the woman's breast cancer.

THE BREAST MANAGEMENT TEAM: DIAGNOSIS, TREATMENT, AND REHABILITATION

JOHN M. BEDWINEK, MD

Before a decision is made regarding treatment, it is essential for a woman to consult, either together or separately, with three members of the breast cancer treatment team: the surgeon, the radiation oncologist, and the medical oncologist. If the team thinks that mastectomy is the best surgical option or if oncoplastic surgery is needed, then she will also consult with the team plastic surgeon before any final treatment recommendations are made.

After all members of the team have seen the woman, they will confer with each other, either in conference if they are all in the same clinic, or by phone, and they then arrive at the treatment plan that best fits that woman's particular clinical and psychological situation. The plan can vary significantly depending on the situation. The first step may be a mastectomy with immediate reconstruction, or it may be lumpectomy and sentinel lymph node sampling. For some women, neoadjuvant chemotherapy followed by lumpectomy or mastectomy is the best choice. The point is that there is no longer a "one plan fits all" in breast cancer treatment today, and to arrive at the best individualized plan requires input from each member of the team.

This team approach is critical to the optimal treatment of breast cancer today. It is essential that she receive the input of all of the team specialists before a definitive treatment is decided on and before she is scheduled for surgery or for adjunctive therapy. Therefore I would recommend to a woman that if her surgeon schedules her for definitive surgery before she has seen the radiation oncologist and medical oncologist and possibly the plastic surgeon as well, she should consult with another surgeon who is more accustomed to working as a member of a team. Likewise, if she is scheduled to begin radiation before seeing the medical oncologist, she should seek another radiation oncologist; and if she is to start chemotherapy before seeing the surgeon and radiation oncologist, she should consult with another medical oncologist.

Cancer centers and clinics have been established to facilitate this team approach and to permit all three members of the team plus the breast radiologist to work elbow to elbow with each other. The woman sees two (and sometimes all three) members of the team on the same appointment day. Seeing every member of the team during one visit is not only convenient, but it also allows all procedures to be immediately coordinated and scheduled so that there is no waiting for scheduling until the next consultant can be seen. Also, the ordering of laboratory studies, imaging studies, and follow-up visits is all coordinated so that there is no redundancy or risk of omitting a test.

• • •

Now let's explore what roles are played by the different members of the breast management team and how they interact to provide you with the best care possible. We begin with the diagnostic radiologist, who bridges the gap between the patient's primary care physician and those members of the breast management team who will treat her breast problem. Screening or diagnostic mammograms may be ordered by any of these physicians, and the radiologist will confer with these specialists and with the woman herself to help screen for or diagnose any breast problems.

The Diagnostic Radiologist's Role in the Detection and Diagnosis of Breast Disease
BARBARA S. MONSEES, MD

The diagnostic radiologist is a physician with special training in interpreting imaging studies such as mammograms, chest x-ray films, computed tomographic scans, ultrasonograms, and magnetic resonance imaging scans. Some diagnostic radiologists specialize in breast imaging and are called breast imagers.

Under most circumstances, the diagnostic radiologist functions as a consultant to physicians who order imaging studies to diagnose and evaluate their patient's problems. In the case of breast imaging, however, unlike other imaging tests, the radiologist assumes a more direct role, consulting with the patient herself and explaining the findings on her mammograms.

Although the radiologist does not position the patient for the mammogram and obtain the actual images (this is done by a radiologic technologist), he determines the number and quality of images obtained, maintains a standard of quality control, and interprets the examination itself.

When a woman has no signs or symptoms of breast problems, she is usually referred for a screening mammogram. Her breast images are then taken by the technologist and later interpreted by the radiologist. In this situation the patient has no contact with the radiologist.

If an abnormality is detected on a screening mammogram, however, the radiologist takes the lead in evaluating the problem, because lacking any signs or symptoms, it isn't observable on physical examination. Other mammographic views or ultrasound studies may then be suggested by the radiologist to fully evaluate the problem so that the radiologist can advise the referring physician as to whether an abnormality is present and whether it is likely to be benign or malignant. Often this information is also communicated directly to the woman herself by the radiologist so that she may seek consultation with a cancer surgeon who deals with breast problems. It is important for the radiologist to be sensitive to the patient's fears and to take the necessary time to explain what has been found on the mammogram and what that means for the patient.

When a woman or her physician finds a suspicious lump or thickening in the breast or a bloody nipple discharge, the woman should not be referred for a screening examination but for a diagnostic mammogram, which is performed under the direct supervision of the diagnostic radiologist. At that time the standard mammographic views will be taken, followed by any extra views necessary to better evaluate the suspicious area. The radiologist may also perform a clinical breast examination to correlate the mammograms with the physical findings. If an abnormality is suspected to be a cyst, ultrasonography (which is effective in distinguishing between a solid lump and a fluid-filled cyst) can be performed. If warranted, the cyst can be aspirated using ultrasound guidance. After all of the necessary images have been taken, the radiologist offers an opinion as to the type of follow-up needed: whether careful surveillance by the referring physician or surgical consultation. Frequently the radiologist will confer directly with the woman's primary care physician to expedite surgical consultation.

When a suspicious abnormality can be seen on the mammogram but cannot be felt, a biopsy is usually warranted. A small hookwire is inserted into the breast (breast needle localization) using mammography to ensure its accurate placement; this is then followed by a surgical biopsy. The advent of accurate equipment capable of placing a needle within even the tiniest lesion that can be seen on a mammogram offers the potential for radiologists (as well as surgeons) to perform minimally invasive biopsies of suspicious areas that are seen only on mammography using either mammographic or ultrasound guidance. (See Chapter 4 for more information on these techniques.)

The radiologist plays a key role in detecting and diagnosing breast problems. This specialist not only interprets the breast x-ray films, but also consults with the woman and her referring physicians, offering solace when necessary and answering questions. The breast imager's role extends from detecting abnormalities that cannot be felt (through screening mammography) to characterization of detected abnormalities using diagnostic mammography, ultrasonography and other adjunctive techniques, and biopsy.

The Surgeon's Role in a Woman's Breast Care

KENNETH J. ARNOLD, MD, and JULIE A. MARGENTHALER, MD

Breast surgeons are experienced in diseases of the breast, and this aspect of patient care represents a significant portion of many surgical practices. When a woman or her primary care physician suspects a lump or abnormality, when a breast examination proves difficult, or when the mammographic results are ambiguous, it is usually the cancer surgeon who is consulted.

After examining the patient and reviewing her x-ray films, it is the surgeon who ultimately decides whether to recommend a breast biopsy. In arriving at that decision the patient's history, risk factors, and mammograms are all taken into consideration. In general, one of three conditions will result in a recommendation for breast biopsy: (1) a dominant lump, (2) a suspicious or indeterminate mammogram, or (3) bloody nipple discharge.

Frequently a mammogram will indicate a need for biopsy, even though a palpable mass cannot be felt. In those cases a stereotactic needle biopsy or a needle-localized excisional biopsy is ordered rather than a surgical biopsy. The surgeon is in the best position to discuss those options with the patient and make recommendations as to which is most appropriate for her situation. When a lump is palpable, the surgeon often can place an ordinary hypodermic needle into the lump and gain valuable information quickly and with minimal discomfort. (This is a fine-needle aspiration biopsy, as described in Chapter 5.) This usually can be done during an office visit.

For the woman who requires a biopsy, the surgeon not only performs the biopsy, but also provides the information and the emotional support she requires. This means explaining the reason for the biopsy and the specifics involved in the procedure. It is important for the woman to know when the definitive pathology report on the result of this procedure will be available and can be discussed with her surgeon.

The surgeon can and should be more than an arbiter of treatment options; he should be a resource to the patient, knowledgeable about various conditions of the breast and their significance and able to answer the many questions that today's informed women have about their breasts. Many women do not require a biopsy, but they do need an expert to provide them with information about their breasts, to answer their questions, and to address their concerns. The breast surgeon uses his expertise to reassure and educate these patients about benign breast conditions and breast cancer, the need for breast self-examination and physician breast examination, and the necessity for cancer screening.

For a woman diagnosed with breast cancer, the surgeon plays a key role in her care. The surgeon must be able to sensitively discuss with the woman and her family the many controversies surrounding the issue of breast cancer and the various choices available to her. Because the woman is faced with so much information and misinformation, it is important for the surgeon to take the time to help her sort through the plethora of fact and fantasy that confronts her.

In general, the surgeon will explain to the patient that there are two basic problems to be dealt with in breast cancer: local control of the disease within the breast itself and control of the disease within the rest of the body. Most women will have choices in these areas, and it is important that the surgeon adequately discuss these with the patient. It is also imperative that the patient, already distressed by her diagnosis, feel comfortable with her surgeon and be unafraid to ask even the most basic questions. Dealing with these issues is time consuming, but it is important for the patient to feel that she has been given sufficient information so that she can make the decisions that are required of her.

For a mastectomy patient, he will also inform the woman of the option of breast reconstruction. Then, if the woman is interested in this option, she and her surgeon can discuss the timing for reconstruction. If she desires immediate breast restoration during the same operation as her mastectomy, the cancer surgeon often will refer her to a plastic surgeon, usually the one on his breast management team.

After fulfilling the role of teacher in educating the woman and her family about breast cancer, the surgeon must be able to make appropriate recommendations for treatment and then skillfully carry out the agreed upon surgical treatment, whether breast-conserving surgery or mastectomy, referring her to other specialists as indicated. At this point the surgeon will often act as the coordinator of a team approach to the woman's breast cancer treatment, coordinating her care and referring her to various other specialists, such as a radiation oncologist, medical oncologist, genetic counselor, plastic surgeon, and support group personnel as needed.

Among the many questions a woman might consider asking her surgeon are the following:

- How should I examine myself? What time of the month is best, and what am I looking for?
- When and how often should I see a physician?
- What are my risks of breast cancer, and what can I do to lessen them?
- When is genetic testing indicated to determine whether I carry a breast cancer gene?
- Is mammography necessary, and will it increase my risk of developing cancer?
- Should I undergo additional imaging tests, such as ultrasound and/or MRI?

When a biopsy is necessary, she might ask:

- Should this procedure be done on an inpatient or outpatient basis, and will I be put under local or general anesthesia?
- Can I have a fine-needle aspiration or a minimally invasive biopsy procedure?
- If I have a surgical biopsy, what will the scar be like?
- Why is this biopsy necessary? Will the whole lump be gone, or just a portion? When will the result be known with certainty?
- After biopsy, how long do I have to make up my mind on treatment if the biopsy reveals cancer?
- What happens if it is cancer? What are my treatment options? What are the benefits and risks associated with each option?

- What are the differences between breast-conserving surgery and mastectomy? Which is safer? Is survival the same? Is the recurrence rate the same?
- What are the aesthetic ramifications of treatment?
- Do I have to lose my breast?
- Can I have breast reconstruction if I need it?
- Will I need chemotherapy, hormonal therapy, or radiation therapy?

For the woman who develops breast cancer or for any woman conferring with a cancer surgeon, no question should be considered too trivial. She deserves a thoughtful answer to every inquiry. Above all, she must feel comfortable not only with the surgeon's ability, but also with his approachability since theirs is a relationship that will last through years of follow-up observation.

The Pathologist's Role in the Diagnosis and Treatment of Breast Problems
JOHN S. MEYER, MD

A pathologist is a medical doctor specializing in the analysis and diagnosis of disease in the laboratory. He analyzes tissues obtained from biopsies or removal of organs and analyzes blood and other body fluids. He is an expert in cytology, which is the analysis of cells from tissues and fluids. In this role he will analyze Papanicolaou (Pap) smears, smears of secretions from the nipple to detect malignant cells, and fine-needle aspirates from breast masses. To effectively diagnose breast cancer, the pathologist must also be thoroughly familiar with the microscopic anatomy of the breast and various disease states that affect it.

Although a woman with a breast lump will talk to and be examined by her personal physician and surgeon, she is not likely to meet the pathologist who is responsible for diagnosing her condition if a biopsy is done. Ordinarily the specimen that the surgeon removes is sent to the laboratory, where the pathologist examines it in light of the surgeon's findings, which are written on a form accompanying the specimen.

This examination involves two steps. First is the gross examination in which the pathologist uses his naked eye to scrutinize the specimen and select portions for microscopic study. After hardening and preserving these portions of tissue in formaldehyde or some other fluid, histotechnologists prepare microscopic slides on which very thin, transparent sections of the tissues are sliced and stained to make them visible under the microscope. Next, during microscopic examination of these slides, the pathologist analyzes the types of cells present and their relationship to each other.

In analyzing a biopsy specimen a pathologist does more than simply diagnose or rule out the presence of cancer. Breast cancer is actually not a single disease, but a classification containing many subtypes that have different implications for the patient and the doctors treating her. First, the pathologist decides whether the cancer is invasive (infiltrating) or intraductal (in situ). In situ cancer, either within the breast duct or lobule, does not metastasize and is virtually 100% curable by lumpectomy and irradiation or mastectomy. If the cancer is invasive, it is classified as to the exact type. Certain invasive cancers are slow growing and usually do not metastasize. The great majority of women with these special types of breast cancer are cured by lumpectomy and irradiation or mastectomy and sentinel node dissection without further treatment.

Most invasive breast cancers are not of the slow-growing type. The pathologist can classify these cancers further by noting the characteristics of their cells (whether well differentiated or poorly differentiated) and their patterns of growth in the breast tissues and axillary lymph nodes. If sentinel node or axillary node dissection has been done, he examines the lymph nodes microscopically to determine the presence or absence of carcinoma. The chances of having a recurrence of cancer or a metastasis depend strongly on the number of lymph nodes that contain cancer.

The pathologist may perform a battery of tests or assays to identify specific oncogenes (genes that play a role in producing cancers) and growth factors that predict breast carcinoma prognosis. One oncogene that he may look at is the oncogene *HER-2/neu*, a protein present on the surface of breast cancer cells that is associated with a high probability of distant cancer spread (metastasis) when a patient has positive axillary lymph nodes. This gene is thought to be abnormal in up to 20% of women with breast cancer (particularly in women with a family history of breast cancer) and is capable of making tumors more aggressive and lethal. Tests are also conducted to measure the presence of epidermal growth factor receptors. Breast cancers with increased numbers of receptors for epidermal growth factor (a protein with growth-stimulating properties) have a relatively high likelihood of metastasis. The pathologist may also conduct tests to measure the enzymes that breast cancers secrete. These enzymes may attack surrounding tissues and help the carcinomas become invasive.

Much of the pathologist's attention focuses on growth rate measurements. Cancers with high rates of growth are more likely to produce recurrences within a few years of treatment than those with slow growth rates. Growth rates (S-phase fraction) may be measured by flow cytometry, which is an automated method for determining the ploidy (the amount of DNA in the cells). Tumors with abnormally high amounts of DNA are called *DNA-aneuploid* and usually have a less favorable prognosis, because they are faster growing than tumors with near-normal DNA content, which are called *DNA-diploid*. Labeling indexes and Ki-67 assays also are used to measure cell growth rate in tumors. Low labeling indexes are associated with a good prognosis and less chance of tumor recurrence.

Tests to measure the estrogen and progesterone receptors in cancer cells are an important means of determining the risk of cancer recurrence, the subsequent need for further therapy (adjuvant chemotherapy, radiation therapy, or hormonal therapy), and which tumors are likely to respond to treatment with tamoxifen (an antiestrogen agent) or other methods of hormonal therapy. Carcinomas that contain large amounts of estrogen and progesterone receptors, in general, are less likely to recur or metastasize within a few years of breast removal than are carcinomas with small amounts of these receptors or no detectable receptors. Thus information about the presence or absence of estrogen and progesterone receptors should be included in the pathologist's report.

The final report issued by the pathologist diagnoses the cancer and classifies it based on the various findings previously mentioned. This report is used by the surgeon and other members of the breast management team in assessing the woman's risk of spread or possible recurrence of cancer and in determining the appropriate treatment and the need for any adjuvant therapies designed to prevent recurrence.

Identification of a breast cancer requires a woman to consult with still other members of the breast management team who will help with her treatment and rehabilitation.

The Role of the Genetic Counselor in Advising a Woman About Her Risk Status

JENNIFER IVANOVICH, MS

A genetic counselor is a health care provider who is specifically trained in clinical genetics and family-based risk. While the master's-level training is directed to the study of general clinical and molecular genetics, many genetic counselors have chosen to specialize in cancer genetics. Cancer genetic counselors educate individuals regarding their family-based cancer risk, coordinate appropriate medical screening, interpret genetic testing, and are uniquely trained to recognize and acknowledge the psychosocial complexities of inherited disease. See the National Society of Genetic Counselor website (*www.nsgc.org*) to find a board-certified genetic counselor in your area.

The three most significant breast cancer risk factors are sex, age, and family history. Although assessment of the first two risk factors is straightforward, evaluation of the family cancer history is often complex. In essence, the genetic counselor estimates how much a woman's breast cancer risk is increased above the risk of the general population based on her personal health history and her family's history of cancer. The reason for identifying women with an increased breast cancer risk is to institute medical recommendations that appropriately address this risk. For many women, their breast cancer risk is *not* significantly higher than the average chance of developing breast cancer. For such women, institution of medical recommendations beyond what is recommended for every woman of the same age is *not* warranted. In contrast, women at high risk for developing breast cancer may benefit from earlier and more extensive breast health screening or taking medications such as tamoxifen to reduce their risk. Families with hereditary cancer have the highest cancer risk. (Detailed information about hereditary breast cancer is provided in Chapter 7.)

Most women with breast cancer will not work with a genetic counselor, since most breast cancer develops sporadically with no inherited genetic contribution; that is, most cancer is *not* hereditary. Women are referred for genetic counseling when one of their physicians, or the woman herself, is concerned that her family may have hereditary cancer. Women who are typically referred for genetic counseling include the following:

- Women diagnosed at a young age (less than 45 years old)
- Women who have a family history suggestive of hereditary cancer

- Women diagnosed with two separate primary cancers (bilateral breast cancer, or breast cancer and another type of cancer), diagnosed at the same time or at two different times
- Women with a family history of a male relative with breast cancer
- Women with a known family history of a cancer gene mutation or genetic condition
- Women with specific questions about their family history of cancer

Before your evaluation with a genetic counselor, it is essential to document your family cancer history. The family history is the tool used to identify whether a woman has an increased family-based cancer risk and to determine the possibility her family has hereditary cancer. The genetic counselor will help you to construct a pedigree or family tree. The pedigree provides a diagram of your family size, relationships among affected family members, and is used to identify patterns of cancer in a family (see the first pedigree). The woman who seeks genetic counseling is considered the *proband*. An arrow is placed by the proband, because all relatives are described by how they are biologically related to the proband.

First Pedigree

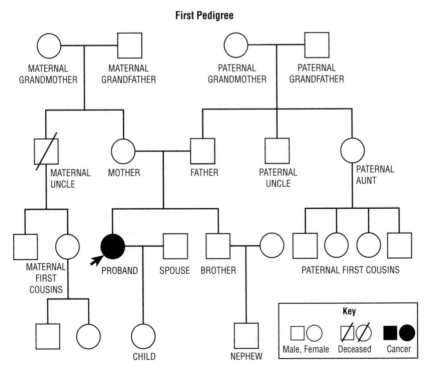

Now examine the other two family pedigrees.

Second Pedigree

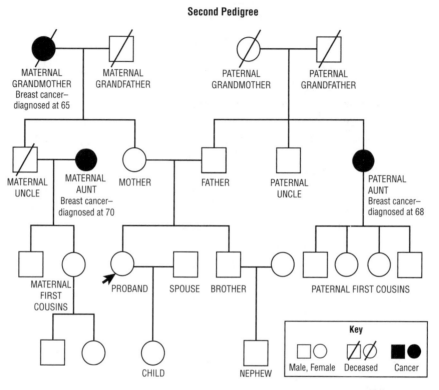

These two families have the same number of women with breast cancer. However, it is easy to see the woman in the third pedigree has a much more significant family history, and consequently a higher family-based breast cancer risk. All of her affected relatives are biologically related to one another, are found in the same family, and have a younger age at diagnosis. In contrast, the women with breast cancer depicted in the second pedigree are not biologically related to one another and are diagnosed at an older age. In fact, one of the affected women is not biologically related to the proband, and as such her diagnosis has no influence on the proband's calculated risk to develop breast cancer.

The following points are important when documenting your family cancer history:

- List all family members, including children, siblings, parents, grandparents, aunts, uncles, and cousins. Knowing the number of *unaffected* family members and family size is also important when assessing the family history.

Third Pedigree

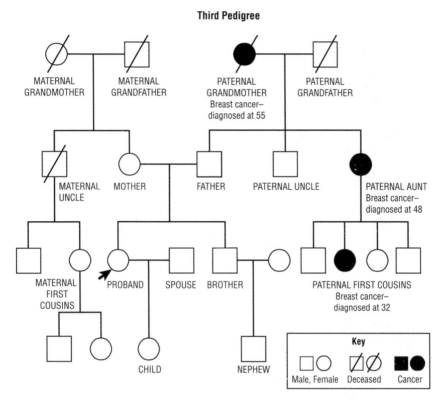

- Include family members from both your mother's and father's family. Many women mistakenly focus only on their mother's family history of breast cancer. The father's side of the family is of equal importance when assessing a woman's family-based cancer risk.
- Indicate the type of cancer and the age at which a person was diagnosed with cancer. The organ or site where the cancer started is considered the *primary cancer site*. Where the cancer has spread to is considered the *metastatic site*. The primary cancer site is the information used in assessing the family-based cancer risk.
- Include family members with any type of cancer, including tumors that develop during childhood. Don't just consider your family's history of breast cancer.
- Collecting medical records or death certificates may be useful in clarifying a family member's specific cancer type. Consider a woman who reports that her paternal grandmother died of a

tumor in the abdomen. The death certificate indicates the paternal grandmother died from ovarian cancer. The ovarian cancer diagnosis is more informative and allows more accurate assessment of the family cancer history than the reported "abdominal tumor."

- Remember, it doesn't matter if a person's cause of death is cancer related. Any cancer diagnosis is relevant, regardless of the individual's eventual cause of death.
- Document your ethnic background. The frequency of some genetic or hereditary conditions varies among different ethnic groups.

In addition to the family cancer history, information from your breast cancer pathology report also provides valuable information. Most women are familiar with the hormone receptors and *HER2-neu* status of their breast cancer. These tumor characteristics are used to establish the treatment plan. Studies that examine hundreds of characteristics of a given breast tumor are being performed in a research setting. Ultimately, it will be possible to characterize the unique features of each woman's breast cancer. This detailed catalog will not only allow us to tailor each woman's treatment, but will also be used to determine whether a woman has hereditary breast cancer.

What Happens During a Genetic Counseling Appointment?

During your evaluation, the genetic counselor will first ask you about your personal medical history. A personal history of a second cancer, as well as a history of benign tumors, cysts, or unusual pigmented skin lesions are information also used in the assessment of your family-based cancer risk. Your medical records of any biopsy or surgery may be requested in advance of your evaluation.

Next, the genetic counselor will review your family history to assess the number of affected relatives with a cancer diagnosis and their age at diagnosis and look for certain patterns of cancer that may exist in your family. The genetic counselor will then provide you with information regarding your family-based cancer risk and the likelihood that your family has a history consistent with hereditary cancer. Many women overestimate their family-based breast cancer risk, and the genetic counselor can provide reassurance to these women about their cancer risk and recommend appropriate screening. Such overestimations may occur because a cancer diagnosis has a significant psychological impact on the whole family. If you watched your mother go through extensive cancer treatment, your intellectual calculation of your breast cancer risk may be influenced by your psychological response to your mother's diagnosis. The genetic counselor will be able to provide an objective evaluation of your family-based risk.

For women with a family cancer history consistent with hereditary cancer, the genetic counselor works to identify the specific hereditary cancer syndrome that explains the family cancer history. A hereditary cancer predisposition syndrome is an inherited condition associated with an increased chance of developing certain types of cancer. Hereditary cancer results from mutations in a specific gene. Information about a specific cancer syndrome is used to determine appropriate cancer screening recommendations and genetic testing options, as well as to identify how the syndrome is passed on in a family. There are well over 100 hereditary cancer predisposition syndromes. Despite this large number, there are many families with hereditary cancer for whom the underlying cancer syndrome or gene abnormality has yet to be identified. For these families, further cancer genetics research is needed to help explain why their family has a history of cancer and how best to care for family members with a high cancer risk.

Many women may have read about genetic counseling as it relates to genetic testing. The genetic counselor will also review the availability of genetic testing, explain how genetic testing may be useful for your specific medical decision-making and your family's medical care, and discuss potential test results. For women who pursue genetic testing, the results are typically reviewed at a follow-up appointment scheduled to disclose the test results, regardless of whether the test results are positive or negative. Genetic testing is complex and requires careful interpretation. No other cancer-related testing will have such a significant impact on your family for generations to come.

After Your Genetic Counseling Appointment

It is important to contact your genetic counselor annually by telephone, regardless of the results of your evaluation or any genetic testing. New advances in the understanding of a hereditary cancer syndrome may be useful in planning the medical follow-up of women found to have a known gene mutation. For example, breast MRI screening has recently been added to the medical follow-up of women known to have a *BRCA1* or *BRCA2* gene mutation. Breast MRI screening was not used in the care of women with a gene mutation when these two genes were discovered in the mid-1990s.

Advances in cancer genetics research are important for tracking women with a family history of hereditary cancer but for whom the results of gene testing have proved equivocal. As other genes associated with breast cancer risk are identified, women may consider undergoing additional testing to examine these newly discovered genes.

Maintaining an ongoing dialog with your genetic counselor allows your family to take advantage of advances that may improve your family's medical care and follow-up.

The Radiation Oncologist's Role in Treating a Woman With Breast Cancer

JOHN M. BEDWINEK, MD

Before describing the specific details of what a radiation oncologist is and does, I want to stress that he is first and foremost a member of the breast cancer treatment team. I cannot stress enough the importance of the team approach in the treatment of breast cancer today. Before treatment decisions are reached, it is absolutely necessary for a woman to be seen in consultation by all 3 team members: the surgeon, radiation oncologist, and medical oncologist. This approach will ensure that she gets the best treatment that is individualized to her particular situation.

The radiation oncologist is a physician who specializes in the study of cancer and its treatment. His particular expertise is in the use of ionizing radiation—a potent killer of malignant cells. The radiation oncologist determines whether and when radiation should be used and in conjunction with the other members of the team, decides on the optimal combination of the three cancer treatment modalities: surgery, irradiation, and chemotherapy. The radiation oncologist also decides how much and what type of radiation therapy should be used and what anatomic areas should receive radiation. He is also directly responsible for delivering the radiation dose effectively and safely.

The radiation oncologist must have a broad range of training. He must have a thorough understanding of all types of cancer and a familiarity with the capabilities, limitations, and side effects of the other two cancer treatment modalities: chemotherapy and surgery. He should be well versed in nuclear physics and the physics of ionizing radiation, understand the effects of radiation both on tumors and on normal human tissue, and know the latest techniques for precisely delivering the right amount of radiation to cancerous tissue while sparing normal tissue. He also should know the side effects and impact of combining radiation with chemotherapy. In addition, he must be knowledgeable in general medicine so he can manage his patient's problems and know when to refer to other physicians if problems arise outside his area of expertise.

The radiation oncologist has a number of different responsibilities, beginning with the initial consultation, when he first sees the patient and studies all aspects of her condition. He reviews her current symptoms and past medical history, performs a physical examination, orders and evaluates all appropriate x-ray studies and blood tests, and reviews the biopsy specimen with the pathologist. Once the necessary data have been assessed, he confers with the surgeon and medical oncologist, and they determine as a team whether radiation is indicated, and if so, where in the overall game plan it should fit.

If radiation treatment is used, it is the radiation oncologist who determines how much radiation to give and what specific areas of the body should be targeted. For example, he must decide whether to treat the breast only or whether to treat the breast and the adjacent lymph node areas. The radiation treatment has to be planned so that a precise and uniform radiation dose is delivered to all tumor-bearing tissue while minimizing the dose to normal tissues as much as possible.

Care of the patient during the course of and after completion of radiation therapy is also the responsibility of the radiation oncologist. He ensures that the daily radiation treatments are being given according to his plan and monitors the effects of the radiation, not only on the cancer, but also on the surrounding normal tissues. He must recognize which symptoms are side effects of the radiation dose and which are not, and manages all side effects and problems that occur during the course of radiation therapy. Once this treatment has been completed, the radiation oncologist assesses the effectiveness of the treatment and monitors the patient at regular intervals to watch for radiation complications, regrowth of the cancer, and/or the development of new cancers.

The team approach should also be used for follow-up of breast cancer patients. Follow-up visits should be coordinated among the members of the team so that the patient is not seen by different members of the team within a short period (such as within the same 3 months). In our clinic, this redundancy of care is avoided by one of the team members dropping out of the follow-up process, and the other two then alternating follow-up visits at appropriate intervals.

Ongoing emotional support for the patient and her family pervades all stages of patient management. The patient needs to know that the radiation oncologist truly cares and will be there to answer all questions and to help with all problems. A radiation oncologist must have compassion and sensitivity, qualities not usually taught in a formal training program. The patient who discovers that she has cancer has special psychological needs, and the radiation oncologist must be sensitive to these needs and be equipped to offer the necessary emotional support and understanding.

Of equal importance is the ability to communicate and teach effectively. Patient education is one of the radiation oncologist's most important functions. It is crucial that the radiation oncologist provide clear and easily understandable answers to the following questions:

- What kind of cancer do I have, and how does it grow and spread?
- What are my treatment options, and how successful is each option? If more than one treatment is to be used, why? How are the different treatments combined?
- What is the specific purpose of each of the treatments?
- What are the potential side effects and complications of each of the proposed treatments, and what are the chances of these occurring?
- What are the consequences of the complications if they occur, and what is the treatment for the complications?
- Will I be able to engage in normal daily activities during the treatment? If not, what are the restrictions, and how soon can normal activity be resumed?
- Are there any alternatives to the proposed treatment, and what are the chances of success and possible side effects of these alternatives?

These questions are the bare minimum that must be explained clearly and simply without the patient having to ask. There will always be more questions, and the patient should be given ample opportunity to ask additional questions after she has had time to reflect. The radiation oncologist must also make every effort to ensure that the patient fully understands what is said. Explanations and answers to questions should be given at least twice. It is the rare patient who can understand and fully grasp unfamiliar facts and concepts on the first explanation, particularly since she may still be in a state of shock and anxiety from recently being told that she has cancer. For this reason, the radiation oncologist should see the woman a second time a few days after the initial visit so that he can repeat earlier explanations and answer any questions that may have arisen since the first appointment. Also, it is helpful for the woman to have a close friend or family member present when explanations are given.

Being able to explain medical facts and concepts in an easily understandable fashion is, in part, a gift, but it is also a skill that can be acquired through patience, effort, and practice. The gift of communication is not possessed by all physicians and not all physicians take the time and effort to develop such skills. This is unfortunate, because being able to help the patient understand all aspects of her disease and treatment will greatly diminish her fear.

Patient education is one of the most important responsibilities of any doctor, not just the radiation oncologist. Unfortunately, most doctors seem to have forgotten that the origin of the title "doctor" comes from the Latin word *doceo*, which means "to teach" or "to explain." A doctor should first and foremost be a good teacher. If he is not, then the patient should find another doctor who is.

To summarize, a good radiation oncologist must not only be knowledgeable and skilled; he must also be compassionate, a good teacher, and a team player.

The Medical Oncologist's Role in Treating a Woman With Breast Cancer

DAN W. LUEDKE, MD

The medical oncologist is a physician who has his MD or DO degree, has had a medical residency, and is certified by the American Board of Internal Medicine. He has completed a fellowship in medical oncology, which provides the training to specialize in cancer therapy. Most now are also board certified in medical oncology.

Medical oncologists participate in the multidisciplinary care of the breast cancer patient. The patient is usually referred to the medical oncologist by the primary care physician or the surgeon once the diagnosis of breast cancer has been made. Referral frequently occurs at the time of diagnosis and before definitive surgery has been performed. This allows the medical oncologist to have input as to what additional studies on the patient or her cancer will be needed to provide the information necessary to determine appropriate systemic therapy, if needed, as well as the timing of that therapy. For patients with metastatic disease, either at the initial diagnosis or later, the medical oncologist usually plays the role of "quarterback," because systemic therapy is the foundation of her treatment. *Systemic therapy* refers to treatment that goes through the bloodstream to all parts of the body to destroy cancer cells wherever they may be (there are exceptions, including the brain, which is protected from chemotherapy by the blood-brain barrier). Systemic therapy may be chemotherapy, hormonal therapy or one of the new so-called targeted therapies. The therapeutic agent may be given by mouth, vein, or injection into the muscle or skin. The medical oncologist gathers the information necessary for the patient to make decisions regarding systemic therapy.

The medical oncologist supervises the administration of the systemic therapy and monitors response to therapy. The medical oncologist also follows the patient closely during systemic therapy, evaluates the patient for side effects, and alters the treatment regimen accordingly.

The medical oncologist must be aware of the latest developments in breast cancer therapy to appropriately integrate them into the patient's regimen. Recently the National Comprehensive Cancer Center Network (NCCN) developed guidelines to assist in selecting the appropriate diagnostic tests and treatments for the various stages of the different cancers, including breast cancer. These guidelines are important for providing a more standardized approach in testing and treatment, whether the patient is being cared for at a National Comprehensive Cancer Center (such as Memorial Sloan-Kettering Cancer Center in New York or M. D. Anderson Cancer Center in Houston) or a community oncologist's private office.

The medical oncologist is also trained to care for the complications of cancer and its treatment. This includes problems associated with pain, nausea, vomiting, diarrhea, fever, and weight loss. Because the effects of cancer can potentially be seen in all organs of the body, the foundation of medical oncology care rests on broad-based internal medicine training, which is a requirement before undertaking a medical oncology fellowship.

Today the role of the medical oncologist is undergoing change in following a breast cancer patient after systemic therapy has been completed and the patient is deemed clinically free of disease. Amid the larger questions of the delivery of health care in America, the issue of how we can offer quality care and at a reasonable cost to the breast cancer patient is being addressed. As a nation, we can no longer afford to have the medical oncologist, the radiation oncologist, and the surgeon all seeing the patient every 3 months. Also, testing the patient for possible disease recurrence must be done cost effectively. Ordering every possible test is not appropriate because of the potential hazards of testing, including false-positive test results and the hazards of unnecessary x-ray exposure.

The primary care physician must play a central role, and this is now being better defined. There is a growing movement toward the so-called *medical home,* in which the primary care physician is at the hub of integrated care for the patient, but what that will mean in the shared care of the cancer patient in general remains to be fully defined, as does the role of the surgeon and the radiation oncologist. I think that the breast cancer patient treated systemically should have lifetime follow-up with the medical oncologist to monitor for long-term toxicities from the medications given and for possible new cancer events, whether a local or systemic recurrence or a new primary cancer. Guidelines for the frequency of follow-up visits and appropriate testing are provided by the NCCN and should at least be loosely followed.

A woman needs to understand why she is seeing an oncologist. Questions about the stage of her disease and the implications it has for her life or prognosis should be addressed to the medical oncologist. In addition, she must understand the goals of the suggested treatment. Further questions about the actual treatment program and how she can assess the effectiveness of treatment are very important. Some of the questions she might ask with anticipated answers include the following.

Why are drugs used to treat cancer?

Cancer cells can escape from the original tumor and spread throughout the body. Chemotherapy or hormonal drugs can travel through the bloodstream to reach the cancer cells wherever they may be.

How do you know which drugs to use?

Medical research has allowed physicians to compile their experience with specific drugs to prove their effectiveness in controlling cancer. Once it is established which chemotherapy or hormonal agents work best, combinations are employed to increase their effectiveness. By combining drugs we hope to obtain additional therapeutic benefit and less toxicity. In general, drugs that work by different mechanisms are additive and produce a synergistic combination (that is, $1 + 1 = 3$ or 4).

Why are there side effects of chemotherapy?

Chemotherapy drugs work to kill or damage cancer cells throughout the body. The cancer cells are thought to be more susceptible to this type of damage, whereas normal cells can heal themselves more easily. Side effects are the temporary effect of the chemotherapy on the normal tissue.

What can be done to prevent side effects of chemotherapy?

Many side effects can be minimized by using drug combinations in more moderate doses. Certain side effects such as nausea can be prevented by using antinausea medications before or after treatment. Simple measures such as holding ice in the mouth while certain drugs are administered intravenously can prevent mouth sores. Patients who receive a drug such as cyclophosphamide, which can irritate the bladder, can prevent these symptoms by drinking adequate amounts of fluids.

Why does my blood cell count have to be checked every time I go for chemotherapy?

Most chemotherapies can lower the red blood cell, white blood cell, or platelet count, which causes problems. If the white blood cell count is very low, the woman might be at high risk for serious infection. A low platelet count makes a person susceptible to bleeding or bruising. Anemia is the effect of a low red blood cell count and might require blood cell transfusions. The intensity of the chemotherapy regimen or the exact combination of medications used determines how severely suppressed the count might be. The patient's blood cell counts are usually allowed to recover before chemotherapy is safely administered again. Growth factors can be given in appropriate cases to stimulate normal white blood cell, platelet, or red blood cell production and recovery.

Are there other generalized effects of which the patient needs to be aware?

Many patients who are being treated with chemotherapy will experience fatigue, which may be worst when the white or red blood cell count is lowest. Depression and anxiety are common symptoms in patients undergoing cancer treatments. Even the end of a preventive chemotherapy program might cause anxiety.

What are the most important side effects?

A suppressed blood cell count is usually the most serious aftermath of chemotherapy. If the white cell count is very low, the patient is at risk of an infection in the bloodstream, which can be life threatening. A severely low platelet count may allow the patient to bleed internally, which could be critical or cause permanent damage to the body.

What should I expect from cancer treatments?

The goal of a cancer treatment should be clear to the patient. Many patients receive adjunctive or preventive treatment with chemotherapy or hormonal medications (usually tamoxifen). The goal of treatment is to eradicate the breast cancer; the intention is to improve the cure rate if possible. There is nothing specific to check, except to look for the absence of symptoms or physical findings. Women with metastatic cancer may have a more specific goal of treatment, since there are symptoms that might be alleviated, x-ray results or laboratory tests that could be assessed, or even physical findings. Physicians hope to improve symptoms and lengthen survival, but cure is unlikely.

● ● ●

The patient needs to understand the benefits and potential ill effects of treatment. Common side effects of chemotherapy must be clearly outlined, along with the means of preventing or minimizing toxicities. The woman then may have specific questions about the drug therapy as it applies to her, its timing, and even its cost. She may also have questions about her activities, job, or exercise. Possible drug interactions should also be explained before chemotherapy or hormonal therapy is started. The oncologist may want to make use of literature designed for patients by the National Cancer Institute about breast cancer, chemotherapy programs, and specific drugs.

The title of this section, "The Medical Oncologist's Role in Treating a Woman With Breast Cancer," is appropriate, because the medical oncologist's role is to treat each woman, singular—not women, plural. A patient with breast cancer is like a snowflake: no two are alike. Guidelines are good, but should only be used to guide and not to dictate, because no two breast cancer patients should be treated alike.

The Oncology Nurse's Role in Caring for Breast Cancer Patients and Their Families
MARY ELLEN HAWF, RN, OCN

An oncology nurse is a professional registered nurse who is committed to providing optimal care to women diagnosed with breast cancer and their families. She is licensed in the state in which she practices and has completed educational training ranging from a diploma nursing program to a doctorate nursing program. He or she may also be certified in oncology nursing (OCN), demonstrating a level of knowledge sufficient to perform the tasks necessary for competent practice. However, the level of education or degree should never be confused with one's level of competence. Frequently the oncology nurse has provided general nursing care before specializing in oncology. Much like physicians, nurses choose a particular area of expertise within the oncology field—surgery, gynecology, medicine, radiation, bone marrow transplantation, pediatrics, research, and hospice. The woman with breast cancer may encounter oncology nurses from several of these specialty areas throughout the course of her care.

Regardless of the nurse's specialty area, she must have extensive knowledge of the disease process, possible treatment modalities, and side effects of treatment and their management. She must also have a thorough understanding of the overall plan of care for each patient.

The nurse may be the woman's first contact when she arrives at the surgeon's office for consultation for a breast lump or for a breast biopsy. The woman is understandably anxious at this time, and the surgical oncology nurse can help alleviate this anxiety by explaining any planned procedures. After the consultation or biopsy, the nurse instructs the patient in care of the biopsy site or assists in coordinating additional tests such as mammography, ultrasonography, or surgery. Once pathology reports, surgical summaries, and x-ray, scan, and laboratory reports are complete, more precise planning for definitive treatment will be recommended. Further discussion with the nurse regarding surgical options, the expected recovery period, and postsurgical care is helpful for the woman and her family and permits them to freely express anxieties, fears, and concerns they may be experiencing during this difficult decision-making process. The surgical oncology nurse will focus on methods to minimize the impact of any subsequent surgery to facilitate a quick return to normal daily activity.

If radiation is recommended, an oncology nurse in the radiation oncology department will explain the plan of treatment (radiation therapy alone or in combination with other therapy), the type of radiation therapy to be used, dates of treatment delivery, overall length of treatment, location of the planned radiation "field" on the body, types of markings used, possible side effects to expect, and testing to be done to monitor tolerance of the treatment (assessing skin reaction, laboratory results, weight change, and so on). The nurse will monitor the patient's skin daily for signs and symptoms of infection or skin breakdown, inquiring about the patient's level of comfort and her ability to manage the symptoms. Suggestions to help the patient maintain healthy skin and to promote comfort will be given as needed.

Referral to a medical oncologist might indicate the need for chemotherapy or hormonal therapy as a form of treatment. Once again, an oncology nurse will play a vital role. In-depth explanations of recommended drug therapy will be provided with ample opportunity before beginning therapy for the patient to ask questions and express concerns regarding expected side effects, scheduling of treatment, and anticipated lifestyle changes. Chemotherapy will be administered by a nurse who has been specifically trained to give chemotherapy drugs safely. This treatment may be given in an ambulatory care facility, hospital, the woman's home, or more frequently, in the physician's office. The decision to administer treatment in one location or another is often determined by the intensity of the chemotherapy regimen prescribed, but it may also be determined based on the physical surroundings and capabilities of the facility or by the insurance policy provider. The nurse, along with the physician, will monitor any toxicities and make recommendations or adjustments in the treatment regimen to safely administer therapy while still maintaining therapeutic efficacy.

The woman may encounter other oncology nurses who work in the hospital. Some hospitals have a designated floor or unit for oncology patients. The nurses who choose to work in these areas are specifically trained to care for patients with cancer and have the appropriate knowledge and experience to minister to their needs. This is not to say that the lack of such an oncology unit indicates that the personnel are less knowledgeable or trained, but frequently a designated floor or unit allows easier coordination of multiple services and more focused attention on the needs of an oncology patient.

Oncology nurses working with a home care agency are available to meet the needs of the woman with breast cancer at various points in her therapy. After surgery, the woman may need assistance with dressing changes or drain care. Some chemotherapy regimens can be given at home instead of in the hospital or an outpatient facility, so teaching the woman and/or her family members and loved ones the basics of self-care ensures that the appropriate care can be safely provided in the home. Nurses may also make referrals to community agencies. If cancer is in an advanced stage, home health or hospice nurses are available to meet the needs of the woman and her loved ones, assisting with long-term care issues, pain control, psychological support, and facilitating arrangements in the face of impending death.

Educating the woman and her family is a major responsibility of oncology nurses in all specialty areas. In addition to the details of a specific treatment modality, the oncology nurse will provide nutritional counseling with recommendations for follow-up care, including frequent physician examinations and breast examinations, as well as early detection methods recommended for the woman, her family, and caring others. Referrals to community agencies, prosthetic suppliers, support groups, and home care services are also initiated and coordinated by the oncology nurse.

In addition to providing hands-on care to these women, the oncology nurse frequently acts as the liaison between the physician and the woman with cancer. Women rely extensively on their nurses as a sounding board for their ideas, concerns, anger, grief, hopes, and fears. Given the predominance of females as nurses and males as physicians, a natural female bonding between patient and nurse frequently evolves. The nurse has the unique opportunity to become the patient's confidant.

Because multimodality therapy is commonplace in the treatment of breast cancer, coordination and timing of testing, surgery, treatment, and follow-up care can be quite a challenge for the woman. That challenge may be compounded by news that a newly diagnosed or recurrent breast cancer has been found, presenting a whole new set of decisions regarding treatment and care that needs to be made promptly. Although not intentional, it too frequently escapes the attention of medical professionals that this woman, regardless of her age, may also have a job that she enjoys (or financially needs), children that need car-pooling to and from school, an invalid spouse or relative dependent on her, or previously arranged engagements and commitments, to say nothing of the endless hopes and dreams she has for the rest of her life. The oncology nurse is uniquely aware of all of these pressures, and it is her responsibility to help coordinate a plan of treatment and care that is medically as well as emotionally therapeutic and accommodates a woman's needs and eases some of her tensions.

The role of the oncology nurse is a particularly rewarding one that enables her to establish lasting bonds with cancer patients that help these women cope with their disease and the problems it imposes. These women share with oncology nurses their joys and hopes, their idiosyncrasies, their family pictures and stories, and their tears of sadness as well as their tears of joy.

The Plastic Surgeon's Role in the Rehabilitation of a Woman With Breast Cancer
GLYN JONES, MD, and JOHN BOSTWICK III, MD

Plastic surgeons treat patients with a wide range of problems and deformities. They perform aesthetic surgical procedures to counteract the effects of the aging process and reconstructive procedures to repair major body defects, such as deformities resulting from birth defects, injuries and scars caused by accidents (including hand injuries and burns), and deformities resulting from cancer treatment.

Breast surgery is a major part of many plastic surgeons' practices. Women consult plastic surgeons for aesthetic breast operations to enlarge, reduce, or elevate their breasts and for reconstructive breast surgery to replace their missing breasts and nipple-areolas after mastectomy or reconstruct the defects after breast-conserving surgery. Recent developments in the field, combined with the skills acquired from treating aesthetic breast problems, enable plastic surgeons to create aesthetic breast reconstructions for patients with all types of lumpectomy or mastectomy deformities.

Plastic surgeons have become an increasingly important part of the breast cancer treatment team. Today a woman consults with the plastic surgeon before she undergoes cancer surgery when she is considering her options for local and systemic therapy and assessing the option of reconstructive breast surgery, either to replace a missing breast or to fill in a defect or correct an asymmetry resulting from a lumpectomy. Many women also come to the plastic surgeon after referral by other women who have been treated by him for similar problems.

When a woman consults with a plastic surgeon about breast reconstruction, he must consider her psychological state, the stage of her disease, and her need for additional therapy. Management of her tumor is a primary concern, and he will confer with the cancer surgeon and other members of the team to determine the best care for each woman and the best timing for reconstruction.

Today, with the use of oncoplastic techniques and skin-sparing mastectomy and immediate reconstruction, women can expect excellent aesthetic outcomes. Immediate breast reconstruction has become the preferred approach and is frequently selected by women who want to avoid permanent breast loss and to achieve the most aesthetic reconstructive result. This should be discussed at the initial plastic surgery consultation, as well as the possibility of incorporating a breast lift or reduction technique into the pattern of the mastectomy incisions. When immediate reconstruction is planned, the plastic surgeon works closely with the cancer surgeon to coordinate the mastectomy and reconstructive procedures.

The plastic surgeon is also aware of the woman's ongoing concerns about her cancer and must deal with her in a sensitive, humane fashion. A woman who is considering breast reconstruction has had to cope with the reality of breast cancer and partial or total breast loss. The emotional trauma she has experienced should never be overlooked by the plastic surgeon in his dealings with her. He must provide support and understanding for the special problems and fears that she is confronting.

The plastic surgeon must be aware of some of the conflicts faced by the woman who inquires about reconstructive breast surgery. Although a woman may want to have her breast restored, she may fear that reconstructive surgery will lead to a recurrence of her cancer. The patient can be reassured that breast reconstruction, whether immediate or delayed, will not jeopardize her survival and has been clearly shown not to increase recurrence rates. The plastic surgeon needs to be sensitive to this fear and discuss it with his prospective patient. She may also worry that this elective surgery will be misconstrued as mere vanity on her part. The plastic surgeon's role is to reassure her that breast reconstruction is not a cosmetic procedure but a beneficial part of her total rehabilitation program, affecting her body image, sexuality, and femininity as well as the fit of her clothes. Consultations should be conducted in a private, quiet atmosphere to enable a woman to feel comfortable and free to speak frankly.

As a counselor, one of the plastic surgeon's chief obligations is to be a good listener as well as a teacher. If he does all of the talking, he will never really know what the woman's expectations are for treatment. He should ask open-ended questions that allow her to communicate her feelings and desires. He must understand what a woman expects so that he can plan an operation that most nearly produces her desired result. If her expectations cannot be met, he needs to explain the limitations of what surgery can accomplish.

The patient's medical history and the status and treatment of her breast cancer provide the plastic surgeon with important information in formulating a plan for breast reconstruction. He will perform a physical examination to assess the options for reconstruction. These options will then be discussed with the woman, covering such topics as the pros and cons, expected results, anticipated hospital stay and recovery period, and the risks of each approach. If a woman chooses reconstruction with an implant or expander, this explanation will also include a full description of these devices and any problems or complications associated with them.

In addition, the patient will be given an informed consent document that comprehensively describes the advantages and disadvantages of these devices and operations. The patient should read those documents and understand them before she signs them and agrees to this operation.

Breast reconstruction is a very personal procedure, and the woman should understand that no one surgical technique is appropriate for all patients. She should be fully advised of all options and directed toward those procedures to which she is most suited. After these explanations, the plastic surgeon can formulate an operative plan that attempts to incorporate the patient's desires and expectations and is designed with her specific needs in mind. He should not assume, however, that a woman will naturally understand the details of her proposed surgery and should carefully review this plan with her.

The actual breast reconstruction is carried out by the plastic surgeon according to the preoperative plan that he, the breast management team, and the patient have discussed and agreed on. After reconstruction, the woman returns to the plastic surgeon for periodic evaluations. On follow-up visits the plastic surgeon will continue to encourage his patient and to contribute to her rehabilitation from breast cancer.

The Plastic Surgery Nurse's Role in Counseling and Caring for the Breast Reconstruction Patient

LYNNE A. McCAIN, BSN, RN

Plastic surgery nurses provide a variety of services for a woman undergoing breast reconstruction. Educating patients about their reconstructive options is an important part of the nurse's role. Nurses serve as a valuable resource for women, answering their questions and addressing their concerns. Once a reconstructive approach has been selected, the nurse provides specific information on the details of the procedure and follow-up care.

In an educational session with the patient and her family, the nurse discusses the tests to be taken, anticipated treatments, medicines that are safe to take and those to be avoided, diet and exercise recommendations before and after surgery, possible complications from surgery, expected pain and recovery, the effects of smoking on healing, and clothing needed after surgery.

The nurse can show diagrams of the procedure, plus photographs of before and after views of women who have had similar reconstructive procedures. Many women request the opportunity to speak with other patients who have had breast reconstruction performed by the plastic surgeon. These names are provided so that she may contact women who have had the procedure that she is going to have and who have agreed to be contacted. By talking to other reconstruction patients, the woman will hear about the experiences of these other individuals and gain personal insights. Although photos and diagrams are important tools to educate patients about various reconstructive techniques, nothing compares with the personal experience of speaking with another woman who has been there. It enables the woman contemplating breast reconstruction to realistically learn what to expect from this operation. It also gives her access to a networking system to share fears and worries and joys. Often women who have had reconstruction are willing to have a show-and-tell session with the new patient so she may visualize and touch a reconstructed breast.

Before the patient meets with the physician, it is helpful to jot down questions on these subjects and others to ensure that nothing of importance is overlooked. Many patients have also found it helpful to write down the answers to their questions so this information is available for ready reference.

The nurse can also discuss insurance provider coverage with the patient. Most states currently have laws mandating insurance coverage for breast reconstruction and for any surgery required for symmetry of the opposite breast.

During the educational session, the nurse may provide input about what clothing to pack to wear home from the hospital and what works best during the first few weeks after surgery. Many women who have had reconstructive surgery mention the importance of loose, baggy clothing. All agree that the best clothes are those that button down the front. These disguise the drains and dressings in the early postoperative phase.

During the reconstructive experience women encounter plastic surgery nurses from different specialties, ranging from operating room and recovery room nurses to hospital and office-based nurses. All contribute to the care and recovery of these women. The operating room nurses are probably the least familiar to the patient, since preoperative medications may have been administered before the patient's encounter with these nurses in the operating room. These nurses are attired in hospital scrubs, caps, and masks; they greet the patient, introduce her to the operating room staff, and try to comfort her, often by tucking the woman in with warm blankets, holding her hand until the anesthesia has taken its effect, and answering questions or calming fears. Once the patient is under general anesthesia, these highly skilled nurses provide assistance to the plastic surgeon, ensuring that all the surgical instruments are available and that the operation proceeds smoothly.

When the surgery is completed, the patient is transferred to the recovery room, where the next team of specialty nurses assumes care of the patient. These recovery room nurses monitor the patient's vital signs, provide pain relief, and reassure the patient that all is well. The recovery room stay may last 1 to 2 hours, depending on the patient's ability to recuperate from the effects of the anesthesia. The nursing staff releases the patient once she is alert, awake, and oriented. Both the operating room and the recovery room nurses are the silent caregivers who provide invaluable assistance to ensure that the operation proceeds smoothly.

The last specialty nurse that the patient encounters during her hospitalization is the bedside nurse. This skilled professional cares for the patient during her time in the hospital and prepares her for discharge by teaching her how to monitor the surgical site, how to change dressings, how to empty a surgical drain, how to take prescribed medications, and what restrictions on physical activity are necessary until her recovery is complete. These nurses provide teaching sessions throughout the patient's hospital stay to facilitate her recuperation. In addition to these verbal instructions, the nurse also provides the patient with written instructions that restate the "how to" of home care and recovery.

Nurses are readily available and attentive to the patient 24 hours a day during her hospitalization and are often the first to detect problems that may arise. These nurses are trained to detect even subtle changes in vital signs, in the surgical site, or in urine output and to respond to these changes before they become problems. The nurse alerts the plastic surgeon to changes and implements alterations in the care plan to ensure optimal care and a speedy recovery.

Nurses who care for breast cancer and breast reconstruction patients are in a unique position to serve as educators, confidants, and support personnel. These nurses and the office-based nurses respond to the patient's physical and emotional needs. Nurses are attuned to their patients' possible psychological responses and are prepared to help the woman adjust. They recognize that the reconstructive process is not complete when the incisions are healed; breast reconstruction after a mastectomy or lumpectomy begins a process of emotional healing. Losing a breast after mastectomy is an emotionally devastating experience. The patient finds herself overwhelmed by emotions ranging from anger, depression, isolation, and sadness and ultimately to acceptance. Women newly diagnosed with breast cancer need to be aware that while the body may be physically healed enough to resume normal activities, the spirit or emotional self takes much longer. Often women say that in retrospect, they feel it takes nearly a full year to adjust to the emotional jolt of being diagnosed with breast cancer and the changes the body undergoes from chemotherapy, radiation, cancer surgery, and reconstructive surgery. Women often turn to their nurses for comfort as they try to cope. Many patients feel that they can open up to a nurse more readily because she has helped other women through the same experience and has worked closely with the woman through the reconstructive process.

Some plastic surgery nurses have become involved in organizing support groups for women undergoing breast reconstruction. These groups are often led by a nurse or social worker, and they help women to educate themselves about what to expect from reconstructive surgery, to share feelings, and to know that they are not alone in this experience. During meetings women discuss issues of self-image, the impact that mastectomy and reconstruction has on sexuality and body image, dating and relationship concerns for the single woman, and other personal concerns that they are hesitant to share with others who have not gone through the same experience. If these groups are available, women undergoing breast reconstruction are often encouraged to attend the meetings, because they provide an accepting, supportive environment and a forum for sharing common experiences during the reconstructive process.

The following poem, adapted from 1 Corinthians 15:44, is an example of the uplifting message and positive reinforcement often provided to women through these groups and through the support of nurses:

What Cancer Can't Do
Cancer is so limited
It cannot cripple love,
It cannot shatter hope,
It cannot corrode faith,
It cannot eat away peace,
It cannot destroy confidence,
It cannot kill friendship,
It cannot shut out memories,
It cannot silence courage,
It cannot invade the soul,
It cannot reduce eternal life,
It cannot quench the Spirit,
It cannot lessen the power of the resurrection.
Our greatest enemy is not disease, but despair.

Plastic surgery nurses are a major source of support to the woman undergoing breast cancer surgery and breast reconstruction. They serve as educators, counselors, and caregivers, ministering to the physical and emotional needs of these women.

The Team Effort

Many specialists are involved in the care of the woman with breast cancer. Most likely she has known her primary care physicians for years. She feels comfortable with them and trusts their judgment. Others, however, are specialists she sees for the first time on referral for treatment of her life-threatening illness. The thought of seeing strange doctors is often intimidating to an already stressed woman. That is why the team approach is so important to a woman faced with a cancer diagnosis. Knowledge of what these specialists do and how they work together as a team to provide her with the best care possible is enormously reassuring and allows her to feel more in control of her own destiny so she can participate fully as a member of the team rather than a passive recipient of care. In addition, knowledge of the role of the genetics counselor in evaluating a patient's risk status and of the support that nurses can provide throughout this ordeal may help in this coping process. This chapter has been designed to provide this information for women and to demonstrate how the team functions at its best and how individual doctors and nurses, regardless of specialty, can deal with their patients with caring and sensitivity.

COMMUNICATING
WITH YOUR DOCTORS

*I*n society we place so much emphasis on "communication" that it is surprising that the doctor-patient relationship is so often marked by frustration and an inability to convey thoughts and feelings effectively. This setting may be the stage for acting out the most significant of life's dramas, yet communication is often halting and bewildering. When a woman develops breast cancer, the difficulties in communicating become magnified by the seriousness of the disease itself. Breast cancer attacks a woman's life as well as her femininity; that makes it a powerful silencer. However, silence is no solution, and women need to be able to relate to their doctors about their health care concerns so they can make reasonable, educated decisions.

Although communication problems are more easily confronted on paper than they are in real life, they are sufficiently important to merit attention and active problem-solving. In the previous chapter we explained ways in which specific doctors can help you and listed some of the questions you might want to ask them. That is only half of the equation. No matter how frightened or intimidated you may be by the specter of your disease, you must bring something to the communication process for it to succeed. With that in mind, this chapter attempts to provide you with concrete suggestions for evaluating and selecting your doctors and with skills to facilitate the communication process. The goal is to ensure that you get the information that will empower you to cope with the decisions you have to make and the therapy you must undergo. As most women have emphasized in our surveys and interviews, the worst part of breast cancer is the feeling of loss of control and helplessness. The goal of this chapter is to enable you to reclaim some of that control.

First let's examine what you as a patient need from the doctor-patient relationship. Those needs are as various as the women who will be reading this book. Some women want the facts presented honestly and in as much detail as possible. They want to know what they have to deal with and then get on with it. Others need a softer, gentler approach, the diagnosis and prognosis presented in a *Chicken Soup for the Soul* format, softened and accompanied by the appropriate handholding and solicitude. Still others don't want to hear what they term the "gory details" and prefer to trust their doctors to do "what is best for them." Obviously, these are stereotypes, and many of us will find ourselves somewhere in between. None of these approaches is to be condemned as inappropriate, but it is beneficial for each woman to understand what her expectations of her doctors are and how much information she really wants. Only then can she establish a satisfactory doctor-patient relationship.

Once you have addressed these needs, some basic questions and considerations will help you select a doctor who will meet your expectations. Even though managed care may limit the pool of doctors a woman may choose from, she should always be aware that it does not eliminate choice.

QUALIFICATIONS AND COMPETENCE
What are your doctor's qualifications and training?

A woman has an obligation to herself to check her doctor out, to find out about his training and credentials, to ask for referrals, and to determine whether this is an area in which this physician has expertise. Information about a doctor's training is readily obtainable online at *info@abms.org* or at your local library reference room in a book entitled *The Directory of Medical Specialists,* which lists only board-certified specialists (see Chapter 12). Board certification is an important credential. It means that after training and an initial period of practice, a doctor has passed a competence test showing that he meets the criteria for practice in the specialty. This directory will list the doctor's year of birth, medical school, the year he was licensed to practice, the year of specialty certification, primary and secondary specialties, and type of practice. Other information on training and hospital and medical affiliations is also included. Doctors are listed geographically, making it easy to locate names of doctors in each community. *The American Medical Directory* is another helpful reference, but unlike *The Directory of Medical Specialists*, it does not indicate whether a physician is board certified.

Is your doctor on staff at a medical school–affiliated hospital? Does he have a teaching appointment with that hospital?

Association with a medical school suggests access to the latest techniques, technology, and developments in the field; knowledge of or participation in research efforts; and involvement in the education of residents. Breast cancer is a complex and life-threatening disease; you deserve the best care possible.

What professional associations and societies does this doctor belong to?

He should belong to one or more professional societies, indicating that he has a focused interest in his specialty area and that he has access to the latest developments in his field.

Does this physician specialize in breast cancer treatment?

It is not enough to just be a good doctor; the physician you choose, whatever his specialty, should have special expertise in treating breast cancer patients. You need to inquire what portion of his practice is devoted to treating breast cancer. How many breast cancer patients does he see in a year? How many has he treated this year? Last year? If you are consulting with a breast surgeon, he should have experience with a variety of surgical techniques for treating breast cancer. You should ask if he performs lumpectomies and modified radical mastectomies and approximately how many of each in a typical year. You want a doctor who has the versatility to provide you with options for care. The same applies to a medical oncologist, radiation oncologist, or plastic surgeon. (More information on selecting a plastic surgeon is included in Chapter 12.)

You should also inquire whether the physician is a member of a breast management team. Comprehensive, coordinated treatment is provided by such a team effort. Members of a team are experienced in working with each other and pool their efforts to consult on your problems, to devise treatment plans that are individualized, and to ease some of the trauma involved in having to see various specialists. This team approach is common at major medical centers and will ensure that your doctors will have access to state-of-the-art technology and have the skills to use it. Ask what specialists are included on the team. At a minimum, an effective team has a cancer/breast surgeon, diagnostic radiologist, pathologist, medical oncologist, radiation oncologist, and plastic surgeon.

REPUTATION

What is this doctor's reputation within the medical community?

Do you know any of his patients? Ask them about their level of satisfaction with this doctor's care. Patient referrals are an excellent way to find out about a doctor. Also, ask other physicians you know and respect for their recommendations and their opinions of this particular physician. The local medical society will have a list of recommended physicians in your area, as will the specialty society for which he is board certified. Check all of these sources.

PERSONALITY AND PROFESSIONAL MANNER

A doctor's presence and style may not be the most important consideration for some patients, but certain characteristics are basic to a sound doctor-patient relationship.

Is he courteous?

Courteous treatment is a minimum standard of care that all patients have a right to expect.

Is he pleasant when he talks to you or examines you?

Has he taken the time and effort to learn something about you? Does he make an honest effort to relate to you? Not all doctors can be "Mr. Personality," but it is important for a patient to feel that her doctor is humane and caring; this makes it easier for her to cope with her disease. After all, as one of the women we interviewed explained, "When a woman develops breast cancer, she goes steady with her doctors. She doesn't have to love them, but it is important that she like them, because she is going to be spending a lot of time with them." How well you relate to your doctor has a bearing on your treatment program and how you respond. Therefore it is important that you respect him and that he regards you as a person, not just a patient.

Does he respect your sense of privacy, dignity, and modesty?

There will be times when your privacy will be invaded; physical examinations and preoperative and postoperative photographs are two cases in point. At such times it is difficult not to feel uncomfortable. But your physician can avoid creating situations that lead to an invasion of privacy and place you at a disadvantage. One such situation is when a doctor tells his patient her prognosis or explains her proposed treatment plan when she is still undressed in his examining room. No woman can think clearly when she is struggling to keep herself covered with a flimsy sheet or gown.

Is he sensitive to your feelings? Does he allow you to express your emotions? Does he make light of your worries?

No matter how insignificant your concerns may seem to someone else, they are important to you; your doctor should never downplay your feelings as trivial. Your emotions warrant similar consideration. Breast cancer is an emotional disease; at times women need to cry, to vent the feelings that tend to surface suddenly and sometimes unexpectedly. It is important to have a doctor who doesn't suppress or discourage these expressions of feelings. (It is also nice if he has a box of Kleenex conveniently located for those moments.)

ADDITIONAL QUESTIONS

Is he prompt, or does he keep you waiting without an explanation? Is he tactful and diplomatic? Does he treat you like an adult? Does he address you by your first name, even though you have just been introduced? Does he seem brusque and hurried? Does he give you his undivided attention during your appointments? Does he refrain from taking phone calls or checking his BlackBerry during your examination and conference?

Unfortunately, far too many physicians lack good bedside manners and are woefully unaware of this deficiency. Many of the women in our surveys complained about their doctors keeping them waiting, sometimes for hours, with no explanation and no apologies. Then when the doctor appeared, it was "business as usual" with no wasted time. Some even informed their patients that they were running behind, "so let's get this over with." In response to such a comment, one woman humorously wrote, "If he was in such a hurry, why couldn't he manage to get his butt in to see me 2 hours earlier, when my appointment was scheduled?" Checking their BlackBerry or taking telephone calls from other patients during their consultations was another source of displeasure and frustration. Not only is this inconsiderate to the patient sitting in the doctor's office, but it is also a violation of privacy for the woman on the phone who thinks she is having a confidential conversation with her doctor.

Although the telephone provides an effective means of contact and communication between doctor and patient, it can be abused. Our surveys provided ample examples of this abuse, but two cited by Mimi Greenberg in her book *Invisible Scars* merit repeating. One concerns a gynecologist who invited a patient into his office, informed her that she had breast cancer, and before she could respond, asked her to step into the waiting room while he answered a call. The other, and one we have heard frequently repeated in various versions, concerns a surgeon who telephoned a patient regarding her breast biopsy results. He cheerfully began, "I have good news and bad news. The bad news is you have breast cancer. The good news is yours is the best kind to get." Unless the patient is from out of town and a personal visit to the doctor would be an inconvenience, most women would appreciate and deserve the courtesy of receiving this highly charged, sensitive information in person.

• • •

There is a lesson to be learned from these vignettes. A diagnosis of breast cancer deserves and demands your doctor's full and undivided attention—in person (when possible) and without interruption. No patient should ever have to settle for anything less.

COMMUNICATION SKILLS
Are his explanations understandable?

Does he confuse you with medical jargon that you cannot understand? Are his explanations filled with statistics? Does he explain how these numbers actually relate to your prognosis?

Does he take the time to inform you of all of your options?

A patient should demand to know her alternatives. It is unwise to make a decision based on partial information. That limits your alternatives right from the start. Learning all you can about your disease and the options means you can control the way your illness is handled.

Does he ask you if you have any questions? Does he answer your questions to your satisfaction, or give them short shrift?

Frequently, particularly in an emotionally charged situation, a patient will not hear everything the doctor tells her during the first explanation. It is important to have a doctor who will take the time to repeat himself and to review his comments until the patient feels that she has a good grasp of what he is trying to tell her.

Is he offended if you inquire about a second opinion?

Second opinions are common in modern medical practice. Many insurance carriers insist on them before authorizing payment. A second opinion is an intelligent way of investigating options thoroughly. It is not meant to be an insult. A doctor who implies that you are disloyal or says that he won't treat you if you get a second opinion is doing you a disservice.

Is he honest with you?

Your physician cannot always say what you want to hear, but you should expect honesty. He should tell you the truth and not circumvent the issue. A physician cannot promise a cure; what he can do, however, is bring honesty, integrity, and skill to bear on the problem. In all of our surveys with patients, a perceived lack of honesty on the part of the doctor was judged to be the most damaging to the patient's well-being and was the main reason many women gave for changing doctors. *Fear of the unknown is far worse than fear of the worst known.*

Does your doctor respect your confidentiality and the private nature of your health records, conversations, and medical treatments?

A patient has a right to expect confidentiality from her physician. It is her health problem, and no one else should be informed of it unless she agrees that this information can be divulged.

Does he listen to you?

Some of the most satisfied patients we have heard from are those who describe their doctors as good listeners. As one woman explained to us, "The best way a doctor can make you feel important is just to listen to you. Sometimes I just need to vent some of my frustrations or fears. I don't want someone to lecture to me; I just want someone to hear me. My doctor is very quiet, but he looks at me when I talk to him, he smiles and nods at the appropriate moments, and he makes me feel that he cares about me and about what I am saying. That makes all the difference to me; it also makes me more receptive to what he needs to tell me."

ACCESSIBILITY

How accessible is your doctor?

Is it difficult to get in to see him, or can you arrange appointments with relative ease? Does he have regular and convenient office hours? Is he genuinely interested in having you as a patient, or do you have the feeling that he is overbooked and too busy to see you? Is his office within reasonable travel distance?

Does he return your phone calls promptly? The same day? Does he set aside enough time for you to ask questions at the end of each visit?

Does he encourage you to ask questions? Does he seem rushed when he is with you? Does he sit down to talk to you and establish eye contact, or do you get the impression that he is in a hurry to get to his next patient? It is important to feel that your doctor is willing to invest the time that you need.

When you have problems, is your doctor willing to accommodate you, to fit you into his schedule?

It isn't reasonable to expect your doctor to spend hours with you every time you have an appointment, but if you need more time and you ask for it, your physician should be able to schedule it. You should check to see if your doctor has designated someone in his office to assist patients when he is not available, and you should make an effort to meet this individual and talk with him or her.

The following list summarizes some of the fundamentals that you should look for and expect in your doctors:

- He should be willing to answer your questions.
- He should explain what you do not understand.
- He should spend a reasonable amount of time with you when you need it.
- He should treat you as an adult.
- He should not suppress your expressions of emotion.
- He should not discourage a second opinion.
- He should respect your confidentiality.
- He should always be honest with you.
- He should be sensitive to your feelings.
- He should treat you as a person as well as a patient.

Basically, you are looking for a doctor who is competent, caring, and informative. In turn, you as a patient also must bring something to this interaction. What can you do to facilitate communication? What is your responsibility?

THE PATIENT'S RESPONSIBILITIES*

MIMI GREENBERG, PhD

Let's take a look at the patient's responsibilities in the doctor-patient relationship. Following are some suggestions to help you improve the quality of this interaction:

Be prompt. If you want or expect your doctor to respect your time commitments, you must be willing to respect his.

Try not to cancel an appointment. Apart from the fact that cancellations, especially at the last minute, are usually annoying because they leave a big hole in the doctor's appointment schedule (and are not likely to increase your popularity with the nurses, technicians, and office staff), you may also wind up sabotaging your own treatment. Certain procedures are on timed schedules or doses (chemotherapy, radiation, and some surgical procedures), and you may be compromising your own prognosis and health. A good rule of thumb is this—don't cancel unless you are too sick to crawl out of bed. And frankly, if you are that sick, you need to be seen.

*Excerpted with permission from Greenberg M. Invisible Scars: A Guide to Coping With the Emotional Impact of Breast Cancer. New York: Walker & Co, 1988.

If you have several questions or wish extra time to speak with your doctor, tell the person at the front desk when you set up the appointment. You will be given a time that is mutually convenient. Don't wait until the day of your appointment to request extra time. In all probability you won't get it, because the schedule will be full. You will be disappointed and feel unnecessarily rejected.

Write down your questions ahead of time rather than trying to retrieve them from memory while you are talking with the doctor. If you don't, you will probably forget them and then remember just as soon as you leave the doctor's office.

Take notes and write down the answers to your questions. This will save you many anxious hours and sleepless nights of wondering whether you are accurately remembering what was said.

Be direct in your communications. If you have a request, a problem, or a complaint, let your doctor know so that it can be resolved right away. Most physicians value your feedback and are genuinely interested in improving their services and meeting their patients' needs, but you have to let them know what your concerns are. Unfortunately, many of us insist on playing the role of the perfect patient who never complains and is always nice. This is not to suggest that you become nasty, but if you are unhappy with your doctor, his staff, the treatment, and/or anything else that is breast cancer related, you owe it to yourself and your emotional well-being to make your concerns heard.

Follow the doctor's instructions. Don't improvise. If the instructions seem unreasonable, check to make certain you understood them correctly and discuss the possibility of modification or change. For example, if you are told not to drive for 2 weeks following breast surgery and axillary node dissection but you feel up to driving within a week, get the medical okay before you take matters into your own hands. Without it you may be compromising your treatment and cosmetic results as well as irritating the doctor, who may see you as a difficult and noncompliant patient.

A difficult patient is one who creates unnecessary problems that complicate treatment and/or recovery and are time consuming to the physician and staff. One misunderstanding will not earn you the reputation of being a difficult patient, but certainly habitual and chronic disregard for instructions will. For instance, if your doctor tells you it will take 6 to 8 weeks before you can safely return to work, it is pointless to call his office every few days to report that you feel fine and

wonder if he has changed his mind. Why not use the time construc-
tively to give yourself a special treat—like going to museums, art gal-
leries, concerts, or catching up on your reading or movies you have
missed? Physicians call it "patient compliance" and patients call it
"following doctor's orders." One reason some women find it a problem
is that they tend to feel so controlled by their doctors and/or breast
cancer that they grasp (sometimes mistakenly) for any little bit of
power that will prove to them and their doctors that they are not
helpless. Rushing back to work and driving prematurely are two cases
in point.

**Be businesslike with your bill payments and with your health
insurance refunds.** If your company mistakenly sends the reimbursement check to you instead of your physician, present the check immediately to your doctor's office. Also, unless you have been advised
to the contrary, you are expected to pay for whatever your insurance
does not cover.

Your doctor is only human. Avoid placing him on a pedestal.
Once there, the only place to go is down . . . and with a thud! The
main problem with idealizing your doctor is that he cannot possibly
live up to your expectations and fantasies. Once the bubble bursts,
you are apt to feel disappointed, angry, and anxious to switch physicians. And if you do switch, you are likely to repeat the same pattern
all over again.

Even in the best doctor-patient relationships there are awkward,
embarrassing, and comical situations. One such awkward situation is
the fear or belief that your doctor has made a mistake or isn't giving
you the right treatment. This is a universal fear: everyone experiences
this at some point. This is not the initial reaction of "Not me . . .
there must be some mistake." This is the wave of panic that washes
over you at the moment you decide a serious and irreversible error
has been made. When these panicky thoughts hit you, ask yourself
two questions: (1) Why am I having these thoughts now? Usually you
are upset at something or someone else, and without realizing it you
seize the most convenient target. (2) What can I do to alleviate my
panic? If you are certain you are not upset with someone else and are
not transferring your feelings to your doctor or your treatment, then
the healthiest and smartest course of action is to present your concerns to the doctor. This will give both of you a chance to examine
the reality of the situation.

There is no point in keeping your fears to yourself, because it will only upset you and cause distance and mistrust in the doctor-patient relationship. There is also no point in seeking a second opinion without first discussing the problem with the doctor who is treating you. Why? Because doctor No. 2 will need your records from doctor No. 1 to intelligently assess your diagnosis and treatment. In other words, doctor No. 1 is going to find out anyway, so why not give him the courtesy of finding out from you?

How does this affect the relationship? Most competent doctors will not try to talk you out of a second opinion. This is not to say that they love it, either. They don't. They may see it as a big red flag that something is wrong in the relationship. Sometimes it isn't treatment competency at all, but rather the doctor's availability or bedside manner or a communication breakdown that is at the root of the problem.

In any case, you are not the first patient to feel that your doctor has made an error (or that you just feel more secure with another opinion), nor will you be the last. Doctors expect it. It comes with the territory. So take a deep breath, talk to doctor No. 1, and then for your own peace of mind talk to doctor No. 2 as well. You will sleep better for it. And if it turns out that it was all in your imagination, you needn't feel bad.

BUILDING A RELATIONSHIP

Much of what you feel about your disease depends on the kind of relationship you have with your doctors and their attitudes toward treatment and toward you. It is important to approach this relationship with realistic expectations and with a commitment to be an active partner with your doctors in your own care. Just as you will experience bad days, doctors will too, and they are as individual and various in their personalities as the patients they minister to. Therefore it is important to keep in mind that your doctors will have off days. Furthermore, not all physicians are good communicators. Some are quieter than others; some tend to overwhelm you with information; others only offer it if they are prompted. The patient has to bring something to the communication process. You have to help your doctors understand what you need. If your doctor is one of the reticent ones and you still feel he is the doctor for you, then it is your responsibility to ask the questions and probe for information. If you don't know what to say, if you are stunned or upset by his diagnosis or plans for treatment, it is your responsibility to say so. It is okay to ask to have someone accompany you to your appointments if you want someone else to listen to what the doctor has to say as a backup. You may also want to take a list of questions with you for your visit so you don't waste time trying to remember what you wanted to ask. Some people suggest taking a tape recorder to the doctor's appointment to record what is said. Personally, we feel this would tend to create an artificial barrier between the patient and her doctor. And considering the litigious environment we live in, it may even make your doctor hesitate to speak openly with you. Let your doctor know if you need more help and information. Ask for information on support groups and the names of other patients with similar problems whom you can talk to.

One woman we talked to felt her doctor didn't spend enough time with her. She described him as "a butterfly, flitting in and out of the room before I had time to ask him what I wanted." Her solution was a simple one. During one appointment she placed her hand on his arm as he was exiting the room and asked if he could please sit down, slow down, and give her some more time. Surprisingly, he hadn't realized how rushed he had seemed. His response was to smile, sit down, and talk to her. From then on their relationship improved. The point is this relationship is one worth working on.

In the years that we have been interviewing women on this topic, we have seen attitudes change. Women have become more assertive about their own health care needs, less passive and accepting, and more consumer oriented. This new attitude puts them more in control and contributes positively to their ability to cope with their treatment. They are demanding that their doctors consider the psychological as well as the physical aspects of their disease. Women are asking questions and expecting answers. When they don't get them and they don't feel comfortable with their doctors, they are making the necessary changes. Sometimes this means changing doctors; other times it means concentrating their efforts to salvage and improve the situation. Similar to a marriage, the doctor-patient relationship requires mutual participation; it is an active partnership in which both members contribute and ultimately benefit.

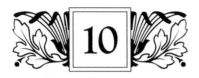

WHY WOMEN SEEK
BREAST RECONSTRUCTION

My breast was an essential part of my femaleness (not femininity), and I wanted to be breasted.

I was only 17, an oddity for breast cancer patients. I had a long life to live, and I wanted to live it whole.

I was planting seedlings one day, and my prosthesis fell out while I was bending over. Crying, I picked it up out of the muddy water. I called a plastic surgeon that same day.

I desperately wanted to preserve my breast, but my tumor was so large that my breast looked deformed after my lumpectomy. It didn't match my other breast and just wasn't what I expected. I needed to have my breast back.

I ached to once again be able to put on a beautiful nightgown and fill it all out. I wanted to shop for pretty things and feel feminine and sexy again.

I began to feel good about life again. I decided that I was going to live and beat cancer. I wanted to look as good as I felt.

This chapter opens with just six of the many different responses that we received when we surveyed and interviewed women who had undergone breast reconstruction. Some had oncoplastic procedures to improve lumpectomy results, while others sought immediate or delayed breast reconstruction after mastectomy. Their reasons for seeking reconstructive surgery were diverse, but all were touching manifestations of the need to preserve a normal body image in the face of a devastating cancer diagnosis. The desire for "wholeness" was pervasive. For these women, breast reconstruction represented a means of putting life into perspective—removing concerns about breast loss or breast deformity and focusing fully on cancer recovery.

Today breast-conserving surgery (lumpectomy with irradiation) is standard therapy for early breast cancer. For some women, however, lumpectomy or breast conservation does not deliver the aesthetic result they anticipated. The preserved breast may not match the normal breast, requiring the woman to wear a prosthesis for symmetry, or the removal of a large tumor from a small breast can produce a substantial defect. In addition, radiation therapy may cause shrinkage, redness, and hardening of breast tissues. Newer oncoplastic reconstructive techniques offer a solution to these problems. As one woman explained, "I wanted breast preservation, but this is not the breast that I wanted to preserve. Reconstruction was a godsend in allowing me to fill in the hollow left by my lumpectomy."

Another woman talked about the unexpected bonus she got when her surgeon suggested an oncoplastic reduction technique instead of the standard lumpectomy that she requested. As she related, "My friend had a lumpectomy and her breast looked just fine. You could hardly tell that anything had been done. So when I was diagnosed with breast cancer, that was what I wanted. However, because my breasts are so large (DDD bra size), my surgeon felt that the results would be disappointing and the delivery of appropriate radiation therapy problematic. I was delighted when he and the plastic surgeon suggested an immediate oncoplastic procedure whereby my lump was removed and both my breasts were reduced during the same operation. It was an unbelievable choice. My breasts had always been too large, causing back aches and neck pain. I had no idea that I could fix two problems at once. Now my breasts look better than they did before surgery, my tumor is gone, and I have more clothing choices. It was a win-win situation."

For women who require or prefer mastectomy, immediate reconstruction done at the time of their breast cancer surgery has a definite appeal. These women want to totally avoid the mastectomy appearance and are particularly appreciative of being able to wake up after surgery with their breast intact. As one women explained, "I couldn't imagine waking up without my breast. I am only 42, and breast cancer is tough enough to deal with. A flat chest would have just done me in. Immediate breast reconstruction was the only choice for me, and it has made all the difference." For these women, immediate reconstruction is a positive means of avoiding the mastectomy deformity and the associated trauma of an altered body image.

Newer reconstructive techniques combined with skin-sparing mastectomy have remarkably improved the results of immediate reconstruction, and women are the beneficiaries. Today immediate breast reconstruction is a frequently chosen option. One woman who had immediate reconstructive surgery proudly boasted about how her doctor could not tell which breast had been reconstructed when she went for her yearly gynecologic checkup. "He thought my breasts were gorgeous . . . and so do I. If he hadn't known that I had immediate breast reconstruction, he would never have guessed." Another exclaimed, "Why not do it immediately? It seems like the only logical choice."

Women who had delayed reconstruction often expressed unhappiness with the mastectomy experience that left them feeling "ugly" and "lopsided." For them, reconstruction represented a means of regaining beauty and wholeness. For these women, femininity was a core issue, and they felt that their "mastectomy appearance" deprived them of feeling fully female. The mirror had become a fearsome presence in their homes. They hated looking at their bodies and found the simple act of bathing to be repugnant. Furthermore, they avoided any situation in which they might have to disrobe in front of others— dressing rooms, locker rooms, the beach. For a good number of these women, dressing and undressing had become a strictly private act, conducted in closed bedrooms, closets, or bathrooms, until they had their breasts reconstructed and no longer felt the need to hide their bodies.

As one woman explained, "I am again a woman in my own mind. I don't look down anymore and cringe. I just know that something is there, and it has changed my whole life." Clearly, an improved self-image was one of the chief reasons for desiring breast reconstruction expressed by all of the women we surveyed. This elective plastic surgery allowed them to feel more relaxed and happier about the future.

Relatively few of the women in our survey sought breast reconstruction because it would improve the quality of their sex lives or help to save their marriages or relationships. Motivation for reconstructive surgery was usually self-inspired. Breast reconstruction, however, often had a positive impact on a woman's ability to contribute to and feel good in a relationship. By making her feel better about herself, this operation allowed the woman to relate to others, especially loved ones, with increased confidence and self-assurance.

Many women alluded to their children as a powerful motivating factor. Young women, in particular, worried that their small children would be frightened by their scarred or lopsided chests, would ask uncomfortable questions, or would fear for themselves. They did not want their children to see them "deformed." For them immediate breast reconstruction was a wonderful solution.

They also wanted to set an example for their daughters if they too must face breast cancer one day—to give them hope for restitution. Other older women said they had breast reconstruction to encourage their daughters to consider the same option. As one woman explained, "My daughter had breast cancer at the age of 28. She and I had our breasts removed during the same year—first me and then her. We both had immediate reconstruction. I led the way and set an example for her to follow when she had her mastectomy. I figured if this old broad could do it, then my daughter was a natural. We are both delighted with our decision, and it has helped us to be more optimistic about the future."

A family history of breast cancer also figured into women's decision for breast reconstruction. It was sobering to see how many of the women who answered our surveys had mothers, sisters, grandmothers, and aunts who had breast cancer. They had witnessed their loved ones' struggles firsthand. They sought to avoid some of the traumas that their relatives had experienced when reconstructive techniques were far less advanced. As one woman related, "I grew up seeing my mother with a radical mastectomy on one side and a modified on the other; I saw her struggle getting clothes so that she would look 'normal.' I didn't want to spend the rest of my life going through the same thing that she did." Other women referred to the successful reconstructive experiences of close relatives. One woman's identical twin had immediate breast reconstruction, and she laughingly related that when she also received a breast cancer diagnosis, she needed breast reconstruction to maintain their lifelong symmetry. "After all," she said, "if I were breastless, my sister and I would no longer be identical." For these women, reconstruction represented a positive way to confront their heritage.

The desire for "wholeness" was a strong motivating factor for all of the women we interviewed, and this reason also pervaded the answers to our questionnaire. Even when the results of reconstruction were not perfect, the woman's dissatisfaction seemed to be minimal, because the breast was now a part of her body and could be incorporated into her self-image. As one woman said, "The reconstruction is not like a normal breast; there are some problems. It is too hard and it shifts around, but I wouldn't go back to the way I was for anything. I love my new breast, hardness and all. I am not embarrassed to undress in front of someone now. I feel like a sexual person again. I am whole again."

Elimination of the need for an external prosthesis was another important reason that many women elected to have reconstructive surgery. Women seemed to feel constantly aware of the presence of a false breast, worrying that it would become dislodged and the lopsided chest would be exposed. In their attempts to hide their deformity, some women even resorted to using surgical tape to secure their false breasts to their chests.

Other women who were large-breasted objected to the size and weight of the prosthesis necessary for symmetry with their remaining breast. For these women, the weight of the prosthesis created a physical imbalance, and they felt as if they were being pulled to one side. Furthermore, the heavier the prosthesis, the greater its tendency to pull away from the woman's body, resulting in her attempt to counterbalance this force by holding herself very straight. Some women actually said that they developed back problems and were unable to function without pain and disability. One woman, whose remaining breast was a bra size 42, had to be helped up from bed in the morning because the strain on her back had become so severe and debilitating.

Because a woman's prosthesis is fitted to provide breast symmetry when she is upright with her arms at her side, it does not move with her and is often unsuitable for an athletic woman who actively participates in sports. Accounts of prostheses that fell out on the tennis court or slipped over to a woman's armpit during running or aerobic exercise were prevalent in our interviews and the source of much embarrassment to the women involved. With strenuous activity, this artificial breast was easily displaced or dislodged and could even float out of a bathing suit during swimming. It also could prevent the escape of heat from a woman's chest and cause skin irritation and rashes. Thus, for practical reasons of movement and comfort, many women felt that an external prosthesis was a nuisance and an inconvenience. "My prosthesis gets in my way. It interferes when I clean, exercise, or bend over," one woman explained. "Prosthetic devices may be great in the beginning, but they are not totally comfortable. With breast reconstruction, one can feel whole again with no shifting of the prosthesis." The freedom afforded by reconstruction was emphasized by another woman, who complained, "I enjoy being active; I am a swimmer and a golfer. My first prosthesis was large to match the existing breast, and it was cumbersome and floated when I dived."

For many women, one of the real bonuses of breast reconstruction was the increased variety of style and cut it allowed them in clothing. Reconstruction eliminated their need "to shop for clothes with higher necklines and specially designed swim wear." They now gained pleasure from the very act of shopping for clothing and once again felt excited about the possibility of purchasing lacy lingerie, pretty bras, and attractive blouses. Proud of their newfound ability to display a cleavage if they desired, they were also secure in the knowledge that when they were dressed, there was absolutely no way that anyone could tell that their breasts had been reconstructed.

Before they had breast reconstruction, none of these women regarded their prosthesis as a part of them or as a new breast. It was never incorporated into their body image, but instead was regarded as a necessity, a symbol of something missing and a constant reminder of the real breast. These women repeatedly emphasized their need to feel less obsessed with the cancer experience and a desire to rid themselves of their sense of deformity, which had resulted from having a mastectomy. Some felt that breast reconstruction relieved them of a cancer "stigma."

Interesting also was the reaction of older women we surveyed. Some of these individuals, in their late sixties and seventies, did not have reconstructive surgery because it was not a viable alternative when they had their mastectomies years earlier. They had lived so long without breasts they felt they were too old to bother with additional surgery. These women readily agreed, however, that if their daughters were to develop breast cancer and require mastectomies (and their daughters had an increased risk), they would urge them to have their breasts restored. Other women, in their seventies and eighties, had only recently developed breast cancer and their reaction was very different. They readily embraced the option of breast reconstruction, proclaiming that they had lived this long with breasts and intended to live the rest of their lives with them as well. Age was not a deterrent, and these women expressed extreme satisfaction with their decision and were quick to recommend this option to their friends, who increasingly were being touched by this disease. For all of these women, breast reconstruction represented an exciting option, and they felt that it would be "wonderful to have two breasts again."

In further examining motivations for seeking breast reconstruction, we noticed a definite correlation between age and marital status of a woman and her corresponding interest in reconstructive breast surgery.

The incidence of breast cancer is increasing in young women. Moreover, breast cancer occurs with greater frequency in women who have never had children. Concomitantly, there are more childless women who are single than married. A mastectomy and the resultant deformity pose a number of especially uncomfortable and difficult questions for single women in the early stages of an intimate relationship.

How does one explain a missing breast to a potential lover? Some of the questions raised by women facing this situation include the following:

- Do I tell my date I had a mastectomy?
- What is the right timing for this disclosure? Before or after discovery?
- Do I keep my body covered while we are having sex?
- Will I continue to be seen as desirable after I admit to a deformity?
- Can I feel sexy and good about myself with a deformity? Or is it easier to avoid sexual situations?

Many women choose the last option, preferring to steer clear of relationships that might lead to sexual intimacy. As one woman expressed it, "I could not face my life with just one breast. I was 42 years old and single when I had my mastectomy. I buried my sexuality for 13 months until I had the reconstruction."

Just as single and divorced women interested in meeting men and beginning new relationships often cite reconstruction as an attractive option, some widows reported feeling that breast surgery might be one step in a personal program of "starting over." Although many women who have had mastectomies after age 65 decide not to have additional elective surgery, age alone has no relationship to how women feel about themselves. Women at any age feel the sense of loss when they have a mastectomy. They still want to return to wholeness. Many of the breast reconstruction patients we interviewed were over 50, and they felt that this surgery had renewed and invigorated them. In fact, some of the happiest and most satisfied women who have had breast reconstruction have been in these older age groups.

For many women, reconstruction is a symbol that they are completing the treatment and rehabilitation phase of their lives and are ready to get back to living. When the surgeon recommends reconstruction (whether immediate or delayed), he is saying that he feels optimistic about the woman's chances for survival. In these cases, reconstruction represents a positive and reassuring statement from the breast surgeon.

Reasons women seek reconstruction are as varied and individual as are the women themselves. Some women focus on the practical considerations of comfort and convenience, whereas others have psychological and aesthetic concerns; reconstruction bolsters their sense of femininity, self-confidence, and sexual attractiveness. Still other women seek peace of mind about the cancer experience, a realignment of their body image, and a return to wholeness. No one answer is better or more important than any other. The fact remains that after a woman's breast has been removed, a deformity exists, and many women feel a deep sense of loss. The desire for restitution is a healthy reaction to this problem. It helps a woman to reconfirm her body image and bring her self-awareness back into harmony. For those women who feel the need to rebuild their bodies and replace their missing breast or breasts, reconstruction offers a positive source of hope for the future.

QUESTIONS FREQUENTLY ASKED ABOUT BREAST RECONSTRUCTION AND BREAST IMPLANTS

Over the past 25 years, the approach to breast cancer treatment has undergone considerable change. Whereas once the emphasis was primarily on cancer removal, today treatment has a broader focus, including local tumor removal and quality of life issues such as breast preservation or breast restoration. Lumpectomy followed by irradiation has withstood the test of time as a viable and effective primary treatment for breast cancer; women who choose this option can do so with confidence that survival rates are equivalent to those expected after mastectomy. As a consequence, lumpectomy and irradiation as well as immediate breast reconstruction following mastectomy have become the norm, enabling women to have the most effective cancer treatment while preserving their breasts. In this context the value of breast reconstruction, particularly immediate breast restoration, with its considerable aesthetic and psychological benefits, is no longer questioned after mastectomy or after lumpectomy or partial mastectomy (when tumor removal will produce breast asymmetry or deformity). Women considering this option, however, continue to have numerous questions about the specifics and safety of breast reconstruction and whether they are appropriate candidates. Some worry that reconstruction can cause cancer or mask a recurrence; they may be concerned about the use of implants, which are foreign materials, and may be unaware of newer types of implants as well as newer reconstructive techniques that allow women to have breast reconstruction using their own natural tissue. Others have anxieties about the appearance of the new breast, the prominence of breast scars, or the development of complications. Still others are concerned about the costs and the correct timing of surgery.

Some queries are so frequently posed that we have compiled the following list of questions and answers to serve as a primer.

Why is it important for women to know about the option of breast reconstruction?

Many cancer specialists believe and our experience would suggest that knowing that breast reconstruction is an option will save many women's lives because they will not procrastinate in seeking care for breast problems for fear of breast loss.

What are the psychological benefits of breast reconstruction?

Each woman benefits from breast reconstruction in her own personal and individual manner. Patients having immediate breast reconstruction often say they appreciate not having to deal emotionally and physically with the mastectomy deformity. Many women who have had their breasts rebuilt have said that this operation made them "feel better about themselves . . . normal or whole again." Some women indicated that it relieved them of a constant reminder of the cancer and the mastectomy. Other women were pleased at the freedom it afforded them compared to wearing an external prosthesis.

Who is a candidate for breast restoration?

Today, most breast cancer patients can have their breasts rebuilt, and this option is frequently mentioned during the initial discussions about primary treatment so that women can avail themselves of an immediate procedure with skin-sparing mastectomy (provided there is no skin involvement) at the time of their mastectomy. Age is not a factor in determining a woman's suitability nor is her type of mastectomy or the placement of her mastectomy scar. Women who have had modified radical mastectomies (removal of the breast with chest wall muscles left intact), or lumpectomies or partial mastectomies can now have satisfactory breast reconstructions. Although breast reconstruction is increasingly being done at the time of the mastectomy, it does not matter how much time has elapsed since a woman's original cancer surgery. There is no statute of limitations for reconstruction and no disadvantage to waiting. Women have had successful reconstructive breast surgery 15 to 20 years after mastectomy.

How does a person's age affect the success of reconstructive surgery? Are you ever too old?

A woman's age is not as important a factor in determining the ultimate success of her breast reconstruction as is her motivation for the operation and her general health. Many women in their seventies have had successful reconstructive breast surgery and are very pleased with the results of this operation. A woman is never too old if she is in good health, is motivated to have breast reconstruction, and selects a type of reconstruction compatible with her general physical condition.

Does the size and extent of a woman's cancer have any influence on whether she should have her breast reconstructed?

Women with small tumors have the best prognosis for survival, and breast reconstruction is most frequently performed for these individuals. Immediate breast reconstruction is a viable and appealing option for women who select a mastectomy and whose tumors have been discovered in the earlier stages. Women with larger tumors that have spread to the lymph nodes also may have their breasts restored, but the timing of their operation is influenced by the type and sequencing of the chemotherapy and radiation therapy they require. Women with larger tumors may have their tumors shrunk with preoperative chemotherapy, allowing them to become suitable candidates for immediate or staged breast reconstruction.

Are women with advanced disease eligible for this operation?

Occasionally a woman whose breast cancer has spread beyond her breast region requests this surgery. When this happens, the surgeon must reconcile the woman's present health status with her desire for "wholeness." For this woman, reconstruction is discussed and performed in the context of improving the quality of her remaining life. Many women desire this procedure despite the presence of systemic disease. As one woman explained, "Even if I die tomorrow, it was worth it. I want to go out just like I came in." If the woman's motivation is strong and if she is fully informed about this surgery, then her psychological and emotional needs are an important consideration. The decision for breast reconstruction cannot be made in isolation and requires consultation and follow-up with the breast management team. The final decision must be made by a well-informed patient.

Are there some women who are not suitable for breast reconstruction?

Yes, some women should not have breast reconstruction. Their emotional state, motivations, or personal circumstances may indicate that they cannot effectively cope with a major operation and recuperation. Women also may not be suitable candidates for this operation if their general health status is poor. For example, if a woman has advanced diabetes mellitus, a recent stroke or heart attack, severe chronic lung disease, or Alzheimer's disease, she should not be considered for this procedure.

Are there health considerations that would have a negative impact on the success of breast reconstruction?

The effects of smoking can have a detrimental effect on the success of any reconstructive procedure. This is primarily because nicotine dramatically reduces blood flow to the skin and underlying tissues. Skin and autologous tissues can fail to heal and infection is more common. Implants may have to be removed and flaps may fail to survive. All smokers are strongly advised to discontinue smoking before and after surgery.

Obesity is associated with an increased complication rate from anesthesia, blood clots from the legs, as well as pneumonia. Implant reconstructions are often unsatisfactory in obese patients. There is also an increased risk of flap failure in these patients.

Autoimmune diseases that cause healing problems may impair potential reconstructive and radiation results. Women with these problems who decide to pursue breast reconstruction may want to avoid implants, but they should be aware that their condition will also make them more prone to possible flap failures. Consultation with their rheumatologist is important before considering any type of reconstructive surgery. Prior radiation therapy reduces the blood supply of the skin and underlying tissues and increases the possibility of poor healing or complications. Medications that affect blood clotting must also be discontinued.

What are the timing options for breast reconstruction?

Reconstruction can be performed immediately, that is, right after the lumpectomy or mastectomy or during the same hospital stay, or it can be performed on a delayed basis, that is, a few days, several months, or many years after the initial lumpectomy or mastectomy. There is also the possibility for *delayed-immediate* reconstruction whereby tissue expanders are placed temporarily in patients who may require radiation therapy.

Most medical centers now have breast management teams experienced in performing immediate breast reconstruction and able to offer this option to women who are having a lumpectomy or mastectomy. Frequently their surgeons will refer them to the plastic surgeon in the team before the cancer surgery so that they can investigate the option of breast reconstruction and the best timing for this operation. Although immediate breast reconstruction is now most frequently performed, the ultimate decision about the timing of reconstruction must be made by a fully informed patient in consultation and agreement with her cancer surgeon and her plastic surgeon to ensure the best treatment for her cancer.

Who are suitable candidates for immediate reconstruction?

Although immediate breast reconstruction is not appropriate for every patient it is widely regarded as the approach of choice, regardless of the stage of disease. It has been shown to provide the best aesthetic results regardless of the technique used to reconstruct the breast. More breast cancers are being discovered at an early, more curable stage. Women with early breast cancer are the natural and obvious choices for immediate breast reconstruction should breast-conserving surgery not be selected; this would include women in general good health with small tumors (about 1 inch in diameter or less) and no involved axillary (armpit) lymph nodes (indicating less likelihood that the cancer has spread beyond their breast tissue). Of these early cancer patients, young women, women with a strong desire for breast preservation, women with small breasts, and women who require bilateral (both breasts) reconstruction are particularly appropriate for an immediate procedure. Patients who require partial reconstruction after lumpectomy are also candidates for immediate surgery.

Who are suitable candidates for delayed reconstruction?

A woman who had a mastectomy before reconstructive procedures were offered or readily available is a natural candidate for delayed reconstruction. The woman with positive lymph nodes, indicating the disease has spread and additional therapy is necessary to treat her cancer, also is an appropriate candidate for a delayed procedure after chemotherapy and radiation therapy. Another candidate is the woman who needs time to evaluate whether she wants breast reconstruction. The delay between the mastectomy and the reconstruction gives her the opportunity to get acquainted with her plastic surgeon and decide on the best approach for her.

Delayed-immediate reconstruction allows a woman to have the appearance of an immediate breast mound reconstruction while deferring the definitive reconstruction until after other treatments are complete. With this approach, a tissue expander is inserted and initial inflation is performed at the time of mastectomy to provide her with a semblance of a breast during her chemotherapy and radiation. This device is then removed and a definitive reconstruction with an implant or with her own tissue can be performed after her recovery from radiation therapy.

What are the advantages of immediate reconstruction?

Immediate reconstruction, or reconstructive surgery performed at the same time as the cancer surgery, has a definite psychological appeal for many women and offers major advantages for obtaining an optimal result. Dealing with a life-threatening disease and simultaneously coping with the loss of a breast are devastating to most women. Some women even delay seeking medical help because they fear losing a breast. Others will not consider a mastectomy unless they can have immediate breast reconstruction to avoid the mastectomy deformity. In interviews with young women in their twenties and thirties who had chosen mastectomy and immediate breast reconstruction, many explained that they felt that immediate reconstruction was a compelling necessity for them in order to adjust to their diagnosis and to continue to conduct normal social lives. The desire to be seen as "normal" among their peers and to be able to interact comfortably with the opposite sex was crucially important to them.

Obvious psychological and aesthetic advantages are associated with an immediate procedure; the patient who requests it is usually pleased with her decision. The breast management team is sending her a message that her prognosis is positive enough to justify beginning her rehabilitation without delay. She feels that her doctors are addressing not only her tumor but also her overall concerns and well-being.

Studies by Schain et al and Noone et al reveal that immediate reconstruction has positive psychological benefits for women who wish to avoid breast loss and rid themselves of their preoccupation with cancer. Furthermore, these women are, for the most part, satisfied with the results of their immediate surgery. They experience less overall psychological trauma and have less recall of the pain associated with their mastectomy. Their new breasts are incorporated more quickly into a redefined body image and they exhibit a lower level of distress, probably because they awaken from the mastectomy with a breast contour intact and thus do not see the mastectomy deformity and experience the sense of mutilation that so often accompanies breast amputation. These studies and others have also shown that the survival rate of immediate breast reconstruction patients is comparable to that of patients who have not had reconstructive surgery and that the local recurrence rate is no higher in this group.

Many plastic surgeons think that the aesthetic results they achieve with immediate reconstruction are better than those attained with delayed reconstruction. Cooperation between the oncologic surgeon and plastic surgeon has led to major advances in technique and to more attractive reconstructed breasts, usually with less scarring than was previously the case. Often immediate reconstruction can permit the surgeon to remove less breast skin than would ordinarily be removed for a mastectomy alone, thus reducing or shortening the breast scar. This technique is called *skin-sparing mastectomy* and is only appropriate if there is no tumor involvement in the skin. With this approach, the surgeon removes the nipple-areola and only as much skin as is needed for ideal tumor treatment. The reduced scar is even less conspicuous later when most of it is covered by the nipple-areola reconstruction. The preserved skin used to cover the new breast reduces the need for skin expansion and requires less skin to be transferred from the abdomen, back, or buttocks if autologous breast reconstruction has been selected. The surgeon can also help preserve the natural landmarks of the breast such as the inframammary fold (where the breast meets the chest wall), medial cleavage, and the lateral (outer limits) area of the breast. These boundaries can then be used to more accurately define breast shape when rebuilding the woman's breast. The result is a reconstructed breast that often has optimal symmetry with the remaining breast.

Immediate breast reconstruction also provides a quicker resolution of the mastectomy deformity and reduces the number of operations a woman has to undergo without significantly lengthening her hospitalization. She benefits from the reduced cost of having one operation under general anesthesia performed during one hospitalization. She can recover from the mastectomy and the breast reconstruction at the same time without the need to schedule additional time for another operation for the reconstruction later.

What are the disadvantages of an immediate procedure?

The major disadvantage is that there are many decisions to be made at once and the time constraints of an immediate procedure may place the woman under even greater stress. She will also have to undergo more surgery at the time of the initial primary cancer treatment, which will increase her hospitalization, recovery time, and initial cost. Immediate breast reconstruction with an implant or expander typically requires about the same amount of time to perform as that of the original mastectomy. When a TRAM flap* or latissimus flap is done, it usually takes twice as long as the mastectomy. Free flaps (transferred by microsurgery) typically take from 4-8 hours of surgery.

The added complexity of the operation means that there is a higher complication rate from skin loss, hematoma, and infection with immediate reconstruction. For implant and expander reconstruction, fluid accumulation (seroma) in the mastectomy wound and low-grade infection add to the potential for fibrous formation around an implant, possibly resulting in capsular contracture or hardening of the reconstructed breast. Infection can pose a problem if a tissue expander is in place; the expander may have to be removed to allow time for the tissues to heal before once again attempting reconstruction, this time on a delayed basis. The reconstructive surgeon may suggest that a portion of the latissimus dorsi muscle be transferred from the back to enhance implant cover and lower the chance of infection or implant exposure.

The woman who elects immediate reconstruction must have realistic expectations about her breast appearance after immediate reconstruction. Even though modern skin-sparing techniques permit remarkably natural reconstructions, there are differences. Her rebuilt breast will not be an exact replica of the breast that she lost. Sensation will be diminished and initially absent and lactation will not be possible. Furthermore, the breast reconstruction will not be complete with this one operation. A second and sometimes a third procedure is necessary to complete the process, depending on the type of breast reconstruction selected, the individual's healing process, and the expectations and preferences of the surgeon and the patient.

Close teamwork between the cancer surgeon and the plastic surgeon is required for this surgical approach. The cancer surgeon should be supportive of the decision for immediate breast reconstruc-

---

*A flap is a portion of tissue (with its blood supply) that is moved from one area of the body to another for reconstructive purposes such as breast reconstruction.

tion, and he must work with the plastic surgeon to plan and perform this operation.

There are obvious benefits and risks to be considered in immediate reconstruction. They are summarized as follows:

Benefits	Risks
Probable improved aesthetic result	More complex procedure to coordinate
Reduction of psychological trauma associated with the mastectomy experience	Less time for a woman to cope with a cancer diagnosis and evaluate her options
Reduced overall cost and hospitalization	Minimally higher complication rate
Reduced overall operative, anesthesia, and recovery time	Longer initial operative, anesthesia, and recovery time
Shorter mastectomy scar and improved sensation	

What are the advantages of delayed reconstruction?

Delayed reconstruction can be performed from a few days to years after the mastectomy. Delayed surgery affords a woman time to cope with her initial cancer. In recent interviews, 14 women who had delayed reconstruction were asked if they would have preferred that their reconstruction be done immediately. Although four admitted that they could have had the procedure earlier than they did, they all felt that a waiting period allowed them to "cope with their cancer, get their emotional lives in order, and separate the negative cancer experience from the very positive reconstruction." In addition, these patients also felt delaying their surgery gave them more time to investigate reconstructive surgery, and thus they had more realistic expectations of the results that could be achieved.

By delaying her reconstructive surgery, a woman has time to fully evaluate her decision to have her breast rebuilt; some women change their minds after a waiting period and decide not to pursue this option. This time also allows her to recover from any additional therapy that might be required and to fully explore the topic of reconstruction, find the right plastic surgeon, get to know him, and decide on the correct reconstructive approach.

For the plastic surgeon, delay offers the psychological benefit of a patient committed to this procedure. In addition, for health considerations, the plastic surgeon and general surgeon often prefer to assess and to help the patient understand the full extent of her disease and the anticipated treatment before she embarks on further surgery.

Delayed reconstruction allows the breast tissues time to heal, soften, and settle. There is less chance of infection, seroma, and implant extrusion. The surgeon has more time to plan his surgery to achieve breast symmetry and accurate placement of the nipple-areola (if it is to be reconstructed). The plastic surgeon may feel he has better control of the variables than when a new operation is initiated at the end of a mastectomy operation.

What are the disadvantages of a delayed procedure?

One of the primary disadvantages of a delayed procedure is the period of time that a woman must live without her breast and the associated psychological and emotional trauma experienced. Because more skin is removed during a delayed reconstruction, the scars are often longer, more skin is required to produce an acceptable result, and the results may not be as good as those achieved with immediate breast reconstruction. A second operation also involves another hospitalization with the associated risks of general anesthesia and additional pain, recuperation time, and cost. Some women who do not have this procedure at the time of their mastectomy may not have the opportunity for breast reconstruction in the future. Again, there are risks and benefits associated with a delayed procedure.

Benefits	Risks
Time to recover from mastectomy	Time to dwell on cancer and on the deformity
Time to recover from adjunctive therapy	Patient may experience depression from mastectomy status
Time to get acquainted with the plastic surgeon	Patient may never "get around" to having reconstruction
Time to make an informed decision	Additional cost of two surgeries (both financial and time)
	Additional potential for problems from two surgeries and two anesthetics
	Probably more skin removal with longer scars from initial mastectomy

What is the correct timing for breast reconstruction if the patient requires chemotherapy or radiation therapy?

Most patients with positive lymph nodes have chemotherapy, hormonal therapy, or radiation therapy after the mastectomy and axillary lymph node dissection. Most adjunctive chemotherapy now lasts for 3 to 6 months. Chemotherapy impairs the body's ability to resist infection by lowering the white blood cell count; therefore it is important to delay breast reconstruction for at least 1 month and preferably 2 to 3 months after the completion of chemotherapy to be sure that the patient's blood count has returned to normal. Because radiation therapy causes some changes in the skin and underlying subcutaneous and fatty tissues, the reconstructive surgeon may also recommend that the patient wait at least 3 months after radiation therapy to reduce the possibility of healing problems after the operation. Many women do not want to wait until the adjunctive therapy has been completed and opt to have immediate reconstruction and then radiation treatment and/or chemotherapy. Implant reconstructions do not perform well after irradiation or when the implants are placed into irradiated breast tissue. There is a high incidence of capsular contracture, firmness, and breast distortion. When postoperative radiation is planned, an immediate-delayed procedure with immediate expander placement or a delayed autologous tissue flap reconstruction should be considered to reduce the possibility of radiation-induced problems.

What timing is suggested for patients with advanced disease?

Once a decision is made to proceed with reconstructive breast surgery, the correct timing for this procedure needs to be determined. On one hand, these women have a less favorable prognosis than if they did not require chemotherapy; thus they often prefer to go ahead with reconstruction without delay. On the other hand, they also have a greater risk of developing local recurrences, and chemotherapy can affect their blood count and modify the wound-healing potential. Most surgeons prefer to delay breast reconstruction until after mastectomy and chemotherapy and/or radiation therapy. Because some patients with advanced disease have earlier recurrences or relapses after cessation of chemotherapy, some oncologists suggest that reconstructive surgery be delayed for 6 months to 1 year after chemotherapy. However, the blood count and other variables that can affect wound healing usually return to normal by 1 month. Each case is individual, and the reconstructive surgeon and medical oncologist should confer concerning the proper interval after chemotherapy.

Patients with larger tumors who are receiving preoperative chemotherapy (also called *induction and neoadjuvant therapy*) can complete this therapy and then have a mastectomy and immediate breast reconstruction with autologous tissue, followed by radiation therapy. This approach has not been associated with compromise of local control or general disease control in the years it has been studied. It does, however, subject the autologous reconstruction to the negative effects of radiation therapy, which can manifest as shrinkage and firmness of the reconstruction in the medium to long term. This effect can be minimized somewhat by reducing the daily dose of radiation from 2 Gy per day down to 1.8 Gy per day. This approach can be discussed with the radiation oncologist, since it does not compromise cancer care. In general, most plastic surgeons prefer to delay autologous reconstruction until after radiation therapy has been completed. As discussed earlier, a temporary adjustable implant or expander can be used to fill the mastectomy space prior to radiation, replacing it after therapy with the final autologous flap. This delayed-immediate approach eliminates the negative effects of radiation on an autologous flap.

How many operations are needed for breast reconstruction after mastectomy?

Aesthetically acceptable reconstructions usually can be completed in two operations. Immediate breast reconstruction allows the first operation to be done at the same time as the mastectomy or partial mastectomy. The first operation includes the reconstruction of the chest wall and breast mound. Operations on the other breast would include enlargement, reduction, or uplifting to eventually achieve breasts of comparable size and position (see Chapter 14). (For the immediate breast reconstruction patient, these adjustments are often accomplished during a second procedure, although they can also be done at the time of the initial operation.) The second procedure is less extensive and includes nipple-areola reconstruction and any additional procedures that improve breast symmetry. When a temporary tissue expander is inserted initially, the permanent implant is placed during the second operation and nipple-areola reconstruction is usually delayed until a third operation on an outpatient basis. One-stage procedures (building both the breast and nipple-areola in one operation) have a higher incidence of malposition of the nipple-areola and breast asymmetries; these problems can be avoided with a two-stage procedure.

How many doctor visits are necessary for each different reconstructive approach?

Before the operation the patient usually sees the reconstructive surgeon once or twice to discuss the details of the surgery and address questions. A follow-up visit is ordinarily scheduled approximately 1 week after the operation, with another visit planned about 6 weeks later. When tissue expansion is done, a woman may need to return for up to three or four additional visits so the saline volume in the tissue expander can be adjusted. No matter which reconstructive procedure has been used, the surgeon will want to see a woman regularly for follow-up visits after her breast reconstruction.

Are blood transfusions necessary for breast reconstruction?

Although blood transfusions are occasionally necessary for flap procedures, microsurgical procedures, and for some immediate bilateral flap breast reconstructions that have a higher risk for blood loss, newer surgical techniques tend to reduce blood loss and the need for transfusion. Simple implant or expander placement usually does not require transfusion. To alleviate patient concern about possible risks from blood-borne viruses, some surgeons request that patients donate 1 to 2 units of their own (autologous) blood for possible reinfusion in the operative and postoperative period. While autologous blood donation is helpful in removing the risk of donor blood, it leaves the patient somewhat anemic, even if blood is donated 2 weeks before surgery, because they cannot regenerate enough hemoglobin to return to normal levels within so short a time. For this reason, many surgeons have stopped using autologous-blood banking almost completely.

Will breast reconstruction cause cancer?

Breast reconstruction patients usually have already had a mastectomy in which the surgical oncologist removed as much breast tissue as possible. After mastectomy, sometimes a few cells from the breast tumor persist in the region of the mastectomy and later grow in this area (called a *local recurrence*). The likelihood of local recurrence is highest in women whose cancer has spread to the axillary lymph nodes. Radiation therapy and chemotherapy help reduce that risk. The rate of local recurrence after a mastectomy for early breast cancer is generally low.

There is no evidence of any kind, however, that breast reconstruction causes cancer to grow or increases the chance of recurrence. Many scientific studies have shown that the incidence of local recurrence after a mastectomy is not increased or the patient's survival affected by breast reconstruction, regardless of the technique used.

Will the reconstruction hide the recurrence of cancer?

The site of local recurrence of breast cancer is usually in the mastectomy scar, in the skin flaps, or in the axillary area. To monitor the woman's breast area for local recurrence after breast reconstruction with implants or tissue expanders, the reconstructive surgeon places the breast implant behind the muscle layer. When reconstructing the breast with a flap of the woman's own tissue, the tissue is placed behind the woman's chest skin. There is usually little difficulty in detecting an early local recurrence because the breast implant or the flap is beneath the skin and therefore does not obscure the most frequent sites of local recurrence. If a small area of recurrence is discovered in the mastectomy skin, this area is surgically removed (often as an outpatient procedure). The implant, expander, or flap does not need to be disturbed or removed. Additional therapy (radiation or chemotherapy) may be required, however, to protect against another recurrence or possible spread of the cancer to other parts of the body.

With the use of autologous flaps (using the woman's own tissues) such as the TRAM flap, DIEP flap, or buttock flaps, tissue is moved from a distant site and blood flow may be decreased, leading to the formation of a condition known as fat necrosis. This manifests itself as small areas of nodularity (firm, thickened areas of fat) that may be confused with a local recurrence. These areas, however, are within the abdominal or buttock tissue and can be differentiated from a local recurrence. Sometimes mammography, ultrasonography, or a biopsy may be necessary for a definitive diagnosis. If a biopsy is needed, it can sometimes be done with a fine needle to avoid a surgical incision.

If recurrence develops in relation to any form of reconstruction, it is almost always around the edge of the flap and not within it, as the flap does not consist of, or contain any breast tissue.

Will a woman be able to detect tumors after reconstruction?

After reconstruction with an implant or expander placed beneath the muscle layer or with a flap from the back, abdomen, buttock or thigh, the skin and scar are actually pushed forward and thus new tumors usually can be felt easily on breast self-examination (BSE). That is why it is equally as important for women to continue to perform BSE after a mastectomy or lumpectomy whether they have had breast reconstruction or not.

Does breast reconstruction compromise a woman's immune system?

There is no medical evidence that breast reconstruction or general anesthesia compromises a woman's immune system. Some believe, however, that a woman who has breast cancer may already have a compromised immune system.

What is the best placement of a mastectomy scar for the woman who desires breast reconstruction?

When skin-sparing mastectomy is to be done for immediate reconstruction, the best placement for this scar is usually around the areola with a 1- to 2-inch (3 to 5 cm) extension of the scar to the side or below the areola. For delayed reconstruction, the best placement of the mastectomy scar is in a low oblique position, extending from below the axilla (armpit) to the inner lower breast area. Either of these scars is easily covered by a brassiere.

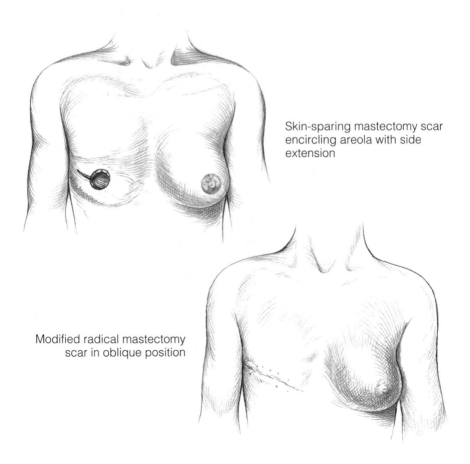

Skin-sparing mastectomy scar encircling areola with side extension

Modified radical mastectomy scar in oblique position

When immediate breast reconstruction is done after a modified radical mastectomy, the general surgeon and the reconstructive surgeon can plan the location of the incisions to ensure the best placement for the breast reconstruction. They may be able to minimize the incisions and preserve more skin, which improves the final breast appearance. Sometimes these incisions can resemble those used for a breast reduction in a woman with large, droopy breasts (see Chapter 14). Sometimes a separate, shorter incision is also made to remove the tumor in the upper breast region.

For delayed reconstruction, frequently a portion of the scar can be reopened and an implant placed through it to avoid creating a new incision and thus a new scar. Sometimes, however, the primary cancer is located in an area of the breast that makes it impossible for the surgeon to leave an oblique scar, especially when it is high and medial in the breast area.

What can be done if the mastectomy scar is in a bad location?

Breast reconstruction can be done with a mastectomy scar in any position. The scar position cannot be changed, but the reconstructive implant or flap can be positioned through this scar and the scar revised to provide the best possible appearance.

Can the plastic surgeon totally remove the mastectomy scars from the cancer surgery when he restores the breast?

The scars from the cancer surgery cannot be removed, although they sometimes can be reduced or made less obvious by a plastic surgery procedure called scar revision. A scar line will always be present where the original skin incision for the cancer surgery was performed. Initially the scars will be red and raised, a condition that will persist for several months after the operation. This redness (indicative of increased blood flow during the healing process) and thickness will subside over the next 1 or 2 years as the scars improve in appearance and become less obvious. Scars in fair-skinned women tend to remain red for a longer period of time. It takes less time for the scars of older women to fade. Some women heal with thick scars, and this tendency is obvious from the appearance of the mastectomy scar as well as any other scars that they may have. The postoperative use of silicone-containing creams or silicone sheets may significantly improve the appearance of the scars.

What type of new scars are created by reconstruction?

Reconstruction using the existing tissues or by expanding the existing tissues is most frequently accomplished through the mastectomy scar. No new scar is created. Sometimes, if additional skin is needed to reconstruct the breast, other scars will be created when this skin is inset into the breast. New scars on the breast will encircle the areola and extend into the underarm for immediate reconstruction after skin-sparing procedures and will usually extend along the lower breast crease and either up to the old scar or up to the nipple level for delayed reconstruction.

Whenever new distant tissue is added, scars will usually be left where the tissue is obtained (the donor site). Common donor sites are the lower abdomen, back, side, and buttocks. Scars will either be left across the back or under the arm if the back is the donor site. The abdominal scar will usually extend across the lower abdomen just above the pubic hairline. The buttock scar will be in the crease or across the midportion of the buttock region.

TYPES OF BREAST SCARS FROM FLAP RECONSTRUCTION

Skin-Sparing Mastectomy

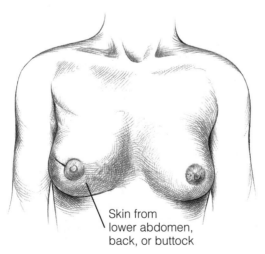

Skin from lower abdomen, back, or buttock

Immediate breast reconstruction with a flap of tissue from the lower abdomen (TRAM, DIEP, or SIEA flap), back (latissimus dorsi flap), or buttock (gluteus maximus, IGAP, or SGAP flap) after skin-sparing mastectomy

TYPES OF BREAST SCARS FROM FLAP RECONSTRUCTION—cont'd

Modified Radical Mastectomy

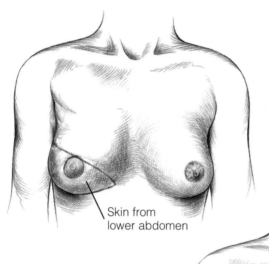

Breast reconstruction with a flap of tissue from the lower abdomen (TRAM, DIEP, or SIEA flap) after modified radical mastectomy

Skin from lower abdomen

Breast reconstruction with a flap of tissue from the back (latissimus dorsi) after modified radical mastectomy

Skin from back

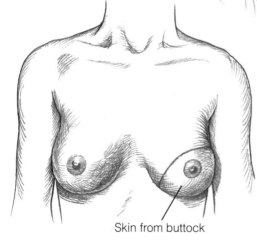

Breast reconstruction with a flap of tissue from the buttock—gluteus maximus, IGAP (inferior gluteus maximus), or SGAP (superior gluteus maximus) flap—after modified radical mastectomy

Skin from buttock

TYPES OF DONOR SCARS CREATED BY FLAP RECONSTRUCTION

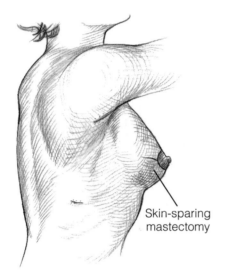

Skin-sparing
mastectomy

Donor scar left on back from
immediate endoscopic latissimus
dorsi reconstruction

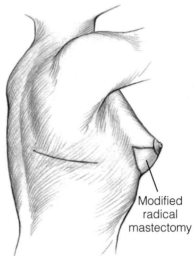

Modified
radical
mastectomy

Donor scar left on back from
latissimus dorsi reconstruction

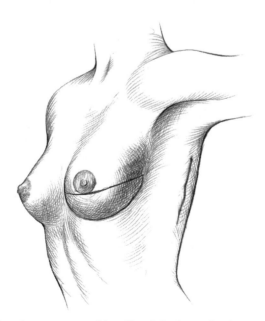

Alternative donor scar on side with a latissimus dorsi reconstruction

TYPES OF DONOR SCARS CREATED BY FLAP RECONSTRUCTION—cont'd

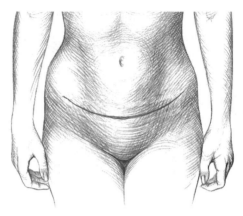

Donor scar on lower abdomen from TRAM, DIEP, or SIEA flap reconstruction

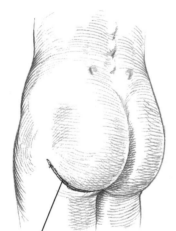 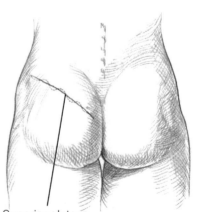

Inferior gluteus
maximus flap
and IGAP flap

Superior gluteus
maximus flap
and SGAP flap

Donor scar left on buttock from gluteus maximus flap,
IGAP flap *(left)* or SGAP flap *(right)*

How much skin is removed during mastectomy and can you be sure enough can be preserved for breast reconstruction?

When a woman has a mastectomy to treat her breast cancer, the oncologic surgeon usually removes some skin around the biopsy site as well as the nipple-areola. Many surgeons can perform the operation through these incisions. The incision may need to be extended to the axillary region to gain access to the lymph nodes. Studies have shown that it is not necessary to remove additional skin from the breast region as was done in the past. Therefore more skin can be spared and preserved for breast reconstruction. In some instances, particularly when a flap of the patient's own tissue is available for the reconstruction, the skin at the biopsy site and area of nipple-areola removal is replaced with the skin on the flap. Any additional skin that is needed is supplied from the remaining skin at the mastectomy site. With this approach, the skin of the restored breast has the same consistency and appearance as the skin of the opposite breast. Furthermore, when less skin is removed initially, the mastectomy scars are shorter and the extra skin that is left is filled out by the transferred tissue or the breast implant or expander that is inserted.

Actually, a woman's breast can be reconstructed regardless of the amount of tissue remaining after the mastectomy. When the pectoralis major muscle and sufficient breast skin are present, a simple reconstruction with an implant or expander can usually be done. When much of the skin or pectoralis major muscle is missing and there is a significant skin deficiency, a flap, either from the back, lower abdomen, or buttock area, is usually necessary.

If a woman knows that she would like to have breast reconstruction before her mastectomy, her general surgeon should be informed so that he can confer with a plastic surgeon to ensure the best possible plan to facilitate the reconstruction.

Is it necessary for the normal breast to be modified to match the new one?

Many times a good match can be achieved with breast reconstruction if the opposite normal breast is not too large or droopy. This approach leaves the normal breast untouched. Tissue expansion and implant placement tends to achieve better results in smaller breasted women who do not have much sagging of the normal opposite breast. If the patient has a larger or more droopy opposite breast, a flap procedure can often result in good symmetry without touching the woman's normal breast. When the normal breast is very large and sags or is very flat and small, the surgeon may not be able to match it and some modification might be required such as a breast lift, breast reduction or breast augmentation.

What areas can be reconstructed? Can large deformities and chest hollowness be filled in?

Predictably good restoration of the breast shape, contour, and size can now be achieved though breast reconstruction. It often improves the appearance of (but may not eliminate) scars, skin grafts, or radiation-damaged skin. Fat injections using the patient's own fat can be used to fill small hollows or indentations that exist next to the reconstructed breast.

Can partial defects after lumpectomy and quadrantectomy be reconstructed?

After completion of the lumpectomy or quadrantectomy, the general or oncologic surgeon checks the margins of resection to ensure complete tumor removal. He also assesses the area of tumor excision to determine if it will leave an unsatisfactory breast shape or size after healing and/or radiation therapy. If this is the case, the volume of the breast may be restored using oncoplastic surgical techniques or with injections of the woman's own fatty tissue.

What is oncoplastic surgery? Is this another method for breast restoration and when is it used?

Oncoplastic operations combine cancer therapy with breast reduction techniques. These procedures are used in conjunction with breast conservation therapy (lumpectomy, quadrantectomy) when the removal of an appropriately sized amount of breast tissue to provide adequate margins for surgical clearance may result in significant breast volume loss and even breast deformity.

Generally, lumpectomy will create some degree of tissue loss at the tumor removal site. This defect can be filled by rotating local flaps of breast tissue into the empty area to fill it, using breast reduction techniques that lift and reduce the shape and size of the breast. The result is a better cosmetic appearance to the breast after treatment. These procedures are covered by insurance.

The benefits from oncoplastic surgery are far greater than the cosmetic results they deliver. Women undergoing lumpectomy require postoperative radiation therapy. The larger the breast being radiated, the greater the risk of tissue becoming hard, shrunken and deformed. If a large breast is reduced prior to radiation therapy, it is easier and safer for the radiation oncologist to treat the breast with lower complication rates. However, it is essential that the oncoplastic procedure be performed prior to the administration of radiation therapy.

What are endoscopic techniques, and can they be used for oncoplastic reconstruction of lumpectomy deformities?

With the endoscopic technique for harvesting the latissimus dorsi back muscle and fat, the surgeon uses the incisions made at the time of primary cancer treatment, which are usually in the lateral breast region and in the underarm area (where the axillary lymph node dissection was done). A video camera is attached to the endoscope so the image can be viewed on the TV monitor by the surgeon while he operates using special long instruments that are inserted through the small incisions. The endoscope permits a video image of tissues beneath the skin to be projected on the video monitor via fiberoptic light. Sometimes separate incisions about an inch long are also needed in the middle to lower back. Through these small incisions the surgeon visualizes the area with the use of the endoscope, dissects the flap that contains the fat and muscle, preserves the blood supply to the tissue, and moves the flap through the incisions used for the primary local cancer treatment. This flap is then used to fill and contour the defect remaining after the breast-conserving procedure. This technique is also useful for secondary breast deformities that require some additional tissue.

What is the role of fat grafting in reconstructing lumpectomy or mastectomy defects?

Fat injections taken from areas of tissue excess (such as the abdomen, buttocks, and thigh) and then reinjected into the breasts after the fat has been filtered of blood and other elements, represent an exciting new option for improving the results of breast restoration after lumpectomy and mastectomy. These grafts are used to fill hollows, to soften the tissues around breast implants and to improve skin quality after radiation therapy because of the stem cells that they contain which have a regenerative effect on the overlying skin.

Can the missing nipple-areola be reconstructed?

Both the central projecting nipple and the darker surrounding areola can be reconstructed. This procedure is usually done as a second operation after the proper breast shape and size have been obtained. Although there are several different methods for reconstructing the nipple, some of the most effective techniques use tissue available at the site of the new nipple in the form of local skin and fat flaps. Earlier techniques primarily used tissues from other areas of the body. The areola can be reconstructed from a circular graft of excess skin near the mastectomy scar or from the abdominal scar if an abdominal (TRAM) flap has been used for the reconstruction. Most commonly, the areola is recreated using a surgical tattoo performed 4-6 weeks after nipple reconstruction. This allows for the areola and reconstructed nipple to be colored to the proper shade in order to match the opposite nipple. (See Chapter 16 for more detailed information on the different techniques for nipple-areola reconstruction.)

What are the different options for breast reconstruction?

Basically, breast reconstruction can be performed with implants and tissue expanders or with flaps of the patient's own tissues (autologous tissues). Implant and expander reconstructions are simpler, shorter, less expensive procedures with less downtime. However maintenance surgery is required over time. Autologous flap procedures are more extensive, bigger procedures that take longer to perform and have a longer recovery period. However, they have no long-term maintenance. Both types of reconstructive surgery can produce very satisfactory results.

How do the risks involved with flap surgery compare to those encountered in implant surgery?

The decision to have breast reconstruction with a flap or with a breast implant involves an analysis of the risks and benefits of the two approaches. Flap operations take longer, which means increased risks of major surgical complications such as deep vein thrombosis (DVT), pulmonary complications, and fluid retention. The success of flap procedures depends on the blood supply of the flaps; if this is compromised, part or all of the flap can be lost. Fortunately, this is a rare occurrence. The shaping of the flap tissue into a breast form also requires more skill and artistry on the part of the surgeon than that required for placement of a breast implant or expander. The obvious benefit of autologous flap reconstruction is that it creates a lasting, more natural breast symmetry that is usually maintained for a lifetime and uses the woman's own tissues, generally without the need for an implant.

The perioperative risks of implant reconstruction are less serious and pose a lower chance of major complications. The benefits of breast reconstruction with breast implants are also significant for the patient who can have a successful procedure with minimal inconvenience and cost. The drawback of this approach is that a deflation or rupture can occur or a capsular contracture can develop around the breast implant and may require additional procedures in the future. Furthermore, implants are not considered lifetime devices and may have to be replaced at some point in the future. The average lifespan of implants is about 10 to 20 years.

RECONSTRUCTION WITH IMPLANTS AND TISSUE EXPANDERS

What is the value of breast implants?

Breast implants have been an integral part of breast surgery for almost 45 years. They have been successfully used to restore breast shape and contour after mastectomy, correct breast and chest wall deformities and asymmetries, augment small breasts, and lift sagging ones.

How are breast implants and tissue expanders used for breast reconstruction?

These devices are inserted under a woman's skin and pectoralis major muscle to create a breast mound during breast reconstruction. For breast reconstruction with implants to be successful, the implant must provide volume, projection, and size that approximates that of the opposite breast. Just as the appearance of the normal female breast changes with age, breast implants may also need to be changed or adjusted over time to maintain the best results. Expanders are temporary devices used to stretch the overlying chest wall and breast skin to reach a final volume that will accommodate an implant similar in size to that of the normal opposite breast. The use of tissue expanders makes obtaining the proper size for the breast reconstruction more likely. The size of the expander can be adjusted if the fill valve is left in place.

Why do women choose reconstruction with implants? Why don't they just have breast reconstruction with their own natural tissues?

Many women want an operation that can be done either as an outpatient procedure or with minimal down time, expense, and inconvenience. For them, implant and expander reconstruction is the best choice because it affords the convenience, short recovery period, and reduced cost they desire. This is also the procedure of choice for a woman who does not want any additional scars, a necessary consequence of most flap procedures. Implant surgery is a good choice for a slender woman who may not have enough fatty tissue for a flap procedure or for a woman with a medical condition that places her at increased risk if she has a more complex operation such as a TRAM (abdominal) flap, latissimus dorsi (back) flap, or a free flap. Furthermore, many surgeons experienced in breast reconstruction techniques with implants and expanders prefer these operations for most patients over the more involved flap procedures.

What are the physical benefits of implant surgery?

Implants can be used to correct breast or chest wall asymmetries associated with developmental conditions or trauma. They are also used for breast reconstruction after mastectomy. Many women who have had mastectomies report that the implant helps restore a feeling of balance. For women with a large opposite breast, it may also alleviate back and shoulder pain and postural problems caused by attempts to disguise the uneven chest with a heavy external prosthesis. The implant can provide cover for the exposed chest wall, which may be sensitive after breast removal. It can also be used to replace an external prosthesis, thereby affording a woman greater freedom in selecting clothing styles and avoiding the discomfort and skin irritation that sometime accompany use of an external breast prosthesis.

What types of breast implants are currently available and what shapes do they come in?

Basically, there are two broad categories of implants: fixed-volume breast implants and implants in which the volume can be changed after they are implanted (tissue expanders). All of the currently available implants have an outer layer or envelope of silicone that is in contact with the body tissues. This envelope is available in a smooth or textured surface. The textured surface results in a thicker implant wall. In some patients these textured-surface implants are more visible and may exhibit a rippled appearance through the skin.

Implant shapes are described in terms of projection or profile (low, high, and medium) and overall design: round versus anatomic or shaped.

What types of filling materials are used in implants? What are the "gummy bear" implants?

Implants are filled with saline (saltwater) or with silicone gel. Gel-filled devices may contain the original, more fluid silicone gel or the newer more solid, heavily vulcanized, cohesive silicone gel, which has the consistency of Jell-O; hence their nickname of "gummy-bear" implants. These cohesive gel-filled implants have a somewhat firmer consistency than their older counterparts. (See Chapter 13 for more information on implants and expanders.)

How do the aesthetic results of operations with saline-filled implants compare to those achieved with silicone gel–filled implants?

Certain characteristics of silicone gel–filled breast implants make them preferable to saline-filled implants. The gel has a more natural consistency than saltwater and feels and flows more like a natural breast. These implants also offer flexibility in designing different breast shapes—some wider, some with additional projection to allow for individualization. Saline-filled implants are more limited in their shape; they are also slightly heavier than silicone gel–filled implants and when overfilled are firm, almost spherical, and therefore feel and look unnatural. When underfilled they can be soft, and their envelopes, which are generally thicker than those containing silicone gel, can develop noticeable and palpable folds and ripples, particularly through thin skin at the mastectomy site. Some of the newer models of saline implants have "shaped" contours that seem to help improve the shape of the reconstructed breast. The newer generation of cohesive gel implants comes in a wide range of profiles and shapes to optimize the choices available for a given patient. These may vary from almost round devices to strongly tear-drop shaped implants.

Is silicone safe to use in humans?

Silicone, a commonly used substance for various implantable devices, is considered by many to be one of the least reactive biomaterials. Initially introduced for evaluation in medical applications in the 1940s, silicone is used for artificial joints, implantable pumps, shunts, drains, ocular implants, and other devices that require a material that is relatively nonreactive, non-allergenic, and easily tolerated by the body. Implantable silicone devices include pacemakers, hydrocephalus shunts, breast implants, penile implants, and testicular implants. Anyone who has ever taken a capsule medication has probably ingested silicone, because it is used to coat many capsules so they can be swallowed more easily. Silicone is also present in processed foods, in cosmetics, and in many drugs (especially antacids). Silicone is used to lubricate syringes, in intravenous tubing, and in shunts used for chemotherapy. Anyone who has had blood drawn or been given an injection has had some silicone introduced into his or her body. Many infant pacifiers are made of silicone. As Dr. James Potchen, a radiologist at the University of Michigan explains, "Some systemic levels of silicone will be found in every patient with an implant. The fact is that a very low level of silicone is present in everyone." If silicone represents a serious chemical hazard to the human body, this should already be apparent because of this chemical's widespread use. The fact is, it doesn't. Nevertheless, studies continue to rule out the possibility of currently unrecognized and rare problems. New silicone devices are regularly receiving FDA approval.

What problems are associated with implants, and how often do they occur?

As with all devices, implants are not without problems. They are subject to local complications such as rupture, possible leakage, deflation, displacement, deformation, and capsular contracture, the latter being the most common problem. They also may interfere with mammograms and cause calcium deposits to accumulate in the capsule tissue that forms around implants. Breast implant surgery may cause changes in breast and nipple sensation. These problems are not life threatening, however, and are usually correctable.

What is capsular contracture? Does this pose a serious risk for women who have implant surgery?

A capsule is firm, fibrous scar tissue that forms around a breast implant. This is a characteristic response of the body to isolate any foreign substance; similar scar formation can be observed around most other implants, regardless of whether they contain silicone, including hip implants, artificial joints, hydrocephalus shunts, heart valves, and pacemakers. For unknown reasons, in some cases, the scar tissue capsule may become thick and constrict a soft implant. This phenomenon is referred to as capsular contracture. This condition can make the breast feel harder and firmer than desirable, producing a rounded or spherical breast appearance; sometimes it can also cause pain. The severity of this problem varies with each individual. Ideally, the capsular layer surrounding the implant does not contract and affect the shape of the breast. In some women it manifests itself as a slight breast firmness. Mild contracture requires no treatment. Most women find this minimal firmness acceptable and are not motivated to undergo further adjustments of their reconstructed or augmented breasts.

In more severe cases of capsular contracture, however, a woman may experience significant discomfort and elect to have a procedure to improve this situation. Today, fat grafting is a newer method for improving capsular contracture deformities and softening the breast appearance. Operative solutions focus on releasing some or all of the scar tissue (capsulotomy) or removing it (capsulectomy). During this secondary operation the surgeon may reposition the implant under the pectoralis major muscle if previously placed over the muscle or he may replace it with a textured-surface implant after releasing or removing the capsule. It is usually necessary to remove the scar capsule around the smooth implant before replacing it with the textured-surface implant.

Patients who continue to experience problems after surgical correction may decide to have their implants removed. After implant removal an aesthetic correction such as a breast lift may be necessary to achieve an optimal breast appearance. A woman should be informed of this possibility. Some women with firm breasts decide to have the implant and scar tissue removed and replaced or covered with fatty and muscle flap tissue from the back, lower abdomen, thigh, or buttocks.

Although capsular contracture may be uncomfortable and produce breast distortion and asymmetry, it is not a health hazard. It does not threaten a woman's life or health, and most women who experience this problem can have satisfactory surgical correction. (See Chapter 13 for a more detailed discussion of potential complications associated with these devices.)

How do the risks associated with saline-filled implants compare to those associated with silicone gel–filled implants?

Shrinkage of the scar tissue (capsular contracture) and calcium deposit formation occur with both saline-filled and silicone gel–filled implants. Deflation of the implant may be more likely with the saline-filled type and occurs with an incidence of about 2% per annum on average. When a saline-filled implant develops a leak, it is likely to deflate over a period of hours to days or even weeks, requiring surgical replacement within a month or two or when the implant has lost most of its volume and become flat. Some saline-filled implants will deflate spontaneously, losing all the saline solution at once and requiring reoperation for implant replacement.

Does a woman who has an implant breast reconstruction still need to have mammograms?

Mammograms are usually not necessary after a mastectomy and breast reconstruction. However, if an implant is placed in the opposite breast for symmetry or balance, this breast still needs to be monitored. Women should inform the breast imager that they have a breast implant or expander so that additional displacement views can be taken to help visualize the extent of the breast tissue.

If a woman has implants, what is the proper way to examine her breasts?

Like all women, those with breast implants should perform regular breast self-examination (BSE) and have regular physician examinations. These examinations take on added significance for women with breast implants because they can also help to reveal any problems that may develop with their implants. Women with implants should become fully acquainted with the feel of the implants under their breast skin so that they do not confuse any implant ripples or folds with a breast mass.

Can implants slip, shift, or become displaced?

During the initial operation the plastic surgeon places the implant in the best position to provide the desired breast appearance. During the process of healing, with the development of capsular contracture, and over time the implants can shift or become displaced. This can occur because of the pull of gravity on a smooth implant or subsequent to a capsular contracture, which can elevate the implant. This problem may occur less frequently when a textured breast implant has been used because the rough surface usually adheres to the surrounding tissue, thereby minimizing the chance of displacement.

Can the implant be rejected by a woman's body?

Rejection means an allergic or immune response that causes the body to literally reject a foreign substance. In this sense implants are not rejected. However, the overlying breast skin may become thinned, infection can develop, or healing may be incomplete, leading to exposure and necessitating removal of the implant. Although these are complications, they are not tantamount to rejection.

Can an implant be removed?

Yes. When an implant is not performing the function for which it was intended, or if the woman feels that she would be better off without the implant, it can be removed. In most cases this is a relatively minor operation that can often be performed on an outpatient basis. She should ask her plastic surgeon if the capsule should also be removed. The procedure for capsule removal is called capsulectomy. The patient should decide, in consultation with the plastic surgeon, if additional aesthetic corrections will be necessary after removal.

How long do breast implants last?

The silicone breast implant has been available for use in patients since 1964, and many of the original devices are still in place. Just as human and artificial organs can fail and require transplantation, breast implants also may have to be replaced. These are manmade devices and will eventually fail. No precise figures on the life span of silicone gel–filled or saline-filled implants are available at present. It is known that implants can last from a very short time to many years, depending on the surgical technique used, the patient, and her implant. The average lifespan of implants appears to be between 10 and 20 years after insertion. In any case, breast implants should not be considered "lifetime" devices. Women should be followed up by their physicians over the long term so their breasts can be monitored for possible problems as a part of their general health care regimen.

How strong are implants? Will they break on impact? Can they be broken during mammography?

Breast implants are manufactured to specific standards requiring that they resist breast compression as well as multiple and long-term physical stress. These devices, however, are not indestructible. Although the outer shell of the implant is quite sturdy, it can break if subjected to severe physical trauma. A sharp or blunt injury to the chest wall and breast, such as pressure from a seat belt during a car accident, can cause this problem. Compression views taken during mammography are calibrated to avoid undue pressure that could rupture a breast implant.

What factors increase the chance that an implant will rupture?

The chance for rupture may increase with the length of time the implant has been in the body and with normal wear and tear. The incidence of rupture is increased when the implant develops folds or rippling on the outer surface. Trauma or injury to the breast also increases the chance of rupture.

What happens if a saline-filled implant deflates?

There is a possibility of deflation with saline-filled implants if a leak develops in the implant covering and will require possible reoperation with implant replacement. Currently available saline-filled inflatable implants have a relatively low deflation rate.

What happens if a silicone gel–filled implant leaks?

When the cover of a silicone gel–filled implant is pierced or ruptures, the gel usually remains within the fibrous capsule or membrane that develops naturally around the implant and does not travel to other parts of the body. Significant trauma can cause tears in the surrounding capsule, and the gel can migrate into the breast and possibly beyond the breast to form lumps (granulomas) nearby. Some of this silicone can cause enlarged lymph nodes in the armpit area (lymphadenopathy). When silicone escapes to other parts of the body, such as the arm or upper abdomen, removal can be difficult. Gel migration outside the capsule rarely occurs, however, and, if it does, the viscosity (or thickness) of the gel seems to reduce its ability to migrate. There appears to be even less potential for migration with the "gummy bear" (cohesive gel) implants, which have an even thicker consistency.

How can a woman tell if she has a ruptured or deflated implant?

Any noticeable change in the shape, size, feel, or comfort of the breast could signal implant rupture. For women with saline-filled implants, this change in breast size and shape is often more noticeable when leakage and absorption of the saltwater solution by the surrounding tissues causes implant deflation. When such symptoms occur, a patient should see her plastic surgeon for evaluation.

Can breast implants cause cancer?

Breast implants have been available for more than 40 years and during that time have been studied extensively by plastic surgeons, implant manufacturers, scientists, and government regulatory agencies such as the FDA. In all of that time no scientific studies have documented an increased risk of breast cancer attributable to breast implants nor is there any evidence that these devices have adversely affected the course of breast cancer when they are used for breast reconstruction. The FDA's current informed consent document serves to underscore these findings. It states, "There is presently no scientific evidence that links either silicone gel–filled or saline-filled breast implants with cancer." Research from cancer experts and institutions throughout the world indicates a general consensus that breast implants do not increase a woman's risk of developing breast cancer.

There are some data to indicate a potential benefit associated with breast implants in cancer detection. It indicates that women with breast implants tend to detect breast cancers presenting as breast lumps earlier than their non-augmented counterparts. This may be due to the fact that implants stretch the breast tissue over the underlying device making it easier to feel a mass. Data also indicates that women who develop breast cancers with a background of having had implants have identical survival outcomes to their non-augmented counterparts in the general population.

What are connective tissue disorders? Is there any scientific evidence to show that implants cause autoimmune or connective tissue diseases?

These are rare disorders, such as lupus erythematosus, dermatomyositis, scleroderma, and rheumatoid arthritis, in which the body reacts to its own tissue as though it were a foreign material. A combination of symptoms may characterize these disorders, including the generalized symptoms of joint pain and swelling; tight, red, or swollen skin; swollen glands and lymph nodes; extreme fatigue; local symptoms of swelling of the hands and feet; skin rashes; and unusual hair loss.

The FDA advises a woman who experiences these symptoms to "see her regular doctor if the symptoms do not subside, because these complaints could be indicators of a variety of health problems, not just immune-related disorders." After studying the information about silicone gel–filled breast implants provided by its consultants, the FDA has stated that there is no evidence that implants cause autoimmune or connective tissue diseases.

Should women diagnosed with connective tissue diseases or autoimmune diseases have reconstruction with breast implants?

These diseases are rare, and scientific studies are under way to define and better understand these conditions. As a precaution, however, if a woman has any of these conditions or has a family history of these conditions, she should probably not have breast implant surgery. As Dr. John Sergent, a noted rheumatologist explains, "My recommendation for patients with scleroderma is to minimize trauma of any kind and avoid all elective surgery, not just implants." Women with these problems are also poor candidates for radiation therapy and musculocutaneous flaps.

Is it possible to be allergic to silicone implants or to the silicone gel within them?

As mentioned earlier, silicone has been used in medical devices and oral and parenteral medications for more than 40 years, and there is no scientific evidence that individuals can develop allergies to these devices. It may be possible, however, to develop antibodies to the element, silicon; there is no good test for antibodies to silicone, which is derived from silicon. The mere presence of antibodies, however, does not indicate the presence of disease. The body's normal process of dealing with foreign bodies is an immune response with subsequent development of antibodies. Further studies will need to be conducted to determine if there are actually any allergic reactions.

What possible complications can occur with implant surgery?

As with any surgical procedure, there is the potential for complications, including reactions to anesthesia as well as infection, hematoma, bleeding, seroma, and delayed wound healing with possible implant exposure requiring removal. There are no reports in the medical literature of breast implants being responsible for a single death. There is an inherent risk of serious complications and even death from any operation, but this is usually related to the risk of anesthesia for a period of time. This risk is somewhat higher for longer operations, particularly if the operation lasts for more than 4 hours. However, the risk is still considered very small.

How does the incidence of complications from implant surgery compare to the incidence of complications from other common operations such as appendectomies, mastectomies, and hysterectomies?

The rate of complications experienced after breast implantation is comparable to and sometimes lower than the rate of complications from other commonly performed operations. Patients having breast implant surgery generally have a lower incidence of conditions such as infection, hematoma, pulmonary emboli, and deep vein thrombosis. However, reoperation because of capsular contracture or to achieve a better final breast appearance is necessary in a number of cases.

What is the FDA's role in testing and evaluating implants and expanders?

The FDA has been charged with regulating all medical devices since 1976 and is involved in an ongoing evaluation of the safety and efficacy of breast implants. The FDA designates these devices as class III, which means that they must have premarket approval of their safety and efficacy.

If a woman wants to have breast implants for reconstruction, what should she do to make certain they are covered by insurance?

Most insurance companies do not cover "cosmetic" surgery; however, they do reimburse breast cancer patients for the costs of breast reconstruction after mastectomy, including the cost of breast implants. As a precaution, it is best to contact your insurance company before any anticipated operation. Your physician can often provide essential information to give to the insurance company related to the specific medical diagnosis, the specifics of the procedure, and the computer code numbers necessary for predetermination of coverage and an explanation of your benefits under the policy. In addition, the FDA advises women to get written answers from their insurance company to the following questions:

- Does my policy cover the costs of the implant surgery, the implant, the anesthesia, and other related hospital costs?
- Does it cover treatments for medical problems that may be caused by either the implant or the reconstruction?
- Does it cover removal of the implants if this becomes necessary?

AUTOLOGOUS FLAP BREAST RECONSTRUCTION

What options does a woman have if she wants to have her breast reconstructed with her own natural tissue without the need for breast implants or expanders?

Reconstruction using flaps of the patient's own tissue (autologous breast reconstruction) is a viable and popular option for many women who wish to avoid breast implants but still have the most natural result possible. The consistency and feel of the reconstructed breast closely resemble a normal breast; this reconstructed breast ages similar to the opposite breast because it is the woman's own tissue and therefore is most likely to provide lasting symmetry. In many cases the reconstructed breast actually appears more natural over time. Sources of donor tissue are areas of excess tissue such as the lower abdomen, the back, the hips, the inner thigh, or the buttocks. The donor scar can also be hidden so that a significant deformity is not created. Many women who have gained some weight over the years find this an excellent opportunity to accomplish two goals at one time: rebuilding a full and natural breast while contouring an area of abundant fatty tissue, usually in the lower abdomen. Most women have also noted some return of sensation to their breasts after they are rebuilt with their own tissue. The chance of sensory return is increased with the newer techniques that use shorter incisions and skin sparing at the time of the mastectomy.

It is also possible for a woman to have her breast rebuilt using fat injections following external expansion of the breast tissues at the mastectomy or lumpectomy site. This approach avoids a major flap operation and still has the benefit of using the woman's own fatty tissue. This is a new procedure that is still considered investigational. It is appropriate for small breasted women who are willing to undergo a somewhat tedious expansion regimen that involves wearing an external expansion device prior to the fat injections. The technique requires repeated large volume fat injections; some degree of fat graft loss is unavoidable after this procedure.

When breasts are reconstructed with the patient's own tissue, breast implants are usually not necessary. One of the prime reasons that many women choose this approach is to avoid the insertion of a foreign material in the body. If a woman is very slender and lacks the excess fatty tissue necessary to build a breast without the need for a supplementary implant, particularly if she needs to have both of her breasts reconstructed (bilateral breast reconstruction), she may want to consider selecting a procedure involving implant or expander placement. (Autologous breast reconstruction techniques are discussed in detail in Chapter 13.)

What is the TRAM flap? Is it the same as a "tummy tuck"?

The TRAM (transverse rectus abdominis musculocutaneous) flap is a method of breast reconstruction in which a woman's lower abdominal tissue is transferred to the breast region and reshaped to form a breast that is symmetric with her opposite breast. When this transverse ellipse of tissue is moved from the lower abdomen to the breast region, the blood supply is maintained because the tissue is left attached to strips or "pedicles" of the central abdominal muscle. The name "TRAM flap" is derived in part from the muscle to which it is attached—the rectus abdominis muscle. This operation is often referred to as the "tummy tuck" procedure because the abdominal portion of the procedure in which the donor tissue is taken from the woman's abdomen is similar to the "tummy tuck" operation (abdominoplasty) to improve lower abdominal contour. In both procedures the excess lower abdominal tissue is removed, the abdominal area is closed and tightened, and the resulting scar extends across the lower abdomen.

How are microsurgical techniques used for breast reconstruction?

Microsurgical procedures are performed while visualizing the operative field through the magnification of an operating microscope, thereby permitting the repair and suture of tiny vessels and nerves. Microsurgical techniques are particularly helpful when tissue needs to be moved from a distant part of the body to an area to be reconstructed. These operations are called "free flaps" because the tissue is freed completely and separated from the donor area, moved to the reconstructive area, and the blood supply is reattached under the operating microscope. Donor sites for breast free flaps include the abdomen, buttocks, hip, upper inner thigh, and back.

What are perforator flaps and how are they used for breast reconstruction?

A perforator flap is a flap composed of skin and fat that is based on a single set of blood vessels (the perforator vessels) that pass through the underlying muscle. For breast reconstruction, these flaps are taken from the patient's abdomen (DIEP and SIEA flaps) or buttocks (IGAP or SGAP flaps). Unlike conventional pedicle and microsurgical flap techniques (like the TRAM flap), perforator flap techniques preserve the patient's underlying musculature. The tissue is then transferred to the patient's chest, reconnected using microsurgery and shaped to create the new breast.

What is the DIEP perforator flap and what are its advantages?

The DIEP (deep inferior epigastric perforator) flap is a variation of a free TRAM (abdominal flap) described earlier except that **all the abdominal muscle is preserved.** Only abdominal skin and fat are removed, similar to a "tummy tuck."

What is a muscle-sparing free TRAM flap?

A muscle-sparing free TRAM flap is a hybrid of the DIEP flap and the free TRAM flap. With this procedure a small but relatively insignificant piece of muscle is taken with the flap, permitting more perforators to be incorporated in the flap.

What autologous flaps are the most popular for breast reconstruction?

The most commonly used tissue is the lower abdominal skin and fat attached to the rectus abdominis muscle in the form of the TRAM flap. This flap may be left attached above (pedicled) or detached and reattached using microsurgery (free TRAM flap or DIEP flap). The TRAM flap incorporates varying amounts of muscle from the belly. A pedicled TRAM uses the entire rectus abdominis muscle. A free TRAM flap uses about 10% of the muscle surface area, whereas a DIEP flap or perforator flap uses no muscle. Theoretically, the perforator flap option provides for the strongest abdominal wall after surgery. In practice, patients who have had any of these three abdominal surgical options tend to return to normal activities of daily living over a period of 3 to 6 months. The other procedure that has seen a resurgence of interest in recent years is the latissimus dorsi (back) flap. If there is enough fat overlying this muscle on the back, an autologous reconstruction may be achieved without the necessity of inserting an implant to provide breast fill. If the patient is thin, an implant may need to be added for volume correction. Upper arm power loss is negligible with this procedure.

Can a woman's breast be reconstructed with injections of her own fatty tissue?

It is now possible to combine external breast expansion with serial autologous fat injections of the woman's own fatty tissue that has been suctioned from areas of excess in her hips, abdomen, or buttocks. This approach is only appropriate for women whose breasts are small. This is a less invasive approach than a flap of the woman's own tissue, but it requires a patient who is compliant and willing to wear a somewhat cumbersome external, bra-like expansion device for a number of weeks (10 hours a day) while her tissues are stretched sufficiently to accept a series of fat grafts for rebuilding her breast. This approach may not be appropriate for women with large breasts or for those who have irradiated tissues, which are firmer, tighter, and less compliant or subject to mechanical stretching.

Does chest wall irradiation affect the success of breast recon-struction? Which techniques work best after radiation therapy?

Radiation therapy is designed to destroy cancer cells. Unfortunately the high energy of the radiation beam also damages normal tissue, re-ducing the blood supply to the chest wall skin and muscle as well as damaging skin, and reducing its elasticity and healing potential. Lymphedema is also increased on the chest wall as well as in the arm. After radiation therapy to the chest wall, breast reconstruction with tissue expansion is often not as successful because the skin may be damaged and less resilient; this means that the potential for com-plications is greater. Radiation can also affect the success of a breast implant or flap reconstruction by causing fibrosis (or thickening), capsular contracture, and breast firmness. Therefore, if radiation is anticipated, breast reconstruction may be delayed until after this treat-ment is completed, or an expander may be placed and slightly ex-panded immediately after her cancer surgery to stretch the tissues before radiation therapy. The best and least complicated breast re-constructions after radiation are done with autologous tissue—the TRAM, DIEP, or SIEA (abdominal) flaps, latissimus dorsi (back) flap, or gluteus maximus, IGAP, or SGAP (buttock) flaps.

What is the role of fat grafting in improving breast appearance after radiation therapy?

Fat grafting using the patient's own fat, is a relatively new approach to treating the damage incurred by radiation. It has been found that in-jecting autologous fat in small quantities under the irradiated skin causes improvements in skin quality, elasticity, and blood supply, even to the point of potentially healing chronic wounds over time. There are instances in which preconditioning of the skin with fat injections (done on an outpatient basis) may render previously tight, inelastic skin amenable to successful tissue expansion. This field is in its in-fancy, but initial results are very encouraging.

How will a woman's breasts look over the long term, say 5 or 10 years after reconstruction? Which type of breast reconstruction produces the most aesthetic long-term results?

Although it is impossible to predict with certainty how results will look in 5 to 10 years, generally some degree of capsular contracture will form after implant or expander reconstruction with each passing year. This usually results in some breast asymmetry as the recon-structed breast becomes elevated with time and the natural opposite breast droops subsequent to the aging process. With autologous reconstructions using flaps of the patient's own tissue, the result is more lasting and the breasts are more likely to age in a similar manner.

How does aging or weight loss affect the results of breast reconstruction?

Every woman's breasts age differently. Generally, however, there is gradual settling and lowering of the breast with time. Breast size also changes with aging; these changes are influenced by weight loss or gain, body fat content, and hormonal changes. When a woman's breast has been rebuilt with her own tissues, it tends to age more like her natural breast ages, with better long-term symmetry. This symmetry is not as predictable over the long term with implant reconstruction.

What is the long-term appearance of a rebuilt nipple? Does it keep its projection?

If possible, the nipple built from a flap of chest wall skin is usually made longer than the remaining nipple to counter the tendency of nipple reconstructions to become shorter and flatter over time. When the nipple is built over a flap reconstruction, there is often more tissue available than when it is built over thin, expanded skin. Most of these chest wall flap nipple reconstructions can be expected to lose about one half of their initial projection over time. When built with a graft from the other nipple, symmetry is usually easier to maintain.

Can another person tell if a woman has had breast reconstruction?

A woman who has had breast reconstruction can dress normally without anyone realizing that her breast has been rebuilt. Unless she is naked, her scars will not be noticeable to anyone. (The newer skin-sparing techniques minimize the scars from reconstruction.) When she is clothed, her breasts will appear the same as any other woman's.

How do the results of breast reconstruction compare with a woman's expectations? Do her breasts look and feel normal?

It is important for a woman to carefully define her expectations before she has this operation to make sure that the plastic surgeon knows what she wants and can tell her if it is possible. She also needs to understand the limitations of the operation. Breast reconstruction can fill in and rebuild the deformities resulting from mastectomy. A woman may be disappointed, however, if she expects her new breast to be the same as the one it is meant to replace. Her new breast with an implant will often be cooler, firmer, and more rounded than her remaining one. The shape may be more natural with a shaped anatomic implant. It will not move as naturally with changes in position or posture. Firmness is often associated with the use of implants.

When the skin and overlying tissue cover is thin or irradiated, any irregularities or ripples in the breast implant can show through the skin. This rippling can give an unattractive contour to the reconstructed breast. In addition, the lower portion of the breast implant can sometimes be felt through the breast skin; this is not bothersome to most women and is considered a natural accompaniment of breast reconstruction with implants. (See next question.) A more normal breast "feel" and flow may be obtained by using the patient's own tissue from the lower abdomen, back, or buttocks or with the use of fat grafting.

What are acellular dermal matrices? How are these used to camouflage implant or expander irregularities or rippling?

As mentioned earlier, one of the problems associated with expander or implant insertion is the fact that the lower half of these devices is only covered with skin, while muscle covers the upper half. This allows the implant to be easily felt under the skin, showing ripples and wrinkles if they occur. In addition, the risk of capsular contracture tightening around the expander or implant is higher after reconstruction than after cosmetic breast augmentation. In an effort to solve some of these problems, surgeons now use acellular dermal matrices (such as AlloDerm, Strattice, and FlexHD) to cover the lower half of these devices. These matrices are sheets of human or pig skin that have had their cells removed, leaving a framework of collagen and elastin for support and implant cover. The body's tissues gradually grow into these materials, ultimately replacing them with the patient's own collagen and blood vessels. Thus this can be thought of as a method for new tissue regeneration. These materials have a long track record of safety and provide good camouflage for the lower half of the implant. In addition, preliminary evidence seems to suggest that they may contribute to a reduction in capsular contracture. These materials have been valuable in helping improve the results of breast reconstruction with expanders and implants.

In what ways will a woman's rebuilt breast differ from her original breast?

It will be less mobile and have less sensation. It cannot produce milk. There are scars from the mastectomy and reconstruction. Furthermore, the nipple-areola does not totally match the other natural one and does not respond to stimuli.

What are the chances of achieving breast symmetry?

The chances for acceptable breast symmetry are good. Each reconstruction must be individualized. Preoperatively the surgeon must determine if symmetry can be achieved with or without modification of the other breast. Bilateral reconstructions are often the most symmetrical.

How is fat injection used to improve symmetry?

Fat injection using the patient's own body fat can be used to improve symmetry and fill minor contour defects. Fat is suctioned from the hips, abdomen, or buttocks using a liposuction device, then the fat is spun in a centrifuge to remove impurities. Next the strained fat is loaded into small syringes attached to fine, blunt-tipped needles for injection. Tiny quantities of fat are injected at multiple levels throughout an area of hollowing, for example, to fill the defect. Some of the fat will dissolve, but much of it survives to become a permanent part of the patient's breast shape. The procedure is simple, safe, and effective and is usually covered by insurance.

Will the reconstructed breast have projection?

The reconstructed breast often has a similar projection to the opposite normal breast. However, reconstructed breasts can be flatter and thus have less projection than natural breasts. Occasionally an implant is used to optimize projection after a flap reconstruction. Sometimes, when an implant breast reconstruction develops capsular contracture, the breast becomes rounder and firmer and the projection can actually increase.

Is the reconstructed breast sensitive to touch and to sexual stimulation?

Because sensation or feeling in the chest wall area is lost during the mastectomy, the reconstructed breast can feel numb or at least have less sensation than the normal side. The skin-sparing mastectomy tends to result in more residual sensitivity to touch. The underarm may also be numb and feel strange to the touch. Some women say that shaving their underarms becomes a rather unpleasant, uncomfortable experience. The underside of the upper arm is usually also numb; however, surgeons often attempt to preserve the sensation to this area. Sometimes, as some of these nerves grow back after the mastectomy, the woman may notice some radiating, "shooting," or "tingling" pains in the area where these nerves are located, particularly in her underarm or breast area.

This lack of sensation is more common when an implant has been used for breast reconstruction. Many of the women whose breasts are reconstructed with their own tissue (autologous tissue) from the lower abdomen will develop some sensation to touch in the region of their reconstructed breasts. Their chances for developing additional breast sensation are further enhanced when the reconstruction with autologous tissue is performed immediately after a skin-sparing mastectomy. The patient can maximize return of sensation by reeducating the involved area of numbness with daily massage. The special, pleasant sensation associated with the nipple-areola area with its responsiveness to sexual stimulation is usually lost and does not return.

If a woman has breast reconstruction with implants, will her breast be warm like a normal breast?

Usually the temperature of a reconstructed breast is determined by the thickness of the skin cover and adequacy of the blood supply. When the cover is thin and the ambient air is cold, a cooler temperature of the implant will be noticeable and the breast can feel cold. Flap reconstructions usually are not affected in this manner because they are nourished and warmed by their own blood supply.

Will there be nerve loss?

No additional nerve loss is to be expected after breast reconstruction with implants. With a TRAM flap reconstruction, the area just above the abdominal wall donor site scar is usually numb for a few months. With a latissimus dorsi flap, it is below the back incision; and with a gluteus maximus flap, down the back of the leg.

What is the expected hospitalization for the different reconstructive procedures?

The usual hospital stay for simple implant placement or tissue expansion is 1 to 2 days, although many women can have these operations as outpatient procedures. For the pedicled latissimus dorsi (back) flap, hospitalization is 2 to 3 days; for the pedicled TRAM (lower abdominal) flap, 3 to 6 days; for a microsurgical TRAM flap, 3 to 5 days; for DIEP or SIEA abdominal perforator flaps, 3 to 5 days; and for IGAP or SGAP buttock perforator flaps, 5 to 6 days.

What is the anticipated pain and recovery time?

After breast reconstruction a woman will experience pain in her chest area as well as in any donor sites where additional tissue was taken to build her new breast. The degree of pain and length of the recuperative period will vary with the individual patient, the extent of her defect, and the operative procedure chosen. The postoperative pain comes from the effects of the cut nerves in the breast region. As these nerves grow back, they can often be reeducated by massage of the skin a few weeks after the operation. (Specific information on these matters is provided in Chapter 13.)

An advance in pain control after an operation, the patient-controlled analgesia (PCA) unit, is now available to alleviate some of the patient's pain and discomfort during her hospital stay. It is safe, provides excellent pain relief, and the patient is in control. The PCA unit is connected to the patient's intravenous tubing, the proper pain-relieving drug and dosage are determined, and the machine is set so that the patient can press a button and administer the pain-relieving medication as she needs it. With this device, the pain medication can also be given much more often than when a nurse administers shots to the patient. In 2 to 3 days the patient's pain is usually controlled with analgesics taken by mouth.

Some women do not handle pain medication well, even the relatively small doses delivered by the PCA. A potentially distressing side effect for these women is nausea and vomiting from the effects of the anesthesia and the medication given immediately after surgery. This can be alleviated by reducing the dosage of the pain relief medication to the absolute minimum that the patient needs and can tolerate, or by changing the medication. A patient who does not tolerate medication well should alert the anesthesiologist and surgeon of this problem preoperatively so that some accommodation can be made to avoid nausea following the operation. Alternatively, an epidural spinal catheter can be inserted to administer medication to control pain.

More recently, the use of continuous low-dose local anesthetic infusion into the operative site (ON-Q and Stryker pain pumps, for example) has provided dramatic pain relief to many patients. These pain pumps represent a new generation of pain-control devices that infuse small quantities of long-acting local anesthetic into the wound sites on a continuous basis over 3 to 4 days. The pumps are composed of a central reservoir containing local anesthetic that slowly empties into the wound through very fine epidural-like catheters inserted through the skin. The benefit of these devices is their ability to control pain quite well without heavy narcotic use, reducing the unwanted side effects of morphine-like drugs. They allow the patient to ambulate early with minimal discomfort.

Is it painful when the tissue expander is inflated? What does expansion feel like?

Most women describe a "full, tight feeling" during tissue expansion. For a minority of patients, expansion can be painful. To relieve the discomfort for these individuals the expansion process is paced more slowly, which means more frequent visits and lower volume expansion. In some cases some of the saline solution may even be removed temporarily until the patient feels more comfortable. When expansion is begun soon after the mastectomy, there is less pain because the nerves have not grown back yet. Expansion is usually begun at least 3 weeks after surgery in order to allow time for the mastectomy skin flaps to heal well over the underlying expander.

What after-effects and adjustments should a woman expect after breast reconstruction?

Following breast reconstruction a woman's breast may be swollen and bruised. These are expected and natural responses to healing and the patient should not be alarmed; the swelling will subside in a few days and the bruising will fade and disappear over a period of weeks, leaving her breast with a far more acceptable appearance. Her breast may also appear smaller or larger than expected and may not be completely symmetric with the opposite breast. Some asymmetries will lessen with time. If they persist, the breast usually can be adjusted a few months later during a second procedure and at the time of the nipple-areola reconstruction.

When an expander is used, the reconstructed breast will look smaller and flatter at first. It will become enlarged after several postoperative visits as additional saline solution is added to the expander.

If muscles are used for reconstruction, how will it affect movement and physical strength in the future?

The muscles and portions of muscles used for breast reconstruction are considered functionally expendable; other muscle groups usually take over when one of these muscles has been transferred. Therefore muscle flap reconstructions normally do not impose significant functional restrictions on a woman after the healing period is over. A postoperative exercise program can contribute to rebuilding strength. Practically all patients can expect to return to their normal preoperative activities after the healing process. Perforator flaps have the least impact on muscle function.

What limitations or weaknesses does a woman experience after a musculocutaneous flap reconstruction?

Most of the activities of daily living, including sports activities, are not affected by breast reconstruction with a muscle or muscle and skin flap. However, a woman's ability to perform sit-ups may be somewhat reduced after a TRAM flap. This problem can be more noticeable if both rectus abdominis muscles (bipedicle or bilateral) are used. Some activities that rely heavily on upper extremity strength, such as cross-country skiing, may also be more difficult after a latissimus dorsi flap procedure. Perforator flaps impose the least impact on these functions but are not suitable for all patients.

Will a woman have full use of her arm after breast reconstruction?

Breast reconstruction will not impose any permanent restrictions on arm mobility or strength. Because some free flap breast reconstructions and the latissimus dorsi flap require surgery in the arm area, a woman will be instructed to limit arm activity for a few weeks after surgery to avoid complications. Most women regain full upper arm mobility and physical therapy is rarely required postoperatively.

If a muscle is used for reconstruction, will it still function when it has been transferred?

When the latissimus dorsi back muscle is used, some patients notice that certain movements of the arm cause the transferred muscle to contract, thereby causing the reconstructed breast to move (the so-called dancing breast phenomenon). This can be disconcerting. If this proves a major problem for a woman, it can be remedied during a later procedure that divides the nerve to the muscle. Many surgeons deliberately cut the nerve to the latissimus dorsi muscle during the operation to limit unwanted muscle activity after surgery. The muscles moved from the abdomen are usually not functional after they are moved, because their motor nerves are routinely divided.

When can a woman resume an exercise program after breast reconstruction? Will any activities be permanently restricted?

Although each patient recovers at a different rate, most women who have implant reconstruction can resume normal upper extremity activity after 3 to 4 weeks. After a flap procedure, activity can be resumed in 6 to 8 weeks.

Do women experience any depression after this operation?

Many women go through a limited but normal period of depression after breast reconstruction. The operation, general anesthesia, postoperative pain, and medications may combine to produce these feelings. Because this operation represents a major step for a woman, there is an emotional buildup to prepare for it as well as heightened expectations for a lovely result. Therefore a woman may feel a letdown once the operation is over because the postoperative appearance will not reflect the final result. Instead, her breast may look bruised and possibly flat, far removed from the result she expected. This depression usually subsides in a few days as the patient recovers and the appearance of her breast improves.

What are possible complications from breast reconstruction? When do they occur, and why?

Complications of breast reconstruction appear either immediately after the operation or develop later. The type and degree of complications relate to the method of reconstruction used.

When an implant or expander is used to reconstruct the breast with existing tissues, a blood collection (hematoma) can develop around the implant; this problem usually requires drainage, often in the operating room. When the skin is thin or irradiated, actual exposure of the implant can occur because of the poor cover; the implant must be removed, the wound allowed to heal, and reconstruction restarted a few months later. Infection and delayed healing also may occur. The implant or expander can deflate. Capsular contracture is the most frequent late problem associated with implant and expander reconstruction.

Complications are also possible after flap reconstructions, particularly after the more complex microsurgical procedures. Hematoma may occur in both the site of the reconstruction and in the donor site. If the flap tissue that is moved does not have an adequate blood supply, a portion or occasionally the entire flap may be lost. With microsurgical reconstruction, sometimes the microanastomosis (where the blood vessels are connected) develops a blood clot and the patient may need to return to the operating room immediately for a second procedure to remove the clot and re-suture the blood vessels. (A more detailed discussion of the potential complications associated with the different breast reconstruction operations is included in Chapter 13.)

Is infection a serious problem after breast reconstruction?

Infection is an infrequent problem after breast reconstruction. It is more likely to occur after an immediate implant or expander reconstruction (a 2% to 10% chance). If infection occurs, the implant or expander usually must be removed to control the infection. Reconstruction can begin again a few months later. Infection after a flap procedure is very rare but if it occurs may result in partial flap loss, which would require revision of the flap during another procedure.

Do flaps used in breast reconstruction ever die or fail? If so, what can be done to complete the reconstruction?

Flaps are an essential component of some reconstructions. A flap is a portion of tissue that is moved from one area of the body to another. For the flap to be successful, transferred tissue must have a plentiful blood supply. If this blood supply is marginal or partially insufficient, a portion of the flap can die; this portion of the flap is therefore lost as a source of tissue for reconstruction.

Reconstruction usually can be completed after partial flap loss. Rarely is the blood supply to the flap so impaired that the entire flap is lost. Potential flap loss usually can be identified during the operation and appropriate measures taken by the surgeon to avoid this problem. Certain general health conditions can impair blood supply to flaps and result in flap loss; for instance, if a woman has diabetes, has received radiation to the flap vessels, has an autoimmune disease, or is a cigarette smoker, blood flow may be reduced. It is important to understand that once a flap is healed and viable, it will not die at a later stage; it remains stable.

What is a worst case scenario for each of the different reconstructive procedures?

Implants and expanders can become exposed and infected, requiring removal. In this instance reconstruction must begin again at a later date. The implant can be reinserted or a flap procedure may be needed. Flaps can fail because of partial or total loss of the blood supply. When a flap fails, another reconstructive technique, either a different flap or an implant procedure, usually will be necessary to complete the reconstruction. More serious complications such as deep vein thrombosis (blood clots in the leg veins or pelvic veins) and pulmonary embolus (blood clots to the lungs) can develop, usually after longer operations; these are rare occurrences, but they are life threatening.

Can a woman die from breast reconstruction?

The risks to life from breast reconstruction are very low. One obvious risk is from anesthetic complications; however, administration of anesthetics is safe in the hands of well-trained anesthesiologists. Reconstruction with implants is also safe. Flap reconstructions, especially with the lower abdominal flap and buttock flap, carry somewhat more risk because of the length of these operations and the risk of blood loss and the development of venous blood clots in the woman's legs. It is possible for these clots to go from the legs (deep vein thrombosis) to the blood vessels of the lungs (pulmonary embolus), a potentially life-threatening condition. The development of blood clots is linked to the length of the operative procedure; these clots are more likely to occur when the operation lasts more than 4 or 5 hours. The use of compression stockings enhances the blood flow and venous return from the legs during the procedure and in the postoperative period and thus decreases the possibility that this problem will develop. Portable compression devices for home use can also be incorporated into patient care if deemed necessary. The surgeon may decide to use an anticoagulant in a low dosage to reduce the possibility of a blood clot. Commonly used medications include Lovenox or Arixtra, both of which require injection beneath the skin; these can be used at home after surgery.

What are the costs of breast reconstruction?

The costs of breast reconstruction depend on the extent of surgical repair needed, the type of reconstructive operation a woman selects, whether this surgery is performed as an immediate or a delayed procedure, and the number of operations required. Insertion of an implant costs less than a procedure requiring a flap of additional tissue supplied from the back, buttocks, or abdomen. Creating a nipple-areola further increases the price. These decisions affect the length of hospitalization, the length of the operation, and the anesthesia that is required. Costs include the plastic surgeon's fees, anesthesia, and the hospital charges. In addition, costs for breast reconstruction may vary depending on the region of the country. The cost of surgery, as with the cost of living, seems to be higher on the East or West Coast than in other areas of the country.

Immediate breast reconstruction usually costs less. The patient is already hospitalized for a mastectomy and is only anesthetized one time. She recovers from the mastectomy and reconstruction simultaneously. If the breast reconstruction is delayed, costs are usually greater to account for two anesthesias and two different hospitalizations.

A surgeon's fee for implant and expander reconstruction with the tissues remaining after the mastectomy usually begins at $2500 to $3000 and goes up from there. The cost for the implant is additional and now ranges from approximately $1500 to $3500. Flap operations start at $5000; microsurgical flap procedures are higher, starting at $8000. A second procedure to restore a woman's nipple-areola usually costs upward from $1500 and can be done on an outpatient basis. Costs for managed care contracts, preferred provider organizations, and Medicare are predetermined by contracts and by insurance policies. Oncoplastic procedural fees are the same as the fees for a conventional breast reduction.

These costs are approximate and reflect a range seen in the country today. They are offered merely to give women an idea of the expenses to be anticipated when considering breast reconstruction. Your reconstructive surgeon will tell you the specific costs.

Will the insurance carrier, HMO, or Medicare cover the costs of breast reconstruction?

Most major medical carriers cover the costs of breast reconstruction after mastectomy based on the restrictions, co-pays, and deductibles specified in their individual policies. This usually includes nipple reconstruction as well as revision of an opposite breast for symmetry. This surgery is not considered cosmetic, but rather reconstructive, and many states have passed laws to ensure coverage by any company delivering health insurance within the state. Coverage varies, however, from state to state. Most surgeons accept the insurance company reimbursement rates. However, some surgeons have declined insurance company reimbursement rates and charge higher out-of-network fees ranging from $5000 for an implant reconstruction to as much as $30,000 for a complex microsurgical flap reconstruction.

Before a woman decides on reconstructive breast surgery, she should carefully read her health care policy. It is wise to check with your insurance carrier before you have breast reconstruction to be sure that part or all of your expenses will be reimbursed. Persistence and assertiveness will sometimes be necessary to get the needed information. If only a portion of the cost is covered, you need to inquire what percentage is covered and if this coverage is based on the actual cost of the surgery or on a pre-assigned payment schedule that identifies the "usual and customary fee" for a particular operation as determined by the insurance company. If there is a "usual and customary fee," you need to know what that fee is and how much of your anticipated bill will not be covered so that you can plan accordingly.

Dealing with the medical carrier can be a frustrating experience. It may require additional letters and phone calls, but you should not become discouraged. This is a legitimate reconstructive procedure that qualifies for coverage. It is your right to insist on information and specifically to know the extent of coverage before the operation. A letter from the doctor to the third-party provider may be needed to explain your condition and the need for surgery. Although some carriers still do not cover rehabilitation of any kind, fortunately, they are the exception, not the rule. However, some insurance carriers may not be familiar with some of the more recently developed breast reconstruction techniques, such as fat grafting, and will have to be educated about the technique that has been selected. The plastic surgeon can assist in this process with a telephone call to the insurance provider and a follow-up letter.

In deciding whether she can afford breast reconstruction, a woman needs to assess all aspects of her reconstructive surgery. What type of procedure does she plan to have done? Is it going to be done on an immediate or delayed basis? Is her other breast going to be modified? What is her insurance coverage? Does it cover modification of the other breast? Many policies will cover prophylactic (risk-reducing) mastectomies (the removal of breast tissue as a preventive therapy against the development of cancer in the future), but some will not cover what they consider to be aesthetic changes such as augmentation (enlargement), mastopexy (tightening and lifting of the breast), and reduction (reducing the size of the breast).

If a woman has implants from a former cosmetic breast procedure, she should check to ensure that this will not affect her insurance coverage. Some insurance carriers have restrictions on coverage for women with implants.

For women with no health care coverage and/or limited assets, breast reconstruction is often available through the plastic surgery divisions of university teaching hospitals.

I have heard that I can get my reconstructive surgery more economically if I travel to another country that offers special discounts for medical tourists? Is this safe to do?

Medical tourism is a growing trend in medicine today. There is no doubt that surgery can be performed more cheaply outside of the United States. This is a reflection of lower malpractice costs but may also reflect differences in quality, particularly in the developing world. Among the greatest concerns with medical tourism are these: What happens when complications set in? Who takes responsibility when the primary surgeon is 5000 miles away and has effectively washed his hands of the case? What is the medicolegal recourse? Will insurance cover the costs of out-of-country surgery? It is often difficult to get coverage even for out-of-state procedures, let alone surgery performed in a foreign country. Breast reconstruction is complex surgery, performed in stages, with the potential for short- and long-term complications. It is disconcerting to conceive of a woman having such complex surgery without ready access to her surgeon on a regular basis.

What does informed consent really mean?

"Informed consent" is a legal term that means that the individual contemplating a certain treatment be fully informed of all of the goals and specifics of the treatment as well as its possible consequences. To be truly "informed" this patient must be provided with this information in verbal and in written form and in terms that are clear and understandable. Risks and benefits of the procedure as well as possible complications and their consequences must be fully described and explained.

If considering breast surgery, how should a woman become informed?

When a woman is considering an operation to restructure or reconstruct her breasts, she needs to obtain as much information as possible about the proposed procedure and to consult with a board-certified plastic surgeon with special expertise in breast surgery. (See Chapter 12 for more information on selecting a plastic surgeon.) During the consultation the plastic surgeon should review the patient's condition, discuss her options, and answer any questions she may have. If breast implants and tissue expanders are being considered, the plastic surgeon should describe these devices, detail all potential benefits and risks, and answer questions concerning them or the implant surgery itself. He should also provide the patient with the manufacturer's informed consent documents (these are also approved by the FDA) and have the patient read these documents carefully and ask questions. The plastic surgeon can often provide reading materials to explain the different procedures. A woman should also discuss the operation with her other physicians, and if additional questions need addressing, a second opinion is in order. A woman should make her decision only after all her questions are answered and she understands all of the possible risks and benefits.

How does breast reconstruction affect survival rates from breast cancer?

Many breast cancer experts believe that knowledge about breast reconstruction will save thousands of women's lives. Some women will come for treatment earlier on discovering a mass in their breast if they are aware of the chance for reconstruction after mastectomy. As one expert explains, "This procedure could conceivably have an immense impact upon the entire problem of early detection and treatment of breast cancer."

As breast reconstruction techniques become increasingly sophisticated and widely accepted, more women are seeking information about them. Before deciding for or against breast reconstruction, a woman needs to be apprised of the essential facts concerning this surgery. Her questions should be answered and her doubts should be addressed. This chapter has attempted to provide some of these answers.

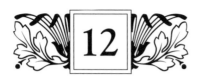

SELECTING AND COMMUNICATING WITH A PLASTIC SURGEON

Having made a decision to seek breast reconstruction, a woman needs to choose her plastic surgeon carefully. Although newspapers, the Yellow Pages, and magazines on the newsstand feature ads for plastic surgery, these provide no valid basis for comparison and therefore are not the best means for selecting a plastic surgeon to perform breast reconstruction—or any procedure, for that matter. Furthermore, in many cases a woman's degree of freedom in making such a choice is limited by her circumstances. If she is already under the care of a cancer or breast surgeon who is a member of a breast team, he will probably recommend one of the plastic surgeons he works with regularly. This is particularly true when immediate breast reconstruction is planned and the cancer surgeon and plastic surgeon must work together closely. The patient's choice also may be directly affected by her insurance provider's list of approved physicians. If she is under a managed care program, she will have to select from that list, or there may be an additional co-payment if she selects someone who is not on the approved list.

When selecting a plastic surgeon, a prospective patient should consider the following guidelines.

TRAINING

The physician a woman selects should be trained in plastic surgery and have met the qualifications of the American Board of Plastic Surgery, which grants board certification in this specialty. To be able to take the board examination, a surgeon must have 3 to 5 years of training in general surgery or in a surgical subspecialty and an additional 2 to 3 years of specialized training in the broad aspects of plastic surgery. Furthermore, he must demonstrate competence by completing an approved residency training program; this means the doctor's peers have approved his moral and ethical qualifications as well as his knowledge, training, and experience in the field. Approximately 1 to 2 years after residency training is completed, he is eligible to take board examinations and once again subject himself to the scrutiny of peers to obtain board certification. Once certified, he may apply for membership in the American Society of Plastic Surgeons (ASPS).

EXPERIENCE

The plastic surgeon a woman chooses should have a special interest in breast reconstruction and should regularly operate with cancer surgeons as a part of the breast team. In addition, he should be experienced with the different techniques appropriate for breast reconstruction and have a record of successful operations. If he has a teaching appointment at a medical school–affiliated hospital, this association suggests access to the latest surgical techniques, involvement in the education of residents, and awareness of recent developments in the field. It is not enough just to be a well-trained plastic surgeon; a good doctor must know about the specific procedures that apply to the patient's problem if he is to render optimal care.

HOW DO YOU INVESTIGATE A DOCTOR'S CREDENTIALS?

Getting information about a doctor's training is easy to do and worth the effort. This information is available online at *info@abms.org* or in the reference room at the local library; look for *The Directory of Medical Specialists*, a book that lists only board-certified specialists. It gives each doctor's year of birth, medical school, the year he was licensed to practice, the year of specialty certification, primary and secondary specialties, and type of practice. It includes other information on training and hospital and medical affiliations. Doctors are listed geographically, so it is easy to locate the names of surgeons in each community. The *American Medical Directory* is another helpful reference, but, unlike *The Directory of Medical Specialists*, it does not indicate whether a physician is board certified. Doctors who are on the staff of hospitals accredited by the Joint Commission in a specific specialty have had their credentials approved by their peers representing the hospital and meet their criteria to practice the specialty.

FINDING A PLASTIC SURGEON

How do you find out whose surgical competence is highly regarded? How do you know who is experienced in breast reconstruction? Most people do not know where to go for reliable information. However, this information can be obtained from numerous sources. One of the best sources of referral is another physician in the community or another member of the breast management team. The cancer surgeon is a knowledgeable person to ask; frequently he works with a plastic surgeon as part of a breast team and feels comfortable with this expert's skill and his ability to work with the other team members to achieve the best result for the patient. He also may have patients who have had breast reconstruction and are willing to discuss this topic and recommend their doctors. Other women who have had breast reconstruction provide an excellent source of information and reliable recommendations about their plastic surgeons; they have firsthand knowledge of this surgery and can personally relate to the surgeon's skill and bedside manner. A woman's gynecologist or family physician also may know the names of plastic surgeons who have performed successful breast reconstructions.

The American Society of Plastic Surgeons (444 E. Algonquin Rd., Arlington Heights, IL 60005; *www.plasticsurgery.org*) provides information on breast reconstruction; it also will supply a list of board-certified plastic surgeons performing reconstructive breast surgery in different communities throughout the United States. The American Cancer Society, through its "Reach to Recovery" Program, also provides information on breast reconstruction. By contacting this organization through the local chapter of the American Cancer Society, the woman desiring information on breast reconstruction will be placed in touch with a woman who has had her breast reconstructed and will share her experiences. Breast cancer and breast reconstruction support groups also provide valuable information and access to other women of similar age and background who have had breast reconstruction. Many times these support groups are affiliated with local hospitals. The local medical society is another source of information; it often has lists of specialists in the community and their areas of interest. (See Appendix B for more information on support services.)

FINDING THE RIGHT PLASTIC SURGEON

Locating a qualified plastic surgeon does not necessarily mean a woman has found the right surgeon for her. She needs to determine whether this physician will meet both her physical and emotional needs. Breast reconstruction is a very emotional experience; a woman's breasts have far greater psychological implications than their anatomy and physiology would suggest. A woman needs a doctor who listens, who treats her as an individual, and who has time to deal with her concerns.

As with any anticipated surgery, a woman should consider a second opinion before finally selecting a surgeon. Some women hesitate to request another opinion for fear it will offend their doctors; they are intimidated by their doctors and are reluctant to question their statements and seek more information. However, time spent in finding the right plastic surgeon is well invested. Unfortunately, most people do not devote the necessary effort to making this important choice. As one woman in our survey so aptly explained, "Most women devote more attention to buying a car than they do to selecting a doctor."

QUESTIONS TO ASK A PLASTIC SURGEON

Before selecting a plastic surgeon, a woman needs to know that he is receptive to her questions and concerns. To assist in making a satisfactory choice of a plastic surgeon, we have included some questions a woman might ask during her consultation*:

- How many breast reconstructions have you done, and what type of results have you achieved?
- May I talk with several of your patients who have had this surgery?
- What are the different options for breast reconstruction?
- What is the best timing for reconstructive surgery? Can I have immediate breast reconstruction at the time of my cancer surgery?
- What are the benefits and risks associated with the different reconstructive techniques?
- What are the benefits and risks associated with breast implants? With tissue expanders?

*Chapters 9 through 13 and 18 are devoted to answering women's frequently asked questions about breast reconstruction.

- Is it possible to have reconstruction with my own tissues and without an implant?
- Is it possible to have endoscopic-assisted breast reconstruction?
- Which reconstructive approach is appropriate for me and why?
- What is involved in this surgery?
- What type of anesthesia will be used: local or general?
- How many different procedures and hospitalizations will be needed? How long will I be in surgery for each operation?
- What type of scars will I have, and exactly where will they be placed?
- What are the expected results of surgery? Can I expect good long-term results?
- Will my breasts be symmetrical?
- How long will it take me to recuperate?
- What are the anticipated costs of surgery?
- Will you help me file for insurance coverage?
- What are the possible complications associated with this surgery?

Most plastic surgeons can show photographs of some of their previous breast reconstruction patients. These might help the patient understand the results that can be achieved for a deformity such as hers. It is important for the patient to make certain that these pictures are of the surgeon's own patients and not just examples of potential results taken from other sources.

QUESTIONS TO ASK YOURSELF BEFORE YOU SCHEDULE SURGERY

It is equally important to take the time to consider the following questions before making a decision about a plastic surgeon:

- Is this the plastic surgeon I want to do my breast reconstruction?
- Is he properly trained and qualified?
- Does this surgeon seem to understand how I feel, and is he sensitive to my needs?
- Has he taken the time to understand what I want done?
- Has he provided me with enough information so that I can make an informed decision?
- Is he going to spend the necessary time with me to answer my questions and deal with my concerns?

- Does he have the necessary skill and experience to perform this surgery?
- Has he explained what he plans to do in terms that I can understand?
- Does he treat me as a responsible adult?
- Does his plan for surgery agree with my expectations for what I would like done?
- If there is a problem, do I feel comfortable with this surgeon's handling it?

COMMUNICATING WITH A PLASTIC SURGEON

Good communication not only helps the patient find the best plastic surgeon to perform her breast restoration, but also enables her to work with him to achieve the result she desires. (See Chapter 9 for more information on communicating with physicians.) Preoperative consultations provide the patient and surgeon with an ideal setting for discussing their thoughts and exploring their expectations for a final result.

A typical consultation with a plastic surgeon about breast reconstruction should begin with an explanation of the woman's concerns and expectations for this operation and a complete review of her medical and surgical history. It is in a woman's best interest to have a plastic surgeon who is well informed about all aspects of her health and tumor care so that he can consider these factors in discussing reconstructive options with her. It is helpful if he has copies of the cancer surgeon's operative report and the pathologist's report or has communicated directly with the other physicians. He also needs to be aware of the radiation therapy and chemotherapy that is planned or that has already been administered, the status of her opposite breast, and her feelings about it.

After this initial discussion the plastic surgeon will need to physically examine the woman's chest, back, thigh, and abdomen to determine the reconstructive approaches that are appropriate for her physical situation.

Preoperative photographs are taken during this initial consultation; the patient should expect to be photographed. If she visits more than one doctor, usually each doctor will take photographs. Although these photographs do not show the patient's face, sometimes this picture-taking process is unsettling for the woman. These photographs are important, however, because the plastic surgeon will use them to evaluate her condition and plan her operation. They also provide a record of her treatment. He may eventually use them (with the woman's permission) for educational purposes to demonstrate the results of this surgery to other patients and physicians and for publication in the professional literature.

Once this examination has been concluded, the woman can again meet with the plastic surgeon to review the various options for breast reconstruction. Final determination of the operative plan must often wait until the plastic surgeon has consulted with the other members of the breast management team.

If a woman has a spouse or significant other in her life, it is often helpful for this person to accompany her on her preoperative visits with the plastic surgeon. Mutual expectations can then be aired and discussed, and the influence of the spouse's feelings on the woman can be observed and evaluated. Although the woman and her spouse or significant other share in the learning process, the final decision about surgery must be made by the woman herself. At no time should a woman feel pressured into this surgery by a relative, friend, spouse, or even the plastic surgeon with whom she is consulting.

If a woman has a consultation with her plastic surgeon before her cancer surgery, they should discuss the correct timing of reconstructive surgery, whether immediate or delayed. If she desires an immediate reconstruction, the cancer surgeon and plastic surgeon need to confer and agree on the suitability of this approach for her. Before an immediate breast reconstruction is done, the details of timing, operative care, and team cooperation must be carefully planned.

The woman who consults with a plastic surgeon after her mastectomy or lumpectomy should remember that reconstructive breast surgery is never an emergency procedure. In the interest of good communication, she may require several visits to her plastic surgeon to get answers to all of her questions, to clearly explain her expectations for reconstruction, and to work with him to define a specific surgical plan appropriate for her. There are many methods for reconstructing breasts today, and a well-trained plastic surgeon will probably be knowledgeable about a number of different procedures. It is important, however, that the type of reconstruction the woman selects be the simplest and safest procedure, yet still be the most likely to meet her expectations for a good result.

INDEX OF BREAST RECONSTRUCTION TECHNIQUES

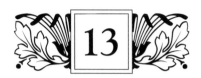

SURGICAL OPTIONS FOR BREAST RECONSTRUCTION

A s recently as 30 years ago, a woman who had a mastectomy had few options if she desired breast restoration. Breast reconstruction techniques had not been perfected, and the most a woman could expect was the creation of a breast mound that bore little resemblance to her remaining breast. Most breast reconstructions were done months to years after the mastectomy. Without reconstructive surgery, she faced the prospect of living with a lopsided chest or wearing a breast prosthesis to hide her deformity. A prosthesis, however, was not always the solution to the problem. Sometimes it made a woman feel increasingly self-conscious because she worried that her artificial breast would become dislodged and be obvious to others.

Today, with the development and refinement of techniques to satisfy the requests of women seeking breast preservation or breast restoration, the results of reconstructive surgery have improved dramatically. The focus now is on breast preservation and avoidance of a mastectomy deformity. Oncoplastic techniques (for partial breast reconstruction), skin-sparing mastectomy, tissue expansion, endoscopic techniques, and autologous tissue refinements have enhanced the results of immediate reconstruction, which is now often the preferred timing for breast reconstruction. Women who require or choose a mastectomy or women who choose a lumpectomy with radiation but require reconstructive surgery to prevent breast asymmetry or contour defects can now select from a number of reliable procedures that meet their psychological and aesthetic expectations for breast restoration. Breasts can be rebuilt with implants or expanders and the tissue remaining after the mastectomy; with flaps of muscle, muscle and skin, or skin and fat (from the abdomen, back, hips, or buttocks); and with external expansion and fat grafting. The choice of reconstructive method depends on the amount and quality of the tissue remaining after the mastectomy or in the case of lumpectomy deformities, on the size of the defect and the corresponding size of the remaining breast. Other important considerations are the surgeon's experience with each technique, and the patient's preferences and expectations. In addition to these basic operations, the patient may request additional procedures to enhance breast appearance and symmetry.

THE OPPOSITE BREAST

In deciding which surgical option is appropriate for her, a woman must resolve her feelings about her remaining breast. Does she like the way it looks and want the rebuilt breast to match it? (With the new reconstructive techniques available, it is often possible to achieve breast symmetry without altering the opposite breast.) Is she willing to consider an operation on her normal breast if this will make both breasts appear symmetrical? If her remaining breast is large and full and she does not want it modified, will she agree to a flap procedure that will provide sufficient tissue to match her large breast but will also result in an abdominal, buttock, thigh, or back scar? Many women have strong feelings about preserving their remaining breast intact. Her feelings about her remaining breast will affect the type of procedure chosen and the ultimate success of the reconstructive effort. (See Chapter 14 for more information on procedures to alter the opposite breast for symmetry.)

OPERATIVE TECHNIQUES

This chapter is designed to serve as a woman's guide to the different techniques available for breast reconstruction, their indications for use, and their advantages and disadvantages. It describes *oncoplastic* techniques for partial breast reconstruction after lumpectomy as well as the range of implant and *autologous* (with a woman's own tissue) flap operations for reconstruction after mastectomy. The various types of implants and expanders and their applications are also described. In addition, we have included information on a relatively new technique that combines external expansion with fat grafting. This procedure is still somewhat investigational, but we wanted our readers to be aware of the latest developments in the field. No one procedure is advocated above any other. The particular approach must be selected with the individual woman's needs and her deformity in mind.

ONCOPLASTIC TECHNIQUES FOR PARTIAL RECONSTRUCTION AFTER LUMPECTOMY

Oncoplastic techniques combine cancer therapy with aesthetic breast reshaping. Increasingly plastic surgeons are being called in to help improve the appearance of lumpectomy defects associated with breast conserving surgery. There are three major reasons to reshape a breast following a lumpectomy: (1) when the lumpectomy creates a substantial deformity in the breast, (2) because a smaller breast is easier to irradiate than a large, droopy breast, and (3) because smaller breasts have a much lower risk of complications from radiation than larger breasts which tend to develop more shrinkage and fibrosis (tissue hardening) over time.

Given these factors, it is preferable to perform a breast reduction and/or breast reshaping at the time of (immediately) or just after the lumpectomy, but definitely *before the radiation therapy*; this timing is critical to achieving a safe outcome. In this situation, the surgeon either moves tissue from A to B and rearranges the same breast volume into a better shape, or he reduces the patient's breasts to produce a better cosmetic appearance. Standard breast reduction techniques are used resulting in smaller more uplifted breasts. (See Chapter 14 for a discussion of breast reduction.) As a result, patients have reduced complication rates from their radiation and breast aesthetics are better in the long term.

A lumpectomy defect can also be filled with a latissimus dorsi muscle flap, which is brought from the back through the underarm to the front of the chest where it is placed in the lumpectomy defect. This procedure, however, is performed less frequently now for immediate partial breast reconstruction; today surgeons are increasingly using local breast flaps and breast reduction techniques to achieve the same results. However, when a patient has already had lumpectomy and radiation, breast reduction or local flap techniques may prove more risky for a delayed reconstruction. In that situation, reconstruction can be accomplished with a latissimus flap or alternatively, with a regional perforator flap. Many reconstructive surgeons prefer to preserve the latissimus flap in case it is needed for a later mastectomy reconstruction in the event of a recurrence. (See p. 303 for a description of this technique.)

BREAST REDUCTION/RESHAPING

Surgical Procedure and Postoperative Appearance

Oncoplastic procedures are generally performed either at the time of lumpectomy or 1 week after lumpectomy when surgical margins are known to be clear (no indication of cancer). The procedure takes approximately 1 to 2 hours to perform, in addition to the time required for the lumpectomy. Before the lumpectomy begins, the plastic surgeon marks the breast to indicate the planned breast reduction approach and to guide the oncologic surgeon's placement of skin incisions. Once the tumor is removed and the margins are confirmed clear, the plastic surgeon develops the appropriate breast flaps, removing excess tissue as needed. A strip of breast tissue is moved up into the lumpectomy defect to fill it and the remaining breast tissue is reshaped and contoured, just as would be done in a conventional breast reduction or breast lift. (See Chapter 14 for a description of breast reduction technique.)

The opposite breast is also reduced so that the breasts are symmetrical. The breast incisions result in scars that encircle the areola and extend in a vertical line down to the inframammary fold (where the breast and chest wall meet). In some situations a short horizontal incision may be placed in the fold. Frequently the lumpectomy side is left a little larger than the opposite breast to compensate for the shrinkage associated with radiation therapy over the long term. Radiation treatments are usually initiated 4 to 6 weeks after surgery, unless chemotherapy is also planned.

Postoperative Care

A suction drain is often inserted into each breast after surgery and is left in place for 2 to 5 days to remove any excess fluid from the operative sites. Antibiotics and oral pain medications are also administered. The patient usually wears a soft bra for support and comfort.

Problems and Complications

Oncoplastic procedures have a low rate of problems and complications. Swelling is an expected side effect; women should be aware that it will take approximately 6 weeks for their breast swelling to fully resolve. Other possible complications include seromas (fluid collections), hematomas (blood collections), and infection, although these problems are rarely encountered after oncoplastic procedures.

Oncoloplastic Breast Reduction/Reshaping

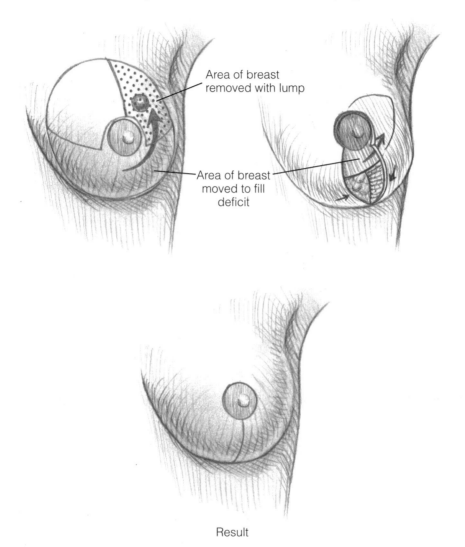

Area of breast removed with lump

Area of breast moved to fill deficit

Result

Compromise of blood flow to the nipple during the lumpectomy is a potential complication that is of greater concern. To avoid this problem, the oncologic surgeon will try to preserve the blood flow to the nipple during the cancer surgery and will not interrupt it unless it is necessary to completely remove the cancer. In such circumstances, a nipple with a poor blood supply can be removed and immediately grafted back onto the breast. A radiation burn is another potential complication; however, this is not related to the reconstruction but to later radiation therapy.

Hospitalization, Pain, and Recuperation

These procedures may be done on an outpatient basis for young to middle-aged patients with no other medical risk factors. Patients over 45 years of age or those with conditions such as diabetes or hypertension should stay in the hospital overnight. Most women who undergo oncoplastic procedures report that their pain is minimal; it is most severe during the initial 24 hours after surgery. Oral pain medications are typically adequate for pain control.

Recovery from this operation is rapid. Some patients are able to return to work as early as 5 to 7 days after surgery. However, many women report that they need 2 to 3 weeks off from work to fully recover both emotionally and physically. They can usually resume nonstrenuous activity, such as walking, in 2 to 3 weeks, and exercise and sports activities in 6 weeks. However, this time frame may be longer if there are side effects from postoperative radiation.

Results of Oncoplastic Techniques

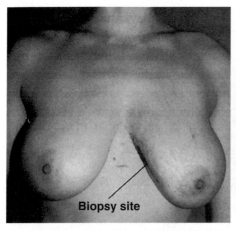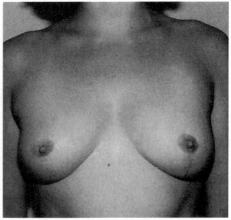

Biopsy site

This 28-year-old woman requested a lumpectomy to treat cancer of her left breast. Because she wanted smaller breasts, the lumpectomy was combined with reduction of both breasts in an immediate procedure. Her result is shown 3 years after breast reduction.

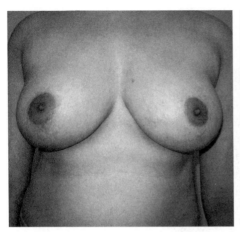 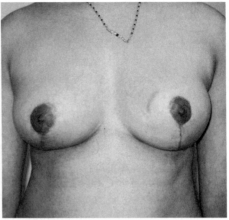

This young woman had a large amount of tissue removed from her lower breast area during a lumpectomy to treat her right breast cancer. She was left with a breast asymmetry. An oncoplastic breast reduction was performed on both breasts to balance her breasts and improve their appearance.

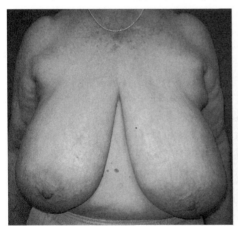 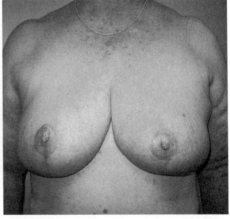

This elderly woman developed a left breast cancer and a lumpectomy with postoperative radiation was planned. Because her breasts were very large, her nipples were removed completely during the lumpectomy, then reconstructed at the time of her breast reduction. She is shown after radiation therapy with smaller, more manageable breasts and reconstructed nipples.

IMPLANT AND EXPANDER RECONSTRUCTION

Despite their desire for breast restoration after treatment for breast cancer, many women will forego reconstructive surgery if it means a lengthy or complicated operation, convalescence, and rehabilitation. Constraints of time and money or psychological needs often limit their choices to a simple procedure or to no procedure at all. Women who choose these simpler procedures do not object to the use of a foreign material in their bodies and do not express overriding concerns about breast implants; their chief goal is the simplest and most convenient method of breast restoration. For these women, implant or expander reconstruction provides the perfect solution. Unlike the more complex flap techniques, the operative variables are not increased, new scars are not created, and the potential for perioperative complications is minimized. Furthermore, these procedures do not preclude the use of other procedures, especially flap operations, if they become necessary in the future. A patient who chooses implant reconstruction should be aware, however, that this reconstructive approach usually is not a one-stage procedure; a second operation will be required to reconstruct the nipple-areola, and, if necessary, to adjust the implant size, shape, and position or to release scar tissue (capsular contracture release). Similarly, tissue expansion will require additional office visits to inflate the expander, place or adjust an implant, and reconstruct the nipple-areola. Under most circumstances, these secondary procedures can be performed on an outpatient basis.

Before we discuss implant and expander reconstruction techniques and the anticipated postoperative care and recuperation, a brief review of available implant and tissue expander options is appropriate.

TYPES OF IMPLANTS AND EXPANDERS

There are two broad categories of breast implants: fixed-volume implants and implants in which the volume can be changed after they are implanted (the latter are called *tissue expanders*). All current implants have a silicone elastomer layer or envelope that contains the filling material; this covering is the outer material in contact with the body tissues. It has a smooth or textured surface, is filled with saline solution (saltwater) or silicone gel, and is either round or anatomically shaped.

Implant Envelope

The implant envelope is available with a smooth or textured surface. The textured surface results in a thicker implant wall with a greater tendency for the edges of the implant to be palpable and may result in more visible rippling and wrinkling of the wall of the implant beneath the skin in some patients.

Implant Fill

Although alternative filling materials have been proposed over the years, the only two that have stood the test of time have been saline solution and silicone gel.

Saline has the obvious advantage of being readily available, entirely safe and inert. If the implant ruptures, the saline is simply absorbed into the body and secreted without problem. The surgeon can fill the device at the time of surgery. Saline-filled implants are more limited in their shape; they are also slightly heavier than silicone gel–filled implants and when overfilled are firm and almost spherical, and therefore feel and look unnatural. When underfilled they can be soft, and their envelopes, which are generally thicker than those containing silicone gel, can develop noticeable and palpable folds and ripples, particularly through thin skin at the mastectomy site. Some models of saline implants have shaped contours that seem to help minimize wrinkling problems and improve the contour of the reconstructed breast.

Silicone gel has a much more inherent *cohesivity* (density), producing a softer, more natural feel to the reconstructed breast. Gel-filled devices may contain a more fluid silicone gel or the newer, more solid, heavily vulcanized cohesive silicone gel, which has the consistency of Jell-O; hence their nickname, "gummy-bear" implants. These cohesive gel–filled implants have a somewhat firmer consistency than their older counterparts. Silicone gel–filled implants also offer flexibility in designing different breast shapes—some wider, some with additional projection—to facilitate individualization.

Cohesive gel implants were developed partially to correct the problem of wrinkling in implants as well as to reduce the potential for migration of silicone gel. To a large extent both of these goals have been achieved. The implants are stiffer than their original gel-filled counterparts, although newer-generation cohesive gel implants are more pliable and feel softer. They require a slightly longer incision for insertion than regular gel devices, because they are not as compressible. Too much manipulation of the device during insertion or attempts to insert these implants through very small incisions can result in fracturing the contained gel, with a higher risk of implant failure. These cohesive gel implants are less prone to leakage outside the breast, have a natural appearance, and are more resistant to capsular contracture. If a cohesive gel implant is cut with a knife, the silicone remains within the device. They are the implants of choice for most surgeons internationally, who have been using them routinely for more than a decade, with excellent results. They are not widely available in the United States for aesthetic breast procedures at this time, but they are available for breast reconstruction.

Implant Shape

Implants are available in round or anatomic shapes.

Round Implants

The original breast implants were round, and they remain the most widely used implants in many surgeons' practices in this country. All round implants have a horizontal and vertical dimension that is symmetrical. Some models are available with different amounts of projection and are generally categorized as having a low, moderate, or high profile. Moderate profile implants have wider bases with less projection, whereas high profile implants have narrower bases, enabling them to project more for a given volume of fill material. Moderate profile implants tend to be used more frequently in breast augmentation surgery, while high profile implants are often a better choice in postmastectomy reconstruction. A breast augmentation patient already has some natural breast tissue present to shape the final breast mound, whereas in a mastectomy patient, the surgeon must rely almost

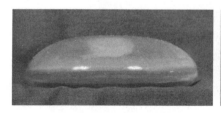
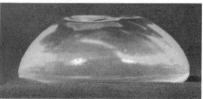

Moderate profile implant   High profile implant

exclusively on the shape of the implant to provide the final breast shape. An attractive, natural breast has a peak centrally beneath the nipple, and for reconstruction of a mastectomy patient's breast, a high profile implant will often provide the correct central projection.

Anatomic or Shaped Implants

Shaped or anatomic implants have a teardrop form that mimics the contours of a normal female breast, which tapers gently onto the chest wall below the clavicle (collarbone). When a mastectomy is performed, the area below the collarbone is extremely difficult to reconstruct unless a flap of the patient's own tissue is used, or unless fat injections are used to fill this area. These shaped devices were designed to provide some fill in the upper aspect (*pole*) of the breast when mastectomy defects are reconstructed.

Many of the new more cohesive gel–filled implants have a contoured profile as well as surface texturing. Shaped implants have to be placed very precisely, and the implant pocket must be accurately created to prevent rotation of the implant. Rotation is not an issue when using round implants. All anatomic implants are constructed with a firmer, denser gel that supports the shell to better maintain the shape of the implant and resist wrinkling.

Anatomic implants also may be filled with saline. The advantage of this design is that the volume can be modified within a range of fill volumes. However, because of the fluidity of saline, this fill provides little support for the implant shell, so if the implant is underfilled, it will result in wrinkling and loss of implant shape.

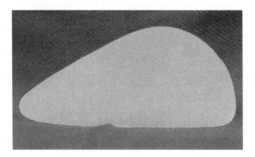

Anatomic implant

Tissue Expanders

Tissue expanders are adjustable implants that can be inflated with saline solution to stretch the tissues at the mastectomy site. All of these devices have a textured silicone shell that is filled with saline solution and adjusted after the implants are placed. The saline is injected through the skin and into a valve leading to the implant. This temporary expander is left in place until the breast has been expanded and adjusted to the optimal volume and shape; the expander is then exchanged for a permanent fixed-volume implant, usually after 4 to 6 months or longer.

Expander Valves

There are two basic designs of tissue expander valves through which the saline is injected to inflate the expander and stretch the tissues. One type is connected to the tissue expander through silicone tubing. This valve may be removed, or in the case of the smaller valves (less than ½ inch in diameter), it can be left in for an extended period to permit future adjustments in breast size. Another type of valve is an integral part of the tissue expander. A metal disk is incorporated in the back of this integral valve, and a magnetic finder is then used to locate the site for injection of the saline solution. This valve is often palpable and can sometimes be felt through thin skin cover.

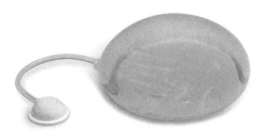
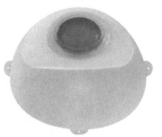

Tissue expander with
remote valve

Tissue expander with
integral valve

Postoperatively Adjustable Implant

A postoperatively adjustable implant is an alternative to the temporary expander. This device permits postoperative adjustments in breast size over a relatively narrow range of volumes. The postoperatively adjustable implant contains only saline solution; it is basically a saline implant that has separate tubing connecting it to a small fill valve, usually located in the underarm area. With this model of adjustable implant, the small, separate fill valve can remain in place for months or even years so that breast size can be altered over a long period, or it can be removed when breast volume is judged ideal. Most women tolerate the small valve without a problem and appreciate the option of changing their breast size and volume if it is necessary or desirable. Once the valve has been removed, this device becomes a permanent fixed-volume implant.

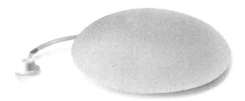

Postoperatively adjustable implant with remote valve

BREAST RECONSTRUCTION WITH IMPLANTS

Implant reconstruction using the tissue that remains after the mastectomy is an option for a woman who has sufficient healthy tissue at the mastectomy site to adequately cover a breast implant or a postoperatively adjustable implant. This method is appropriate for a woman who has had a total mastectomy in which her breast is removed but her chest muscles are preserved. Skin-sparing mastectomy increases the probability that the skin remaining at the mastectomy site will not be tightly stretched. For immediate or delayed reconstruction with an implant, the surgeon should be able to move the skin over the muscle, which indicates the presence of tissue beneath the skin that can be used to provide a smooth contour for a pleasing breast shape. Reconstruction with this technique is suitable for creating a symmetrical appearance in a woman whose remaining breast is small or of normal size and does not sag. It is also suitable for bilateral reconstructions.

There are limitations to the size of the breast implant that can be placed at the time of the mastectomy to avoid complications and not compromise healing. These size limitations make tissue expansion—which permits more flexibility, accuracy, and safety in sizing the reconstructed breast for larger reconstructions—an appealing option for an immediate operation, one that is more frequently chosen today when implant reconstruction is selected.

Surgical Procedure and Postoperative Appearance

Breast restoration using the tissue remaining after the mastectomy is the simplest technique available today. This operation normally takes 1 to 2 hours to perform. If the remaining breast is to be altered, this modification can be made during a second operation to rebuild the nipple-areola. Either a general (the most common) or local anesthetic can be used with adequate sedation.

For immediate implant breast reconstruction, the implant can be placed through the mastectomy incision at the conclusion of the cancer surgery. The plastic surgeon may even remove the entire mastectomy scar and resuture it to produce a thinner scar line. When the mastectomy scar is not in the best location, a small incision can be made near the new inframammary fold (where the lower part of the breast joins the chest wall). The implant is then placed through this new incision. Because this inframammary scar falls in a crease, it will be barely noticeable. When a skin-sparing mastectomy has been performed, it is possible to shorten the length of the scars during immediate breast reconstruction.

After the general surgeon removes the breast and the pathologist examines it, the plastic surgeon begins the breast reconstruction. He elevates the layer of muscular tissue just under the breast, selects a breast implant, and positions it beneath the patient's skin and upper chest muscles to produce a breast shape that has the best symmetry with the other breast. He then closes the muscle layer and sutures the skin incision.

If the surgeon predicts preoperatively that there will not be sufficient cover for the lower portion of the implant, he has a number of strategies to provide additional cover and reduce potential postoperative complications. These include the use of acellular dermal matrix material to cover the bottom of the implant, fat injections, or sometimes a strip of latissimus dorsi (back) muscle can be harvested endoscopically and tunneled through the mastectomy incision for better implant cover. (See Chapter 11 for more information about acellular dermal matrix materials.)

With delayed reconstruction, to avoid creating new breast scars, the surgeon will frequently reopen a portion of the mastectomy scar and insert the implant through this incision. The rest of the operation is the same as described for immediate reconstruction.

Although immediate reconstruction with implants is designed to produce a reconstructed breast of the correct volume and shape at the initial procedure, in practice this goal is not always attainable in one operation, especially if the breast is to appear as natural and symmetrical as possible. It is sometimes necessary to adjust or change the implant during a second procedure. If the adjustments are minor, nipple-areola reconstruction is done during the same operation; otherwise, it is best to wait until a third operation to ensure proper positioning. Adjustments to the opposite breast can be made during the second procedure.

The newly restored breast often appears flattened immediately after reconstruction with available tissue (immediate or delayed). This flatness results from the implant's being positioned behind tissues that are relatively tight, restricting normal projection. These tissues stretch and soften over the next few weeks and months to provide better breast projection and shape. When a postoperatively adjustable implant is used, further adjustments can be made later to improve projection and give the patient some control over final breast size.

Breast Reconstruction With Implants

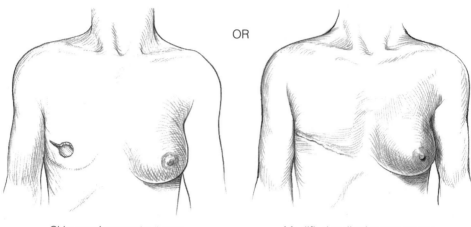

OR

Skin-sparing mastectomy

Modified radical mastectomy

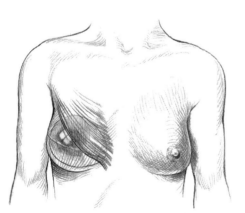

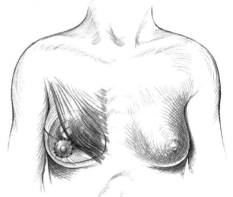

Implant placed under muscle
and through existing scar

Nipple-areola reconstructed
several months later

Postoperative Care

A suction drain is often inserted into the reconstructed breast after surgery and left for 1 to 3 days to remove any excess fluid from the operative sites. The drain may need to be in place longer if there is increased drainage from the removal of axillary lymph nodes. The postoperative dressing selected should provide the best support for the new breast. A brassiere is chosen if the implant needs to be guided upward; an elastic "tube top" or light dressing is selected if it is to be maintained in place or allowed to move downward. Today most reconstructive surgeons use absorbable sutures that do not require removal. If nonabsorbable stitches are used, they are removed approximately 1 week after surgery. This is usually not painful, because the skin in that area is numb and relatively insensitive.

Since the breast has decreased sensitivity, the patient should not use a heating pad at the site of the operation to relieve breast discomfort; this area will be numb, and she could accidentally burn herself. After the stitches have dissolved or are removed, the surgeon may suggest that the patient massage and move her new breast around to keep it as soft and natural as possible. Massage is not needed, however, if textured implants have been used for reconstruction.

In a few weeks the scars will become red; this is a natural healing response and should not alarm the patient. This redness will fade with time. When the woman has fair, translucent skin, the increased blood flow into the healing scars will make them appear red longer, sometimes for several years. Some patients naturally tend to heal with thick, raised scars. (A woman can get some idea of how she will heal by checking the appearance of any other scars she has.) There are various recommendations for improving the appearance of these thickened scars, even though time is often the best solution; they will often fade and soften naturally over a period of months to years. Some surgeons recommend that surgical tapes be placed over the scars for several weeks or months to support the scars and reduce the likelihood that they will widen and thicken. These scars may also be treated by injecting a cortisone solution into them or using silicone sheeting over them to provide gentle pressure to flatten and help fade them. In more severe cases the surgeon may reexcise, revise, and resuture the scars. When the scars are tight, they can be lengthened by a technique called a *Z-plasty*. With this technique, the skin is cut in the shape of a Z and then reshifted and sutured to relieve some of the skin tightness.

After reconstruction the patient's breast skin may be dry because of contact with the dressings. A nonallergenic skin moisturizer can help relieve dryness. In addition, if there are no drainage problems, some surgeons may suggest the use of topical silicone containing creams or cocoa butter; the patient can lightly massage this oil into her scars to help them soften and fade. Vitamin E oil massage has been shown to be of little value, and prolonged use of vitamin E oil can cause a rash.

Problems and Complications

Implant reconstruction with available tissue has a low rate of complications. The most troublesome problem is excessive formation of hard, fibrous tissue around the implant—the body's normal reaction to all foreign material. This reaction is called *capsular contracture*. There is some scar formation around all implants, and most reconstructed breasts feel firmer than normal breasts do. To reduce breast firmness some surgeons use implants that have a textured surface. However, there is no scientific evidence that this texturing helps to reduce the incidence of capsular contracture. Surgeons recommend placement of smooth-surface implants under the chest wall muscle to help avoid this problem; in this location the implant is covered and protected by a layer of muscle. Although textured implants work equally well in either location (above or below the muscle), most surgeons feel that they are best placed under thicker cover so that their texture and ripples are not visible under thin skin.

When a smooth-surface implant is placed, many surgeons suggest that the woman massage her breasts regularly to keep them soft and natural in appearance. Massage is not necessary for women with textured-surface implants; in fact, it may disturb the tissue adherence that the texturing promotes. Sometimes a smooth-surface permanent saline implant is used to replace a textured expander or implant if the first device produces rippling.

In some cases this fibrous formation around the implant becomes tight, the implant becomes hard, and the breast appears deformed. Placement of an implant into an irradiated mastectomy site or subsequent irradiation of a breast with an implant after reconstructive surgery often causes capsular contracture to develop. This problem is often managed by a capsulectomy, a procedure in which the thickened capsule and implant are surgically removed and the implant repositioned or replaced (for example, a smooth-surface implant may be exchanged for an implant with a textured surface). Alternatively, fat injections can be used to cushion the implant and improve the contracture, or a layer of latissimus dorsi muscle may be inserted between the breast skin and implant to cover and cushion the implant. For some patients, the implant is removed, a flap of autologous tissue from the abdomen or buttocks is substituted for the implant, and the breast is thereby reconstructed entirely with the woman's own tissues.

Problems with implant leakage and displacement may also occur and are usually treated by removing the implant and replacing it during an outpatient procedure. Patients should be advised that implants are not lifetime devices; their life spans vary and they may have to be exchanged or replaced at some later date. (See Chapter 11 for more information on implants and possible complications.)

Bleeding and infection rarely occur after this operation. If the patient has had radiation therapy or her breast skin is thin or taut, infection may develop, or, in an immediate breast reconstruction, some of the skin may die because of poor blood supply, thereby exposing the implant. This complication is managed by removing the implant temporarily and transferring additional tissue to cover the implant or occasionally by resuturing the wound. Breast reconstruction is then started over a few months later; the technique selected at this time depends on the individual's situation.

Women who smoke can have more difficulty with healing of the mastectomy skin flaps and experience a higher incidence of infection and exposure of the breast implant or tissue expander at the time of immediate breast reconstruction. In fact, smoking is a detriment to any surgical or reconstructive procedure. It reduces blood flow to the tissues, impairs healing, is associated with increased coughing, lung complications, and infections, and may severely compromise the result of any reconstructive attempt. *All smokers are strongly advised to discontinue smoking for at least 4 weeks and preferably several months before and after surgery. They should also not be around other cigarette smokers to avoid being exposed to second-hand smoke.*

Hospitalization, Pain, and Recuperation

This operation may be done on an outpatient basis or during a brief hospitalization of 1 or 2 days. Most women who select implant reconstruction with available tissue say that it is not as painful or debilitating as the original mastectomy. The breast area is somewhat numb after the operation, but this lack of sensation is a residual effect from the mastectomy. The reconstruction avoids the armpit area, so pain in this region and shoulder stiffness are not concerns, as they were after the mastectomy.

Women recover quickly from this procedure; they are usually out of bed the afternoon of the surgery or the next day and may return to work or normal activity within a week. The patient may take a tub bath the day after the operation, but the incision should be kept dry and the dressing intact. Showers may be resumed 1 to 3 days after the operation if healing is progressing well. Some surgeons place water-proof surgical tapes over the incisions to protect them, allowing the patient to shower the day after the operation. The patient may lift her arms enough to comb her hair 1 or 2 days after surgery. It is possible to drive a car after 1 to 2 weeks, but the patient should not take any pain medications or sleeping pills that could impair her alertness and reflexes. Before driving, the woman should attempt turning the wheel while the car is still parked in the garage or driveway to see if this causes discomfort. It is best to wait 4 to 6 weeks before gradually resuming upper extremity exercise and sports activities. Although the woman may feel fine, she has been inactive for a period of time, and even the muscles not affected by the operation need to be gradually retrained and stretched to regain their suppleness and strength.

Results With Implant Reconstruction

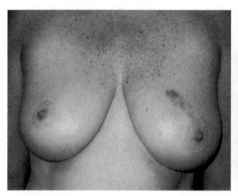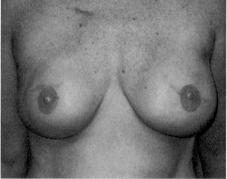

This 55-year-old woman was diagnosed with breast cancer in her left breast. She had bilateral mastectomies (a prophylactic mastectomy on the right) followed by immediate reconstruction of both breasts with high profile gel-filled implants placed in each breast. The implants were covered with acellular dermal matrix to provide additional cover. She is shown 6 months after completion of her reconstruction, including nipple reconstructions.

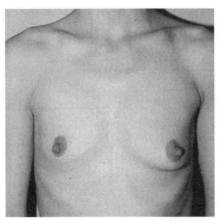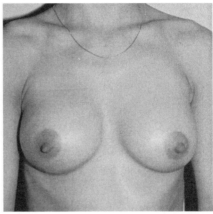

This 26-year-old woman wanted fuller breasts with minimal incisions and requested immediate breast reconstruction after a partial mastectomy. Implants were placed under the muscle in both breasts to achieve symmetry.

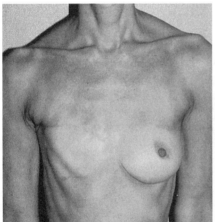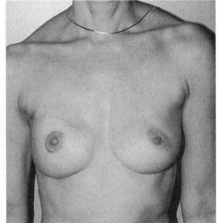

This 52-year-old woman had a modified radical mastectomy. Her breast was reconstructed using intraoperative tissue expansion and immediate implant placement. Her opposite breast was not modified. She is shown 1 year after breast reconstruction.

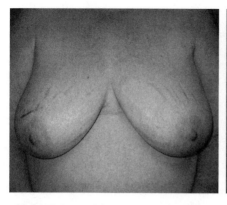 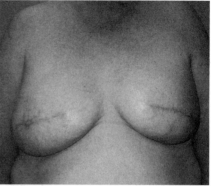

This 65-year-old woman had bilateral mastectomies to treat her cancer with immediate reconstruction of both breasts. She wanted simple implant reconstructions without tissue expansion and did not wish to undergo nipple reconstruction. Large silicone gel implants were inserted beneath her chest wall muscles at the time of mastectomy, providing her with a single-stage reconstruction. She is shown well healed after surgery.

TISSUE EXPANSION

Despite tight skin at their mastectomy site, some women prefer to have simple reconstruction with available tissues rather than a more complicated flap procedure. For these women, the tissue expansion method is a good alternative. It is a simpler reconstructive approach that affords some flexibility in breast size. Today it is chosen much more frequently than simple implant placement. With this approach, the taut skin in the area of the mastectomy is stretched and expanded, thus avoiding a more complex flap operation and permitting placement of a permanent breast implant of suitable size and shape. Although this operation is similar to the approach described in the previous section, it differs in the type of implant used and the postoperative management.

Tissue expansion has a number of advantages for the patient and the reconstructive surgeon. The reconstruction can usually be accomplished without additional breast scars, and the patient can help make the final determination of the volume and size of her reconstructed breast. She has input into decisions about final breast symmetry and the timing of inflation and second-stage breast reconstruction. This approach is particularly applicable for immediate-delayed reconstruction to stretch the tissues before radiation therapy and for bilateral breast reconstruction; it permits the woman to determine final breast volume without the tissue restrictions she might encounter if she were depending on donor tissue from a flap from her abdomen, back, or buttocks, which could be insufficient to build two breasts.

Breast reconstruction with tissue expansion has its drawbacks; it is time intensive, and the woman who wants the quickest approach should understand that usually two or even three procedures may be required. Although the hospital stay necessary for the initial placement of the device is not long, and the procedure can even be done on an outpatient basis in many cases, the patient will require a number of additional postoperative visits for the stretching of the tissues. These office visits and procedures can be inconvenient, may require traveling long distances, and interfere with the demands of family and work. The procedure takes longer than breast reconstruction with other techniques, often a matter of months. Although the desired breast volume is usually attained within a few weeks, additional time is required to complete the reconstruction. For the best results, the breast tissue should be overexpanded, the expanded reconstructed breast allowed time to heal, and the breast evaluated for any further adjustments before second-stage breast reconstruction when the tissue expander is exchanged for a breast implant or the postoperatively adjustable implant is converted to a permanent implant by removing its valves.

Today, in most patients undergoing immediate breast reconstruction with available tissue, a temporary expander or a postoperatively adjustable implant is placed rather than a fixed-volume implant. These expandable devices permit a larger breast to be built and adjusted as it is inflated, avoiding the problem of placing an implant that is not symmetrical or is initially too large for the tissues and could complicate the healing process. The expander enables the surgeon to fine-tune this volume for each individual before placement of the permanent implant. When tissue expansion is used after skin-sparing mastectomy for immediate breast reconstruction, it also has the advantage of avoiding skin tension over an implant while accurately achieving symmetry with the opposite breast.

Surgical Procedure and Postoperative Appearance

Tissue expansion usually requires two operations. The first operation normally takes 1 to 2 hours to perform. It may be done under local or general (the most common) anesthesia. During the first procedure the surgeon inserts a temporary expander or a postoperatively adjustable implant through the mastectomy incision or an inframammary incision. The upper part of the expander is usually positioned below the chest wall muscle, with the lower part just under the skin. The surgeon often manually stretches the breast skin during this initial operation to permit more rapid expansion later, or he may use some volume expansion to stretch the overlying skin intraoperatively. He then positions the valve to allow injection of saline solution for enlargement of the implant. In this early postoperative period the breast skin is still tight, and the reconstructed breast appears flattened and smaller than the remaining breast on the opposite side.

Once the tissue expander is in place and the valve is positioned under the skin for easy access, the woman schedules office visits to the plastic surgeon to have her tissue expander gradually inflated. A typical expansion session lasts 5 to 15 minutes. The saline is injected through the skin into the valve, which is often on the upper front surface of the expander and is found by palpation or by using a magnet. The rate of inflation is influenced by the quality of the healing and the tightness and discomfort being experienced by the patient. This gradual enlargement of the tissue expander produces pressure on the woman's skin, causing it to become tense, stretch, and eventually expand to larger dimensions. Much the same phenomenon occurs when the abdominal skin stretches during pregnancy. This process can be painful for some women, and the volume and timing of the injection and filling process must be individualized. After the breast skin has been distended sufficiently, which is somewhat larger than the other breast (this is called *overexpansion*), and the optimal breast size has been obtained, during a second outpatient procedure the temporary expander is replaced with a permanent implant, or the postoperatively adjustable implant will be converted to a permanent fixed-volume implant by removing the fill tube and valve. (Alternatively, these can be left in place if future changes are anticipated.) After this second operation, the reconstructed breast usually has a more natural appearance and the nipple-areola can be reconstructed in a final operation.

Postoperative Care

Postoperative care is the same as that described for implant reconstruction on p. 273.

Problems and Complications

Capsular contracture, device failure, expander exposure (requiring removal), and implant displacement are potential problems associated with tissue expanders. The use of textured-surface expanders that adhere to the surrounding tissue may help to reduce the possibility of implant displacement. The incidence of device failure and leakage is greater with tissue expanders than it is with implants because of valve problems, displacement of a remote fill port, inadvertent puncture of the tissue expander during inflation with saline, and possible introduction of bacteria that can lead to infection. If this occurs, the device or the fill port may need to be removed and the wound allowed to heal before the expander is replaced.

Tissue expansion can lead to thinning of the stretched skin. If the skin at the mastectomy site is already thin, healing problems may occur. To lower the chance of exposure of the tissue expander through this thin skin, necessitating removal, the reconstructive surgeon may decide to place the tissue expander under the muscle and fascial layer or, as described earlier, he may sew a sheet of acellular dermal matrix to the lower edge of the pectoralis major muscle to provide additional support and cover for the device. These materials are being used with far greater frequency today, because they appear to reduce visible ripples from the implants or expanders; some preliminary data suggest that they may reduce capsular contracture rates. As another alternative, the surgeon can shift a layer of muscle from the latissimus dorsi (back) muscle to the lower portion of the reconstructed breast at the time of the mastectomy. This technique can be performed without additional incisions or scars and without significant functional impairment.

As with implant reconstruction, women who are cigarette smokers may have an increased incidence of healing problems after tissue expansion.

Breast Reconstruction With Tissue Expansion

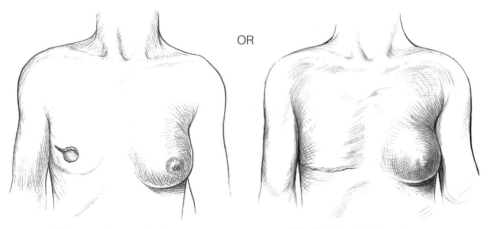

OR

Skin-sparing mastectomy

Modified radical mastectomy

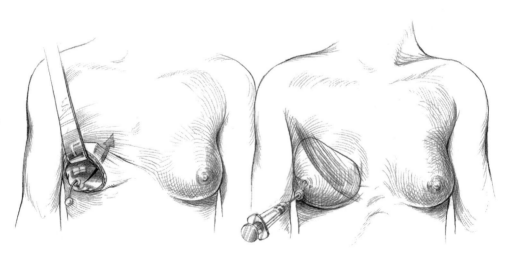

Tissue expander inserted
under skin and muscle

Expander inflated with saline solution
during postoperative visits

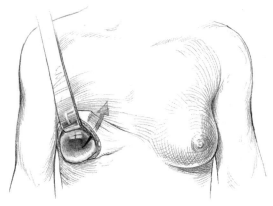

Expander removed and permanent implant inserted
in stretched pocket (with the permanent expander implant,
only the fill tube and valve are removed)

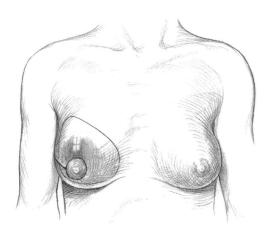

Nipple-areola reconstructed several months later

Hospitalization, Pain, and Recuperation

This operation may be done on an outpatient basis or during a brief hospital stay. If performed in a hospital, the usual stay is 1 or 2 days. The pain associated with tissue expansion is similar to that described previously for implant reconstruction. When tissue expansion is done at the time of the mastectomy, the patient has additional pain from the stretching of healing tissues, which are undergoing wound contraction. Patients often describe a tight, pulling sensation following inflation. Usually this pain is not severe. If it is, the tissue expansion is terminated temporarily to allow the tissues to heal for a week or two and then resumed. If it is too tight, some saline solution can be removed for a few days. The fill valve site is usually in an area where some nerves were removed during the mastectomy and thus this region is relatively numb.

Recovery from this operation is reasonably quick. The patient can usually return to nonstrenuous activity in 2 to 3 weeks and resume sports in 6 to 8 weeks. All other aspects of recovery are the same as those described for implant reconstruction.

Results With Tissue Expansion

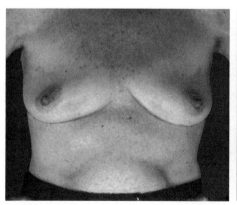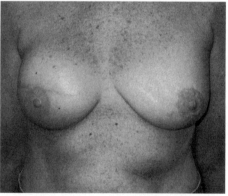

This 45-year-old woman had immediate reconstruction with tissue expander placement beneath acellular dermal matrix material. After her breast was expanded sufficiently, the expander was replaced with a high profile gel implant, and she had a breast lift on the opposite breast. Her nipple was reconstructed with a nipple-sharing technique and was later tattooed.

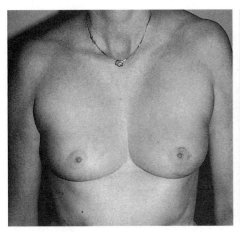
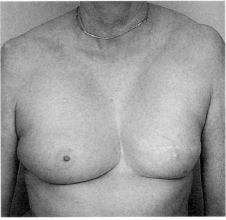

This 52-year-old woman with cancer of the left breast had a modified radical mastectomy and immediate breast reconstruction with tissue expansion and implant placement, which made it possible to match her opposite breast. She is shown 1 year after breast reconstruction. Her nipple-areola was reconstructed with a local flap and a tattoo.

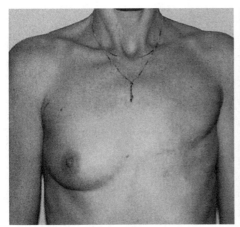
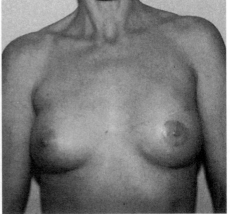

This 35-year-old woman had a left modified radical mastectomy that left tight local tissue. She requested breast reconstruction with tissue expanders and a right breast augmentation. She did not want to have a flap procedure. She is shown 2 years after breast reconstruction.

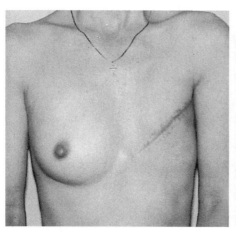 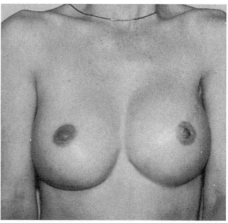

This 34-year-old woman had delayed breast reconstruction after a modified radical mastectomy. Postoperatively adjustable implants were used for reconstruction and for augmentation of her opposite breast. She is shown 1 year after breast reconstruction.

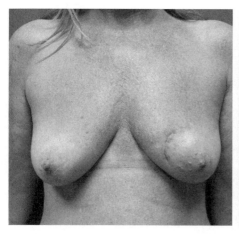 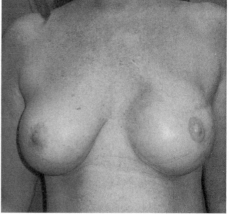

This 42-year-old woman had a skin-sparing mastectomy followed by immediate expander reconstruction. In a subsequent procedure, her expander was exchanged for a high profile gel implant and her opposite breast was augmented with a moderate profile implant. She is shown after nipple reconstruction. She has some breast hollowing that will be corrected with fat injections.

When Available Tissue Reconstruction Is Not the Right Choice

Because reconstruction with available tissues and implants or tissue expanders with implant placement are the simplest of breast reconstruction techniques and offer excellent results, you might assume that these techniques would be the best choice for every patient. Some circumstances, however, prompt a woman to consider other reconstructive options. For instance, when her remaining breast is large and she does not want it changed, reconstruction with these methods will produce breasts of an unequal size, because there will not be enough tissue to build a large breast. Although she might be initially satisfied with the newly reconstructed breast, eventually she will feel lopsided and will probably still need to wear a prosthesis to make her breasts appear equal in size. Consequently, unless the normal large breast is reduced to match the rebuilt breast, reconstruction with the available tissue may not be a permanent solution for this patient, because it will not produce symmetrical breasts. The experienced surgeon can predict in advance whether the other breast will need to be modified or whether a flap is needed.

Although breast implants and tissue expanders have a good track record when used for aesthetic and reconstructive breast surgery, some women prefer not to have a foreign material permanently placed in their reconstructed breast. For them, breast reconstruction with their own tissue is the only logical choice.

If a patient has tight, thin, irradiated, or grafted skin, she also may have limited or unsatisfactory results, because the skin remaining at the mastectomy site, even with tissue expansion, is insufficient to cover the implant and to provide her with a breast that looks and feels natural. A flap reconstruction technique is a more logical choice for a patient with major skin, muscle, and contour deficiencies.

Sometimes an implant or expander must be used in conjunction with a flap. This may be necessary when a woman needs to have both breasts rebuilt and has insufficient flap tissue or when the surgeon needs to design a smaller but necessary flap with a shorter donor scar. For example, a TRAM (abdominal) flap or latissimus dorsi (back) flap may be combined with a tissue expander. The flap can then provide muscle or skin and muscle for the reconstruction, and the tissue expander can be used to create a new breast of the correct size. When the latissimus dorsi muscle is being used for immediate breast reconstruction, it can be obtained through the mastectomy incision using endoscopic techniques. This approach allows the surgeon to harvest the flap tissue with shorter scars, often improving the result and causing less pain. A flap of tissue is also used to provide good cover for the breast implant or tissue expander.

FLAP RECONSTRUCTION

The use of flaps of muscle, skin and muscle (musculocutaneous), or skin and fat to supplement the tissue remaining after a mastectomy represents a major advance in breast reconstruction. With these flap techniques, most women's breasts can now be rebuilt with their own tissue and usually without a breast implant. Furthermore, because the donor sites are often areas of tissue excess, such as the lower abdomen, buttocks, or thighs, these women can expect a full and natural breast that closely resembles the size and shape of their opposite breast. As a benefit, the area from which the donor tissue is taken can sometimes be contoured to produce a more aesthetic appearance. Now even women with radiation injuries or recurrences after lumpectomy with irradiation can have their deformities filled in and rebuilt. The patient's own tissue is often preferred in these situations.

The most frequently used sources of tissue for breast reconstruction with the patient's own tissue (autologous) are the lower abdominal wall and the back. The buttocks or lateral hip areas can also be used as donor sites, although some women and surgeons find hip scars objectionable. More recently, use of the upper inner thigh has become a popular option for some women. When tissue from the abdominal wall or back is used, it is left attached (pedicled) to the blood supply of the muscle beneath it. When tissue from the buttocks, lateral hip, or upper inner thigh is used, microsurgical techniques are necessary to restore the blood supply of the flap by reattaching the vessels supplying this tissue to those in the breast region. The TRAM flap, described previously as a pedicle flap (one that is transferred while still attached to its blood supply), can also be transferred microsurgically as a free flap. Abdominal tissue remains the best source of free tissue flaps, because it is softer and can be shaped far more easily than hip, buttock, thigh, or lateral flank tissue (Rubens flap). The TRAM flap is a highly versatile flap for breast reconstruction, and whether it is transferred as a pedicle flap or by microsurgery often depends on the surgeon's expertise and the patient's preference.

To perform a microsurgical flap reconstruction, the surgeon uses an operating microscope and special fine instruments and sutures to disconnect the tissue and vessels from the donor area and reattach them to tiny vessels in the breast region, usually in the axilla and occasionally in the inner breast area.

Microsurgical breast reconstruction techniques using *perforator flaps* represent the latest advance in breast reconstruction. A perforator flap is composed of skin and fatty tissue and is based on a single set of perforator blood vessels that pass through (that is, "perforate") the underlying muscle. For breast reconstruction, perforator flaps are taken from the patient's abdomen (DIEP and SIEA flaps) or buttocks (IGAP or SGAP flaps). Unlike conventional pedicle and microsurgical flap techniques (such as the TRAM flap), these perforator flap techniques preserve the patient's underlying musculature. The tissue is then transferred to the patient's chest, reconnected using microsurgery, and shaped to create the new breast.

PEDICLE FLAP BREAST RECONSTRUCTION
Reconstruction With the Lower Abdominal (TRAM) Flap

Creation of the breast with a flap of lower abdominal skin and fat over a strip of rectus abdominis muscle is a major contribution to breast reconstruction. This operation, developed in the early 1980s, is now the most frequently used flap procedure and provides some of the most attractive and realistic breast reconstructions. This technique allows the surgeon to restore a woman's breast with her own tissues, usually without the need for a silicone breast implant, and at the same time to give her a slimmer abdomen. With this approach, the surgeon uses excess abdominal tissue to rebuild the breast after a skin-sparing mastectomy or a modified radical mastectomy.

The transverse rectus abdominis musculocutaneous flap, also known as the TRAM flap, is recommended for a woman who requires the extra tissue supplied by a flap reconstruction. She prefers a breast reconstruction without a breast implant and is pleased by or will accept the prospect of having a "tummy tuck" as a bonus. Sometimes the patient's lower abdominal tissue is insufficient to create a breast of satisfactory volume. This most often occurs with bilateral reconstruction. The patient should discuss her preferences and thoughts with the reconstructive surgeon and get his opinion of whether implants will be needed. As with the other flap operations, this is major surgery, and the woman who selects this operation should be in good health.

Her tissue is moved a long distance (from the lower abdomen to the chest), and its blood supply must be healthy and sufficient to nourish the new tissue for breast reconstruction.

It has been found that the TRAM flap blood supply is particularly sensitive and precarious in an overweight woman, a hypertensive woman, a woman who has had radiation therapy, a woman with certain types of abdominal scars, and a woman who is a cigarette smoker. Because cigarette smoking can constrict and narrow blood vessels and precipitate flap failure, the plastic surgeon will insist that the patient avoid cigarettes for at least 4 weeks before and after the operation. The surgeon might also suggest an exercise program consisting of sit-ups and modified sit-ups for several weeks before surgery to increase blood flow and strengthen her abdominal area. If there is evidence that the blood supply may be impaired from many years of cigarette smoking, another method of breast reconstruction should be selected, either tissue expansion, the latissimus dorsi flap, or a microsurgical TRAM flap, a DIEP perforator flap, or a muscle-sparing TRAM flap. A TRAM flap delay is another strategy to increase blood flow to the TRAM flap tissues. (The TRAM flap delay is discussed in the next section.)

A TRAM flap is not appropriate for every patient. When the woman's abdominal wall is very thin or she does not want scars in this region, another procedure should be considered. Patients with medical problems such as diabetes mellitus or heart disease, and women who have had abdominal irradiation, have abdominal scars, or have had lower abdominal liposuction should strongly consider other techniques, because these issues can increase the complication rate of the TRAM flap.

The TRAM flap is now frequently used for immediate breast reconstruction with a skin-sparing mastectomy when there is no tumor involvement in the skin. An immediate TRAM flap reconstruction offers a number of advantages. By combining the mastectomy and the breast reconstruction in one operation, the general surgeon is able to limit the amount of skin removed to only that which is necessary to properly treat the breast cancer. The removed skin is then replaced with the abdominal skin supplied by the TRAM flap. When the nipple-areola has a small diameter, the entire TRAM flap can be buried, thus further reducing the breast scars. By preserving the remaining breast skin and restoring the important landmarks of the breast, such as the inframammary fold and the lateral breast, immediate breast reconstruction with the TRAM flap creates a natural, well-contoured breast with minimal breast scars. This operation can only be done once, and the patient should be advised that if the need arises in the future for another breast reconstruction, another technique will have to be used.

When immediate breast reconstruction with the TRAM flap is planned, close cooperation between the cancer surgeon and the reconstructive surgeon is essential, and the patient must be fully informed about the specifics of the procedure, its possible complications, and the expected recuperation period.

Surgical Procedure and Postoperative Appearance

TRAM flap breast reconstruction is major surgery and usually takes approximately 3 to 6 hours in the operating room compared with the 1 to 2 hours required for implant or expander reconstruction. Using this reconstructive method the surgeon designs a transverse flap of skin and fat on the middle to lower abdomen. The tissue for the new breast is surgically freed from the abdomen but left attached to a strip of the vertical abdominal wall muscle (the rectus abdominis). Sometimes strips of both rectus abdominis muscles (bipedicle TRAM flap) are used to ensure a better blood supply to the flap. The donor site is closed by bringing the remaining muscles together and tightening the entire central abdomen to restore abdominal wall strength. The scar that is left on the abdomen is similar but may not be quite as low and inconspicuous as the horizontal scar left from an abdominoplasty (tummy tuck), which removes excess abdominal tissue for aesthetic reasons. The flap is then ready for transfer to the chest.

When an immediate reconstruction is being performed, the recipient mastectomy site has already been prepared to accept the flap, and more breast skin can be preserved to help shape the new breast and shorten the mastectomy scar. For a delayed reconstruction, the plastic surgeon must first remove the mastectomy scar (if it is in an inconspicuous position) or create a new incision to accept the flap and permit a more aesthetic reconstruction. The flap is then elevated and transferred to the chest wall area through a tunnel under the upper abdominal skin, extending to the new incision in the breast area. The upper part of the flap is sutured into position to give the best contour for the upper breast area, and the lower portion of the flap is positioned, folded under, and contoured to form a breast mound. The breasts are then checked for symmetry and form with the patient positioned upright, and the flap is carefully stitched in place. If the patient has sufficient excess abdominal fat, there ordinarily is no need for a breast implant.

Flap Delay for High-Risk Patients

If the surgeon is concerned preoperatively about the adequacy of the blood supply of the abdominal flap (usually in patients with a combination of findings such as obesity, cigarette smoking, previous abdominal scars, and/or chest wall irradiation), he may decide on an operative delay. In this approach the operation is sequenced into two procedures. One to 2 weeks before the definitive flap operation, the patient has a minor procedure in which the surgeon divides some of the blood vessels going into the lower portion of the TRAM flap. He does this through two short incisions placed in the lower abdomen along the lower line of the planned TRAM flap. Later, during the major operation, these short incisions will be incorporated into the TRAM flap incisions. This so-called delay of the vessels redirects and increases the flap's blood flow and venous drainage and is designed to improve its blood supply and therefore help ensure flap survival.

Several months after the TRAM flap procedure, the plastic surgeon restores the nipple-areola in a second or third procedure (if a TRAM flap delay has been used) with a local anesthetic, followed later by a tattoo if additional pigmentation is desirable. Frequently the flap shape is altered and the abdominal wall is contoured with liposuction or ultrasound-assisted liposuction during a second operation. Ultrasound energy causes the fat to be cavitated (hollows or pockets are created), emulsified (globules are broken into tiny, suspended particles), and loosened so that it can more readily be suctioned out.

A patient who decides on a TRAM flap procedure needs to be fully prepared for the donor deformity and scar and the breast scars required for placing the TRAM flap. After an immediate reconstruction, the skin incision extends around the area of the areola and sometimes laterally toward the axilla, or there is only a short breast scar after the skin-sparing mastectomy. If the breast reconstruction is to be delayed, the new breast usually has an elliptical pattern of stitches running along the lower breast crease and up toward the nipple area. A donor scar extends across the lower abdomen between the pubic area and umbilicus (navel). In addition, there is often some fullness on the inner portion of the new breast because of the addition of the rectus abdominis muscle, which supplies nourishment to the flap. This fullness usually subsides in the first 2 to 3 months after the operation as the transferred, unexercised muscle becomes thinner. If this fullness persists, if the reconstructed breast is larger than the opposite breast, or if there are other areas of fat accumulation in the lateral or lower abdomen, these areas can be contoured later using liposuction to remove the excess fat.

Postoperative Care

Surgical drains are placed in the breast and abdomen; the breast drain is often removed before the patient goes home unless an extensive lymph node dissection (axillary dissection) has been performed. Abdominal drains are best left in longer, since early removal may predispose the patient to fluid collections known as *seromas*. The hospital bed is flexed to relieve abdominal tension caused by the removal of lower abdominal tissue and muscle during the operation. The patient is usually asked to get out of bed the next day and walk. Even though her abdomen may be tight, it is important for a safe recovery; activity enhances the blood flow throughout the body and can lower the chance of developing blood clots in the legs, which could travel to the lungs. The reconstructive surgeon may ask the patient to wear support hose before the operation and for the first few days after the operation to use sequential compression stockings or to wear support hose to further enhance the blood return from the legs and lessen the chance of deep venous thrombosis. When the patient first gets out of bed, she may be unable to stand up straight; this is to be expected. It often takes days to weeks for the patient to be able to stand erect, depending on the tightness of the abdomen. This tightness may also make her feel full after eating only a small amount of food, and she may find that smaller, more frequent meals are better. The other specifics of postoperative care are described in the section on implant reconstruction on p. 273.

Problems and Complications

Because this is major surgery, there are more possibilities for complications. About 1 in 10 patients experiences some healing problems, resulting in an area of skin loss, fat drainage, or firmness of the fatty tissue on the flap. This hard, thickened tissue can be frightening to a woman because of its resemblance to her original tumor. It sometimes softens in 6 to 18 months. This thickening can be differentiated from a tumor by examination, mammography, and sometimes fine-needle aspiration. These thick areas can be removed surgically or with standard liposuction or ultrasound-assisted liposuction techniques. Delayed healing or even loss of some or rarely all of the flap because of insufficient blood supply is a potential complication. Sometimes a portion of the skin edge or fat will have a reduced blood supply, causing drainage from the new breast for a few weeks. To avoid this drainage, the surgeon may want to remove this strip of tissue in a minor outpatient procedure. If fluid accumulates beneath the abdominal skin, it may need to be aspirated or a small drain placed through the incision to allow this liquid to be removed.

Other less frequent complications include bleeding (hematoma) and infection. If blood accumulates at the operative or donor site, a brief trip to the operating room is necessary to drain the hematoma. Antibiotics are frequently used to minimize the problem of infection. The development of venous clots in the legs or pelvic region is a rare but serious complication. These clots can potentially travel to the lungs (pulmonary embolus). If clots develop, the woman will be placed on *anticoagulants* (blood thinners). In addition, the patient should be encouraged to resume some activity right away, actively exercising her leg muscles when she is in bed and getting out of bed and attempting to walk the day after surgery. While she is inactive in bed, compression stockings are recommended.

Because the TRAM flap is obtained from the abdominal wall, there is some chance of a hernia developing. This complication is now reported to occur in less than 2% of patients having this operation. As a preventive measure to strengthen the abdominal wall and reduce the possibility of hernia, the reconstructive surgeon may place a sheet of mesh or of acellular dermal matrix over the site where the strip of abdominal muscle is removed. Mesh substantially reduces the risk of a bulge or hernia developing. If a hernia does develop, mesh may also be used to repair it, and this can be done at the time of the nipple reconstruction.

Hospitalization, Pain, and Recuperation

This procedure is done with the patient under general anesthesia and requires a hospital stay of 3 to 6 days. This operation is potentially more painful and uncomfortable than any of the other methods of breast reconstruction, especially in the abdominal area. The recent improvements in pain management using thin catheters placed into the wound through which local anesthetic can be administered, have made a major difference in the recovery from these operations.

Because the surgeon removes a strip of lower abdominal tissue during surgery, the abdomen is tighter and the woman feels a distinct pull. It may be difficult for the patient to stand upright until the muscle is stretched out again. A day or two after the operation when she is ready to eat, she may notice that she gets full quickly, because the abdomen is tighter. During the first week after surgery, most patients report soreness and pain in the abdominal area; movement is initially difficult and quite uncomfortable, but most patients are able to cope with basic activities of daily living within a few days. As with most operations, each patient has a different tolerance level for pain; some patients take very little if any pain medication, whereas others may experience a great deal of pain and require analgesics for several weeks. The discomfort involved in a TRAM flap has been compared by patients to the pain experienced after an abdominal hysterectomy or a cesarean section.

The patient usually can get out of bed the first day after the operation, but it takes another 1 to 2 weeks before she can stand fully upright. Recuperation is somewhat slower with this operation than with the implant procedures discussed earlier. Most women find that they can gradually resume normal basic activities within the first 4 weeks after returning home but that it takes 4 to 6 weeks before they are ready to return to work. Usually they are able to participate in sporting activities within 3 to 6 months.

Few functional problems exist after transfer of the rectus abdominis muscle. Most patients can return to the same level of activity as before the operation. They can also usually perform athletic activities at the same level and intensity as before. A preoperative and postoperative exercise program helps strengthen the abdominal wall muscles and makes recovery less difficult. Although sit-ups sometimes may be difficult and women may have to push up when rising from the reclining position, most athletic activities can be continued without difficulty, and many women have returned to tennis, golf, swimming and jogging.

Skin-Sparing Mastectomy and Immediate Breast Reconstruction With a TRAM Flap

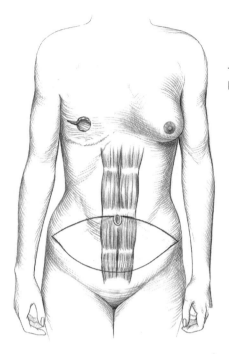

TRAM flap designed on lower abdomen

Abdominal tissue transferred to breast area while still attached to abdominal muscle (rectus abdominis)

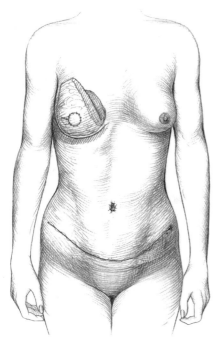

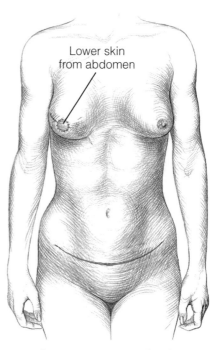

Abdominal tissue fashioned into
a breast and lower abdomen closed
as a transverse scar

Lower skin
from abdomen

Breast reconstructed and
short incision (encircling areola
with side extension) closed

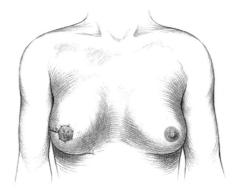

Nipple-areola reconstructed several months later

Modified Radical Mastectomy and Breast Reconstruction
With a TRAM Flap

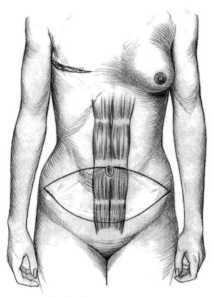

TRAM flap designed on
the lower abdomen

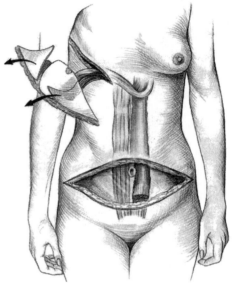

Abdominal tissue transferred to
breast area while still attached
to abdominal muscle

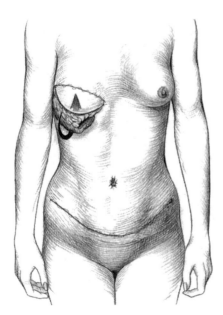

Abdominal tissue fashioned into a
breast and lower abdomen closed
with a transverse (tummy tuck) scar

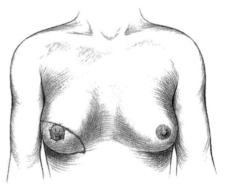

Nipple-areola reconstructed
several months later

Results With the TRAM Flap

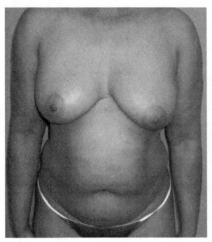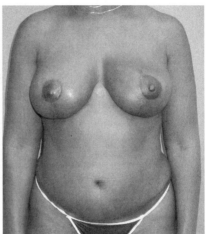

After being diagnosed with right breast cancer, this 40-year-old woman had a right modified radical mastectomy using a skin-sparing technique and immediate breast reconstruction with a TRAM flap. She subsequently had a left breast lift and right nipple reconstruction. The reconstructed left nipple was tattooed to create the areola. She is shown 1 year later.

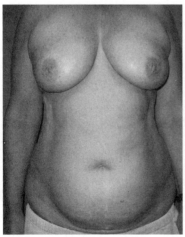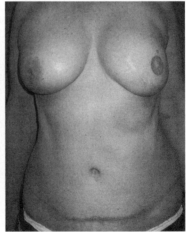

This 54-year-old woman had a modified radical mastectomy to treat the breast cancer in her left breast followed by immediate breast reconstruction with a TRAM flap. Although her opposite breast was heavy, she did not wish to have any corrective surgery on it. She is shown 1 year later. Her nipple-areola was re-constructed with a local flap and a tattoo.

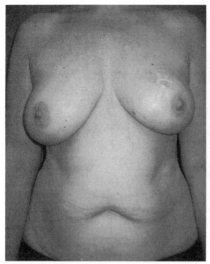 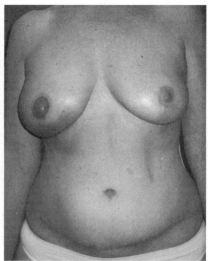

This 55-year-old woman had cancer of the right breast. She had a modified radical mastectomy with skin-sparing incisions and immediate reconstruction with a TRAM flap. The TRAM flap was shaped to match her normal opposite breast. She is shown 1 year after breast reconstruction. Her nipple-areola was reconstructed with a local flap and a tattoo.

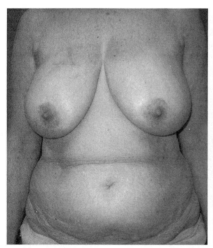 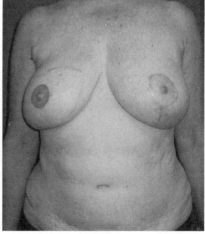

After cancer of the right breast was diagnosed, this 58-year-old woman had a skin-sparing mastectomy with shorter incisions and immediate breast reconstruction with a TRAM flap. The tissue from the abdomen was used to replace the breast tissue and a round piece of the abdominal wall skin was used to fill the defect left after the nipple-areola was removed. She is shown 6 months after breast reconstruction. Her droopy left breast was reduced and lifted to match the reconstructed right side.

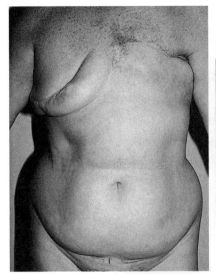

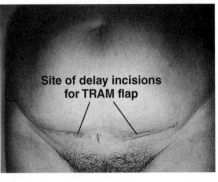

Site of delay incisions for TRAM flap

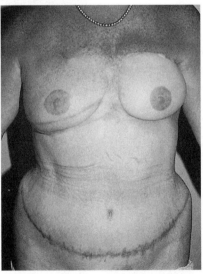

This 58-year-old woman had a modified radical mastectomy and postoperative radiation therapy for cancer of the left breast. She had a history of cigarette smoking and was somewhat overweight. Subsequently, a second breast cancer developed and she had a left modified radical mastectomy. She decided to have delayed breast reconstruction. Because of her risk factors, she had a TRAM flap vascular delay in which two lower abdominal wall incisions were made 1 week before the main TRAM flap breast reconstruction. She is shown 1 year after bilateral reconstruction. Her nipple-areolas were reconstructed with local flaps and tattoos.

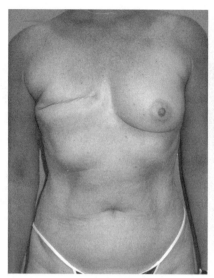 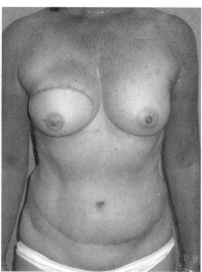

This 40-year-old woman had a right modified radical mastectomy followed by chemotherapy and radiation. She requested breast reconstruction with her own tissues. She had delayed reconstruction of her right breast with a TRAM flap to match her remaining breast. She is shown 1 year after breast reconstruction.

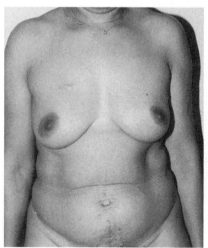 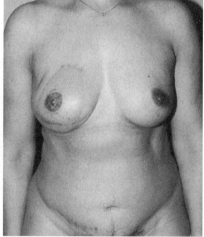

This 48-year-old woman had a modified radical mastectomy of her right breast followed by immediate TRAM breast reconstruction. Three months later liposuction was used to contour her upper abdomen and breast. Her nipple-areola was also reconstructed and later tattooed. She is shown 2 years after breast reconstruction.

RECONSTRUCTION WITH THE
LATISSIMUS DORSI (BACK) FLAP

A latissimus dorsi flap technique is selected when additional tissue is needed to rebuild mastectomy defects. This is a safe, reliable flap with a good blood supply, and endoscopic surgery offers the advantage of leaving minimal scars. The latissimus dorsi flap is most often used when the reconstructed breast needs to be large or ptotic to match the opposite one, the patient does not want a TRAM flap or a TRAM flap would pose too much risk and prolonged recovery. Because it has a long track record of safety and predictability, many surgeons feel comfortable recommending it.

With this procedure, a skin and muscle (musculocutaneous) flap or sometimes only muscle is transferred from a woman's back around to the breast area to replace the skin and chest muscle removed during mastectomy or partial mastectomy. The latissimus dorsi flap provides functioning, healthy muscle tissue for covering an implant or expander, for filling the hollow areas in the chest wall area, and for recreating the anterior axillary fold.

Adding additional skin to the chest wall area also permits the formation of a more naturally shaped, fuller, larger breast than could be created by just implant placement or tissue expansion. The healthy skin added is often thicker and of better quality than the thin, expanded skin. This muscle and skin (musculocutaneous) flap is also useful for patients who have skin grafts or very tight or irradiated skin. Many women prefer a donor scar on their back or side to a scar on their remaining breast, which would be necessary to adjust it to match the expanded breast reconstruction.

Extended Autologous Latissimus Dorsi Flap

Sometimes a woman's breast can be reconstructed entirely with the back tissue without a breast implant. This autologous latissimus dorsi flap reconstruction is used when the woman has excess back tissue, especially in her midback, or if she does not have a particularly large breast. In the past additional volume was harvested by using a progressively larger skin island. It is now appreciated that in heavier patients, a significant part of the fat between the skin and the muscle can be safely harvested (or removed) with the muscle as an extended autologous latissimus dorsi flap. A modest skin island is raised but the fat is then preserved for a varying thickness over most of the muscle to allow for a substantial increase in volume without the use of an implant. This results in a less tight back donor site closure as well as providing an implant-free reconstruction. The procedure has been widely accepted and has resulted in a resurgence of interest in this very reliable muscle flap reconstruction. It is particularly suitable for a patient who is too heavy for a TRAM flap or another abdominal flap procedure. The latissimus dorsi muscle alone can be used for immediate breast reconstruction to enhance implant cover or can be transferred with some additional skin to replace missing skin.

Oncoplastic Technique With Latissimus Dorsi Muscle and Fat Flap

Latissimus dorsi muscle (back) and fat flaps may also be used to fill localized defects within the breast after lumpectomy and quadrantectomy. (See p. 259 for a discussion of oncoplastic procedures.) This reconstructive procedure extends the application of breast preservation to women who require larger areas of breast tissue removed during breast-conserving surgery. After the lumpectomy or quadrantectomy is done, the breast surgeon or oncologic surgeon checks the margins of resection to ensure complete tumor removal. He also assesses the area of tumor excision to determine whether it will leave an unsatisfactory breast shape or size after healing and/or radiation therapy. If so, the volume of the breast may be restored with the latissimus dorsi back tissues. In this situation, the reconstructive surgeon uses an endoscopic technique to harvest a flap of latissimus muscle and its overlying fat through the incisions used for the primary local cancer treatment. This flap is then used to fill and contour the defect remaining after the breast-conserving procedure. This technique is also useful for secondary breast deformities that require some additional tissue.

Surgical Procedure and Postoperative Appearance

Reconstruction with the latissimus dorsi flap is a longer, more complex procedure than techniques using local tissue or tissue expansion. This operation takes between 2 to 4 hours to perform. Since the operation is longer and there is additional back pain, it is done with the patient under general anesthesia, and hospitalization is required.

When using the latissimus dorsi flap for breast replacement, the plastic surgeon designs a skin island over the muscle or midback, hidden in the natural skin lines. He then separates the latissimus dorsi muscle from its deep attachments and frees it with its attached skin from the back. This muscle-skin flap remains attached to its nourishing vessel, a main artery in the armpit area that the surgical oncologist saves during the mastectomy. The flap is now ready to be transferred to the chest area.

When an immediate reconstruction is being performed, the recipient mastectomy site has already been prepared to accept the flap, and more skin can be preserved to shape the new breast and shorten the mastectomy scar. For a delayed reconstruction, the plastic surgeon must first remove the mastectomy scar (if it is in an inconspicuous position) or create a new incision to accept the flap and permit a more aesthetic reconstruction. Next the flap is rotated to the front of the chest through a tunnel created high in the underarm so that it extends through to the opening left by the mastectomy incision or by removal of the mastectomy scar. The incision on the back donor site is then closed. The flap is adjusted for the most aesthetic appearance and sutured to the front of the chest; the latissimus dorsi muscle is stitched to the pectoralis major muscle, and back skin is stitched to breast skin to supplement deficient tissue in this area. An opening is left in the outer part of the incision for the insertion of a breast implant or tissue expander to provide a breast shape symmetrical with the opposite remaining breast. The surgeon positions the upper part of the expander under the chest wall muscle (pectoralis major) above and the lower part is covered by the back muscle (latissimus dorsi). When skin is needed, it replaces the skin removed during the mastectomy. If necessary, a postoperatively adjustable implant is placed to permit accurate postoperative sizing. The surgeon then closes the incision. The nipple-areola is created during a later operation that is performed with a local anesthetic.

Endoscopic Technique for Flap Harvest

With the endoscopic technique for harvesting latissimus dorsi back muscle and fat, the surgeon uses the incisions made at the time of primary cancer treatment, which are usually in the lateral breast region and in the underarm area (where the axillary lymph node dissection was done). A video camera is attached to the endoscope and the image is displayed on the monitor for the surgeon to see while he operates using special long instruments that are inserted through the small incisions. The endoscope permits a video image of tissues beneath the skin to be projected on the video monitor through fiberoptic light. Separate incisions about 1 inch long may also be needed in the mid to lower back. Through these small incisions the surgeon visualizes the area with the use of the endoscope, dissects the flap, which contains fat and muscle, preserves the blood supply to the tissue, and moves the flap through the underarm to the front of the chest for the breast reconstruction.

Skin-Sparing Mastectomy and Immediate Latissimus Dorsi Flap Breast Reconstruction With Tissue Expansion

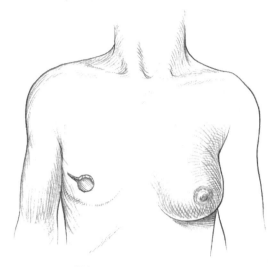

Skin-sparing mastectomy

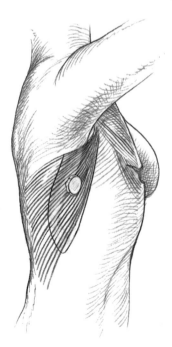

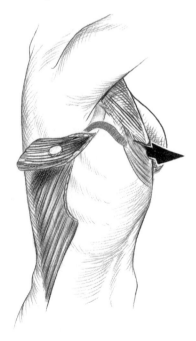

Latissimus dorsi flap designed
on the side for harvest of
latissimus dorsi muscle

Latissimus dorsi muscle
elevated for transfer to the chest
wall for coverage of the
tissue expander

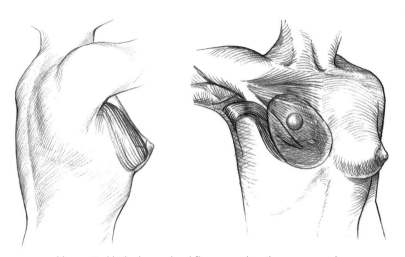

Harvested latissimus dorsi flap covering tissue expander

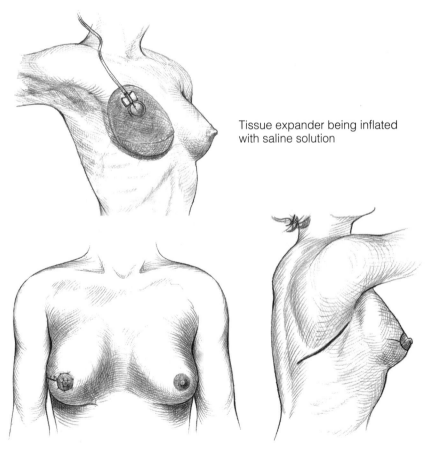

Tissue expander being inflated with saline solution

Nipple-areola reconstructed several months later

Skin-Sparing Mastectomy and Immediate Endoscopic Latissimus Dorsi Flap Reconstruction With Tissue Expansion

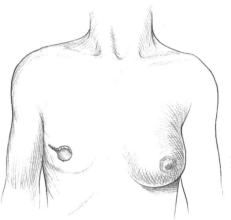

Skin-sparing mastectomy

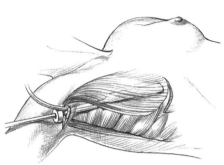

Endoscope used for pectoral muscle release through an axillary incision for breast reconstruction with expander or implant

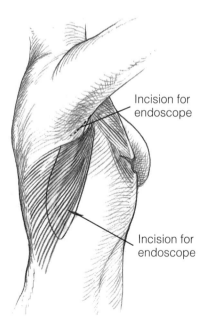

Incision for endoscope

Incision for endoscope

Latissimus dorsi flap designed on the side with incisions shown for endoscopic harvest of latissimus dorsi muscle

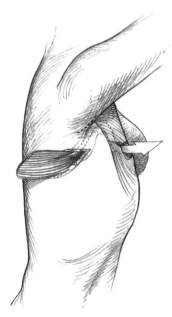

Latissimus dorsi muscle elevated for transfer to the chest wall for coverage of the tissue expander

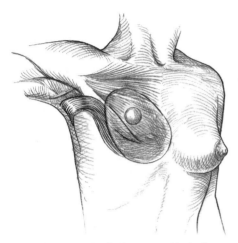

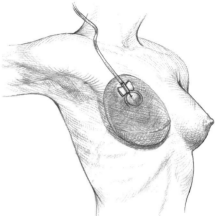

Endoscopically harvested latissimus
dorsi flap covering tissue expander

Tissue expander being inflated
with saline solution

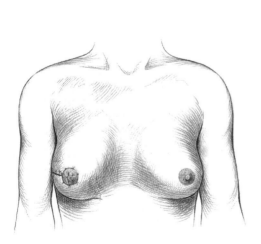

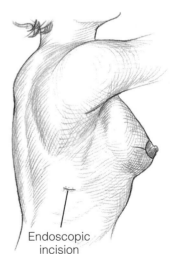

Endoscopic
incision

Nipple-areola reconstructed several months later

Breast Reconstruction With Latissimus Dorsi Flap and Tissue Expansion

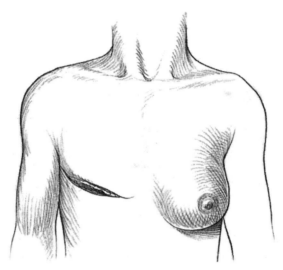

Modified radical mastectomy scar opened

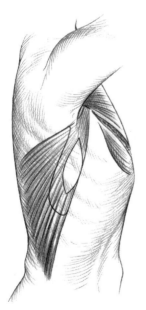

Latissimus dorsi flap designed
on the back

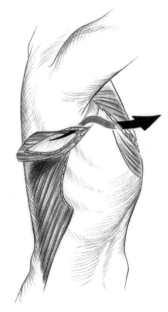

Skin and strip of latissimus dorsi
muscle elevated on side of chest

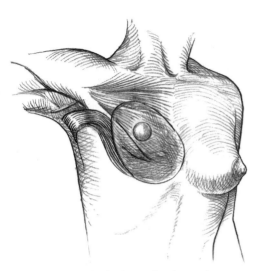

Latissimus dorsi muscle
covering a textured anatomic-shaped
expander

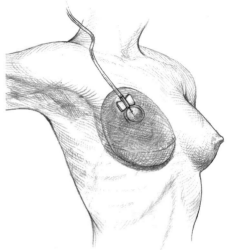

Textured anatomic-shaped expander
with integral valve inflated
with saline solution

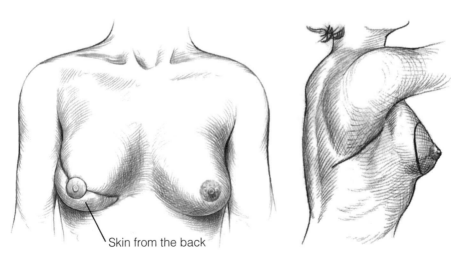

Skin from the back

Nipple-areola reconstructed several months later

Breast Reconstruction With Extended Autologous Latissimus Dorsi Flap Without an Implant

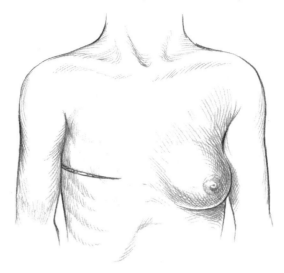

Modified radical mastectomy

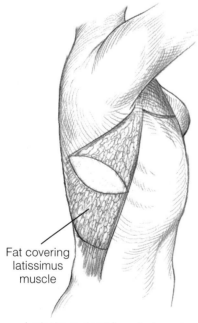

Fat covering
latissimus
muscle

Latissimus dorsi flap designed
on the back

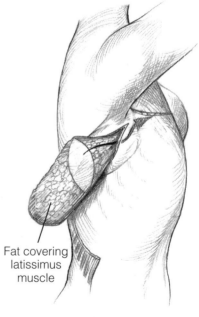

Fat covering
latissimus
muscle

Autologous latissimus dorsi skin and
muscle flap elevated from the back

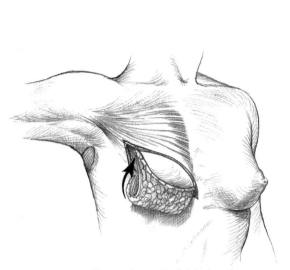

Fat and muscle folded under
and fashioned into a breast

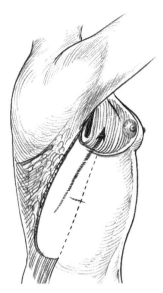

Autologous latissimus dorsi
flap inset

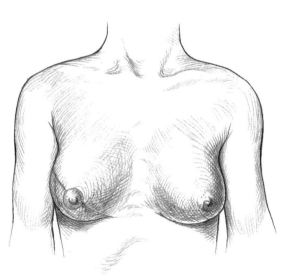

Nipple-areola reconstructed several months later

Partial Oncoplastic Breast Reconstruction With an Endoscopic Latissimus Dorsi Flap

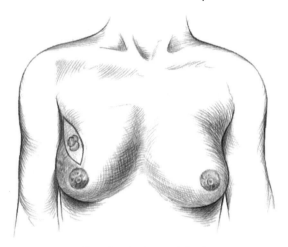

Quadrantectomy defect

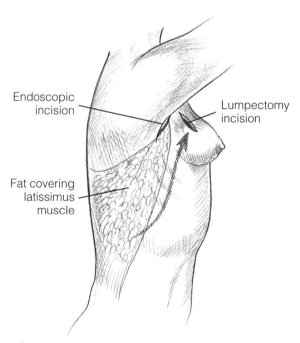

Harvesting of the latissimus dorsi muscle and fat through short endoscopic incisions to fill in a large lumpectomy or quadrantectomy defect

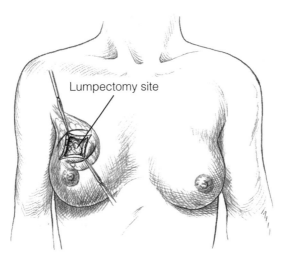

Endoscopically harvested latissimus dorsi flap in place in the upper quadrant of the breast after a large partial mastectomy

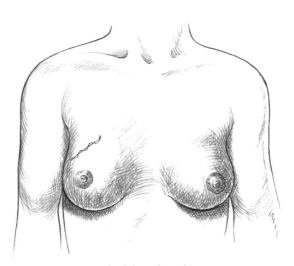

Incision closed

Reconstruction with a latissimus dorsi flap leaves a donor scar on the patient's back (under her bra line) or on her side (in a diagonal line under her upper arm) and additional scars on her breast when the flap is placed into the breast area. When an immediate reconstruction is performed, the skin island can be used to replace the missing nipple-areola skin as a circular skin disk from which the nipple can be fashioned subsequently. In delayed reconstructions, the entire almond-shaped skin island from the back is used to recreate the front of the breast, resulting in longer scars.

The reconstructed breast may be somewhat rounder and firmer than the normal breast. In addition, the woman may have a slight bulge under her arm where the latissimus dorsi flap was tunneled through to her chest area. This bulge will shrink with time as the muscle atrophies with inactivity, but it will not completely disappear. This fullness is usually positioned in the axillary region to reduce the hollowness after axillary lymph node removal.

Postoperative Care

After the operation, the plastic surgeon inserts surgical drains into the reconstructed breast and back area to remove excess fluid from the operative site. Patients are advised to expect significant drainage as a normal part of the recovery process, particularly with this flap. The reconstructive surgeon usually recommends that the back drain remain in place even after the patient goes home and until the drainage is less than an ounce (30 ml) a day. This drainage can sometimes last several weeks. It is advisable for the woman to limit shoulder or arm activity, because this tends to increase the fluid drainage. The other specifics of postoperative care such as stitches, dressings, and restrictions on activity are similar to the postoperative instructions for patients whose breasts are reconstructed with implants (see p. 273).

Problems and Complications

Fluid collection in the back is a common problem after latissimus dorsi flap surgery. Sometimes fluid can accumulate after the drains are removed; it usually is reabsorbed by the body and disappears after several weeks. When this fluid buildup becomes uncomfortable, the surgeon may need to drain it with a syringe or reinsert a drain. Blood accumulation (hematoma) in the operative sites of the breast or back is an unusual complication. When it occurs, usually during the first 24 hours after the operation, the patient needs to be returned to the operating room to correct this by removing the blood. Infection is also rare, and the surgeon will ordinarily prescribe antibiotics to lessen the chance of infection. Problems with the blood supply to a portion of the latissimus dorsi flap have occurred in about 2% of patients, usually in women who have had radiation treatments after mastectomy. When this complication occurs, it may require delaying implant placement or selection of another reconstructive technique. Complete loss of the latissimus dorsi flap because of poor blood supply has been seen in less than 1% of patients. In such a case, another method of breast reconstruction will be necessary.

Jumping Breast Phenomenon

When the latissimus flap is brought around to the chest from the back, it is attached by its blood vessels as well as its motor nerve, which enables the muscle to move. Many surgeons cut the nerve routinely, leaving the blood vessels intact. Others leave the nerve intact as well as the vessels in an effort to prevent the muscle from shrinking too much, which can result in a progressive volume loss and asymmetry over time. Unfortunately, an intact nerve means that in some patients, arm motion, such as pulling the arm backward, stimulates the nerve to the latissimus dorsi and causes it to twitch or contract on the front of the chest wall. This looks like a "jumping breast." If it continues to be a problem, it is possible for the surgeon to go back under the armpit, find the nerve, and cut it to eliminate the problem. Some muscle shrinkage will then occur, however, and the size of the reconstructed breast may decrease a little.

Hospitalization, Pain, and Recuperation

Hospitalization of 2 to 3 days is required. This operation is more painful than reconstruction with implant placement. There is normally some pain in the back and underarm area where the flap was taken. The back and arm areas are sore for 2 to 3 weeks; the pain subsides as the arm regains motion. The drains are also usually uncomfortable and occasionally painful, particularly when they are removed. This discomfort is similar to that experienced after a mastectomy.

The patient requires 3 to 6 weeks before returning to work and 2 to 4 months before resuming exercise or sports such as aerobics, tennis, and golf. If the woman's anterior axillary fold has been re-created, she needs to avoid strenuous arm activity for 6 to 8 weeks while this area heals.

Latissimus dorsi flap reconstruction generally does not cause loss of arm and shoulder function, even though a muscle has been used. The muscle is still functional. It is simply transferred to the front of the body to provide tissue for rebuilding the breast. Some women report, however, that the muscle transfer makes it more difficult for them to keep their shoulder erect on the side of the muscle transfer. Exercise will help alleviate but may not totally eliminate this problem.

Results With the Latissimus Dorsi Flap

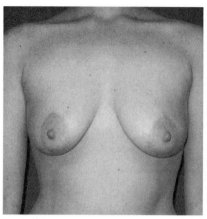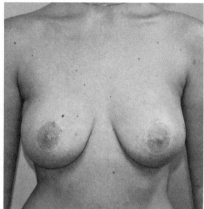

Because this young woman was found to have the *BRCA1* gene, she opted for bilateral prophylactic mastectomies and immediate reconstruction using bilateral latissimus flaps with implant insertion. She is shown 18 months after surgery with excellent breast shape and symmetry.

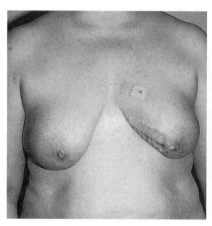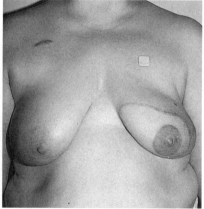

When cancer was detected in the upper-inner quadrant of this 48-year-old woman's left breast, she requested treatment with a lumpectomy. However, after two local resections were unsuccessful in obtaining clear margins, a mastectomy was performed. She had an immediate breast reconstruction with a latissimus dorsi musculocutaneous flap and the fat over the muscle. No implant was required. Her nipple-areola was later reconstructed with a local flap and a tattoo. She is shown 1 year after breast reconstruction.

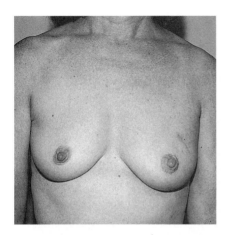

This 38-year-old woman with reasonably symmetrical breasts requested a lumpectomy to treat the cancer in the upper-outer quadrant of her left breast. To get a local resection with clear margins, the entire breast quadrant was removed, as well as some additional tissue from beneath the nipple-areola. The significant deformity that remained was filled in with harvested latissimus dorsi muscle using endoscopic techniques that created no additional breast scars. She is shown 1 year after partial breast reconstruction and subsequent radiation therapy.

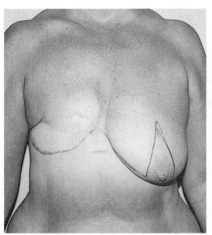

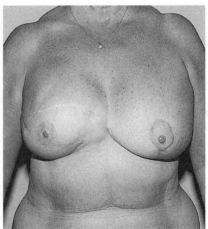

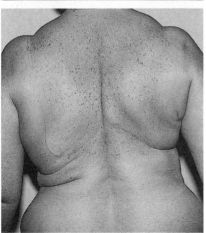

This 58-year-old woman had a modified radical mastectomy of her right breast and delayed breast reconstruction with a latissimus dorsi flap. Her opposite breast was ptotic and heavy, and she requested a reduction mammaplasty for symmetry. She is shown 1 year after breast reconstruction and reduction mammaplasty of her opposite breast. Her nipple-areola was reconstructed with a local flap and a tattoo.

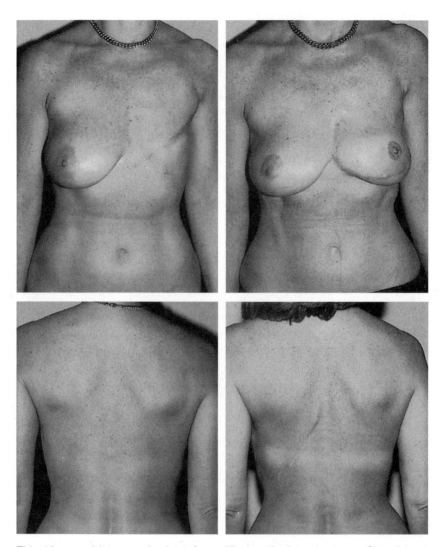

This 42-year-old woman had a left modified radical mastectomy. She did not want a lower abdominal scar and opted for a delayed breast reconstruction with a latissimus dorsi flap and a tissue expander. Her other breast was reduced for symmetry. She is shown 2 years after breast reconstruction.

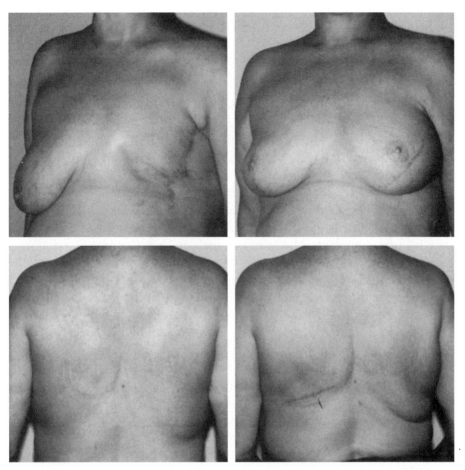

This 48-year-old woman had a left modified radical mastectomy. She is shown 2 years after delayed latissimus dorsi flap breast reconstruction with tissue expansion, nipple-areola reconstruction, and reduction mammaplasty of the right breast.

MICROSURGICAL BREAST RECONSTRUCTION

One of the more significant advances in reconstructive surgery during the past 25 years became a reality when surgeons began to suture and repair tiny blood vessels under the magnification of the operating microscope. This skill enables surgeons to move tissues from one part of the body where there is an excess of tissue to a deficient area that needs rebuilding. Because these flaps of autologous tissue are separated and freed from the donor site and transferred to the new area where the blood vessels are reattached, they are often referred to as free flaps. This technique brings added choices to breast reconstruction. The reconstructive surgeon can rebuild a woman's breast by transferring her own fully mobilized tissues usually without the need for a breast implant. The most common and popular free flap donor tissues are the lower abdominal (TRAM and DIEP) and the buttock skin and muscle (gluteus maximus, SGAP and IGAP) flaps; they provide abundant tissue for a well-contoured reconstructed breast from a donor site that is often enhanced by tissue sculpting. The latissimus dorsi free flap is also a possibility but is used less frequently because abdominal and buttock free flaps provide more abundant tissue with more acceptable donor sites for the patient. The lateral hip region can be used if the TRAM flap tissue has already been used. The upper inner thigh or outer thigh can be used for free flaps. While most women find the donor site contour and visible scars of the outer thigh flap to be objectionable, they are generally very accepting of the inner thigh scars from transverse upper gracilis/transverse myocutaneous gracilis (TUG/TMG) muscle flap harvest.

The freedom and flexibility that microsurgical breast reconstruction offers is balanced in part by the level of surgical support and expertise required. This is the most complex and demanding of all of the reconstructive procedures. It also takes longer to perform with the attendant risks of greater blood loss, and usually requires a more extended hospitalization and recuperation period than implant or expander breast reconstruction. It is not for an inexperienced surgeon or a patient who desires a simple, easy route to breast restoration. The patient should fully understand the extensive nature of this operation before she selects it. She needs to be physically and psychologically prepared for the extended convalescence it requires. Even under the best of circumstances these techniques are not 100% successful. Since the standard pedicle latissimus dorsi flap and TRAM flap have more than 99% reliability, if a free flap is chosen, the surgeon should have a high level of expertise and success with the technique, because if complications of blood flow develop, a reoperation will be needed and the transferred tissue can be lost. The patient should have an idea of the surgeon's success rate with this operation before choosing it. The best centers should quote a success rate of about 98%.

Immediate free flap reconstruction has some advantages over delayed free flap reconstruction: there is less scarring, and the patient goes to sleep with a breast and wakes up with a breast.

For microsurgery to be successful, a woman should be healthy and have normal blood vessels. Excess scarring and radiation to these vessels may reduce the chance of a successful result. Patients with radiation damage to the chest wall and patients in whom previous flaps have failed are prime candidates for free flap breast reconstruction, as are women in whom the traditional pedicle TRAM or latissimus dorsi flap is unavailable or inadequate. This would include women with abdominal scarring that precludes the TRAM flap or patients in whom the nerve and blood supply to the latissimus dorsi muscle has been severed or the area damaged by radiation. Some women choose these techniques simply to preserve as much abdominal muscle function as possible. It is also crucially important for a woman who desires this technique to have a skilled microsurgeon experienced in performing microsurgical breast reconstruction with an equally skillful and experienced breast management team.

TRAM FREE FLAP

The TRAM flap is usually the first choice when additional tissue is needed for breast reconstruction. Sometimes the TRAM flap cannot be transferred safely in the usual manner; that is, by moving the lower abdominal tissue to the breast region while maintaining its blood supply within the strips of the rectus abdominis muscle. When the abdominal wall is scarred or when the upper abdominal vessels are judged not to have sufficient blood supply to keep the lower abdominal tissues alive, as in the woman with a long-standing history of cigarette smoking or the woman who is overweight with evidence of diminished flow from the vessels from the upper abdominal muscle (rectus abdominis), then a TRAM free flap is indicated. Some surgeons experienced with this technique advocate it for most TRAM flaps.

Surgical Procedure and Postoperative Appearance

Reconstruction with the TRAM free flap is a major operation and takes approximately 3 to 8 hours in the operating room, on some occasions even longer. As with the pedicle TRAM flap, this operation can only be done once, and the patient should be advised that if another breast reconstruction is needed at a later date, another technique and tissue source will have to be used.

The operation for an immediate breast reconstruction with a TRAM free flap is basically the same as that for the delayed TRAM free flap reconstruction. Technically it is an easier operation because the axillary vessels are already freed up and there is no scarring.

The TRAM free flap is designed on the lower abdomen, similar to the design used for the standard TRAM flap. After the flap from the lower abdomen is transferred to the breast region, the vessels in the lower portion of the abdominal flap are sutured into the blood vessels of the armpit region under the operating microscope. When an immediate reconstruction is being performed, the recipient mastectomy site has already been prepared to accept the flap and more skin can be preserved to shape the new breast and shorten the mastectomy scar. For a delayed reconstruction, the chest wall is prepared by removing and reopening the mastectomy incision (if it is in an inconspicuous position) or creating a new incision that will permit a more aesthetic reconstruction. The flap is then transferred to the chest wall area. The highly technical hookup of the small vessels of the flap to the breast region is performed under the magnification of the operating microscope.

The skin and fatty tissue of the flap is shaped and inset to form a breast mound to match the other breast. The breasts are checked for symmetry and shape, and the flap is stitched into place. The nipple-areola reconstruction is performed in a second or a third procedure, depending on the amount of contouring that still needs to be done to the reconstructed breast.

Microsurgery can also be combined with the pedicle TRAM flap. This has been called the "supercharged" or "turbo" TRAM flap. With this procedure the lower blood vessels, along with a strip of lower abdominal muscle, are transferred for the reconstruction, and these blood vessels are hooked into the blood vessels of the armpit region or under the ribs next to the breast bone, using an operating microscope. Sometimes just suturing a vein or artery in conjunction with a standard TRAM flap is adequate for this supercharged approach. The results of this procedure are similar to those of the traditional TRAM flap with its pedicle intact.

Results of this procedure are quite acceptable, but as with the immediate pedicle TRAM flap, the woman must be fully prepared for the donor deformity and scar and the additional breast scars required for placing the TRAM flap.

The description of the scars and postoperative appearance for a free TRAM flap is similar to that described on pp. 292-293 for the standard pedicle TRAM flap.

Skin-Sparing Mastectomy and Immediate Breast Reconstruction With a TRAM Free Flap

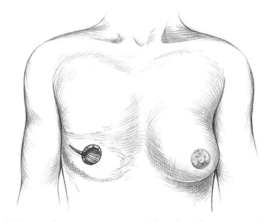

Skin-sparing mastectomy deformity after removal of the breast and nipple-areola

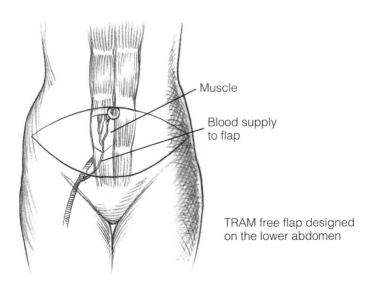

Muscle

Blood supply to flap

TRAM free flap designed on the lower abdomen

Skin-Sparing Mastectomy and Immediate Breast Reconstruction With a TRAM Free Flap—cont'd

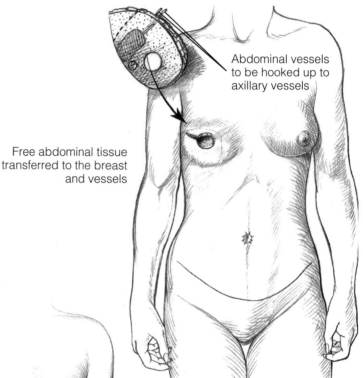

Abdominal vessels to be hooked up to axillary vessels

Free abdominal tissue transferred to the breast and vessels

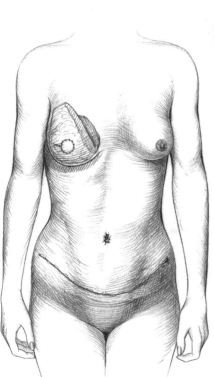

Abdominal tissue fashioned into a breast and lower abdomen closed as a transverse scar

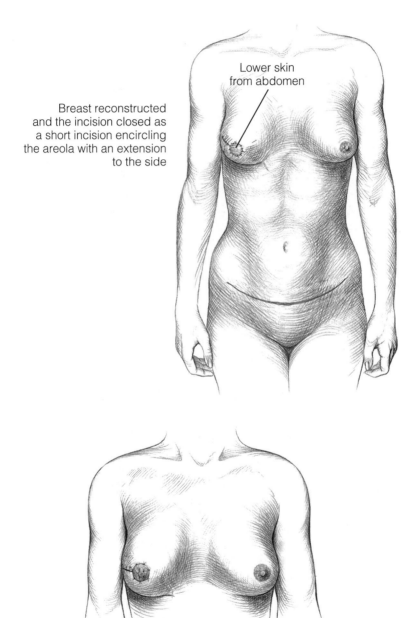

Breast reconstructed
and the incision closed as
a short incision encircling
the areola with an extension
to the side

Lower skin
from abdomen

Nipple-areola reconstructed several months later

Delayed Breast Reconstruction With a TRAM Free Flap

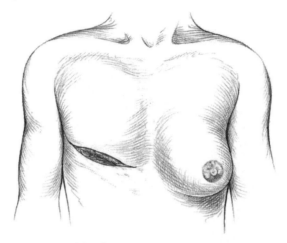

Modified radical mastectomy

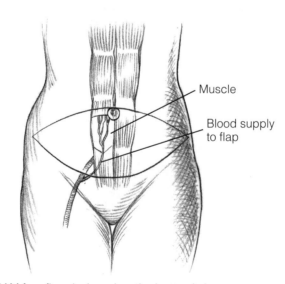

TRAM free flap designed on the lower abdomen

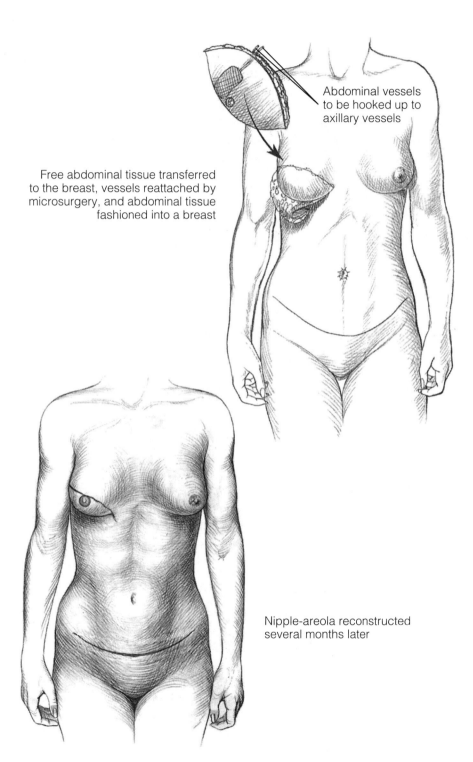

Abdominal vessels to be hooked up to axillary vessels

Free abdominal tissue transferred to the breast, vessels reattached by microsurgery, and abdominal tissue fashioned into a breast

Nipple-areola reconstructed several months later

Postoperative Care

As with the standard TRAM flap, drains are placed in the breast and abdominal areas for 3 to 4 days after the operation. The drains are usually removed before the patient leaves the hospital and after the antibiotics have been discontinued. Sometimes serum accumulates in the donor defects and may need to be drained during a subsequent office visit after the patient has been released from the hospital. For the first few days postoperatively, antibiotics are administered to all patients undergoing microsurgical breast reconstruction. Cigarette smoking and exposure to environmental tobacco smoke are prohibited during the postoperative period.

A primary concern of the reconstructive surgeon in the postoperative period after a TRAM free flap is that the vessels are open and the transferred tissue is maintaining a good blood supply. The color, blood supply, and temperature of the flap are carefully monitored postoperatively. Many surgeons will implant a Doppler probe (a device that measures blood flow) near the blood vessels of the flap so that blood flow can be checked postoperatively with an audible signal it produces. The probe is simply pulled out before the patient leaves the hospital. The blood supply to the flap can also be assessed by checking the appearance of the flap and by pricking the flap with needles to test for blood flow. If it is determined that the flow to the flap has stopped, this necessitates an immediate return to the operating room to reexplore the vessels and repair the problem.

Problems and Complications

The potential for blood clots in the leg may be somewhat greater with microsurgical reconstruction because of the length of this operation and the fact that the dissection is nearer the veins in the pelvis. To protect the transferred vessels the patient's upper extremity movements are restricted for 5 to 6 days after the operation.

Hospitalization, Pain, and Recuperation

A hospital stay of 3 to 5 days is required. Since the muscle is not attached and less muscle is removed with a TRAM free flap, there is usually less abdominal pain. The patient usually can get out of bed 1 to 2 days after the operation, but it can take several weeks before she can stand fully upright. Most women gradually resume normal, basic activities over the next 4 to 6 weeks. They can often return to work in 4 to 6 weeks and participate in sports in 3 to 6 months.

All other aspects of postoperative care, potential complications, and recuperation for the TRAM free flap are similar to those described for the standard TRAM flap and implant reconstruction.

Results With the TRAM Free Flap

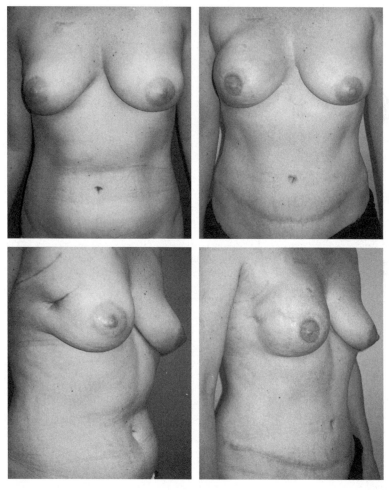

This young woman had a skin-sparing mastectomy for a breast cancer in the lateral aspect of her right breast. This was followed by immediate reconstruction with a free TRAM flap. She later had radiation therapy to the breast. She is shown one year after completion of radiation therapy.

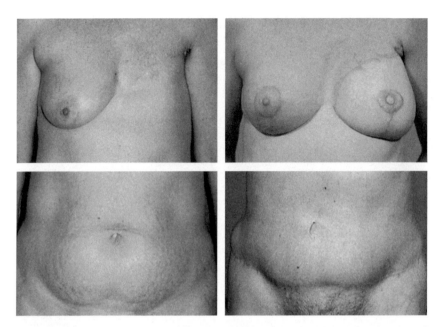

After a left modified radical mastectomy, this 52-year-old woman requested delayed breast reconstruction with a TRAM flap. Because most of her lower abdominal fat and skin would be required to match her opposite breast, a TRAM free flap was selected to provide additional volume. At a second operation her nipple-areola was reconstructed, and a mastopexy (breast lift) was performed on the opposite breast to improve breast symmetry. She is shown 10 months after her nipple-areola reconstruction and mastopexy.

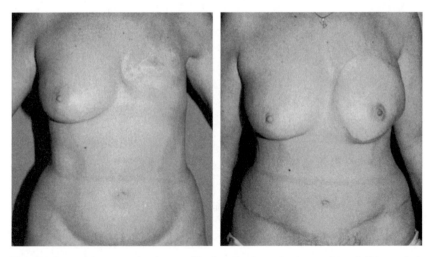

This 54-year-old woman had a modified radical mastectomy of her left breast. A pedicle TRAM flap breast reconstruction was ruled out because she was a heavy smoker. She is shown 1 year after delayed TRAM free flap breast reconstruction.

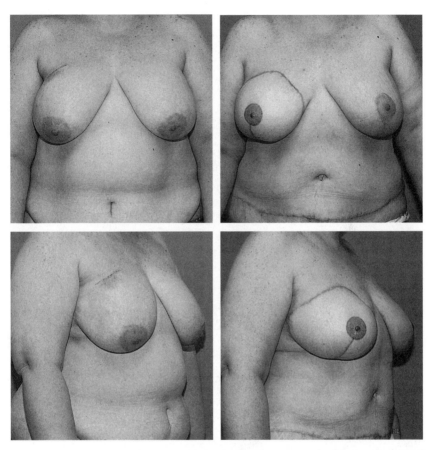

This 36-year-old overweight woman had a breast cancer in the upper pole of her right breast. She had a modified radical mastectomy, followed by immediate free TRAM flap breast reconstruction. Her risk factors included smoking and obesity, and the need for a large skin surface and breast volume. She healed with excellent breast symmetry after opposite breast reduction.

MUSCLE-SPARING FREE TRAM FLAP

Many surgeons are now using a hybrid of the DIEP (abdominal perfora-tor) flap and the free TRAM flap that is known as a muscle-sparing free TRAM flap. This is particularly appropriate for smokers and patients with diabetes or other high risk factors. With this approach, a small but insignificant piece of muscle is used; this technique enables several perforators to be incorporated into the flap without as much time-consuming dissection. This variant tends to be predictable and less prone to fat necrosis. Recovery, pain, postoperative care and complications are similar to that experienced with a free TRAM flap.

Skin-Sparing Mastectomy and Immediate Breast Reconstruction With a Muscle-Sparing Free TRAM Flap

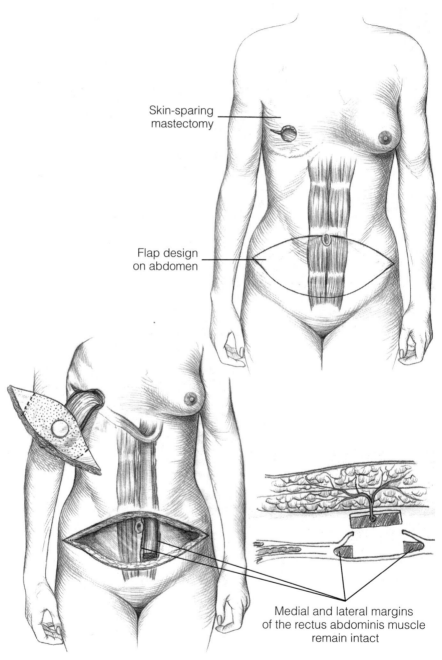

Skin-sparing
mastectomy

Flap design
on abdomen

Medial and lateral margins
of the rectus abdominis muscle
remain intact

Flap transferred to the breast area

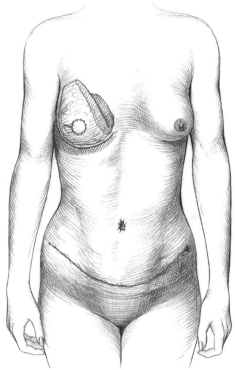

Abdominal tissue
fashioned into a breast

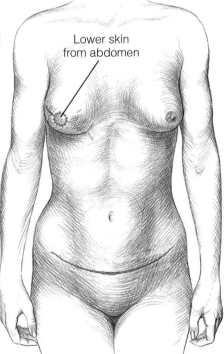

Lower skin
from abdomen

Nipple-areola reconstructed
several months later

Results With the Muscle-Sparing Free TRAM Flap

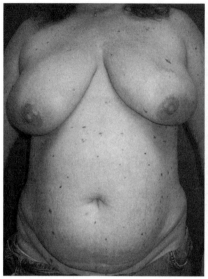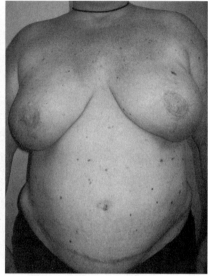

This 30-year-old woman had a modified radical mastectomy for left breast cancer and a prophylactic mastectomy of the right breast. She wanted bilateral DIEP flaps, but the anatomy on one side was not appropriate. Therefore she had a muscle-sparing free TRAM performed on that side, with a DIEP on the other. She is shown 9 months after surgery with a well-healed abdominal donor site. Her breasts have similar breast volume to her preoperative situation per her request. Preoperative CT angiography was used to locate the perforators.

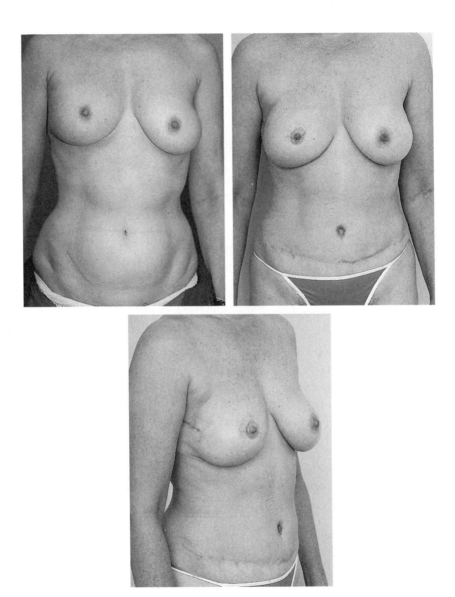

This 46-year-old woman had a modified radical mastectomy to treat the breast cancer in her right breast. She had an immediate muscle-sparing free TRAM flap in which only a wide strip of muscle was removed to capture the two main perforators supplying the skin island to be used in her breast reconstruction. She is shown 1 year after the procedure and nipple-areola reconstruction.

THE GLUTEUS MAXIMUS FREE FLAP

The buttocks were one of the first distant areas used for breast reconstruction with microsurgery. Since the blood supply cannot be preserved when moving buttock tissue this great a distance, a microvascular (involving the small blood vessels) technique is used to hook up the blood vessels of the buttocks to the blood vessels in the woman's breast region.

When the DIEP or TRAM flaps are unavailable or of insufficient size, the tissue for the breast reconstruction can be supplied by transferring a portion of the buttock skin and muscle to the breast region and resuturing the vessels of the buttock tissue to the vessels in the axilla or in the midchest region under the ribs. The buttock skin and muscle can be taken from either the midportion of the buttock (superior gluteus free flap) or more often from the lower buttock crease (inferior gluteus free flap). The advantage of using the lower crease is that this is usually the region of greatest excess tissue. Removal of the tissue from the lower buttocks can actually reduce and flatten a large buttock, and the scar can be placed in the crease, where it is less obvious and can be covered by a woman's undergarments. In addition, the vessels of the lower gluteus flap are often better suited for microsurgical hookup.

While some surgeons still perform gluteus myocutaneous flap reconstruction, many microsurgeons have now switched to using the gluteal perforator flaps the superior gluteal artery perforator (SGAP) and the inferior (IGAP) flap. (These are discussed on p. 362).

Surgical Procedure and Postoperative Appearance

Patients selected for this technique must be healthy and able to undergo a procedure that takes a minimum of 4 to 8 hours and possibly longer. This operation is done with the patient under general anesthesia and requires hospitalization. The success of the operation depends on the microsurgeon's skill and artistry in designing and shaping the buttocks into the new breast.

The operation for an immediate gluteus maximus free flap is basically the same as that for the delayed reconstruction. Technically it is an easier operation because the axillary vessels are already freed up and there is no scarring.

The gluteus maximus free flap is designed as an ellipse along the buttock crease, either along the fold, where the buttocks meets the thigh, or slightly higher on the mid-portion of the buttocks, depending on where the greatest concentration of fatty tissue is located and on the vessels to be used. The inferior gluteal flap is designed along the buttock crease while the superior gluteal flap is designed obliquely, much higher on the buttock. The flap of skin, fat, and a small portion of the gluteus muscle is obtained along with the small blood vessels going into the muscle that nourish the tissue. The flap is then transferred to the chest wall where the mastectomy incision has been opened and extended and the recipient vessels have been located. Next, the flap is connected to the vessels in the underarm or occasionally in the midchest region using microvascular techniques performed under the operating microscope. The vessels and flap are checked to ensure that there is good blood flow. Then the transferred muscle is sutured to the underlying chest wall and the flap of skin and fat is shaped and inset to match the opposite breast. Buttock fat is very much stiffer than abdominal or breast fat, making it more difficult to shape. During a second procedure it is sometimes necessary to further perfect the breast shape and contour both buttock and hip regions with additional surgical revisions and/or liposuction.

Postoperatively, after skin-sparing mastectomy and immediate reconstruction, the incisions on the breast extend around the areola and toward the underarm area. After delayed breast reconstruction, the rebuilt breast usually has an elliptic pattern of stitches running along the lower breast crease and up toward the nipple area. The resulting donor scar is positioned across the lower crease of the buttocks or across the midportion of the buttock. It is usually hidden by the patient's undergarments.

Postoperative Care

Drains remain in the breast for 3 to 4 days and in the buttock for 7 to 10 days after the operation. The breast drain is usually removed before the patient leaves the hospital, and the buttock drain is left in place until the fluid loss is less than 1 ounce (30 ml) per day. This may take several weeks. The reconstructive surgeon avoids removing the drain too early, because fluid accumulation (*seroma*) would require aspiration or replacement of the drain. To protect the transferred vessels, the patient's upper extremity movements are restricted for 5 to 6 days after surgery. Antibiotics are administered for the first 4 days postoperatively. Cigarette smoking and exposure to environmental tobacco smoke are prohibited during the postoperative period. All other aspects of postoperative care are similar to those described on p. 330 for the TRAM free flap, p. 293 for the pedicle TRAM flap, and p. 273 for implant reconstruction.

Skin-Sparing Mastectomy and Immediate Breast Reconstruction With a Gluteus Maximus Free Flap

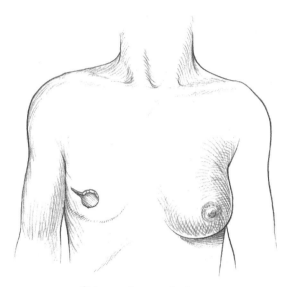

Skin-sparing mastectomy

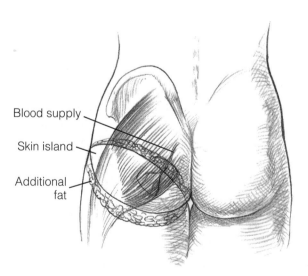

Blood supply

Skin island

Additional fat

Gluteus maximus free flap designed on the buttock

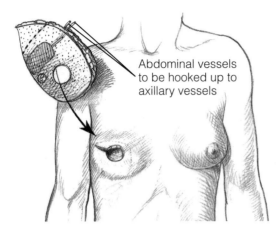

Abdominal vessels
to be hooked up to
axillary vessels

Free buttock tissue transferred
to the breast, vessels reattached
by microsurgery, and buttock
tissue fashioned into a breast

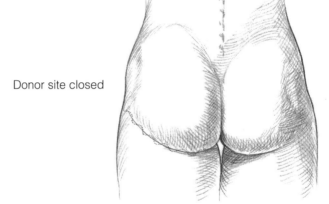

Donor site closed

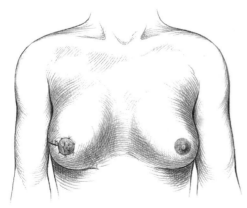

Nipple-areola reconstructed
several months later

Delayed Breast Reconstruction With a Gluteus Maximus Free Flap

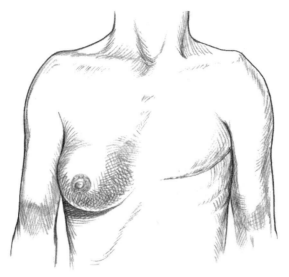

Modified radical mastectomy

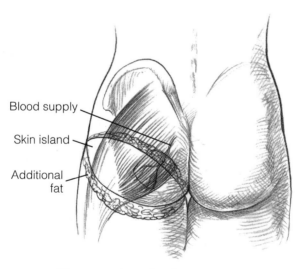

Blood supply

Skin island

Additional
fat

Gluteus maximus free flap designed on the buttock

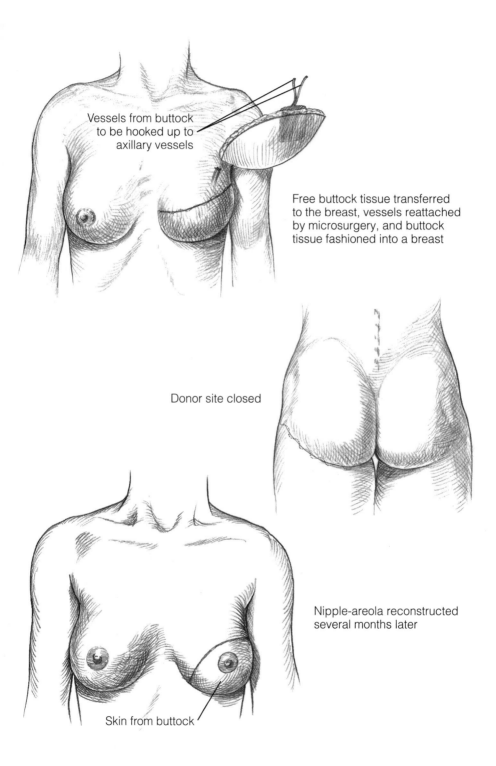

Vessels from buttock to be hooked up to axillary vessels

Free buttock tissue transferred to the breast, vessels reattached by microsurgery, and buttock tissue fashioned into a breast

Donor site closed

Nipple-areola reconstructed several months later

Skin from buttock

Problems and Complications

The greatest risk is that the blood flow into the transferred buttock tissue that forms the new breast will fail or occlude (become blocked). If this occurs, the surgeon will need to reoperate to restore the blood flow. Because a nerve in the back of the leg has to be divided with the buttock flap, a portion of the back part of the thigh is numb after this operation. This nerve can also develop a sensitive swelling (*neuroma*), which could necessitate another operation. The accumulation of fluid in the buttocks can require drainage, either intermittently with a syringe and needle or by replacement of the drain. Antibiotics are usually prescribed in the postoperative period, and it is unusual for an infection to develop after the operation.

Hospitalization, Pain, and Recuperation

A hospital stay of 6 to 7 days is required. Since the donor site is in the buttock region, the patient will have to lie face down or on her opposite side after the operation. The pain and discomfort from this operation are usually not as severe as that experienced with the TRAM flap, but more than that experienced after breast reconstruction with implants and expanders. A patient-controlled analgesia (PCA) pump or ON-Q pain system is used to relieve the postoperative pain. A pain pump delivers local anesthetic into the wound through a fine tube that is placed at the time of surgery. This has the effect of numbing the area and thereby reducing the amount of pain medications the patient requires. To alleviate pressure on the buttock area where the flap was taken, some surgeons use a low-air-loss type of bed. Pain when sitting can be relieved by using an inflatable donut pillow for the first few weeks after surgery. As with other free flap breast reconstructions, care is taken to monitor the flap after surgery to ascertain that there is good blood flow to the transferred tissue.

The patient can get out of bed the following day. Most women gradually resume normal basic activities over the next 4 to 6 weeks. They can return to work in 4 to 6 weeks and can participate in sports in 3 to 6 months.

Results With the Gluteus Maximus Free Flap

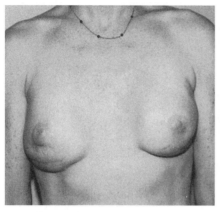 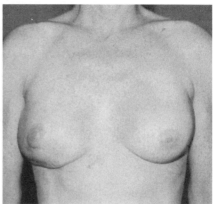

This 39-year-old woman requested bilateral flap breast reconstruction because she was dissatisfied with the results of her previous implant reconstruction. She is shown 6 months after reconstruction with lower gluteus maximus free flaps.

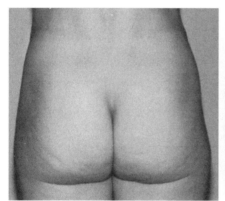 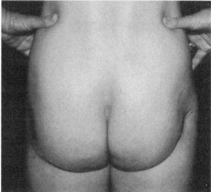

The buttocks region is shown before and after the procedure.

Results With the Gluteus Maximus Free Flap—cont'd

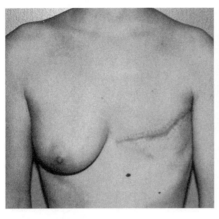 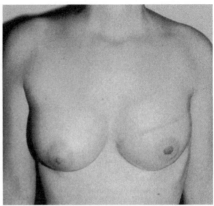

This 24-year-old patient had a left modified radical mastectomy. She wanted a breast reconstruction to match her unmodified opposite breast. Since her lower abdomen was thin, scarred, and irradiated, an abdominal flap could not be used. The patient did not want a back scar. She is shown 18 months after an inferior gluteus maximus free flap reconstruction.

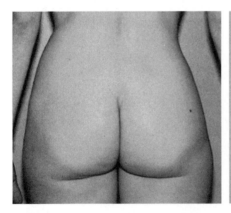 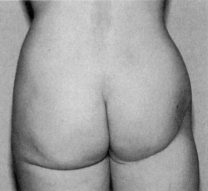

Her donor scar is located in the right buttock crease. Liposuction was performed on the opposite buttock at the time of nipple reconstruction.

THE RUBENS FREE FLAP

The lateral hip or Rubens free flap is an alternative when the TRAM or buttocks flaps are not available. The technique, complications, and postoperative care and recovery are similar to that described for the TRAM free flap and the gluteus maximus free flap. This flap does not provide the abundance of tissue supplied by some of the other donor sites, and many patients find the donor scars objectionable. It is a technically demanding procedure and takes tissue from only one hip area. With the advent of perforator flaps, this type of flap is less commonly used today.

The Rubens flap was devised for use in patients who had had a previous tummy tuck but had residual fat available in the hip area. It is a difficult operation requiring very careful donor site repair to minimize the risk of hernia formation. Very few surgeons have experience with this procedure, and patients should seek out someone who knows how to perform it safely. If only one side is used, the patient may need the opposite hip suctioned down for symmetry at a later stage.

Result With the Rubens Flap

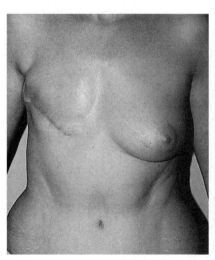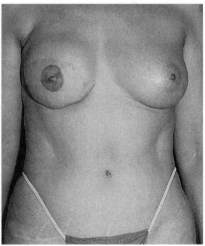

This 48-year-old woman was referred for breast reconstruction salvage after two failed attempts at gluteal free flap reconstruction elsewhere. She was not a candidate for TRAM flap reconstruction, because she had previously had a tummy tuck. A Rubens free flap reconstruction from her left hip provided satisfactory volume to create symmetry with her opposite breast. She is shown after nipple-areola reconstruction with local tissue.

GRACILIS FLAP BREAST RECONSTRUCTION

PETER C. NELIGAN, MD

The TUG flap, also known as the TMG flap, has become a popular option in recent years as an alternative to the abdominal and buttock flap techniques. Some women have a tendency to accumulate fat in the upper inner thigh, and this flap uses that inner thigh fat. The flap also includes the gracilis muscle, through which the blood supply reaches the skin. The scar is placed in or just below the groin crease and is very acceptable for most women.

Surgical Procedure and Postoperative Appearance

The surgical procedure is similar to the free TRAM flap or the DIEP flap procedure; in fact, the breast segment of the procedure is the same. Where the procedure differs is in the harvesting of the flap. The donor site is in the upper inner thigh, and one of the advantages of this flap, as opposed to buttock flaps, is that the patient doesn't have to be turned during the procedure. As with the DIEP flap, two teams of surgeons can work together, one preparing the breast while the other concentrates on flap harvest. The scar is placed as close as possible to the groin crease and is similar to the scar of a thigh lift.

Skin-Sparing Mastectomy and Immediate Breast Reconstruction With the TUG Flap

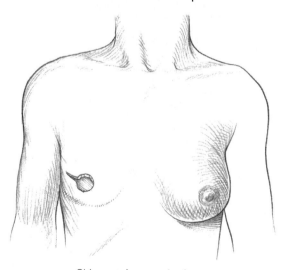

Skin-sparing mastectomy

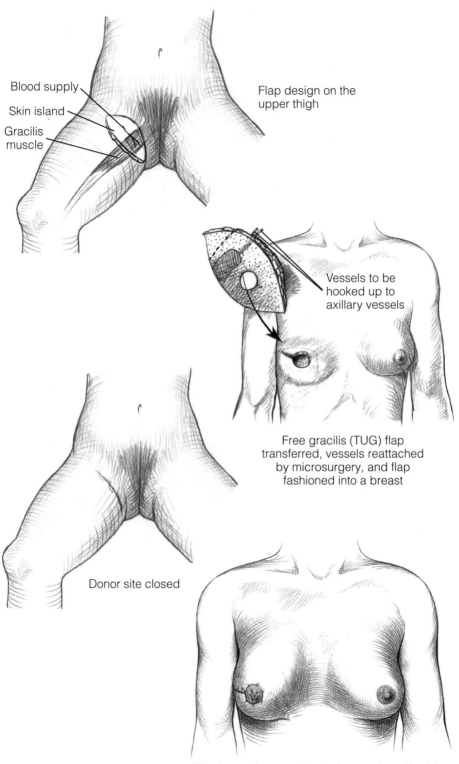

Blood supply

Skin island

Gracilis muscle

Flap design on the upper thigh

Vessels to be hooked up to axillary vessels

Free gracilis (TUG) flap transferred, vessels reattached by microsurgery, and flap fashioned into a breast

Donor site closed

Nipple-areola reconstructed several months later

Postoperative Care

Closure of the donor area on the thigh is necessarily tight, and in the postoperative period it is important that the patient be aware of this. Frequently, a pain pump is used in the immediate postoperative period to minimize donor pain. A drain is also routinely used and typically stays in for approximately 7 days.

Problems and Complications

Because of the tightness of the closure, there is a danger of wound separation known as wound dehiscence. To avoid this, the patient needs to be careful about postoperative mobilization and should be aware of the importance of listening to instructions on postoperative activity. Another consequence of tight closure is that the scar will often stretch, however, because of the placement of the scar in the upper inner thigh, this is rarely an issue. One of the problems with this flap is that the amount of tissue available for reconstruction is relatively small, so the patient must understand the limitation of reconstruction in terms of breast size.

Hospitalization, Pain, and Recuperation

The hospital stay is typically 3 to 5 days. Often the patient will go home with drains (in both the thigh and breast) still in place. Postoperative pain is moderate. Use of a pain pump at the donor site is helpful. Before hospital discharge, the patient will be reasonably mobile and once she goes home, she can generally increase her level of activity over the next several weeks. As with the DIEP flap, the patient's total down time is approximately 4 to 6 weeks.

Result With the TUG flap

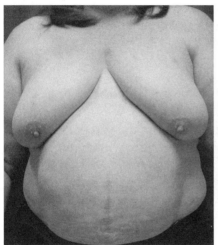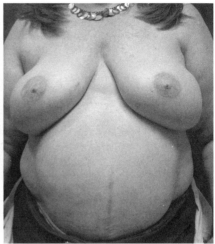

This patient is shown before and after bilateral mastectomy with immediate TUG flap reconstruction. She had previous abdominal surgery and therefore was not a candidate for a DIEP flap.

PERFORATOR FLAP RECONSTRUCTION

PETER C. NELIGAN, MD, and GLYN JONES, MD

Microsurgical breast reconstruction techniques using perforator flaps represent the latest advance in breast reconstruction. A perforator flap is composed of skin and fatty tissue and is based on a single set of blood vessels (the perforator vessels) that pass through the underlying muscle. Donor sites for perforator flap breast reconstruction include the abdomen (DIEP and SIEA flaps) or buttocks (IGAP or SGAP flaps). Unlike conventional pedicle and microsurgical flap techniques, perforator flaps spare the patient's underlying musculature. The tissue is then transferred to the patient's chest, reconnected using micro-surgery and shaped to create the new breast.

Because perforator flap procedures preserve the underlying mus-cles as well as the motor nerves to the muscle, they do not compro-mise muscle function; thus maximal muscle strength is preserved. This is particularly important for active individuals.

Perforator flaps can provide natural, aesthetic breast reconstructions in patients with no major risk factors (such as smokers, obese patients, and those with health problems). These operations are technically demanding and should only be performed by surgeons experienced with perforator flap technique.

DIEP FLAP RECONSTRUCTION

The DIEP (deep inferior epigastric perforator) flap is a variation of the free TRAM (abdominal), flap described earlier, except that *all the abdominal muscle is preserved*. Only abdominal skin and fat are removed, similar to a tummy tuck. This is a major, somewhat tedious procedure for the surgical team, because it requires carefully teasing out of the perforating blood vessels from the muscle.

The procedure thereafter is identical to that of the free TRAM flap, and in the hands of an experienced microsurgeon takes the same amount of time to perform as a TRAM flap reconstruction. The DIEP flap is a viable option for women desiring autologous reconstruction, particularly young and athletic individuals, those requiring smaller-volume reconstructions, and lower-risk patients, such as nonsmokers and thin patients.

Advantages of the DIEP flap include optimized abdominal strength, reduced risk of muscle bulges or hernia, a good flap blood supply, and an improved abdominal contour. The recovery time is shorter and post operative discomfort is less. Disadvantages include a technically demanding procedure with greater risk of fat necrosis when compared with a muscle-sparing free TRAM flap.

This technique produces excellent results in most patients; however, it is essential that the surgeon performing this complex procedure be a skilled microsurgeon who is experienced in performing this operation, with an equally experienced surgical team. Today more women are requesting these operations because of the perceived benefit on abdominal wall function. Although a difference has been shown between abdominal wall function in patients having pedicle TRAM procedures compared with muscle-sparing TRAM procedures, no real difference has been shown between a muscle-sparing TRAM and DIEP procedure.

Surgical Procedure and Postoperative Appearance

Reconstruction with the DIEP flap is a major operation and takes approximately 5 to 10 hours. Before surgery, most patients have a CT angiogram taken so the surgeon can identify where the largest vessels enter the flap and how many vessels do so. This reduces the duration of the operation and helps the surgeon identify the best vessels to use. Today many surgeons are beginning to use newer intraoperative imaging systems that involve dye injection to determine the best blood vessels to use. A single, very large vessel is safer to use than multiple tiny vessels. If there are multiple small vessels, a muscle-sparing free TRAM flap is preferable.

During surgery, a skin island identical to that used for any type of TRAM flap is designed on the abdomen and raised. The perforator to be used is identified and then followed through the muscle to its parent vessel by splitting the vertical fibers of the rectus muscle along their length. The parent vessels are then cut in the groin and delivered through the split muscle for transfer to the chest with the skin island. Once on the chest, the vessels are rejoined to a suitable recipient vessel under the ribs or, less commonly, in the armpit. This involves complex microsurgery. After blood flow is reestablished, the flap is shaped in exactly the same way as any other TRAM flap (see p. 291) and looks just the same. Abdominal closure is a little easier as the muscle split is repaired with a simple double layer of internal stitches following which the tummy tuck component of the operation proceeds exactly like a conventional TRAM flap.

The postoperative appearance of a DIEP flap breast reconstruction is identical to that of any pedicle or free TRAM flap in terms of breast shape and abdominal scarring. The difference lies within the donor site. No muscle is taken whatsoever. The muscle fibers are simply split to allow the vessels leading to the flap, to be freed from deep within the abdomen. The concept of the flap is that if the flap is supplied by one or two large perforators, then only these vessels are necessary for successful transfer of the flap from the abdomen to the breast where these vessels will be reconnected by microsurgical technique. The abdominal muscles are minimally disturbed, thereby maintaining maximum strength and function postoperatively. Once healed, these flaps perform just like TRAM flaps, whether pedicle or free.

Skin-Sparing Mastectomy and Immediate Breast Reconstruction With the DIEP Flap

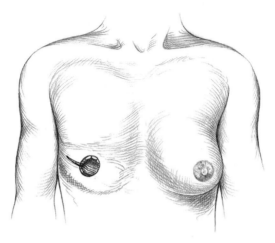

Skin-sparing mastectomy deformity after removal
of the breast and nipple-areola

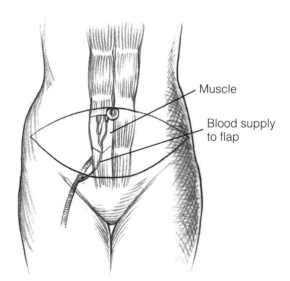

Muscle

Blood supply
to flap

TRAM free DIEP flap designed on the lower abdomen
coming up through the muscle

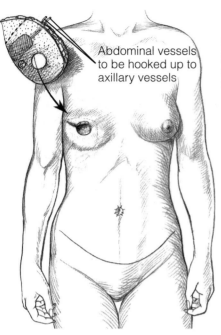

Abdominal vessels to be hooked up to axillary vessels

Free abdominal tissue transferred to the breast and vessels reattached by microsurgery

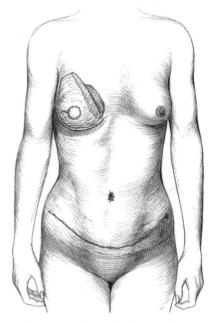

Abdominal tissue fashioned into a breast and the lower abdomen closed as a transverse scar

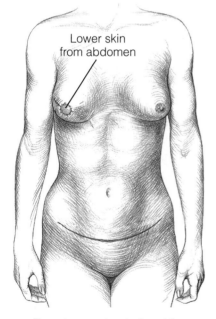

Lower skin from abdomen

Breast reconstructed and the incision closed as a short incision encircling the areola with an extension to the side

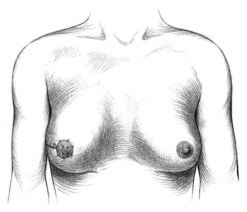

Nipple-areola reconstructed several months later

Postoperative Care

Patients are encouraged to ambulate on the first day after surgery. Deep venous thrombosis prophylaxis with drugs such as enoxaparin (Lovenox) by injection are used routinely, as are sequential compression stockings. Patients are usually eating well by 2 or 3 days after surgery and can often leave the hospital by the third day. All other aspects of postoperative care are similar to those described on p. 330 for the TRAM free flap, p. 293 for the pedicle TRAM flap, and p. 273 for implant reconstruction.

Problems and Complications

Complications are similar to those described for free and pedicle TRAM flaps. Total flap loss is a potential but rare complication. If this occurs, a new reconstruction has to be performed using alternative tissue donor sites. To prevent the possible development of deep venous thrombosis, a serious complication, blood thinners are administered and compression stockings and compression devices are used to stimulate the circulation. Given the length of these operations, pneumonia and retained secretions in the airways is a potential problem that requires respiratory treatments as needed. Fat necrosis is slightly more common in perforator flaps than in muscle-sparing free TRAM flaps because of the smaller number of vessels that are incorporated into the flap. However, the new intraoperative imaging techniques are helping to address this problem. These problems are encountered more frequently in higher-risk patients, such as smokers, obese patients, and patients who have undergone radiation therapy. In these high-risk patients, a muscle-sparing free TRAM flap may be preferable to a DIEP flap. (See p. 333 for a description of this technique.) Although abdominal strength is well preserved in many of these patients who have DIEP flaps, abdominal bulges can still sometimes occur. When this happens, treatment is identical to that for repairing a TRAM flap donor site bulge; mesh is inserted into the defect to repair and strengthen the abdominal wall.

Hospitalization, Pain, and Recuperation

A hospital stay of 3 to 5 days is usually required. Pain is similar to that of a free TRAM flap. However, because the abdominal muscles are not disturbed, as they are with the pedicle TRAM flap, recovery is usually a little faster because there is less pain and tightness at the closure site. Pain is most intense during the initial 24 to 48 hours, decreasing gradually after that. The use of PCA pumps and local anesthetic delivery systems such as the ON-Q or Stryker pumps have dramatically improved pain management for patients.

Patients typically take about 6 weeks to recover. Full return to exercise other than walking is usually restricted for the first 2 to 3 months after surgery. The other specifics of pain and recuperation are the same as those described for the pedicle TRAM and free TRAM flaps.

Results With the DIEP Flap

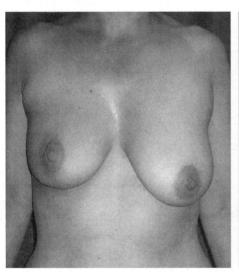 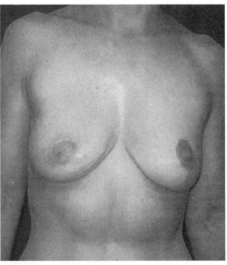

This woman had a skin-sparing mastectomy to treat her right breast cancer. She had an immediate DIEP flap reconstruction and a mastopexy (breast lift) on her opposite breast to produce reasonably symmetrical and soft breasts. (Patient example provided by Peter C. Neligan, MD.)

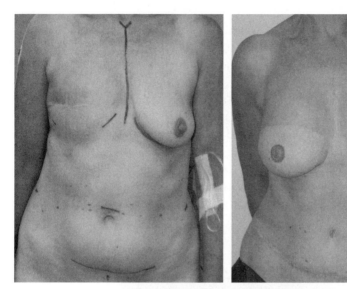

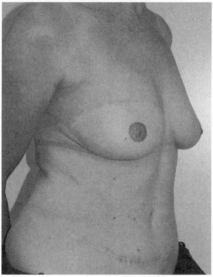

This woman had a delayed DIEP flap to reconstruct her right breast to match her opposite left breast that she did not want altered. Six months later some trimming of excess tissue was done, and the nipple-areola was reconstructed using a free nipple graft from the opposite side. Four months later she had bilateral tattooing of the areola. (Patient example provided by Phillip N. Blondeel, MD.)

SIEA PERFORATOR FLAP RECONSTRUCTION

The superficial inferior epigastric artery (SIEA) flap is similar to the DIEP flap procedure. Both techniques use the lower abdominal skin and fatty tissue to reconstruct a natural, soft breast following mastectomy. The SIEA has all of the advantages mentioned for the DIEP and requires no muscle dissection whatsoever eliminating any risk of hernia or bulging.

Although the SIEA is similar to the DIEP, it is used less frequently, since the arteries required are generally too small to sustain the flap in most patients, and it is not reliable across the midline unless both pedicles are used. The vessels needed to perform a SIEA flap are absent in 15% to 20% of patients. When the vessels are present and usable, it is safe to use only one side of the abdomen based on them. If both sides are needed for volume, the vessels of both sides need to be joined microsurgically.

Surgical Procedure and Postoperative Appearance

The SIEA flap procedure takes 3 to 6 hours. The main difference between the SIEA flap and the DIEP flap is the artery used to supply blood flow to the new breast. The SIEA blood vessels are found in the fatty tissue just below the skin, whereas the DIEP blood vessels run below and within the abdominal muscle (making the surgery more technically challenging). Although the surgical preparation is slightly different, both procedures spare the abdominal muscle and only use the patient's skin and fat to reconstruct the breast.

Postoperative Care

Postoperative care is identical to that for TRAM and DIEP flaps.

Problems and Complications

Problems and complications are similar to those seen with DIEP flaps although abdominal strength problems are virtually nonexistent, and there is no risk whatsoever of hernias or bulges developing.

Skin-Sparing Mastectomy and Immediate Breast Reconstruction With the SIEA Flap

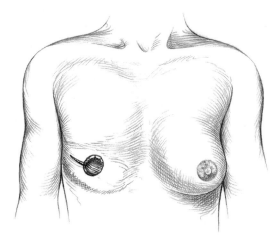

Skin-sparing mastectomy

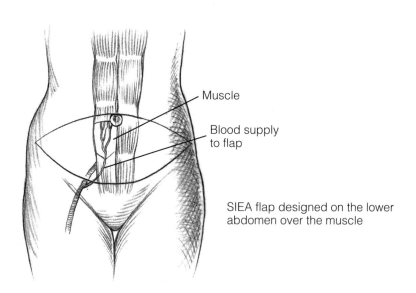

Muscle

Blood supply to flap

SIEA flap designed on the lower abdomen over the muscle

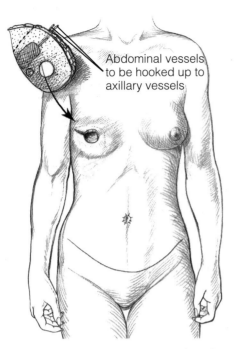

Free abdominal tissue transferred
to the breast and vessels reattached
by microsurgery

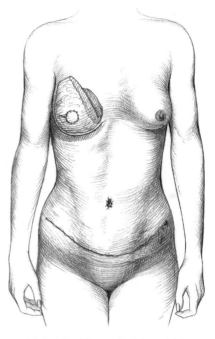

Abdominal tissue fashioned into
a breast and the lower abdomen
closed as a transverse scar

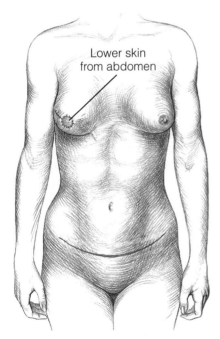

Breast reconstructed and the incision
closed as a short incision encircling
the areola with an extension to the side

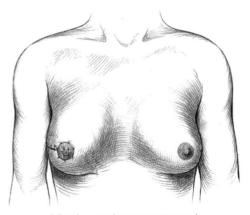

Nipple-areola reconstructed
several months later

Hospitalization, Pain, and Recuperation

The SIEA flap requires hospitalization for 3 to 5 days. The dissection for this procedure is a little quicker with no muscle dissection so there is less pain and recovery is faster than with the DIEP flap. Pain control is managed with PCA pumps, and ON-Q or Stryker pain pumps. These patients are more comfortable than women who have a pedicle or free TRAM flap that takes all or a portion of the abdominal muscle. Return to normal physical activity is much quicker than after pedicle or free flap procedures. Most patients can drive after several weeks and return to active athletic exercise by 3 to 5 weeks.

SUPERIOR AND INFERIOR GLUTEAL ARTERY PERFORATOR (SGAP AND IGAP) FLAPS

The SGAP and IGAP flaps are variations on the superior and inferior gluteus maximus free flaps described earlier (see p. 338), except all buttock muscle is preserved. These flaps have now essentially replaced the superior and inferior gluteus maximus free flaps. This operation is a little more challenging than the DIEP flap, and the fat of the buttock is much stiffer and less pliable than abdominal fat, making shaping of the reconstructed breast somewhat more time consuming. These flaps are also more difficult to harvest. The procedure is indicated when the patient wants an autologous tissue reconstruction but does not have available abdominal tissue.

Surgical Procedure and Postoperative Appearance

Gluteal flap procedures are complex and demanding operations. Operative times are lengthy, usually taking 8 to 10 hours to perform. The patient has to be positioned partially on her side to allow access to the buttock and is then rotated back for the microsurgery on the front to perform the breast reconstruction and achieve the desired breast shape. Two different buttock perforator flaps can be used for breast reconstruction: the superior (upper) gluteus maximus perforator (SGAP) flap and the inferior (lower) gluteus maximus perforator (IGAP) flap. The SGAP flap is designed as an ellipse across the mid-portion of the buttocks, while the IGAP is designed on the lower part of the buttocks.

The flap is raised off of the underlying gluteal muscle until an appropriate-sized perforator is identified. This is then followed down through the thick gluteal muscle onto its undersurface, where the parent vessel is located. This vessel is followed deeper into the buttock until the desired length and size are obtained and the vessels are then clamped and cut. The donor site is closed over a drain and dressings are applied. The patient is then rotated into an acceptable position for the breast reconstruction to be performed. The recipient vessels in the breast area have already been prepared by the other surgical team and the microsurgical repair is performed as usual (as described for the TRAM free flap or gluteus maximus flap). The breast is then shaped and sewn into place.

Postoperative Care

Postoperative care is identical to that of the regular gluteus maximus free (buttock) flap. However, postoperative pain is much less, as no muscle is harvested and patients are able to ambulate very quickly after surgery.

Problems and Complications

Complications specific to this procedure include wound breakdown, pain on sitting and seroma or fluid formation. It is essential to drain these operative and donor sites thoroughly to prevent seroma formation. With the use of the perforator options for this buttock flap breast reconstruction, problems with sciatica have been virtually eliminated. Other complications are the same as those described on p. 344.

Hospitalization, Pain and Recuperation

Hospitalization is typically for 5 to 6 days, or until the patient is able to ambulate comfortably. Potential muscle pain may be less than with the free gluteus maximus (buttock) flap because the muscle is preserved. Pain control is similar to that used for the DIEP flap but sitting can be uncomfortable initially. A walker may be helpful initially to aid with mobilization. Patients may return to normal activity after 6 to 8 weeks, although great care must be taken initially to prevent overstretching the repaired buttock defect to minimize the risk of wound breakdown.

Skin-Sparing Mastectomy and Immediate Breast Reconstruction With the SGAP and IGAP Flaps

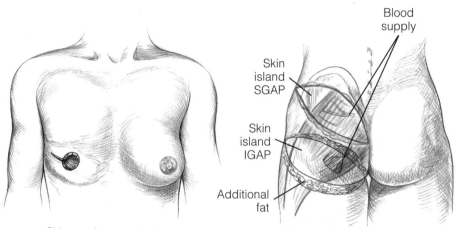

Skin-sparing mastectomy

IGAP or SGAP flap designed
on the buttock

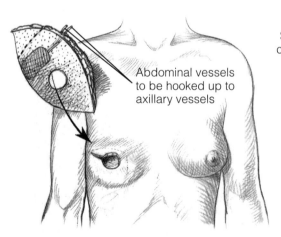

Buttock tissue transferred to the breast,
vessels reattached by microsurgery,
and tissue fashioned into a breast

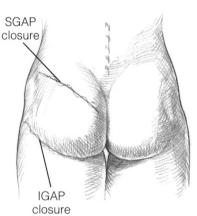

Donor site closed

Results With SGAP and IGAP Perforator Flaps

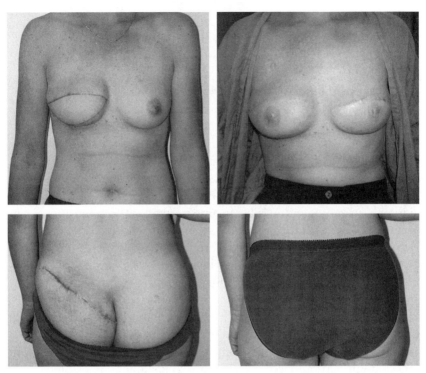

This patient is shown after a right mastectomy and reconstruction with an SGAP flap. The patient is seen 3 years later after developing cancer in her left breast. This breast was also reconstructed with an SGAP flap. Her nipples were reconstructed several months later, and her areolas were subsequently tattooed. An SGAP donor scar is shown. (Patient example provided by Peter C. Neligan, MD.)

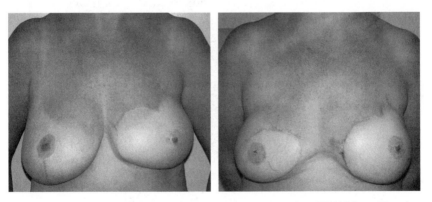

This patient had a left mastectomy reconstructed with a free TRAM flap. She also had a reduction of her right breast. She subsequently presented with an invasive cancer of the right breast requiring a mastectomy. The right breast was reconstructed with an IGAP flap. The left breast mound was revised for symmetry. Her nipples were reconstructed and her areolas were tattooed in a later procedure.

EXTERNAL EXPANSION WITH MEGA-VOLUME FAT GRAFTING FOR BREAST RECONSTRUCTION

It is now possible for a woman to have her breast rebuilt with a procedure that combines external tissue expansion to stretch the skin at the mastectomy site with serial fat injections to fill the enlarged breast envelope.

This is a relatively new procedure that is still considered investigational. There are many questions still to be addressed and there are few data at this stage. We have included this procedure because it holds considerable promise, and it is beginning to attract the attention of surgeons worldwide. This approach avoids a major flap operation and still has the benefit of using the woman's own fatty tissue.

A woman who is interested in having this procedure for breast reconstruction needs to locate a surgeon who has experience with the special external expansion device that is used and with fat grafting technique. She must also be fully informed about the concept of fat grafting. This is a less-invasive operation than autologous flap reconstruction, but it is a time-consuming procedure. It requires a patient who is compliant and willing to wear a somewhat cumbersome external, bralike expansion device daily for a number of weeks while her tissues are stretched sufficiently to accept a series of fat grafts for rebuilding her breast.

This procedure is appropriate for small-breasted women. It may not be appropriate for women with large breasts or for those who have irradiated tissues that are firmer, tighter, and less compliant or subject to mechanical stretching. Smoking is an absolute contraindication to this procedure.

Procedure and Postoperative Appearance

With this approach, a specially designed bralike expander device consisting of a semi-rigid dome with a silicone gel rim cushion is positioned against the skin. A woman wears this device around her breast like a bra. A small, concealed, battery-operated pump maintains a low negative vacuum pressure inside the dome that imparts a constant gentle force on the breast surface to stretch the skin. For adequate expansion, it is recommended that the bralike domes be worn at least 10 to 12 hours per day for 2 to 4 weeks before fat grafting is begun. Fat grafting sessions are started after the expansion process is completed.

The breast is marked in a mapping pattern to indicate the crisscross pattern by which the fat will be infiltrated into the breast. Fat is suctioned from areas of excess, such as the abdomen, buttocks, and hips, and processed for grafting. The fat is then transferred to syringes in preparation for grafting. Tiny amounts of fat are injected through multiple needle entry sites. Gentle, blunt tunneling is done to fill the tissue that has been expanded. The quantity of fat grafted in the first grafting session depends on the amount of expansion achieved and breast edema (swelling) that is created. For subsequent grafting sessions there are more planes to fill, because a larger, thicker space exists. Generally, the more breast tissue that is present, the more fat that can be grafted; however, no more than 200 to 300 cc of grafted fat should be infiltrated at one time. Special care is taken not to overgraft in patients who have irradiated tissues. Following fat grafting, the reconstructed breasts have the same natural feel as those reconstructed with flaps of a woman's own tissue.

Hospitalization, Pain, and Recuperation

A postoperative bra and a simple dressing are applied over the breasts. No hospitalization is required. Local anesthesia plus sedation is used for the fat grafting session. The pain level is low and can be controlled with over-the-counter pain medications.

Problems and Complications

This is still an investigational procedure, so many questions remain. Small areas of fat necrosis are possible. Fat grafting into the breast can result in microcalcifications and oil cysts and concerns have been raised that these could be confused with cancer during breast imaging, even though there is no evidence that this is the case. The size of the breasts will also change with fluctuations in weight.

External Expansion With Mega-Volume Fat Grafting

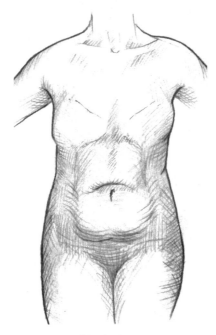

Mastectomy

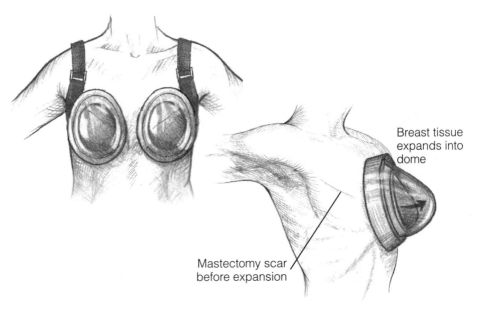

Breast tissue
expands into
dome

Mastectomy scar
before expansion

External expansion bra device
and expansion process

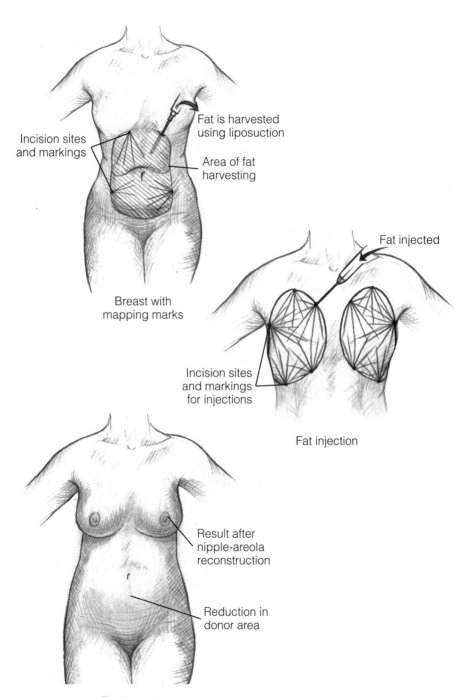

Incision sites and markings

Fat is harvested using liposuction

Area of fat harvesting

Breast with mapping marks

Fat injected

Incision sites and markings for injections

Fat injection

Result after nipple-areola reconstruction

Reduction in donor area

Final result

Results With External Expansion and Fat Grafting

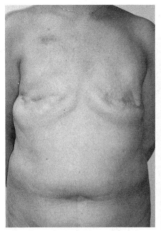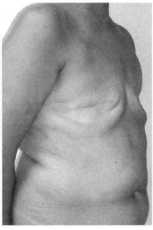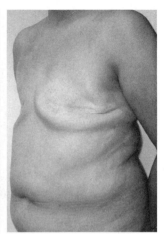

This 42-year-old woman is shown 9 months after bilateral mastectomies and chemotherapy. (Patient example provided by Roger K. Khouri, MD.)

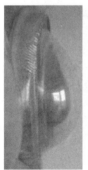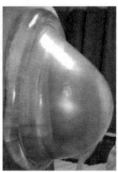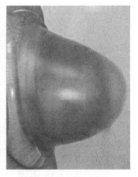

The left breast of this patient is shown in the external expansion device. Her breasts were progressively expanded using increasingly larger expansion domes. Her breast size was then increased with 3 fat grafting sessions. The expansion process took 4 weeks and each of the fat grafting sessions were separated by 6-week intervals. (Patient example provided by Roger K. Khouri, MD.)

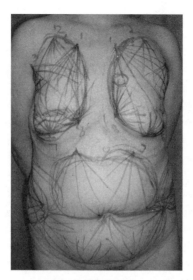

The markings show the mapping pattern on the breast that indicate where fat was injected. (Patient example provided by Roger K. Khouri, MD.)

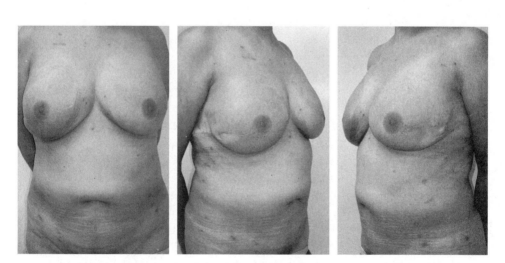

The patient is shown 6 months after the last grafting session. Her breasts are soft and natural. (Patient example provided by Roger K. Khouri, MD.)

FOLLOW-UP OPERATIONS

Although it would be ideal for breast reconstruction to be completed in one operation, thereby creating a superbly shaped, symmetrical breast, in practice this is expecting too much. The usual breast reconstruction can often be enhanced or improved with a second refining procedure. At this time the scars can sometimes be improved, excess tissue can be removed or deficient tissue supplemented, and if necessary, an implant can be inserted. Reconstruction of the nipple-areola is usually accomplished during this second operation. (A detailed explanation of nipple-areola restoration is given in Chapter 16.)

Proper timing for the second operation to place the nipple-areola should be determined once the breast appearance after the first operation is evaluated; the woman's breasts should look as similar as possible. If they are not symmetrical, the surgeon may need to modify the size, shape, and position of the reconstructed breast, either before or at the time he creates the nipple-areola. Usually it is best to have the breasts optimally formed and shaped before placing the nipple. The need for a second operation does not indicate that the first procedure was a failure. The second operation presents the woman and her doctor with an opportunity to obtain the best possible result.

When a significant modification of the reconstructed breast is necessary at the time of the second operation, it is best that the nipple-areola reconstruction be delayed until a third procedure to ensure that it is accurately positioned on a stable breast reconstruction.

The timing of the second operation is also determined by the need for additional treatment such as chemotherapy. This is particularly true for the patient who has immediate breast reconstruction and then must have chemotherapy. Her second operation should usually be delayed until chemotherapy is completed. It is wise to wait at least 2 to 3 months after chemotherapy for the woman to feel her best and her general metabolism and blood count to return to normal. Because of unforeseen complications such as unpredictable healing or an especially extensive mastectomy defect, sometimes additional operations are necessary in addition to the two procedures.

A common secondary operation after implant or expander reconstruction requires the replacement of one implant with another to improve the breast contour, size, or position. The new implant is inserted through the incisions that are already present. Conditions of recovery are similar to those described for the initial implant placement, but pain and recovery time are frequently less than for the initial procedure. If capsular contracture persists after several operations, the implant can be replaced with the fatty tissue from the lower abdominal area, a TRAM flap.

After a TRAM flap reconstruction it is sometimes necessary to shape the breasts further, especially in the lower inner area where the abdominal (rectus abdominis) muscle is transferred. The patient's overall body contour can also be improved at the second operation with some finishing touches. These include liposuction or ultrasound-assisted liposuction of the reconstructed breast if it is larger in some areas than the opposite breast. The abdominal wall and hips may also be recontoured with liposuction or ultrasound-assisted liposuction to give a more aesthetic appearance. Similar corrections may be needed after the gluteus maximus free flap to contour the breast or the buttocks and hip area so that they are symmetrical. When there is not enough tissue to create the ideal size breast reconstruction or the breast lacks projection after a TRAM flap, an implant or expander can be inserted at the time of the second procedure. Many women, however, who choose these procedures do so to avoid implants and prefer the flatness to the use of a foreign material in their breast. The back flap can be used to supplement a TRAM flap if more tissue is needed and the woman does not want an implant. Sometimes thickened areas of fat occur in the reconstructed breast after flap surgery; when this happens, these areas may need to be excised or biopsied both to confirm their diagnosis and to remove them. If the thickened tissue is determined to be thickened fat, then it can be excised or treated with standard or ultrasound-assisted liposuction.

Fat injections are also being used with more frequency as secondary procedures performed on an outpatient basis to fill hollows or defects left after reconstruction, to provide fill under damaged, irradiated tissues, to soften the edges, and to provide a protective layer over implants and expanders.

REOPERATIVE BREAST RECONSTRUCTION SURGERY

Reoperative breast reconstruction is secondary surgery performed to improve a previous breast reconstruction. It may be performed for a variety of reasons. Some women who have had breast reconstruction are disappointed with the results. Others may have had complications or may find that the appearance of the breast reconstruction has deteriorated over time. Some women who had implant reconstruction want their implants removed and their breasts reconstructed with their own tissues.

Reoperative breast reconstruction can include any of the operative approaches or combinations of procedures mentioned in this chapter. Possibilities range from exchanging a breast implant for another of a different size, shape, or texture to replacing a breast implant with the woman's own tissue from her lower abdomen or buttocks. Fat grafting can be used to fill in hollows or to provide cushioning over breast implants. Sometimes a back flap can also be useful for augmenting a breast reconstruction or filling in a defect with additional tissue.

Reoperative breast reconstruction surgery is challenging. Before pursuing this course, a woman should consult with her reconstructive surgeon about her options. Sometimes the plastic surgeon may tell the woman that under the circumstances she has the best possible result that he can achieve and no further operations are advisable. Alternatively, the reconstructive surgeon may suggest that she see another plastic surgeon with extensive experience in reoperative breast reconstruction procedures.

Today a woman requesting breast reconstruction and the plastic surgeon performing this operation have a number of options to choose from. Local tissue reconstruction with implants and expanders and reconstruction with abdominal, back, thigh, and buttock flaps are all means of restoring women's breasts. Perforator flap and muscle-sparing free flap techniques provide new options for autologous breast reconstruction with less compromise to muscle function. Oncoplastic techniques provide an exciting approach for using reduction techniques for filling defects or reshaping the breasts after lumpectomy. A woman's personal needs and the specifics of her deformity dictate which procedures are most suitable. It is very important for the woman to communicate her desires for this surgery to her plastic surgeon so they can examine the different procedures together and decide on the simplest and most reliable operation that can meet these expectations.

WHAT TO DO ABOUT THE OTHER BREAST: AESTHETIC BREAST CORRECTIONS

After losing one breast to mastectomy, a woman finds that her remaining breast assumes a special importance to her. It is a reminder of the breast she lost and a symbol of her once-unscarred chest. She fears the development of a second tumor in her breast, but she is also protective of this lone survivor, not wanting to alter or touch it unless she has no choice.

When a woman contemplates breast reconstruction, her feelings about her remaining breast must be thoroughly discussed with her plastic surgeon, since this will affect the type of reconstructive procedure she chooses and ultimately the success of her operation. Both she and her doctor are understandably concerned about the development of a new tumor in the remaining breast, and this possibility should be discussed with the surgeon. Because the remaining breast will be used as a model for reconstructing the new breast, it must be carefully evaluated. If its appearance is difficult to match or if the woman wants it altered, the plastic surgeon may suggest an aesthetic surgical procedure to change it. Then the woman must decide whether she is comfortable with this suggestion.

Most women having a breast restored want to avoid an operation on their remaining breast. Some women absolutely refuse to submit to any surgery, which always entails some scarring. Usually these women were happy with their breast appearance before the tumor developed, and under ordinary circumstances, they would not have changed their breasts in any way. Therefore they want a reconstructive approach that will leave their remaining breast untouched but will still produce a balanced, aesthetic result. Fortunately, refinements and advances in mastectomy and reconstructive techniques have made this goal attainable for most women. With skin-sparing mastectomies and immediate reconstruction, breasts can be created that closely match the ones they replace. If a woman's remaining breast is of average size (B or C cup brassiere) and the skin at the mastectomy site is not particularly tight, then reconstruction with an expander or implant will be sufficient to match her breast without further surgery. If a woman does not want her existing breast changed and it is relatively large or sags (ptotic), or the tissues at the mastectomy site are tight or irradiated, the missing breast will usually have to be rebuilt with a flap of extra tissue from her lower abdomen or from her back or buttocks, resulting in additional scars in one of these locations. This is also the case for the woman who wants her breast built with her own tissues and prefers not to have a breast implant for breast reconstruction.

Sometimes, however, the size or shape of the remaining breast cannot be easily duplicated, although with newer reconstructive surgery techniques, this does not happen as often as it once did. Or the woman may request that her breast be altered. In this scenario aesthetic alterations of the other breast become more of a positive option for the woman who wishes to incorporate an aesthetic breast alteration into her breast reconstruction. When symmetry is difficult to achieve or when a change is requested, the woman may want to consider an operation on her opposite breast if it will ultimately produce breasts that more closely resemble each other and that she will be happier with. This is preferable to feeling lopsided after her reconstruction and perhaps even having to wear a prosthesis. In this situation, the plastic surgeon uses one of the procedures developed for aesthetic breast surgery to augment, reduce, or lift her other breast. The final decision for breast size is made by the woman herself, and she needs to clearly explain her expectations to her plastic surgeon before undergoing breast reconstruction.

BREAST AUGMENTATION

If the woman's existing breast is small and flattened, she may want to consider having it enlarged to make it fuller. Then her reconstructed breast can be created to resemble this larger breast. This is particularly true if her breast reconstruction will be done with an implant or expander; many of the implantable devices currently on the market tend to produce breasts that are round and full, even though newer anatomic-shaped devices have a more natural teardrop shape. It is therefore difficult for implant reconstructions to match natural breasts that are small, flat, and droopy. Breast augmentation is a relatively simple procedure; however, it does require a breast implant, usually a silicone elastomer envelope filled with silicone gel or saline solution at the time of the operation. As with any operation, the patient should be fully informed about the benefits and risks of implant surgery before choosing this option. (See Chapters 11 and 13 for detailed information on implant surgery.)

To perform this operation the surgeon makes an incision, usually under the breast, in the axilla, or sometimes around the lower portion of the areola, and inserts a breast implant behind the breast tissue, or behind the breast tissue and pectoral muscle layer, thereby enlarging the breast shape. It is then easier for the plastic surgeon to reproduce this larger and fuller breast contour on the reconstructive side.

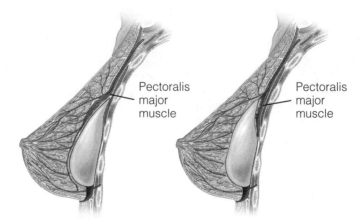

Pectoralis major muscle

Pectoralis major muscle

Breast augmentation with the implant placed partially under the muscle and with the implant placed over the muscle

Breast augmentation may serve a psychological as well as an aesthetic need, giving a woman's self-confidence a boost at a time when she needs an emotional lift. Fears that breast augmentation will hide the development of a new tumor are unwarranted. Because the implant is placed behind a woman's breast tissues and frequently her pectoral muscle layer as well, it does not cover her breast tissue, which still can be accurately and effectively checked for any new lumps or tumors. A baseline mammogram is usually recommended before augmentation mammaplasty and 6 to 12 months after the operation for women over 30 years of age who have developed breast cancer on the opposite side. Mammograms also may be taken, and even a breast biopsy can be done without disturbing the breast implant. Although some have expressed concern that a breast implant can impair mammography, most breast imagers feel that appropriate views of the breast permit satisfactory imaging. (See Chapters 11 and 13 for detailed information on implants and expanders.)

Results

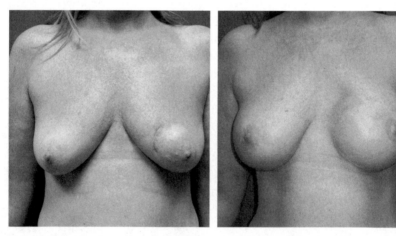

This 42-year-old woman had a left skin-sparing mastectomy. She had immediate expander/implant reconstruction because she wanted larger breasts but did not want a flap procedure. Her opposite breast was augmented with a moderate profile silicone-gel implant for symmetry.

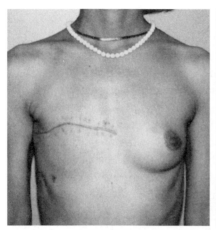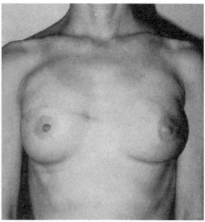

This 30-year-old patient had a right modified radical mastectomy. She requested implant reconstruction and augmentation of her opposite breast. Both procedures were done on an outpatient basis at her request. She is shown 2 years after breast reconstruction.

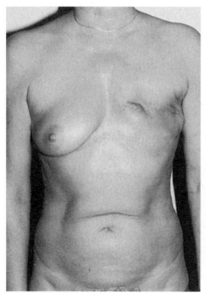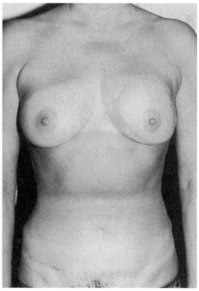

A TRAM flap was used to reconstruct this 52-year-old woman's left breast after a modified radical mastectomy; her right breast was augmented for symmetry. She is shown 15 months after breast reconstruction.

BREAST REDUCTION

When a woman's remaining breast is large, she may require an autologous flap reconstruction to match it. (The TRAM flap often provides enough tissue to produce symmetry with most large breasts.) As an alternative, she may need to have her remaining breast reduced and/or lifted if the rebuilt breast is to match it. A reduction may also make the reconstruction easier to perform, because less tissue will be needed for the new breast, and it can be shaped to better match the reduced breast. Many women with large, heavy breasts that cause problems are only too willing to consider having their normal breast reduced to allow them to feel more comfortable and balanced and to mitigate functional problems caused by large breasts. In addition, tissue removed during a breast reduction is checked for tumors, and this information helps the surgeon assess this breast's status. Current breast reduction techniques are very reliable and have a high level of patient satisfaction and acceptance. A baseline mammogram is recommended before a reduction mammaplasty, for patients over 30, and 6 to 12 months after the operation.

The plastic surgeon does not want to reduce a woman's breast too much; he must know what size to make the breast because, above all, he does not want her to feel as if she is losing another breast. Therefore the expected size of her reduced breast must be carefully explained and the woman must understand how it will look before the reduction of the remaining breast is done. The decision for final breast size should be made by the woman herself and must be clearly communicated to her plastic surgeon. To avoid overreduction, it may occasionally be necessary for the surgeon to perform an extra reconstructive operation later to expand or add an implant to the reconstructed breast. By reducing a woman's existing breast, the plastic surgeon may be able to rebuild her missing breast without a flap procedure; however, a flap should be used if the woman is worried that her breasts will be too small. Most women with a full breast requiring a reduction will have better long-term symmetry if the breast reconstruction is done with a flap of abdominal tissue, but tissue from the back, thigh, or buttocks can be used as well.

The incisions used for breast reduction result in permanent scars. Traditionally these scars resembled an upside-down T. Today there are additional options when breast reduction is needed, newer reduction techniques can produce shorter scars, either around the areola (periareolar) or around the areola with a vertical scar extending down to the inframammary fold (vertical scar). These scars are easily covered when a brassiere is worn. As with all scars, they are often red for the first months after the operation but will usually fade and lighten after 1 to 2 years. Breast function is also a consideration during reduction mammaplasty. The nipple ducts are left intact to permit the possibility of future breast-feeding if this is a consideration. Even though there may be temporary numbness after this procedure, breast sensation and nipple-areolar sensation are usually not permanently affected.

During this procedure, the surgeon removes the excess breast tissue, usually in the lower portion of the breast, to reshape the breast to a smaller size and narrower, more uplifted shape. Extra breast skin is removed, and the final skin closure leaves a scar around the nipple, down to the crease below the breast, and possibly in a line in the crease.

During the postoperative period, the reduced breast is often somewhat swollen and firm. The patient may also note decreased sensation in the breast and nipple-areola. The sensation usually returns during the first few months after the operation. As the sensation returns, the nerves may have heightened sensitivity, occasionally accompanied by shooting pains through the involved breast. When this occurs, the patient is instructed to massage her breast with different textures of cloth and during a bath or shower to use different water temperatures on her breast so that the sensory response can return to normal.

Breast Reduction for Symmetry With the Reconstructed Breast

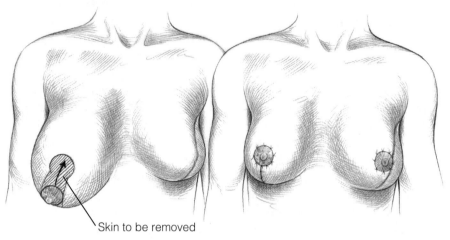

Skin to be removed

Vertical short-scar breast reduction technique without leaving a scar in the inframammary fold

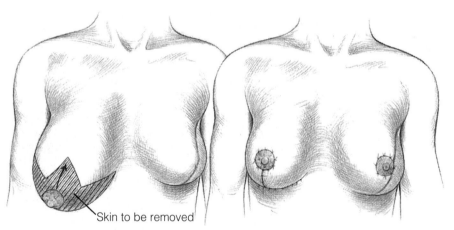

Skin to be removed

Inverted-T-scar reduction technique with a scar in the inframammary fold.

Results

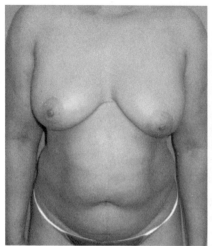 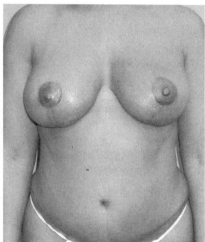

This 40-year-old woman had a modified radical mastectomy followed by an immediate TRAM flap reconstruction on her right breast and a vertical breast reduction for symmetry on her left breast.

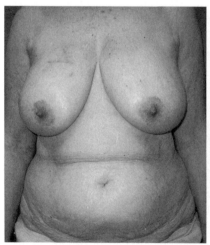 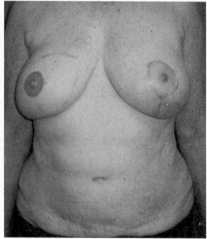

This 58-year-old woman, who wore a 42 E bra, developed cancer in her right breast. She opted for a right skin-sparing mastectomy with TRAM flap breast reconstruction. Her left breast was modestly reduced using a vertical reduction technique with some liposuction of the breast mound. She is shown one year postoperatively; her breasts are soft with improved contour.

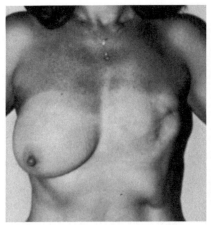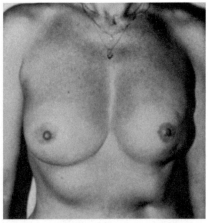

This 38-year-old woman had a modified radical mastectomy. She wanted her large opposite breast reduced and a smaller breast reconstructed to match. She is shown 2 years after implant breast reconstruction and reduction of the other breast.

BREAST LIFT (MASTOPEXY)

If the opposite breast is of reasonable size but sags from the weight of excess skin and loss of support, the surgeon may find that the skin remaining after the mastectomy or available as a flap is insufficient to match this sagging breast. In this case the plastic surgeon may suggest a breast lift, or mastopexy, for the remaining breast. Many women are pleased with the prospect of altering their drooping breasts to give them a fuller, more uplifted, youthful appearance.

In a mastopexy, the surgeon moves the nipple-areola upward on the breast to a new position and removes some skin below the nipple. The breast lift incisions are similar to but often shorter than those used for breast reduction. When the breast does not sag very much, these breast lift (mastopexy) incisions can often be limited to the area around the areola with a vertical line extending to the lower breast crease. Many women who are considering a breast lift have considerable flatness in the upper breast region. Simply lifting the breast will not restore fullness to this area. It is best done with a breast implant. For the woman whose other breast is being reconstructed with an implant or expander implant, insertion of a matching implant behind the normal breast is often a good means of providing the most balanced, aesthetic result because bilateral implants behave more symmetrically over time.

Mastopexy of the Opposite Breast to Obtain Symmetry With the Reconstructed Breast

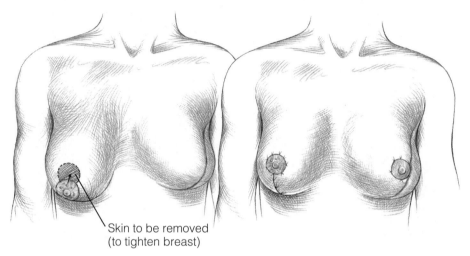

Skin to be removed
(to tighten breast)

Vertical short-scar mastopexy technique with no inframammary scar

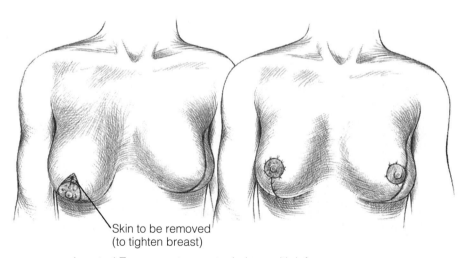

Skin to be removed
(to tighten breast)

Inverted-T-scar mastopexy technique with inframammary scar

Results

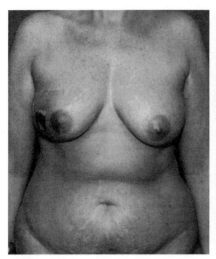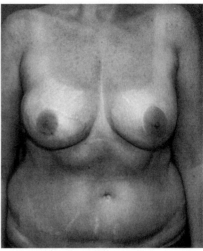

This 48-year-old woman had a right modified radical mastectomy followed by immediate TRAM flap reconstruction. A mastopexy was performed on her left breast for symmetry. She is shown 18 months after breast reconstruction and mastopexy.

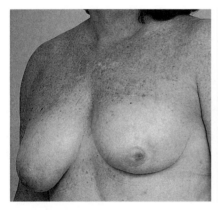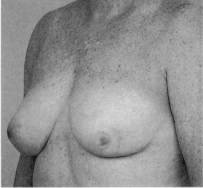

This 39-year-old woman had a lumpectomy of her left breast followed by irradiation. After several years the left breast had become firm, contracted, and somewhat elevated. She was concerned with the asymmetry. She decided to have a vertical scar mastopexy to correct the ptosis of the right breast. She is shown a few months later and is pleased with the improved appearance.

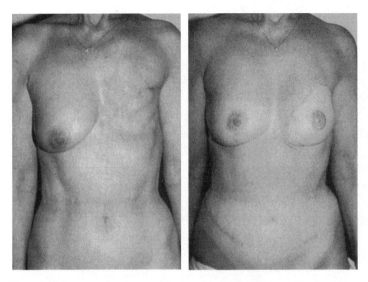

This 46-year-old woman had a modified radical mastectomy. She had breast reconstruction with a TRAM flap, and her opposite breast was lifted for symmetry. She is shown 1 year after breast reconstruction and mastopexy.

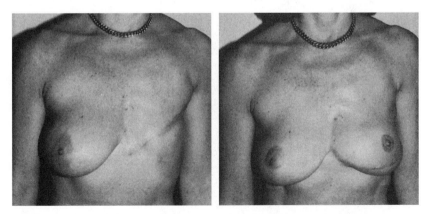

This 48-year-old woman had a left modified radical mastectomy. She is shown 2 years after breast reconstruction with a latissimus dorsi flap and tissue expansion and a mastopexy and small reduction on her right breast for symmetry.

The broad spectrum of techniques currently available to the surgeon permits breast reconstruction that closely approximates a woman's remaining breast without having to alter it. Skin-sparing mastectomy with immediate reconstruction, autologous flap reconstruction, and tissue expansion are all positive methods for creating fuller, more natural, symmetrical breast shapes. When a modification is planned because the patient requests it or the shape and contour of the woman's breast makes it a consideration, the reconstructive surgeon can usually alter the remaining breast and reconstruct the missing breast shape during one operation. The new breast then can be built to match the existing altered breast. If there is some question about the need to operate on the remaining breast or if the woman has doubts about this surgery, the other breast should not be modified at the time of breast reconstruction. In this case only the reconstruction should be performed during the initial operation. Later, after the results of surgery are evaluated, a decision can be made about whether the natural breast should be changed or left alone.

PROPHYLACTIC
MASTECTOMY

Breast cancer is an overriding fear for some women, not merely a statistic. Some have witnessed the suffering and even death of mothers and sisters from this disease; others have themselves been diagnosed with breast cancer. They have become sensitized to the life-threatening danger it poses. We read daily about the growing incidence of breast cancer among women as well as the discovery of breast cancer genes that indicate a strong inherited tendency for breast cancer. This only serves to intensify these fears. Realizing that they are in a high-risk category for developing a malignancy, some women seek a way of reducing the odds.

A *prophylactic* (also called *risk-reducing*) mastectomy with reconstruction is an operation that is performed with the intent of decreasing a woman's risk of developing breast cancer by removing most of her breast tissue and then rebuilding her breasts. According to the National Cancer Institute, existing data suggest that preventive mastectomy may significantly reduce (by approximately 90%) the chance of developing breast cancer in moderate- and high-risk women.

By its very nature, such preventive surgery is controversial and often raises as many questions as it answers. The decision to have this operation with the goal of diminishing a woman's risk of getting breast cancer also involves removing a healthy breast that may in fact never develop a malignancy. The crucial question is whether this operation actually prevents cancer and whether other nonsurgical treatments could accomplish the same purpose.* Unfortunately, there are

*Some doctors are prescribing selective estrogen receptor modulators (SERMs) to help to reduce the risk of breast cancer by blocking the effects of estrogen on breast tissue. Two SERMs, tamoxifen (Nolvadex) and raloxifene (Evista), have been shown in clinical trials to prevent the development of invasive breast cancer in postmenopausal women who are at increased risk of this disease.

no clear-cut answers or definitive scientific data available at present. However, a recent study seems to suggest a benefit for women who carry genetic mutations that put them at high risk for breast and ovarian cancer (see the next section).

Some cancer surgeons are skeptical about the efficacy of this surgery for women with normal risk factors. They believe that many prophylactic mastectomies are unnecessary. As one renowned surgeon stated, "The decision whether to perform a prophylactic mastectomy is difficult for the patient and surgeon, because methods for predicting cancer development are still inadequate and there are no certain methods for preventing cancer." Others question performing a mastectomy (total breast removal) before breast cancer develops to prevent a cancer that could be treated with conservative surgery and irradiation if it occurs. If one waits for cancer to develop, however, there is always the possibility that it may have already spread systemically before it is detected locally within the breast.

THE GROWING INCIDENCE OF PROPHYLACTIC MASTECTOMIES

Despite the skepticism expressed by some experts, there has been a dramatic increase in the number of prophylactic mastectomies performed in this country in the past 11 years. Interestingly, these procedures are being requested by women at all risk levels. A recent report revealed that women diagnosed with ductal carcinoma in situ (DCIS, a noninvasive and highly curable form of breast cancer) in one breast are increasingly choosing to undergo double mastectomy. From 1998 to 2005 the rate of prophylactic mastectomy has more than doubled among women having breast-conserving surgery on one side and almost tripled among women having mastectomy on one side.

Regardless of survival benefit, some patients feel that prophylactic mastectomy of their opposite breast may give them peace of mind. Some women now demand that their opposite breast be removed even though they have no evidence of high-risk disease. They choose this course because they do not want to worry about ongoing mammographic screening or biopsies of the "normal" side. For other women, a small but real 4% risk of developing cancer in the opposite breast is enough to push them toward a prophylactic mastectomy on that side. Unfortunately, no mastectomy can remove all breast tissue at a microscopic level, which still leaves these women at a small but greatly reduced risk of cancer on this side.

Women at high risk for breast cancer are also having more pro-phylactic mastectomies. This may be related to the increased number of women undergoing gene testing today. These tests have resulted in the diagnosis of more individuals who are positive for breast cancer genes (such as BRCA1 and BRCA2) and are therefore at high risk for developing breast cancer. For these women prophylactic mastectomy of the opposite breast or even bilateral prophylactic mastectomies are potentially life-saving procedures that dramatically reduce their sig-nificant risk of developing breast cancer.

A recent study published in the *Journal of the American Medical Association* in 2010 suggests that preventive surgery significantly re-duces the risks of breast and ovarian cancer in women who carry ge-netic mutations that put them at high risk for breast and ovarian can-cer. In this study, scientists followed 2482 women who had been diagnosed with BRCA1 and BRCA2 genetic mutations through ge-netic testing done between 1974 and 2009. These women were tracked through 2009. During 3 years of follow-up, the researchers discovered that 7% of the women who did not have prophylactic mas-tectomies went on to develop breast cancer, while 6% of those who did not have oophorectomies (removal of the ovaries) developed ovarian cancer. The encouraging news was that no breast cancers were diagnosed in the group of women who had prophylactic mastectomies, and only 1% of the women who had their ovaries removed developed ovarian cancer. These women also reduced their risk of breast cancer.

Despite this positive news, it is important for women to under-stand that this preventive surgery does not guarantee 100% that a woman will not develop breast or ovarian cancer, because a very small amount of residual tissue still remains after these procedures. How-ever, for women at high risk, their doctors may recommend these pro-phylactic surgeries as their best opportunity to reduce risk and to max-imize their potential for survival.

Who Is a Candidate for Prophylactic Mastectomy?

Women in a high-risk category with more than one risk factor are potential candidates for prophylactic mastectomy. Their motivation for this operation should be based on their level of concern about can-cer. Are they terrified of malignancy and subsequent death, or can they be reassured that their breasts can be carefully and adequately monitored without surgery? The vast majority of women with risk factors are managed by careful evaluation by their physician, breast self-examination, mammograms, and biopsies of any suspicious breast areas (see Chapters 3, 4, and 5). The use of minimally invasive biopsy techniques is decreasing the need for open biopsy of these suspicious breast masses. Women need to be fully informed about their risks and their options. Although an operation is usually not recommended, it is sometimes presented as an option if the patient's risk is very high and her anxiety level is so overwhelming that it cannot be allayed by continued monitoring.

A prophylactic mastectomy is major surgery. The surgeon should carefully explain the specifics of the operation and make certain that the woman fully understands these details. After surgery, the reconstructed breasts will have less sensation than normal breasts and can actually feel numb. Their appearance may not be as attractive as before surgery, and complications may develop that require additional operations, increasing the potential for disappointment. Some women who undergo prophylactic mastectomies later regret their decision, because the result does not meet their expectations. Physicians are understandably circumspect about an operation that can decrease the aesthetic and functional aspects of a woman's breasts while offering no guarantee that it will prevent breast cancer. A woman considering this approach is already anxiety ridden about her risk of developing cancer; it is therefore crucial that she understand the limitations of this surgery and not expect it to exactly duplicate the breast she is having removed. Most likely, her breasts will not look or feel as they did before. A woman should decide to have a prophylactic mastectomy only after a thorough discussion with her physicians and surgeons. Her doctors need to explain her risk status and the full ramifications of this operation, both positive and negative. A consultation with a genetic counselor may also be helpful in fully evaluating a woman's risk status and understanding its implications for her health. She also needs to discuss this operation with others with whom she is intimate. Finally, input from other physicians involved in her care and second opinions from other surgeons are recommended to ensure that this option is weighed carefully before a final decision is made for or against it.

HIGH RISK FACTORS FOR DEVELOPING BREAST CANCER

Three main factors are believed to contribute to an increased risk of breast cancer. Many women fit into at least one of these categories, but that does not mean they will necessarily develop breast cancer and should consider having their breasts removed. What they do need is good information about their risk status, particularly women who fall into any of the three high-risk categories.

A Strong Family History of Cancer or Hereditary Breast Cancer

Hereditary breast cancer results from the inheritance of a single gene mutation and is associated with a *high* breast cancer risk. Families with hereditary cancer tend to have a strong family history of cancer. Genetics professionals will assess the family history for features consistent with this pattern of inheritance. Some of these features include multiple affected family members who are closely related to one another, multiple generations affected with cancer, different cancer types that may be associated with one another as part of a hereditary cancer syndrome, bilateral breast cancer (in both breasts), or bilateral cancer in paired organs (for example, breasts, kidneys, and ovaries), and young age at diagnosis.

Some women with such family histories also carry a heritable breast cancer tendency, such as women who have tested positive for the breast cancer genes *BRCA1* and/or *BRCA2*. These two genes are thought to account for the majority of instances of breast cancer caused by inherited genetic errors. When these genes are changed or mutated, they lead to an increased susceptibility to breast cancer (in the range of 50% to 70% over a lifetime for women with mutations in *BRCA1*). Increasingly, laboratory testing can define which of these two situations accounts for a particular woman's family history. (See Chapter 7 for a detailed discussion of genetic factors.)

Previous Personal History of Breast Cancer

If cancer develops in one breast, the chance of a new cancer occurring in the woman's other breast increases. If she is over 50, the risk is about 4% for the remaining years, and for those under 50, there is a lifetime risk of approximately 14%. If several cancerous areas are found in the first breast, the risk to the second breast is greater. These risks are further increased if the woman who had one breast cancer also has a family history, especially if her mother or a sister had this disease, and particularly if it occurred before menopause. In addition, women who have a small tumor that has not spread to the lymph nodes are more likely to live longer and therefore are at risk of developing a second tumor over a longer period. The pathologist's report on the first breast cancer can suggest an increased risk for the remaining breast. For instance, if the changes of lobular carcinoma in situ (LCIS) are noted, the patient's risk for another tumor increases by a factor of 2 to 3. The risk of this happening is about 1% for each year of life. If a woman develops breast cancer before the age of 40, the chance that she will develop another cancer in her opposite breast is somewhat increased. Once she reaches the age of 70, her risk increases by 30%.

Advanced Age

Although recent statistics suggest that more younger women are now affected by breast cancer, the overall incidence rises with age. About 85% of breast cancers are clinically detected in patients 45 years old or older. Advances in mammography have made it easier to detect early breast cancer in women over 50 and in postmenopausal women, whose breasts are less dense.

PROPHYLACTIC MASTECTOMY AND RECONSTRUCTION: WHAT TO EXPECT

The objective of a prophylactic mastectomy (also known as *total, preventive,* and *risk-reducing mastectomy*) is to remove as much glandular breast tissue as possible while preserving the skin covering so that the breast may be reconstructed to an attractive appearance. Today these operations are usually done as skin-sparing mastectomies, which seem to provide the best aesthetic results.

Because breast tissue is close to the skin, removal can sometimes impair the blood supply to the skin and nipple-areola. The surgeon will usually request that the patient refrain from smoking cigarettes for 4 to 6 weeks before and after surgery to prevent any further compromise of the blood supply. Heavy cigarette smoking causes the small blood vessels in the skin to constrict, thus increasing the possibility of complications. Problems ranging from changes in the skin, possible scarring, loss of flap tissue, loss of the nipple-areola, or implant exposure (requiring removal) are all possibilities.

When the breast is of normal size, the nipple-areola skin can be left on the breast after the breast tissue beneath the nipple is removed. This is called a *subcutaneous* or *nipple-sparing mastectomy*. The ducts are cut off from deep within the nipple and from the areola complex immediately beneath the skin. This "coring" approach to the nipple can leave very thin skin behind with a poor blood supply, leading to wound-healing problems or color loss in the skin. It also leaves behind more breast tissue than that removed with a total or simple mastectomy. Patients should be warned about the potential complications and the possible need for subsequent revisionary surgery.

From an oncologic point of view, many cancer surgeons prefer to remove the nipple-areola during prophylactic mastectomy (simple or total mastectomy). The plastic surgeon then reconstructs the breast with the woman's own tissue or by placing an implant or expander implant under the pectoralis major muscle layer. This muscle cover will help ensure that the implant remains soft and does not become exposed through the skin. Experience with current implants and textured surface expanders indicates that they provide equally soft results, regardless of whether they are positioned under the remaining skin or muscle. However, for patients with thin skin cover (which includes most of the women who have this prophylactic operation), the implant's contour and folds may be seen and felt through the thin skin; thus it is best placed under the muscle. If the woman is concerned about using breast implants and still requests prophylactic mastectomy, breast reconstruction with bilateral TRAM flaps can be considered. If the woman's breast is large and pendulous, it will require either a flap reconstruction to provide sufficient fill for the remaining breast skin or modification of the remaining breast skin so that the breast appears smaller and more uplifted. In the latter case, the plastic surgeon temporarily removes the nipple-areola and excises the breast tissue and ducts from beneath it. Then he replaces the nipple-areola as a graft in the proper position on the newly reconstructed breast.

After the surgeon removes the breast tissue, he uses one of the methods described in Chapter 13 to reconstruct the breast. Prophylactic mastectomy and the subsequent reconstruction usually are performed in one operation (as described for immediate breast reconstruction), even though some surgeons advise delaying the reconstruction for a few days to months for patients with increased risk factors such as cigarette smoking or breast scars from previous breast biopsies, which could compromise the primary healing of the skin and lead to postoperative complications.

WHERE ARE THE INCISIONS PLACED, AND DO THEY SHOW?

A number of incisions can be used for prophylactic mastectomy; the patient should discuss these variations with her surgeon.

Today many surgeons remove the tissue through a skin-sparing incision that encircles the nipple-areola and may have a slight horizontal extension to ensure complete tissue removal. Some surgeons perform this operation through an opening in the crease beneath the breast (inframammary crease). These incisions produce the least obvious scars. Another option is to use a second axillary incision in addition to the one at the inframammary fold. Other surgeons have difficulty gaining access to the upper axillary breast tissue through this approach and use an incision lateral to the areola. Sometimes this incision is extended over the nipple to elevate it when the breast sags. When a nipple-sparing (subcutaneous) mastectomy is being used, the incision is made around one half of the areola (usually the lower half), with the breast tissue removed through that opening.

The presence of biopsy or other breast scars can influence the safety and position of the prophylactic mastectomy incisions. When the biopsy scars are relatively long, the mastectomy can often be done through these scars, thus avoiding additional breast incisions and causing less risk that some of the breast skin will not survive. When the breasts are large or there is excessive breast skin, the surgeon removes the extra skin from below the nipple-areola and just above the crease, leaving an inverted-T scar, or through the middle of the breast, leaving a scar on the lower midportion of the breast. A woman considering prophylactic mastectomy who has larger breasts that also need to be lifted or made smaller should know that she may have an increased risk of having problems and complications from the operation. The nipple-areolar skin often has to be taken from its low position on the breast and either grafted to its new position or reconstructed at a later operation. Removal of a larger amount of breast tissue and the need for larger skin flaps also increase the risk that the skin will heal poorly.

What If a Breast Cancer Is Found at the Time of Prophylactic Mastectomy?

The surgeon should carefully evaluate the breasts for breast cancer before the decision is made to perform a prophylactic mastectomy. Occasionally, either during the operation or later, after the pathologist evaluates the tissues removed during the mastectomy, a breast cancer is found. Because of this possibility, a total mastectomy should be performed, with breast tissue removed according to recognized cancer treatment standards and guidelines. However, to determine whether the breast cancer has spread, an axillary dissection with removal of a sampling of axillary lymph nodes may still be needed to provide more information about the stage of the tumor and the advisability of chemotherapy or hormonal therapy. These possibilities should be considered before a preventive mastectomy and an agreement reached as to how to proceed if breast cancer is found. When cancer is discovered during the prophylactic mastectomy, the axillary lymph nodes can be removed in the same procedure. If a breast cancer is found later by the pathologist during his evaluation of the mastectomy specimen, a secondary axillary lymph node removal may be advised. If the breast cancer is found near a preserved nipple-areola, it can be removed during a subsequent operation.

It is not possible to totally remove all of a woman's breast tissue during a prophylactic mastectomy; therefore some risk still remains. Estimates put this risk at no more than 0.5% or less—approximately the same risk that men have for developing breast cancer. Therefore a woman who has had a prophylactic mastectomy should continue to monitor her reconstructed breast vigilantly; if any changes are noted, she should report them to her surgeon.

How Will a Woman's Breast Look After Prophylactic Mastectomy and Reconstruction?

Breasts reconstructed with insertion of a breast implant under the muscle after prophylactic mastectomy may not be as soft, sensitive, or mobile as natural breasts. Scars from the operation will be visible, and the re-created breasts often will not exhibit the flow and mobility of natural breasts. They are also usually flatter and do not have normal conical projection in the area under the areola, since the tissue in this area has been removed. This flat appearance often improves during the first few weeks after the operation.

When prophylactic mastectomy is followed by breast reconstruction with the patient's own tissues, the appearance and feel of her breasts are more natural, but she must also endure a more involved flap procedure that usually takes tissue from the lower abdominal wall or back and leaves donor site scars in addition to the breast scars. Breasts reconstructed with autologous tissue often have greater sensation than those reconstructed with implants (which usually feel numb). Up to 70% of these autologous breast reconstructions demonstrate some sensation after a year's time. The unique sensitivity associated with the nipple-areola is not restored with any of the currently used methods of breast reconstruction, which is a major drawback of the procedure for many women.

Despite the obvious limitations of prophylactic mastectomy and reconstruction, women having this procedure usually are satisfied with their decision to have the operation, because their main purpose has been accomplished: they have alleviated their overriding concern about their high-risk status by removing most of the breast tissue at risk.

A woman considering prophylactic mastectomy must be aware that even though only one operation is planned, additional procedures may be needed to correct asymmetry, treat a complication from the initial procedure, or improve breast appearance if it does not meet the patient's expectations as to size or shape.

RESULTS

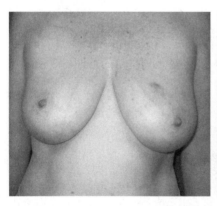 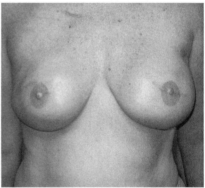

This middle-aged woman was initially seen for cancer of the left breast. She had an overwhelming fear of developing cancer in her right breast that prompted her to request a prophylactic mastectomy. She had a left skin-sparing mastectomy and right prophylactic mastectomy with immediate tissue expander placement in both breasts. When expansion was complete, her expanders were replaced with high profile silicone-gel implants. She is shown 6 months after completion of nipple reconstruction using C-V flaps and tattooing of the areolas.

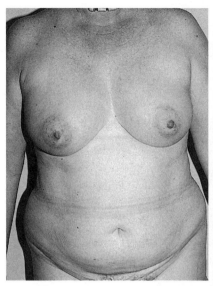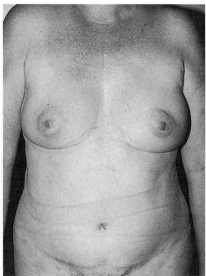

This 46-year-old woman had significant risk factors for breast cancer (her mother and two sisters had developed breast cancer before age 45). She decided to have prophylactic skin- and nipple-sparing bilateral mastectomies with immediate breast reconstruction using TRAM flaps. She is shown 3 years after breast reconstruction. Her anxiety concerning breast cancer is reduced, and she is pleased with the improved abdominal wall contour.

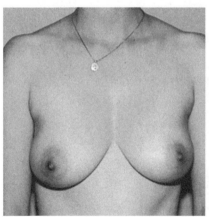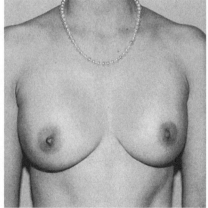

This 32-year-old woman lived in constant fear of breast cancer, because her mother and 38-year-old sister both had premenopausal breast cancer. She is shown 3 years after bilateral prophylactic mastectomies and immediate reconstruction with implants.

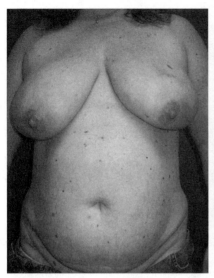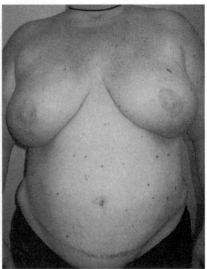

This 30-year-old woman was diagnosed with a left breast cancer; she requested a prophylactic mastectomy to be performed at the time of her left mastectomy for cancer treatment. She had ample abdominal tissue and wanted an autologous procedure because of its long-term benefits. She is shown 9 months after a left DIEP flap and a right muscle-sparing free TRAM flap, since her right-sided anatomy did not favor a safe perforator flap transfer.

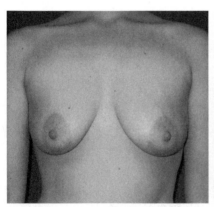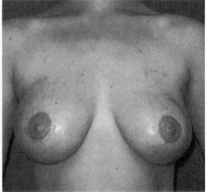

This 28-year-old woman was diagnosed with the *BRCA1* gene; her mother and sister had already had breast cancer. She elected to have bilateral prophylactic mastectomies with immediate reconstruction. The skin of her chest wall was very thin, and her abdomen did not have enough tissue to reconstruct both breasts. She wanted her breasts slightly larger than their preoperative size and was concerned about possible wrinkling of an implant through her thin tissues. Therefore she chose bilateral latissimus dorsi flap reconstruction with immediate implant placement. She is shown 9 months after reconstruction and nipple reconstruction and tattooing.

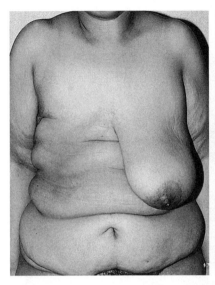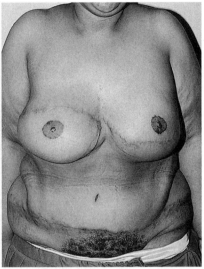

This 36-year-old woman had a right modified radical mastectomy and delayed breast reconstruction. Her opposite breast was quite heavy. Because of her increased risk factors, she requested a prophylactic mastectomy. She had a left total mastectomy and immediate breast reconstruction with bilateral TRAM flaps. She is shown 2 years after reconstruction. Her anxiety about breast cancer has diminished, and she is satisfied with the improved symmetry and abdominal wall contour.

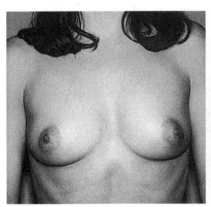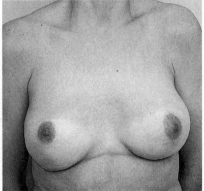

This 32-year-old woman had several significant risk factors for breast cancer. She decided to have bilateral total mastectomies with skin- and nipple-sparing mastectomies and immediate breast reconstruction. She did not want additional scars and elected to have breast implants. She is shown 8 years after breast reconstruction.

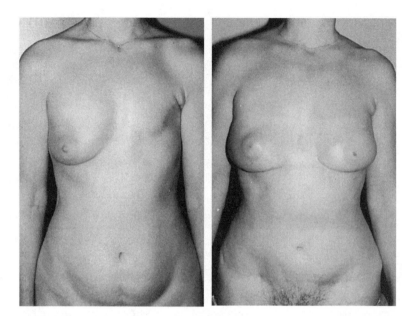

This 34-year-old woman with a strong family history of breast cancer had a modified radical mastectomy several years earlier. She later had a left prophylactic mastectomy and bilateral TRAM flap reconstruction. She is shown 3 years after breast reconstruction.

PROS AND CONS OF PREVENTIVE MASTECTOMY AND RECONSTRUCTION

Although recent advances in technique have made a prophylactic mastectomy and reconstruction more aesthetically predictable, serious complications can still occur. For a woman to make an informed, objective decision, she needs to question her surgeon about the positive and negative aspects of this procedure.

Pros

- Decreases the fear of breast cancer by removing most of the breast tissue.
- Decreases the risk of breast cancer. The effectiveness of this preventive surgery remains a source of controversy. There is no definitive evidence to prove that a prophylactic (total) mastectomy reduces a woman's risk of getting cancer, even though any tumors

occurring in the thin layer of breast tissue remaining after this procedure are usually easier to detect while they are quite small. Available reports do indicate, however, that the incidence of subsequent breast cancer is very low (less than 1%) after prophylactic mastectomy in women initially determined to be at high risk of developing breast cancer.

- A recent study suggests that prophylactic surgery significantly decreases the risk for women who carry a genetic mutation that puts them at risk for breast and ovarian cancer.
- Reduces painful symptoms caused by fibrocystic breast changes. However, breast pain alone should not be the primary indication for the operation. There are many other reasons for breast pain, and these are not improved by prophylactic mastectomy. In fact, some additional pain is always a possibility whenever a breast operation or any operation is performed.

Cons

- Subject to operative risks associated with any major surgical procedure, including those from general anesthesia as well as complications of bleeding, infection, skin loss, nipple loss, capsular contracture, and implant loss. Additional abdominal complications can occur if a TRAM flap is used for breast reconstruction. Correction of these problems often requires additional operations.
- May not produce a reconstructed breast that is as attractive as the original breast. Permanent scars and a lack of normal breast flow and projection can be expected. Additional operations may be needed to improve the appearance of the breasts after prophylactic mastectomy and immediate breast reconstruction.
- Results in decreased sensation or loss of sensation in the reconstructed breast, especially the nipple-areola, because of the division of the sensory nerves when the breast is removed. Even though breast sensation does not return, the woman's breasts may feel uncomfortable, even painful.
- Often requires more than one procedure to achieve the best result or manage complications.
- Still leaves a small percentage of breast tissue as a potential site of breast cancer.

A woman's decision for a preventive mastectomy and reconstruction requires input from the cancer surgeon, other members of the breast management team, and a genetic counselor. These specialists can advise her concerning her particular risks of developing breast cancer as well as the normal, expected results of a prophylactic mastectomy for a woman with her type of breasts. She needs to be examined and counseled by at least two physicians who can evaluate her risk factors and their implications for her future health status. Prophylactic mastectomy is not an emergency procedure. If there is a suspicious breast mass or an indication that breast cancer is present, this question should be resolved before a decision is made for prophylactic mastectomy. Most women at risk are monitored most effectively by breast self-examination and regular physician examinations and mammograms. A woman should carefully consider all of her options and all aspects of her situation before a final decision is made for preventive surgery.

CREATING A
NIPPLE-AREOLA

W hen a woman has her breast reconstructed, she also must decide whether she wants her nipple and areola (the circular pigmented area surrounding the nipple) reconstructed. Some women only want their breast shape restored so they feel balanced and symmetrical. For them, the nipple-areola is of little consequence. To others, however, a nipple-areola is an important component of reconstructive surgery. This represents the finishing touch that makes their breasts look and feel more natural.

In interviews and surveys with women who had breast reconstruction, we discovered an interesting correlation between the success of the initial procedure to build the breast and the woman's subsequent desire for a nipple. When the rebuilt breast does not meet her aesthetic desires, she usually does not want her nipple restored, no matter how simple the procedure, because it merely emphasizes a poor result. The attitude of these women is "enough is enough," and they are content to be able to fill out a bra. Women who have satisfactory aesthetic results frequently have the opposite reaction. They want a nipple-areola reconstruction as the final phase of their operation to create a more natural breast appearance and to provide a good match with their opposite breasts. The fact that simpler techniques are now available makes the option of nipple-areola reconstruction even more appealing. The creation of the nipple-areola seems to complete a rehabilitation program for them. As one woman explained, "It becomes the icing on the cake; it is not absolutely necessary, but it is so beautiful when it's there."

Although reconstruction of the breast and nipple-areola is possible during one operation, the best results are obtained when the ideal breast shape is achieved first. Most plastic surgeons prefer to wait a few months after the first operation or after tissue expansion has been completed until the newly created breast is stable and symmetrical with the remaining breast. Then the plastic surgeon and patient can more accurately determine the proper position, size, and projection of the nipple-areola. It is important for the woman to participate in this decision-making process. Once the nipple has been built, it is very difficult to change its position later without removing and re-grafting it or starting over. She is going to have to live with it, and it should look right to her. Unless additional corrections of the recon-structed breast are needed, the actual reconstruction often can be done on an outpatient basis with the use of a local anesthetic.

Significant advances have been made in nipple-areola recon-struction techniques during the past few years, and there are a number of techniques for women to choose from. It is now possible to rebuild a woman's nipple with the local tissue present at the site of the new nipple-areola on her reconstructed breast. The color of the nipple-areola is defined a few months later with a tattoo. Alternatively, when the skin on the reconstructed breast is thin and the opposite nipple is large, another option is a nipple-sharing technique in which a portion of the large opposite nipple is used for the nipple reconstruction. The areola can be created with excess skin at the lateral portion of the mastectomy scar, or if the patient had a TRAM flap breast recon-struction, it can be grafted from excess tissue at the end of the ab-dominal scar. The circular area of the areola can be simulated with a tattoo of the approximate color and size to match the opposite areola without the need for taking a skin graft to form the areola.

Most women choose to have their nipples reconstructed from the local tissue on the breast and then have their nipple and areola tat-tooed later. These new techniques are often more appealing than pre-vious approaches that created the nipple and areola from two different types of tissue transferred from other areas of a woman's body. These older methods are still used for some patients when appropriate, and they continue to give excellent results. The newer methods, however, are simpler, frequently less painful, and are often preferred because they seem to fit in more readily with most women's active lifestyles.

NIPPLE RECONSTRUCTION

When a woman chooses to have her nipple reconstructed, she does so to complete her reconstruction, to enhance the appearance of her re-constructed breast, and to make the nipple more symmetrical with her remaining breast. Projection seems to be a key issue with many women who elect to have their nipples reconstructed; they want the freedom to wear T-shirts and swimsuits without being self-conscious that one nipple is more prominent than the other. The woman should be advised that creation of a nipple will not provide sensation or the potential for milk production; these functions are impossible for the reconstructed breast.

Presently several primary methods of nipple reconstruction use local tissue at the site of the future nipple-areola to build the new nipple—the C-V flap (thus named because the design of the flap resembles two V's connected by a C), the skate flap, and variants of local flaps that are spiraled or turned to give a projecting nipple. With these techniques, a layer of skin and fat on the reconstructed breast is shifted to the center of the future nipple-areola area and formed into a nipple. The skin is used to create the nipple, and the underlying fat contributes bulk, fullness, and permanent shape. The skate flap uses much of the skin at the site of the future areola for the nipple reconstruction; the areola is then reconstructed from a graft of skin taken

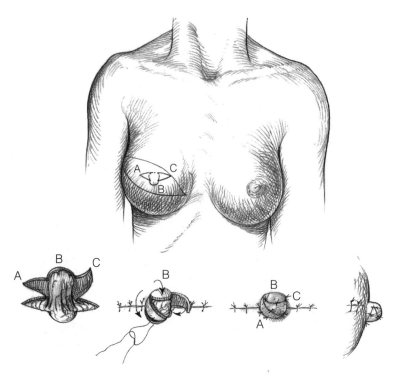

The C-V flap uses tissue of the reconstructed breast to create a nipple, which a few months later will be tattooed along with the surrounding areola.

from another site, such as the outer portion of the mastectomy scar. With the C-V flap, not as much local tissue is used and consequently it may not produce as large and projecting a nipple as the skate flap. However, the donor site for the C-V flap can be closed with two short scars; therefore an areola graft is not always necessary with the C-V flap operation. A tattoo can be done later for nipple color and areola reconstruction.

Although a nice-sized nipple can be created from breast skin, often its color is not dark enough to match the remaining nipple. In this case a tattoo provides a better color match (see p. 411).

The opposite nipple can also be used for nipple reconstruction when there is not enough local tissue to build a symmetrical nipple; however, this is not a popular choice today. It is often not acceptable to either the patient or her husband or significant other, and other sources of tissue for nipple reconstruction are selected. However, when the remaining nipple is very large and projecting, or when the skin over the implant reconstruction is thin and tight and there is not enough extra tissue for a satisfactory nipple reconstruction, this method is still the best way to create a nipple that is symmetrical in size, color, and texture. With this technique, a portion of the lower end of the remaining nipple is used for the nipple reconstruction. The donor area of the normal nipple is not significantly changed or scarred; it usually heals in 1 to 2 weeks without any numbness and little pain. After the nipple has healed, it does not lose its sensitivity or feeling.

AREOLA RECONSTRUCTION

Methods for recreating the areola range from simple tattooing to the more complex graft techniques. The decision as to which technique is appropriate depends on a patient's lifestyle and preferences, although today most women seem to prefer tattooing the areola as the easiest and least time-consuming approach.

Some women do not care if the color is exact; they want the simplest, safest, and least painful method for creating a semblance of an areola. Tattooing, which may not always produce a realistic result, may be the solution that these woman desire. Although the texture and projection of the natural areola will be lacking, the color match of a tattooed areola can be quite good, and an areola graft is not needed. Many women appreciate the convenience of this approach.

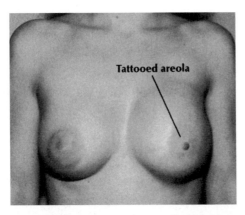

A tattoo without areola grafting was satisfactory for this woman, who preferred a simple, nonsurgical procedure that produced the semblance of an areola.

When local breast skin is used for nipple reconstruction, the tissue for the areola graft can be taken from the lateral portion of the mastectomy scar or the lateral portion of the abdominal scar if the woman had a TRAM flap. (With new skin-sparing mastectomies, the residual scars are now shorter and there is less available scar tissue for areola reconstruction.) When sufficient tissue is available, this technique is very acceptable to most women, and it avoids additional scars; it is also effectively used in combination with the skate flap. The mastectomy scar and the excess skin at the lateral end of the scar can often be improved when the areola graft is removed. Since this area is usually numb from the mastectomy, little pain is experienced when taking the graft or afterward. The main drawback is that the skin graft is not pigmented, and although it will appear pink during the initial weeks to months after grafting, it usually fades, and tattooing may be necessary to obtain a better color match.

A graft of tissue from the upper inner thigh crease is another means of reconstructing the areola. The tissue obtained from this area is pigmented and usually provides a good match with the opposite areola without the need for an areola tattoo. A round areola skin graft is removed from the upper thigh crease, and the remaining thigh skin is brought together as a thin scar line in this crease. This scar is practically invisible when healed; it does not show, even in a bathing suit. The groin area is usually painful after this procedure and will feel tender for about 2 weeks. This technique produces acceptable results, but it involves a painful donor site and is rarely used today with the advent of the newer, less painful techniques just described.

Once the areola graft has been obtained, the actual placement of the new areola onto the breast area can be accomplished. If the upper inner thigh graft has been used, a very thin circular layer of surface skin needs to be removed first to make room for this new areola. (In the skate or C-V flap operation, this skin layer has already been removed to build the nipple.) The areola skin graft is then positioned on this area.

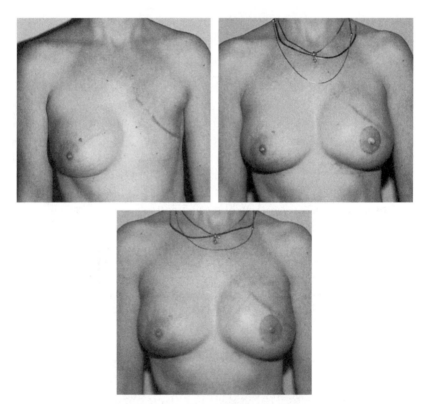

This 33-year-old patient had nipple-areola reconstruction with local skin used for nipple reconstruction and an areola graft taken from the lateral end of the mastectomy scar. Her nipple-areola was tattooed 2 months later. She is shown 1 year after tattooing.

NIPPLE-AREOLA TATTOO

Many times the color of a nipple and areola created from breast skin is not dark enough to match the remaining nipple-areola. In this case a tattoo provides a better color match. A tattoo is the most direct and permanent method for pigmenting the reconstructed nipple-areola. As discussed earlier, it is also effective in creating the appearance of an areola for a woman who does not want to have another surgical procedure or for a woman whose opposite areola is so large that it is not practical to reconstruct a matching areola using a skin graft. Tattooing is used to create a pigmented circle to match the other areola without resorting to a large skin graft.

Many plastic surgeons who do breast reconstruction can perform the tattooing in their office as an outpatient procedure or can arrange to have the tattooing done by a qualified professional. The procedure

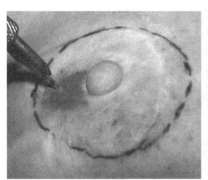 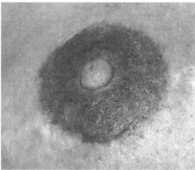

Areola tattoo

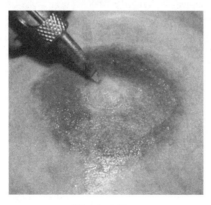

Nipple tattoo

is quite easy. The patient participates in determining the proper color for the new nipple-areola. The natural nipple-areola has a wide spectrum of colors, and the best color match is achieved by blending the pigments.

A local anesthetic is often used before tattooing. The tattoo device is then dipped in the pigment and placed into the outer layers of skin. The pigment is applied until the areola and nipple have been uniformly tattooed. Slightly darker pigments are used for the nipple tattoo. The area will be a little raw for a few days after the procedure; an antibiotic ointment can be applied to keep it moist. If a woman's skin tones have a lot of yellow, the match may not be as close. Newer pigments are providing better matches for these individuals. Over the next few weeks to months, because of the healing process, the tattooed nipple-areola may look darker than the color selected; however, with time it fades, usually to an acceptable color. The woman should be warned of this possibility so that she will not be unnecessarily alarmed. Even so, some women are disturbed by the early disparity in color and are anxious for the color to fade so that it matches the remaining nipple-areola and does not stand out "like a beacon."

To protect the nipple and areola after surgery, a protective dressing is taped over the nipple and stabilized with surgical tape. The reconstructed nipple-areola tends to be dry after surgery; a moisturizing cream can be applied to improve this condition.

Although the creation of a nipple-areola is not an essential component of a breast reconstruction, it adds a realistic finishing touch. By creating a nipple-areola on a woman's new breast, the surgeon can transform her surgically created mound into a natural and aesthetic breast form.

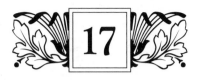

BREAST CANCER AND ITS EFFECT ON RELATIONSHIPS

WHAT WOMEN WANT: MALE SUPPORT

It is always hard on the man. He stands there, outside, and he sees all of the problems down the road. He is both frightened to death and threatened. But the patient, somewhere along the way, comes to terms with herself because she has no choice.

These words express the feelings of one breast cancer patient as she reflected on the predicaments that this disease creates for men and women. Her statement typifies the type of answers we received when we surveyed women about this topic. Drawing on the responses of more than 800 women who had breast cancer, we have summarized their feelings and thoughts about the problems they encountered in their relationships as a result of this disease. Issues addressed include the response to diagnosis, recovery from cancer surgery, the response to lumpectomy, the reaction to mastectomy, issues of intimacy and sexual relationships, common fears of the breast cancer patient, the single woman's special concerns, and male support for breast reconstruction. Although there are no prescribed rules for a man to follow under these circumstances, many of the women we surveyed had suggestions about what had been most helpful for them. This chapter incorporates these suggestions. In addition to information gleaned from our questionnaire, we have included a short section written by a general surgeon on the patient-surgeon relationship, as well as three interviews, two with men and one with a couple.

Facing the Diagnosis

The discovery of breast cancer provokes many fears in a couple, and these fears need to be shared. Both are worried about the prognosis of cancer and its effect on their relationship. They worry about possible treatment options and the effects of chemotherapy, radiation treatment, or surgery. Their concerns may not surface immediately, however, since there seems to be a tendency for couples to hide true feelings behind a cheerful "make the best of it" facade. These true feelings can be damaging to a relationship if they are not brought into the open and examined. All of the women we contacted believed in and stressed the need for open and honest communication. As one woman said, "I asked my husband if he could allow me to feel what I was feeling, and I would try to allow him his feelings. I didn't want pity. I just wanted him to listen when I talked, because it was a release to say how I was feeling." This need for unfettered communication was also echoed by single women who were dating or involved in committed relationships. As one woman explained, "Naturally, when you are dating you are always trying to present yourself in the best light, and sometimes that means not allowing the other person to see all of your hidden flaws. That's why you still wear makeup to bed. But cancer changes that dynamic forever. It gets down to bare essentials. If there is to be any hope for a long-term relationship, subterfuge must go out the window. It is a time for sharing and for honesty. Ultimately, that is the test of a relationship. If a man runs at this point, he probably wasn't worth the investment of time and love in the first place."

Women also stressed the importance of physical closeness and contact accompanying this communication process. The value of hugging and holding was mentioned in virtually all of our surveys and interviews. One woman expressed this feeling most poignantly when she said, "Sometimes when the words wouldn't come, my boyfriend would just hold me, hug me, stroke me, and I would cry. That was real communication. Even though he told me he loved me, and I loved hearing it, his touch revealed all I needed to know. The physical closeness made me feel loved and accepted. Hugging makes a big difference."

Women emphasized the ameliorative effects of talking about their problems with someone else. It was crucial to have someone close to share the burden. Sometimes they just needed someone to listen to them and to hold them without "trying to make things right." As one woman explained, "During the tears, the anger, the insecurity, the fear, the ups and the downs, there is really no need to give advice or try to cheer a woman up. A man just needs to allow her to have all of these feelings and be understanding, even if none of these feelings makes sense. More than anything else, a man needs to listen to a woman's feelings, her fears, her hopes without judging or trying to 'fix' things." Another woman wrote, "There is no way that anybody can really understand what you are feeling when you have cancer, unless that person has experienced it himself. What can you say to someone—'I'm sorry'? Sometimes you just need a one-way conversation with somebody. Men can help us by just letting us get upset and release some of the tension."

The time between the diagnosis of breast cancer and the selection of treatment is a tense one for both a man and a woman. For a man, the fear of his loved one's death from cancer usually far overshadows her possible loss of a breast. Understandably, his priority is the woman's health and survival. It is important, however, for him to acknowledge her concerns and be careful not to minimize her attachment to her breasts. Together they need to define their priorities and investigate her therapy options.

The first priority is for the woman to get the best treatment for her tumor. She often feels confused and depressed by all that is happening to her. By accompanying her to medical consultations, a man can actively demonstrate his concern and help a woman focus on the issues being discussed. Together they can learn about and critically evaluate the various treatment options. Most of the couples we interviewed had taken the time to inform themselves about breast cancer and about breast reconstruction. They had searched the Internet for pertinent information, read articles and books on these topics, attended lectures, and even seen movies and slide presentations. They agreed that this process helped them cope and also gave them a better understanding of what the future held. Repeatedly, in both our surveys and in our discussions with men and women, couples stressed the beneficial value of this educational process. As one man related, "By learning about my girlfriend's cancer, we at least were able to understand our choices and make some decisions based on knowledge instead of fear. I actually think it brought us closer together."

The Patient-Surgeon Relationship

ROGER S. FOSTER, JR., MD

It is normal for a woman diagnosed with breast cancer to react with mixed emotions to her disease and to the surgeon responsible for her treatment. Feelings of desperation, rage, and hopelessness may co-exist with feelings of courage, hope, and determination. She may be angry with fate, God, or even herself. Some of her resentment will naturally focus on her surgeon. Frequently he is the messenger delivering the bad news about her cancer and her prognosis. Furthermore, his treatments inflict pain, create scars, and may deform her body, all good reasons for her to react negatively. In addition to these negative feelings, however, most women also experience positive feelings for their surgeons. Because a woman is dependent on her surgeon, having entrusted her life and body to him, she feels vulnerable and exposed. She needs to reassure herself that he is a skilled professional and that he is a particularly sensitive and caring individual, personally interested in her welfare. Her intense feelings about her cancer and its treatment may lead her to attribute laudatory qualities to her surgeon that are really more reflective of her emotional needs than of the actual character of the surgeon himself.

These conflicting emotions of resentment and admiration are difficult to deal with, particularly for an already stressed woman trying to cope with a life-threatening disease. Her strong feelings are not wrong, but it helps if the woman, her loved ones, and her surgeon are able to recognize these feelings for what they are. Her anger and hostility should not be personalized by the surgeon and taken as an affront. Similarly, a woman should not feel guilty about experiencing these negative reactions. Perhaps the surgeon has been lacking in tact and diplomacy. Maybe his people skills need some polishing. Even so, a woman and her loved ones need to understand that her anger is not necessarily attributable to the surgeon's personality. Much of her rage is situational, a reaction to circumstances beyond her control. The positive feelings of affection and even adulation that she may develop for her surgeon should also be recognized as situational in nature and should not be misinterpreted by the woman experiencing them or the man who cares about her. The patient's affection or even "love" for her cancer surgeon or plastic surgeon is not the same as the love she may feel for a husband or significant other, where reciprocity of affection is expected. Even though a man may experience moments of jealousy or resentment because of his loved one's seeming transference of affection to her doctor, he should realize that with time and recovery, this affection as well as the anger she feels toward her doctor will diminish, and she will view her relationship with him from a more balanced perspective.

Recovery From Lumpectomy

After a lumpectomy a woman's recovery is usually relatively quick and easy. Many times this procedure can be performed on an outpatient basis. She goes home, breast intact and cancer eliminated, without significant pain or the need for a prolonged recuperation and time away from work. This relatively seamless transition between cancer diagnosis, treatment, and return to normal daily activities may cause others to underestimate the seriousness of her situation. Many of the lumpectomy patients who responded to our surveys made mention of their frustration at the seemingly dismissive attitudes they encountered, particularly from the men in their lives. As one woman so aptly explained, "I sometimes feel just like Rodney Dangerfield: 'I get no respect!' For God's sake, I have cancer. I still worry about my life and about the very real possibility of a recurrence. Yes, I have my breast, but that doesn't mean that I don't still worry about it. I don't have to be mutilated or look like I'm dying for people to take me seriously. My boyfriend keeps saying, 'Isn't it great that you are all okay now and it's over.' He treats me as if I'm recovering from a cold. Well, it isn't okay, and it isn't over. Yes, I kept my breast, but the trauma of my cancer diagnosis haunts me every day."

Most of the lumpectomy patients we interviewed stressed the need for a man to be sensitive to the complex emotions that a woman must deal with after lumpectomy and radiation therapy. Although her physical appearance may seem virtually unchanged, it masks an inner turmoil. Whether a woman has had a mastectomy or a lumpectomy, she still has faced the grim reality of breast cancer. The seriousness of her surgery or of her cancer must not be minimized. Her full recovery requires the same grieving process confronted by any patient dealing with a life-threatening disease. Breast cancer will live in her mind, if not in her breast, long after the tumor is removed and the scar has faded. As one woman explained, "People think I shouldn't be upset about having cancer because I only had a lumpectomy." Another woman complained, "My boyfriend keeps telling me, 'Cheer up. You only had a lumpectomy; you are really lucky.' Well, I don't feel cheerful; I need some time to cope with this, to feel sad, to cry. Men sometimes look at lumpectomy as an excuse to avoid emotionally confronting the cancer issue." It is clear from our surveys and interviews that women who choose lumpectomy desire and need the same emotional support and understanding that is afforded to women who have mastectomies.

Recovery From Mastectomy

After a mastectomy or mastectomy with immediate reconstruction, a woman commonly experiences a period of "peak" stress as she attempts to recover from the physical and psychological effects of this operation. Her physical recuperation usually takes 2 to 3 months but may be prolonged if chemotherapy or radiation therapy is necessary. She may be weak, tired, irritable, and possibly ill from the treatments. Lifting a vacuum cleaner or carrying groceries might be too much strain for her, and she may need someone to assume some of her physical responsibilities until she feels better. (Women who have had lumpectomies and are undergoing radiation therapy may experience similar stress and fatigue. They also appreciate help with the daily household responsibilities.) A man's attitude when helping is crucial. Women stressed the importance of a man offering assistance willingly and not begrudgingly so that the woman does not "feel needy or as if she is nagging him to help her." Many women said that their arms felt sore and stiff for the first few weeks after surgery, and they appreciated having someone accompany them on trips to the doctor so they did not have to worry about driving the car and possibly straining themselves. It also was helpful when a man could assist with some of the organizational and parenting responsibilities of the household, seeing to the children's appointments and schedules, attending recitals and athletic events, paying bills, arranging for repairmen, and filling in when necessary. As one woman explained, "My man was there when I needed him most, yet we were thousands of miles apart physically during portions of my treatment. He cared for our children, and his phone calls were sufficient to help me through." By doing the heavy cleaning, driving the carpools, or doing the grocery shopping, a man can provide positive support for a woman during her recovery.

There is a delicate balance between willingly assisting a woman until her strength returns and actually doing everything for her. Most women we surveyed appreciated the physical assistance men provided during their initial recuperation, but they were quick to resist any attempts to take over. Even though some of the men that we interviewed felt that they could best help their wives by relieving them of all worries and responsibilities, their wives did not agree. Most women were uncomfortable with this treatment. "Don't put us on pedestals. Help us, if we need help, but don't cure one thing and start something else. We do not want to be treated as invalids." Getting back into the mainstream of life seemed to be the focus for most of the women we surveyed. They actively feared being left out of life. They wanted to feel useful and to participate as they always had. They did not want people to "whisper and tiptoe around them."

Reactions to a Woman's Changed Physical Appearance After Mastectomy

A man's response to her changed physical appearance worries the woman who has had a mastectomy. Above all, she fears his expressing shock at her missing breast. Many women worry that they will appear less feminine and lovable. Fearing rejection, they desire physical attention, love, and continued reassurance of their desirability. As one woman explained, "No woman is less feminine or intelligent or attractive because she has had a mastectomy, but sometimes it helps to be reminded."

The problem of how to react to a woman's altered appearance is not an easy one. In some cases the woman cannot adjust to her missing breast and does not want the man to see her. Some of the women we surveyed are "still dressing in the closet" so no one sees them. Some have never shown their scars to their husbands or boyfriends for fear they will be disgusted at what they see. Some even avoid intimate relationships and possible exposure of their scarred chests. In other cases the woman is willing to show her missing breast to her loved one and allow him to help her change bandages, rub ointment on her scar, or reassure her that she still looks okay. Many of the women responding to us suggested that problems could be avoided if the scar were seen as soon as possible after surgery. One woman wrote that many of her worries had been eliminated because she and her boyfriend had viewed the scar together in the hospital in the presence of her doctor. They shared the shock together, recovered from it, and went on to concentrate on other matters.

Impact on Relationships

Although many of the women we contacted felt that men were usually supportive of women cancer patients, not all of the stories we heard were positive. Some relationships ended. Boyfriends left and divorces occurred after mastectomy, after breast reconstruction, and even after lumpectomy. Some men could not adjust to their wife's or significant other's status as a cancer victim or to her changed physical appearance. They "could not handle the tumor" or stand to "look at her lopsided chest with a breast on one side and a red scar on the other." Others could not cope with the added responsibility of worrying about a life-threatening illness. Some men found that the woman in their lives had changed and now had difficulty relating to her. They tired of "hearing about her cancer" and found her so inwardly directed after this experience that they did not feel that she could talk about anything else.

The missing breast itself, however, did not seem to be the actual cause of divorce or breakup after a mastectomy. Sometimes it inhibited a woman sexually or made a man more timid in his sexual approaches, but these inhibitions were often overcome with time. Interestingly, both men and women seemed to agree that divorces or breakups after a mastectomy or a lumpectomy were usually the culmination of a history of problems that had previously existed between a couple. These men were temporarily supportive through surgery and recovery, but when the fear of death had subsided and life returned to its status quo, the old unhappiness was evident again, and often the relationship ended. In most cases, where there was good communication, common interests, and a deep, abiding affection, the cancer diagnosis only served to strengthen the ties between the individuals. Relationships that were strong before the surgery became even stronger afterward.

Intimacy and Sexual Relationships

Romance and intimacy is another sensitive area for women after mastectomy and even after breast reconstruction and lumpectomy. Worried about how their identity as breast cancer survivors or their changed appearance will affect their sexual relationship with a man, these women, no matter how close to their husbands or boyfriends, express fears of rejection. Men also have concerns; they worry about making the wrong moves, saying the wrong things, or pushing a woman before she is ready. Most of the women we surveyed desired a return to normal sexual relations as soon as possible. Keeping an element of romance in a relationship was very important to all of the women and men we interviewed. It helped them infuse a feeling of normality into their relationship.

As one woman candidly explained, "Even though I was missing a breast, I still wanted to be treated as a sexy and romantic woman. I wanted to be flirted with. I wanted him to do romantic things to help me to feel loving and sensual. I wanted my man to touch my body, to tenderly caress me, and to look at me in such a way that I knew it didn't make any difference to him. As a woman I needed to know that I was still sexually attractive."

Many of the women we spoke to also agreed that women will differ in their readiness for intimacy and a man should "take the lead from the woman and try to encourage but not to rush sex." That cautionary note also applies to the woman who has had breast reconstruction. As one woman advised, "I think that men should not expect sex too quickly after a woman has had reconstruction. Women need some time to recuperate both mentally and physically. They still feel protective of their bodies. I know that I still protect my body and breasts during intercourse." Obviously this is a problematic situation; a man straddles a line between expressing his affection too forcefully or seeming aloof and standoffish. Each couple needs to work out their own individual method of relating and dealing with questions of intimacy; they need to talk about these problems and understand them.

The value of foreplay and afterplay was frequently reinforced by women as they divulged their personal desires in lovemaking. Many felt that a man should initially be more gentle and stroking, and this caring should continue. "He should not pull away physically after orgasm but should tenderly embrace her and tell her he loves her." A man should not be afraid to touch the woman as he did before. Stroking during lovemaking and after was judged vitally important for a woman's self-esteem, both before and after cancer surgery and reconstruction. "My significant other was and is fantastic. He didn't care if I had reconstruction or not. In fact, my new breast is caressed as lovingly as the old one." One woman suggested the need for a man "to learn new sexual techniques to help a woman achieve arousal." As she explained, "With the loss of a breast and even after reconstruction, a major hot spot is irrevocably gone and all of the sexual sensitivity that accompanies it. Breasts are a 'turn on.' You lose that after a mastectomy, and reconstruction does not fully restore it. You can't get that special sexual sensitivity back; there is a numbness now where you used to feel titillation. You need a good relationship with your sexual partner to compensate for this loss. And sometimes you need to be creative."

A Woman's Fears

Understandably, the mastectomy patient has many questions and fears to cope with. Knowing about her doubts sometimes helps a man to be more sensitive to them. One woman poignantly summarized these worries when she sent us a series of questions that she felt needed to be answered:

- How can I face my husband or male friend?
- Will sex ever be the same?
- Will I be afraid for him to touch me?
- How will I feel about myself?
- Will I be the same person?
- Will I have the same outlook on life?
- Will my sex life be affected?
- Knowing that my man fell in love with my body as well as me, how will he feel about my body now?
- After I get a prosthesis, will people look at me and wonder which breast was cut off?
- Will people pity me, feel sorry for me?
- If I decide to have breast reconstruction, will people think I'm vain and self-centered?

Concerns of the Single Woman

For a single woman involved in dating, her breast cancer status represents a daunting obstacle to a relationship. Many of the single and divorced women we surveyed were frankly perplexed and somewhat distressed over what to tell a man in this circumstance. This confusion reigned regardless of the type of treatment that a woman had.

However, for the mastectomy patient, her missing breast presented special problems, particularly in deciding how to inform a suitor when a more intimate relationship was desired. As one woman revealed, "The worst part of having a mastectomy is that you just don't feel feminine. My male friend didn't make me feel that way; those feelings were self-inflicted. The first time we made love I didn't want to expose myself and I was terribly self-conscious. He just said, 'It doesn't matter to me,' but I said, 'It matters to me.' I always wore a nightgown. I just couldn't do it without it." Many of the single women we spoke to said that they were self-conscious about having a man see them totally undressed or in full light. One woman explained how she "always had a nightgown on and the room was always darkened." Some women, although not as many, even expressed feelings of embarrassment after reconstruction because of their scars, the telltale signs that they had surgery. As one young girl revealed, "For a long time I wore a shirt to bed or I took it off in the dark, but he was patient with me until I reached a point where I didn't feel self-conscious." Learning to relate intimately is not always easy for a couple under the best of circumstances; after a mastectomy, with or without reconstruction, it is particularly challenging.

Most women agreed that a straightforward approach was probably the best. Numerous scenarios were described in which the woman sat the man down and explained about her cancer diagnosis and treatment or her changed physical appearance and what it meant. Generally, men accept this news far better than women anticipate, sometimes even better than the women themselves. This is as true of mastectomy as it is of lumpectomy.

This is a very emotional time for a woman, and in many ways she feels that her femininity and her self-esteem are on the line. Patience and understanding are required of a man, and she in turn must be willing to communicate her feelings and fears to her partner in order to reach a level of comfort and fulfillment.

Fear of rejection was cited by all of the women we surveyed as a reason for not telling. As one woman explained, "The dating scene today is difficult enough without adding breast cancer into the equation. Men are just frightened of commitment. If a man learns that a woman had breast cancer, he may not want to take on the added burden of a possible recurrence or future illness. Not everyone is brave or caring. So I worry about telling someone early on because I don't want him to be scared away before he has a chance to really get to know me and to develop an attachment. On the other hand, if I wait too long, he will think that I am dishonest and may leave anyway. So I just haven't told anyone, and I've been very tentative in forming new relationships until I really decide what to do." This uncertainty was typical of a number of the women we spoke to. There was no one solution for handling this problem. Women were as puzzled about when to tell a man as about how to tell him. Ultimately, much depended on their intuitive sense of the man and their desire to have this relationship grow into something more meaningful. Many of the single women we spoke to chose to avoid disclosure initially, unless they had some special interest in the man. At that point, however, they felt that an honest, heart-to-heart explanation was called for. For the mastectomy or breast reconstruction patient, that disclosure might also involve baring her breasts, although most women felt that verbal communication should always precede any "show and tell." Then, as one woman explained, "I just sit back and see what kind of man I am dealing with." Not all of the responses were what these women had been hoping for, but as one woman explained, "I want to know up front rather than invest a lot of myself in a relationship that is going nowhere. I don't want a jerk in my life. I value myself too much for that."

Support for Breast Reconstruction

When a woman decides that she wants to have her breast reconstructed, whether it is performed immediately at the time of mastectomy or delayed to months or even years after the cancer surgery, she often looks to a man for encouragement. Frequently in our surveys, women explained that despite their strong personal motivation for reconstruction, they still needed a man's emotional support. They wanted to be reassured that reconstruction was okay and that they were not being vain or selfish because they desired more surgery to restore their missing breasts. If a woman seeks breast reconstruction, a man's support helps to enhance this experience and contributes to her rehabilitation.

Some men will resist the idea of breast reconstruction regardless of timing, hoping to shield their loved ones from additional pain, operative risk, and hospitalization. Judging from our questionnaires, we found this initial negative male reaction to be very common. Most of the women we surveyed understood these male concerns but felt that if a woman's commitment to reconstruction was strong, a man should respect her desires and encourage her.* Unlike the mastectomy, breast reconstruction was regarded as positive surgery meant to restore what the mastectomy had removed. As one woman explained, "It is im-

---

*Most plastic surgeons are pleased to see a man accompany a woman for a consultation about breast reconstruction. His presence usually indicates that she is not alone in her decision and has someone to support her.

portant for a man to support a woman's decision about breast recon-struction because it is her body, her feelings, her life. He should avoid making decisions for her. She needs to feel that she is in control."

A woman may not be as pleased with her new breast immediately after breast reconstruction as she had anticipated. It will not fully re-semble the original breast and will bear a scar and feel numb to the touch. At this stage of her recovery she is extremely sensitive and vul-nerable to criticism. She does not want to hear that her new breast is not as nice as her normal breast; she cannot tolerate negative com-ments or criticism of her appearance.

• • •

The man's role in dealing with a woman's breast cancer experience is a difficult one. It requires sensitivity and understanding of the special needs that a woman has as she confronts a life-threatening disease and the physical and mental adjustments that accompany treatment and rehabilitation. There is no way that he can ever really understand the full impact that breast cancer has on a woman's life. Yet his sup-port and empathy are essential to help her cope and heal from this experience. Playing the role of supporting player is the best position he can take. He needs to listen to a woman's concerns, communicate with her, and try to understand her desires. His attitude and assistance can have a beneficial effect and can contribute to a woman's return to good feelings about herself, about him, and about the future.

THE MAN'S ROLE: TWO PERSPECTIVES

The following two interviews further investigate the man's role in the breast cancer experience. Dean Sterling and George Johnson tell their stories and offer suggestions for other men confronting similar situations.

Dean Sterling

Beth Ann* and I have a special relationship and a long involvement with each other. When she was diagnosed with breast cancer 4 years ago, we had been together as friends since 1982, as lovers and compan-ions since 1990, and as a married couple since 1998. We were friends long before we were lovers. We have always tuned in to one another.

*Beth Ann's interview is included in Chapter 18.

Consequently, breast cancer proved an intense bonding experience for us. It was almost as if I had been diagnosed along with my wife; that's how close we are.

My wife's cancer was discovered during a routine physical. It came as a total shock. She takes good care of herself. I am proud of that. She has never smoked and is an extremely light drinker. She has been that way her whole life, sort of wimpy when it came to the college drinking scene, but a great designated driver. She has never done drugs and has always exercised and eaten well. She looks as great now as she did 25 years ago. We were not expecting any difficulty with breast cancer because there was no family history. During her routine physical, her doctor noticed that the consistency of her left breast was different from that of her right breast, so he sent her for a mammogram. The mammogram revealed a tumor and calcifications. He wanted to do a lumpectomy before Christmas to get a definitive diagnosis.

I was working at home the day she got the news. Whenever she comes home she sings out "hello" right away; it is a joy to hear her voice. I heard the door open, but she didn't say anything. All I could hear was the cats meowing. I thought, "Hmm, that's odd." When she came back to where I was, she stood looking at me from the hallway. I said, "How are you doing?" And she said, "I'm not so sure. I went to the doctor and he found something in my breast. They took a mammogram and it was highly suspicious for carcinoma." Then she started crying. That's when I knew that this had really shaken her. She is always upbeat, never dwelling on the negatives. I don't think the full impact really hit her until that moment. We both read the report and understood its seriousness. She cried for several hours. Then she looked at me and said, "Well, there is nothing we can do about it, so let's deal with it." She actually baked cookies that night to keep busy. She doesn't let herself get too down.

I was a wreck, but in her presence I kept a close rein on my emotions to show her that she could depend on me. I also felt that we couldn't afford to lose control now; our energies had to be totally focused on what we would do. We needed to consider all the possible scenarios. That night we started to work up game plans on a big paper tablet. We did decision trees—positive, negative, surgery, no surgery— to eliminate as many unknowns as possible. I also tried to be more attentive to her and more romantic. We went out for supper afterward and then went shopping; she bought a dress. Over the next few weeks

I spent a lot more time with her. Behind the scenes when I was alone, I would get misty-eyed or cry because I knew what was coming up. But when we were together, I was strong and sympathetic so that she felt she could let me absorb some of her pain. I tried to support her by maintaining a confident, upbeat, let's-go-get-em attitude, and that worked well for her.

They did the diagnostic lumpectomy right before Christmas. The pathology report indicated ductal carcinoma in situ. This diagnosis inspired an in-depth research effort on our part to find out as much as we could about this cancer and the treatment options available. We were able to tap into a wealth of breast cancer resources online and the extensive cancer community that is out there. We were never aware of this network before, because breast cancer had not touched us personally. All of a sudden there were magazine and newspaper articles popping up everywhere, and the amount of information on the Internet is almost overwhelming. The mere mention of the topic in casual conversation would elicit a knowing response as well as a story about a mother, sister, or friend who had it. My medical background as a med tech and a physician assistant came in handy. I was familiar with medicine and brought some of that knowledge, along with my computer expertise, to bear on our investigation.

We quickly discovered that a vast array of quality information is available through many different sources. The local library provided articles from popular periodicals, whereas research libraries at local universities or medical schools contained medical books and journal articles on the disease, its prognosis, and more technical information on new drugs, therapies, and operations. The computer terminals in the libraries were really helpful and should not be overlooked. They provided us with access to newspaper articles and other reference materials that were in the library itself or on the Internet. Local bookstores also yielded a wealth of consumer health books, self-help books, and alternative medicine titles.

On the Internet we found a wide range of articles and resources, from popular consumer to highly technical scientific articles. It lists cancer societies, cancer organizations, medical schools, books, and articles. It also has testimonials, chat rooms, and websites with feedback from women who have experienced breast cancer, research findings, information on clinical studies, support groups, you name it. So if someone has the skill and the access (or knows someone who can help), the best place to start is the Internet.

The Internet has search engines to help you locate the information you are seeking. You just type in a subject you want to investigate. For example, you type in *breast cancer* or *cancer* or *breast*. Sometimes you have to be creative and use different types of search criteria. However, if you just want to look up breast cancer, you will probably get over 30 pages' worth of materials, maybe even more. Then you start refining your categories. You can type in *breast cancer surgery, breast cancer chemotherapy, breast cancer mortalities,* or *breast reconstruction* if you want to narrow your focus. The Internet is an amazing resource.

We found that there wasn't just one source that gave us everything we wanted to know. Medical books provided great scientific information, but not the human interest perspective on what women experience. We found that "touchy-feely" input in bookstores and the public library or on the Internet. I found little information directed at the significant other on how to address this problem. I wanted to know what men do. I was forced to develop my own game plan. I spent many hours documenting what I was going to do. So by the time it came time to do it, I would grab my notebook and flip pages to the right stage of therapy. "Let's see. This is surgery day, so I want to make sure I have a medal of St. Michael on her wrist." This helped me keep track of all these little things that needed to be done.

We both felt that the time invested in researching our options was well spent. When we went to see the surgeon, we had a solid knowledge base to help us understand what he was saying. He recommended a modified radical mastectomy with no breast reconstruction. We agreed with his diagnosis, but Beth Ann told him that before she made a decision she wanted a second opinion to explore alternative treatment options.

One of Beth Ann's friends recommended a surgeon at the university hospital and we went to see him. He examined her, took another set of mammograms, and showed them to us. After looking at the breast x-ray films, we were convinced that a modified radical mastectomy was the safest way to remove all the cancerous tissue. The surgeon suggested that Beth Ann might want to consider having a skin-sparing mastectomy with immediate breast reconstruction. That way she could have less skin removed and the reconstruction would provide a very nice result. He felt that she would be a good candidate for this combined procedure. He called a plastic surgeon that he works with in the breast cancer team and had him come over to examine Beth Ann. The plastic surgeon agreed with the surgeon's treatment recommendation and explained the various options for breast reconstruction. Beth Ann was particularly interested in a flap procedure that would not require implants; she was delighted to learn that she had enough fat on her tummy to make her breast look nice and full.

For Beth Ann, the breast reconstruction was very important, more so for her than for me. My first thought was, "Oh gosh, get rid of it, get rid of the cancer. Your breast has never held a good conversation with me, so I don't care. Let's just save you." She is more to me than a breast. But for her it would have been a constant reminder of the cancer that was in her body. Now when she blow-dries her hair in the morning and looks in the mirror, she can see her breasts and she feels whole. She is very pleased with the results. As a man looking at her reconstruction, you know, sexually, it is pleasing also. It looks normal and she is still as much a turn-on after surgery as before.

We debated whether she should have an immediate reconstruction or wait and have a delayed procedure. We shared the same philosophy of attack, attack, attack. That is the way we deal with things. Some people want to sit back and take time to emotionally adjust and work through their feelings of anger and grief; we try to bypass some of the early stuff quickly so that we can get to a resolution. We wanted to attack the cancer just as rapidly as we could. So the debate was do we wait till after the chemotherapy and then go back into surgery and have reconstruction and more hospitalization, or do we do the mastectomy and reconstruction all at the same time and then have the chemotherapy right after? If the breast did not heal properly, they would have to delay the chemotherapy and that might be risky. However, if it did work properly, we would not have to worry about going back to surgery again and would not have that dread hanging over us.

We are very much into positive thinking, so we opted to have the reconstruction at the same time and are very glad that we did. Therefore we were really excited, really pumped after talking to the plastic surgeon and the cancer surgeon. Three weeks later, Beth Ann had the skin-sparing mastectomy and immediate breast reconstruction with a TRAM (abdominal) flap. Next she had chemotherapy, and after a healing process, she had nipple reconstruction and later her nipple and areola were tattooed. Unfortunately, the tattooing did not take well and the breasts are two different colors, but it is close enough so that individually each breast looks normal.

Back to the day of surgery. We arrived early on a Thursday morning, and she stayed in the hospital through Monday, about 5 days total. She went into surgery about 7:30 AM. First, the cancer surgeon did the mastectomy, which took about 3 hours, and then the plastic surgeon took over. She was back in the room by about 1:30 PM. There were no major complications. She was somewhat coherent by 2:30 in the afternoon.

She didn't have a lot of pain. We were very lucky in that. She did have a morphine pump that she could tap whenever she needed a dose of painkiller. Before surgery we listened to a number of CDs by Dr. Bernie Siegal for cancer patients getting ready for surgery. They were very helpful. In addition, we had some subliminal CDs on reducing pain and staying motivated. She had her iPod during the entire surgical process. It played the same music over and over the entire time she was in surgery. I brought it into the hospital room also, and she continued to listen whenever she felt bad. I learned meditation years ago in Southeast Asia. Whenever she had any type of pain, we would focus on where the pain was and then tell it to go away. I think it was the combination of the morphine drip, the iPod, and all the support and positive vibes that helped her. Her attitude was that this discomfort was temporary. We had already spent many hours at home before surgery outlining all of the possibilities of what could happen, ranging from absolutely no pain to death. We left no stone unturned, and we did it in a positive manner. "Well, you could die, you know, or you could come out with no pain at all." We wanted no unknowns. I think the combination of being open about what was happening, along with our confidence in our doctors and the medical staff at the hospital, led to a very easy surgery.

When she came out of surgery, I looked at her breast right away, even though I didn't know if that was okay. I was sort of peeling the bandage off the front of the breast so I could look at it when I got caught by the nurse. She was just great. She laughed and said, "Let's go ahead and take it off." I was fascinated with what I saw, from a mechanical, technical point of view as well as an aesthetic one. Beth Ann had a round white disk of skin where the nipple was before. When you pressed on it, blood flowed back and forth. It didn't look bad; I mean, it just looked like the breast was winking at you, because there was a white circle where the nipple had been. All I could do was heap praises on her and tell her how wonderful it looked. So, I think that Beth Ann felt good that her new breast looked okay. In fact, it looked so good that I got in the habit of wanting to show it to everyone. Beth Ann had to slap my hand and tell me to stop. But it looked great.

While we were in the hospital, I did a lot of her maintenance. I gave her baths. We went into the shower together, and I hosed her off. She even considered trying to make love in the shower, but it wasn't a good idea because she could barely stand up straight. I said maybe we better curtail this activity. Even so, she still wanted to cuddle in bed, so we stayed pretty close.

The surgery didn't pose an intimacy problem for us. However, I understood that she might have concerns about what was happening to her body. I also felt that she knew me well enough to know that this would not be a problem for us. It isn't like some relationships that are already in trouble and this is the last straw for the guy who just can't deal with it. She had enough confidence in me to know that it was not going to affect me one way or the other. However, at the same time my concern was her psychological state; I know that as individuals we tend to be more critical of ourselves than others are of us. So before surgery I talked to her about it. When we found out about the breast cancer, I made sure I spent more time talking with her and not doing the newspaper thing over the dinner table. I bought her dresses that were a little more risqué, a bit more sexy. We had romantic evenings at nice restaurants. We had more private time together, and I tried to reinforce those loving feelings. The night before her surgery I downloaded the Whitney Houston song, "I Will Always Love You," to her iPod. That was our dedication song for the surgery. We actually danced in the living room the night before, and it was great. She was really misty-eyed, and we were both filled with good feelings. We also did an excitement jump. We got pumped up, raised our fists, and literally shouted, "Go, go! We're gonna go get it; let's charge, let's get it!" This was to clear out any negative vibrations.

She had surgery on Thursday morning. She stayed in bed all day on Friday, and I helped her sit up in bed periodically. I got my hand slapped by the nurse for letting Beth Ann sit up too many times. On Saturday she was allowed to get up and sit in the chair for a while. After breakfast I gave her a sponge bath, and then we sneaked her into the bathroom, propped her in a chair, and I washed her hair in the sink, blow-dried it, and washed her face. She was delighted to get her hair done; it made her feel totally clean and refreshed, and it looked great. She wouldn't let me put her makeup on (she said I would make her look like a Kabuki dancer), so she did it herself and put on a bathrobe. Except for the IV and the fact that she was a little bit stooped over, you could not tell that she had anything done 2 days before. She looked totally uplifted and she felt terrific. This is something that I would highly recommend to any man whose loved one is in the hospital. As soon as she is able to get up, help her get cleaned up, wash her hair, and put on makeup. It will do wonders for her spirits. The nursing staff is just too busy to take care of the aesthetics; they do what's required and what's needed. The little niceties like washing your hair or putting on makeup do not fall into the crisis mode, yet these things are really uplifting.

After her bath they told her that she could go for a walk. So we started walking the hallways. She was happy to stretch her legs. We also went down to the cafeteria two or three times before they gave us the go-ahead. The fact that Beth Ann was pushing ahead of schedule on a lot of things was encouraging and inspired confidence in her ability to recover. She knew when she was tiring out and tried not to overdo it.

We developed motivational strategies to help her cope with this experience. I hung posters in her room. One showed a big waterfall in a lush forest and was reminiscent of pleasant experiences we had shared backpacking. Every time she felt any pain she would focus on the waterfall, and it would help her remember the good days. She would put herself there and it would ease the pain. I also taped up posters of colorful birds because she is a bird-watcher, and a poster for people to sign when they came to visit. We had a lot of trinkets in the room to make her feel positive. We made it our environment, not the hospital environment.

Looking back on the hospital experience, I can honestly say that we made the best of it. We converted a difficult situation into a good experience. We actually had some fun with it. We didn't think too much about the negatives; we just concentrated on the positives. We had a special time because we spent 4 or 5 days together in the hospital just talking and laughing and sharing. We really valued that time. The only thing that was bothersome to her was that the morning of surgery she started her menstrual period, which is common after surgery and likely due to stress. I told her not to worry, we'll deal with it, and she said, "Well, now—what else?" So the whole time she was in the hospital I changed her pads and washed her whenever the blood leaked. It was actually pretty funny. She said, "I can't believe you are changing my pads."

After we came home from the hospital it took a few days before she was moving around and going for walks. She was sort of hunkered over, and we didn't push that too hard. I hung a plant hook on the side of the wall and attached a rope to it so that she could tie it to her hand and hoist her affected arm up in the air. She was supposed to elevate her arm to exercise it, but she couldn't, so we used this pulley system to mechanically help her raise her arm up and down.

At home I told her, "It's up to you now. You can either lay in bed and feel sorry for yourself, or you can get off your ass and go get it." We even used the term *carpe diem,* "seize the day." I said that every day is a day of recovery to be seized. She was great; I was so proud of her. I would come home from work and find that she had walked almost a half mile around our entire apartment complex. She continued to do that every day. She would go until she couldn't go any further, and then she would rest and continue to push. The only time she ever got in trouble was when she went a little bit too far and ran out of energy. She actually had to call a taxi cab to bring her home. She didn't allow herself to be restricted very long. Within a week she was out running around doing things. She took 7 weeks off work. She had a lot of sick leave, and her boss encouraged it. That time off gave her a chance to focus on her recovery.

I tried to be helpful whenever I could. There were certain tasks, such as grocery shopping, that were more difficult for her. She couldn't lift the bags, do the dishes, or handle the housework. These are things that women do naturally and most guys don't even notice after a while. But I think the guy needs to take a proactive approach to the housework and laundry and not let things get dirty. One of the best and most appreciated things a man can do for a woman in this condition is to assume responsibility for the household chores. Laundry and cooking are easy enough to do and are things that will prey on her mind unless they are attended to. It is up to the guy to do them before she gets a chance. Otherwise she might overextend herself by trying to do these things.

It is hard for a man to know how to act in these circumstances. One of the problems we encountered early on occurred because for the first time in my life, I couldn't make things better for Beth Ann. I couldn't fix things for her. I have thought about this quite a bit. Previously, if her car broke down or if there was something she couldn't do, even though she tries everything, I could always handle it. But not this time. I could not take her place in surgery, even though

I wanted to, badly. I empathized so strongly that sometimes I would actually eclipse her. I asked the first surgeon more questions than she did. It was as if I were the one that was undergoing the mastectomy, to the point that sometimes I would say, "Do I need to have this done?" I was almost absorbing her psyche, and I had to learn how to back off and let her be the driving force. That was the big challenge, trying to lay back and listen. At the same time she made me aware pretty quickly that she had things to say and thought processes that needed to be respected. She was a little bit steamed at me over that. So for me and for all men dealing with women who are coping with breast cancer, listening is a major thing. You have to understand that you cannot do this for her. That was the only psychological hurdle to overcome. The rest was trial and error. Some things work and some don't. Like having sex. It has to be approached carefully. You must remember that she had an operation and you don't want to hurt her; yet you also don't want to back off too dramatically, because you want her to still feel sexually desired.

We had no problems relating sexually after the surgery. She is probably going to kill me for saying this, but we have always had a hot relationship from the first day I saw her. She was walking down the street with her sister, and she turned me on at that moment. We have always had a super relationship, both as friends and as sexual partners, and it has never changed. There was some concern on her part, but it wasn't whether I would be interested. Her concern was more focused on her ability to have sex, whether she would feel the same, and what body changes she should expect.

Our plastic surgeon told us it was okay to resume sexual intimacy 2 weeks after surgery; that was our official go-ahead. However, we had sex before that time, but we were cautious. I didn't want to be a pig, and she wanted to be careful because of her surgery. She was concerned that uterine contractions during orgasms might cause pain because of her abdominal surgery. So we were very tentative at first. We had to learn new positions to accommodate our special situation. I couldn't be on top of her because she had just had major chest surgery. We had to be creative.

We are cuddlers at night; we have always been. She is just an absolute delight to sleep with. It's like having a teddy bear in bed. It's wonderful to sleep against each other. If she is not cuddling into me, I am cuddling into her, and we are touching all night long. After surgery, however, when you throw that leg over the top or you reach over and just sort of grab, you can do damage or cause pain. We had to figure out a way to prevent me from doing that. I didn't want to sleep in another bed, because we didn't want even the illusion of separation. So we took big bath towels, rolled them up, and put them between us so I would hit them before I bumped her. We could still hold hands, I could still caress her, but I couldn't throw my leg up over her.

After she could almost stand up straight so she didn't feel awkward or uncomfortable going out in public, she got dressed up in a cocktail dress, and we went out to a good restaurant featuring fine dining, nice wine, and good music. Then we came home and had an intimate evening in front of the fireplace. Those romantic touches were very important for her psyche and for mine. I was thrilled to have her back. In a situation like this, it is very important for a man to woo his woman again with the romantic gestures that won her in the first place. Small things like leaving love notes and cards in books for her to find or drawing hearts or smiley faces on her mirror help her to know that things haven't changed; it is even more romantic now than it was before.

It is easy to be overwhelmed by all the concerns associated with the various treatments. To cope, we segregated them into tasks; it was a form of project management. We took one task at a time and just dealt with it. Therefore, as soon as the surgery was over, we put that behind us and turned our attention to the next stage of treatment—chemotherapy and its potential side effects. Again we took an attack approach: "Let's investigate the problem and let's confront it!" We listened to Bernie Siegel during chemotherapy and talked about chemotherapy as our friend, not our enemy. So we got geared up for that too. We took posters into the room where they give chemotherapy, the same ones from the hospital. When we went in for the first treatment, we felt really pumped up. We did another jump up and down and shouted, "Let's get excited, let's do it!" We arrived a half hour early for the blood work and were anxious to get going. Beth Ann took her first treatment without too much difficulty. She was surprised that she did not feel sick right away, only a little tired. So we went out for lunch and shopping. We knew the clock was ticking and the nausea would set in. We got home about 2:00 PM and watched TV. At 3:00 she was feeling a bit light-headed and nauseated, so she went into the bedroom. By 4:00 she was really nauseated, and she listened to music on the iPod; I gave her a heating pad; then I left her alone. She doesn't like me to be in the room when she is vomiting; it's an ego thing. This was the routine we followed for each of the treatments. We viewed it as a day that we spent together rather than a day for chemotherapy.

She was fine after that incident, and she lay there and just zoned out. She slept listening to music. By Saturday morning she was still feeling tired, but she was able to get out. We took it easy the rest of the day. She stayed at home all that week, and there were no major repercussions from the first chemotherapy treatment.

Two weeks later, she started losing her hair. We had talked about the possibility. I was hoping she would lose it because I wanted to see her bald. In the early *Star Trek* movie there was a bald lady who looked great. Beth Ann didn't share my enthusiasm for hair loss. However, she also knew that I would not be repulsed if she did go bald, and we talked about that. She decided that she wanted to save the hair that fell out so that she could match her old hair color in case something changed. She would use it as a reference point. She got ready with a plastic bag for the day she would start shedding her hair.

Before her hair loss we went wig shopping; she wanted a wig to replicate her own hair. For some reason, the wig that we found made her look like Loretta Lynn. I mean, it was like a big hair Momma! Even when she got it cut and trimmed, it looked too big. I thought, "Holy smokes, this wig looks like hell!" The woman at the wig shop recommended a frosted blond wig in a short hairstyle. Beth Ann has never been a blond, so she said, "Let's try it." It looked absolutely great on her. We bought it before her hair fell out so she would be prepared.

Her hair started coming out one weekend when friends were visiting from out of town. She would grab clumps of it and just lift it right off her head and put it in a plastic bag. By Monday she still had a lot of hair, but it was thinning down the middle and on the sides and not looking good. It continued to fall out until Wednesday. Then we decided to shave the rest of her head. She looked great bald. I never could talk her into going public that way, but it looked terrific.

We celebrated after the last treatment. We went out and had a big dinner. Although chemotherapy was not easy for her, we tried to reduce its impact by diverting our attention to more pleasant thoughts.

When something like this happens in a relationship, a man has to look himself in the mirror, put his macho tendencies aside, and recognize that he is a partner in this experience. Most men still engage in old-time role playing. They think that diseases and health problems are for women to worry about, not men. They should grow up, take a more mature attitude, and get involved. Too many of them bail out when a crisis like this occurs; they don't know how to deal with it, so they run. They need to deal with it and participate. That's the big one—participation. Men need to get in touch with their emotions.

One of the regrets I have is that I was too aggressive initially. I was more aggressive than she was during our first visit to her surgeon. (Maybe it was my military training kicking in.) Suddenly I was acting like it was my breast, when it was hers. I thought, "Wait a minute, this is her decision about her treatment; it's not mine." I was ready to do whatever the first surgeon recommended, because my concern was to get rid of the cancer, and that was all I was focusing on. Then I realized that I had overstepped my bounds because this is her life, her decision, her breast. Although I'm a part of it, it is not my place to make the decision. That's when I had to back away; that was the hardest thing for me to do. It was really tough trying not to control things, because I really wanted to help her. I wanted to shield her from as much as I could. But it was still her decision, and afterward, when I thought about it, I was proud that she cut me off and said, "Nope—I want to get a second opinion. I want to see what else is out there." I thought this was great that she was taking charge and not letting me bulldoze her through the situation. If she weren't such a strong person, I might have overshadowed her. For most men, this is one of the hardest parts of dealing with breast cancer. All the guys I've talked to say the same thing: "We feel so helpless; we don't know what to do. You know we have always fixed things before. We want to fix this thing, but we can't do it, and we can't even be involved." But that is not true; a man can be involved, but his role has to change. He has to understand that he is a supporting player now, not the main actor. It is the woman who must take center stage.

George Johnson

Jenny's lump was discovered 1½ years ago during her regular checkup. Her mammogram revealed a possible mass within her breast that had not shown up on her physical examination. She had three other biopsies before, but they had always been benign. When she entered the hospital, the doctor told us that this lump might be cancerous and a decision needed to be made about therapy: whether to go ahead and have a frozen-section biopsy and do a lumpectomy or mastectomy right away or come back later for treatment. Her physician also informed her of other treatment options, including breast reconstruction.

When cancer was diagnosed, it was her decision to have a mastectomy and to do it immediately. I had mixed feelings about having it done right then, but she seemed determined to get it over with. Her decision may have been prompted by her sister's recent death from breast cancer. Her passing created enormous concern on both our parts. Since then, whenever Jenny has any kind of problem, no matter how minor, cancer is the first thought that comes to mind, because it apparently is in the family and has been present all along. Therefore, considering her family history, she was anxious to get rid of the breast and the cancer and to protect herself from her sister's fate.

I tried to be supportive after the mastectomy. I must admit that I was distressed by seeing her body with only one breast on one side and a scar on the other side. She takes such pride in her appearance that I hated for her to have this done to her. It was painful for me to know that she was unhappy. The mastectomy had little effect on our relationship. Initially, maybe, there was some constraint there, particularly in lovemaking, but it was quickly overcome. There really was no problem.

When a couple confronts this type of trying situation, it's important for them to have a deep love for each other, and obviously, after 25 years of marriage, Jenny and I have this feeling. Coping with breast cancer and a mastectomy might be more difficult for a couple who is just dating or in a new relationship. They wouldn't be sure of each other and would be uncertain about what the future would hold for them. I would also think that cancer and mastectomy would be more traumatic for a younger individual because of the sexual implications. If people love each other, however, no matter what their ages or the length of their relationship, they will talk about their problems and try to help each other. If a man leaves a woman over a mastectomy, there wasn't much love there in the first place.

My wife was not happy with her appearance after her mastectomy. She felt that she didn't look right in her clothes, even though with a prosthesis an observer could not tell the difference. But I could tell she felt uncomfortable. When she put on a bathing suit, she would stretch and pull it to make it cover more of her body. Just by looking at her expression, I could see how displeased she was, because she felt her deformity was noticeable. I tried to reassure her that she looked just as good as she always did, which she did. I felt she looked fine in her clothes, but I don't think she really believed me. Her prosthesis was also uncomfortable, and she complained about it. The inconvenience of the prosthesis probably speeded up her decision to have reconstruction. I could tell that she just didn't feel right emotionally. She was not satisfied with the way she looked.

I believe that my wife had already made up her mind to have breast reconstruction even before she had her mastectomy. Almost immediately after she came home from the hospital, she started talking about reconstruction and reading about it. But we really hadn't discussed this topic before.

I had mixed feelings about breast reconstruction, but I didn't make any suggestions one way or the other. My feelings were somewhat negative, because I worried that she wanted this done for my benefit. I also didn't want her to undergo any more surgery, with its pain and discomfort. I felt that she had suffered enough. I gradually changed my mind as she helped me to realize that she was enthusiastic about this operation and wanted it for herself, not for me. After I understood her determination to have breast reconstruction, I got on her side 100%.

If a man feels that reconstruction will make his woman feel happier or as if she were more of a woman, then he should encourage her, be supportive, and go along with her wishes. That's really all he can do, because she will have to make the decision herself, if this is what she wants done. He needs to talk to her about her needs and really listen to what she has to say. If anything, reconstruction might enhance their relationship. If a husband or boyfriend is totally against reconstruction and discourages his loved one from having it done, their relationship might suffer. Once he sees that she is determined to proceed with this operation and that it will make her happy, he should encourage and help her.

To learn more about reconstruction, Jenny got a number of pamphlets, and we read them together to understand the nature of the surgery and the various types of reconstructive procedures. Some of this material was really graphic and showed exactly what the plastic surgeon would be doing and how the new breast would look. It's important for a man and woman to get literature before reconstruction and decide what will be done. They also need to consult with a surgeon together and determine what procedures will be used and what the expected recovery period and restriction on activity will be.

After much research, Jenny got a physician friend of ours to check with a well-known surgeon who could suggest a plastic surgeon for breast reconstruction. We also got a local recommendation for a plastic surgeon. Both doctors recommended the same plastic surgeon, so we felt very comfortable because his name had come up twice. This vote of confidence was particularly reassuring, so Jenny set up an appointment for us to go interview this plastic surgeon.

We were very impressed with him. He seemed concerned for her and interested in doing what she wanted. His first question to us when we came in for the visit was, "Well, what do you want to talk about?" This is really how the conversation started. We discussed our interview at great length later, and I don't think we could have been more pleased with him. He is a gentle person and did not try to push us in any way. After meeting with him, Jenny made arrangements to have the plastic surgery done.

Her breast was reconstructed with a flap of tissue from her back. It was called a latissimus dorsi flap reconstruction. She also had surgery on her other breast as a preventive measure. My wife is at high risk for developing another breast cancer. Over the years she has had breast biopsies for lumps in both of her breasts, and these biopsies have been very anxiety provoking for us. Our plastic surgeon knew of Jenny's cancer status and of the constant fear that we lived with. So he suggested that when her left breast was reconstructed she might also want to consider having the mass of tissue inside her right breast removed and replaced with an implant. He felt that this operation might reduce her risk of developing another cancer. Jenny decided to have this preventive surgery to help alleviate some of her preoccupation with cancer.

Jenny also had a nipple-areola created as a second procedure. She wanted her breast to be complete. Knowing my wife, I don't think that she would have been satisfied without going the full way and having a nipple put on. She has been delighted with it, and so have I.

After reconstruction her recovery was rapid, with no complications. Initially, she could not drive for 2 weeks, but the inconvenience to me was minimal. There were times when I had to chauffeur her somewhere, and I assumed responsibility for certain chores around the house that she could not do physically, but none of this was a problem. A man should plan on offering some extra help during this time.

Jenny's physical condition contributed to her speedy recovery as much as anything. She is conscientious about taking care of herself and has always been in very good shape. She was this way before any problems developed and is even more so now that she has had reconstructive surgery. I think she looks great. Until she healed completely, she was limited initially in what she could do with her arms. Now she is fully recovered and participates in aerobic exercises twice a week. She was never confined much. I think she was determined to recover quickly, because she knew that I did not originally want her to have this surgery, and she was trying to prove something to me.

Breast reconstruction has totally changed Jenny's attitude about herself and her appearance. It makes me feel good to see how pleased she is with herself. For all practical purposes, she is just like she always was before she started having trouble. She is active now with the American Cancer Society as a Reach to Recovery volunteer. She visits and counsels other women about her experiences. She is grateful because her surgery was so successful, and she wants to reassure women who have had mastectomies or who are considering reconstruction that everything will turn out okay.

Her friends around her age and even younger are all interested in her reconstruction. During our vacation with some other couples, the girls got together and they had show and tell. They wanted to see her breast, even though none of them have had breast cancer. One of our friends who lives in Nebraska and might need to have a mastectomy is very interested in Jenny's experiences. Our friends can hardly believe that she went through what she did, because she looks so good. They are impressed with the results, with her great attitude, and, I dare say, that anyone who doesn't know that she had the surgery would not know. There is no way.

I give my wife credit—she changed my attitude about reconstruction. I really think it's something special now.

There is one final point I didn't touch on that might be interesting for people to know, and it has to do with a person's age and what makes you "too old." When Jenny wanted to have this surgery, nobody discouraged her necessarily, but I think there was some feeling, "Why go through with this at your age?" She was 54 years old, and they felt that if she were younger, say in her twenties or thirties, that this would be fine, but at her age, why bother? But that is not so. She is still just as much of a woman as she was when she was 20, and I hope women considering reconstruction will keep this in mind. If you're over 50, so what? Forget about your age; it really doesn't matter. Do it for yourself if it makes you feel good. My wife did, and it has done wonders for her and for us.

HOW COUPLES RELATE

The final interview in this chapter is with a young, unmarried couple: Scott Meyers and Sheila Andrews. Together, they relive their experiences from the diagnosis of Sheila's cancer, through her mastectomy and chemotherapy, to her present decision to have her breast reconstructed. They discuss the problems that a couple faces when the woman develops breast cancer and provide insight into the various methods they have used to help them cope with this disease and the trauma associated with it.

Sheila Andrews and Scott Meyers

Sheila: It all started when I went to my gynecologist for what I thought was a cyst, nothing big. When he checked me and said, "I want you to see someone else," the alarm went off. He assured me that it was nothing to worry about, but when I wanted to wait a month to make the appointment, he wouldn't let me; he insisted I go the next week. I went to see the surgeon he recommended; he did a needle biopsy and said he would call me in a few days with the results. When I didn't hear from him, I called his office because I was getting anxious. It was the day of our Thanksgiving dinner at work. I asked the nurse for the results, and she gave the phone to the doctor who asked me to come in to talk to him. I said, "No, that is worse than you telling me right now, over the telephone. Tell me now, and then I'll come in later today and we can talk." He told me that the lump was malignant. My head was spinning from the news; I felt as if I were in another world. I was just 30, recently divorced with a teenage daughter, and I had no idea that it would be cancer. There was no breast cancer in my family. I was trying to get myself together, so I went into a private office to cry. I was hysterical . . . and then I thought about Scott.

Scott and I had only been going together for 3 months, and we were very new into our relationship. All of a sudden, I was finding out that I had cancer and not only did I have to cope with that, I had to deal with trying to tell someone who I had only known for a short while. I called him on the phone and told him.

Scott: After I got off the phone from talking with Sheila, I fell apart. When I managed to pull myself together, I picked Sheila up from work and we went for a drive. Cancer was something that I had never dealt with or been exposed to before. I'd never known anyone who had it; it was all new to me. I was scared for her, not knowing what she was going to have to experience. Ours was a new relationship at the time, and I didn't know how this was going to affect it and really how I felt about it. I don't know that Sheila knew either. Neither one of us was aware of what was going to happen in the next few months, or even the next year. It was a matter of waiting, talking to doctors, and slowly finding out.

Sheila: When I went to see the doctor, he told me that he was going to put me in the hospital and schedule surgery. Before doing the mastectomy, he would do another biopsy while I was under anesthesia. He had all the consent forms ready for me to sign, because he felt that it was better for me to sign the papers ahead of time so he would not have to wake me to confirm that I had cancer. I signed the papers and went in blindly. I just said, "Yes, yes, yes." I didn't know anything.

After I knew that I had to have a mastectomy, Scott and I were just wasted. Saturday night, before I was to go into the hospital, we went through several bottles of champagne, drowning our sorrows. We decided to have a going-away party for my breast. We put on music, got loud and crazy, and poured a bottle of champagne over my breast. Scott kissed it goodbye. It was a wild thing to do, but it made us feel better. Now that I'm thinking about reconstruction, I guess we will probably have to christen the new one, too, when I get it. It will be like having a new boat, only I'll be getting a new breast. That night we just lay in each other's arms and cried half the night. We hardly said anything. We just got everything out, all the tears that might have been held back. We cried and cried and cried.

Scott: It is essential to be open with each other. You just can't keep your feelings hidden. From a man's perspective, you need to express yourself. You can't be afraid to cry. If you can't cry about this, what can you cry about?

Sheila: I was terrified before surgery. I broke out in hives and went white. I had never had an operation in my life. The only time I was in the hospital was when I had a baby, 13 years earlier. I never had a sick day. This was the first time I had been sick, and that really threw me. It had been such a little problem.

I went to the hospital a week later, and when I woke up, I didn't have a breast. It was that fast. They did a modified radical mastectomy, and I didn't even know what a modified radical was. At that time I didn't know anything. The only thing I knew was what I was told; I put my entire life in the hands of a doctor who I had never met before, and I said, "Just do what you have to do."

Scott: I don't think I thought so much about the mastectomy or her losing a part of her body. I just wanted to see her recover her health. My main concern was her survival.

Sheila: After surgery the doctor told me that my cancer had spread; I had three positive lymph nodes. I was in stage II of my breast cancer, which I didn't understand. Then he started talking about chemotherapy, and that was another whole trip. Everything you hear about chemotherapy is devastating, and all of a sudden, the focus wasn't on losing my breast, but it was on chemotherapy. I thought, "God, how am I going to survive this?" Then the oncology nurse talked to me and gave me brochures on chemotherapy. All of this time when I was in the hospital, Scott took care of my daughter and ran my house. He did all of the cleaning.

Scott: I did all of the housework. There were some habits formed there that are very hard to break.

Sheila: I have a high tolerance for pain, probably abnormally high. The evening of my surgery I took no pain killers, and by the time I was released from the hospital, I was reaching over my head. I was determined to block out what had happened to me. "You know," I said, "there is not a damn thing wrong with me. Life will resume as normal." In fact, I ran the vacuum cleaner when I got home, just to prove that nothing was going to stop me. I caught the wrath of God when Scott got home and found that I had vacuumed the bedroom. After that scene, I just gave up vacuuming forevermore.

Scott: That was a good example of her proving to the world that she wasn't sick. I said, "Don't prove it to me, and don't prove it to the world either. You don't need to be vacuuming this house. You don't need to have that attitude." We talked about that for a long time.

I was asking myself many questions during this period, and I was questioning many values. I had to go back and think about the way I regarded Sheila before she developed cancer. I had to determine how I felt and then ask myself why I should feel any different now. I mean, I love this woman, and at the time I decided that I would see her through this experience, just because of my feelings for her; I didn't think they should change because she had this disease. If anything, this experience probably strengthened my feelings for her in helping me give her the support that she needed.

Sheila: He helped me cope with my problems all the way through. The day after surgery, he said, "Okay, let's see what we're dealing with." He just opened my gown and looked down and said, "Uh, huh." I was the one who looked at my scarred chest and passed out. All he did was go, "Uh, huh, okay." He changed my bandages when I got home and rubbed lotion on my scar when I couldn't do it. He helped me with my bra, he helped me get dressed, he did everything for me. I was never embarrassed or ashamed in front of him.

Scott: It didn't bother me at all. It was just something she had to go through. I knew she didn't want it; who would? I certainly didn't enjoy it, but we had to live with it. I'm also not a squeamish person. Scars don't really bother me. I wanted to see her scar, not merely from curiosity, but from a real interest in her.

I also knew that she was worried about how I would feel about her body, but it really didn't affect our sex life. We had sex the day after she came home from the hospital. I was worried about hurting her, sure, but it worked out just fine.

Sheila: Even though Scott never made me feel ashamed, I was self-conscious about my body, and I probably still feel some self-consciousness. It's hard, even now, to have a romantic candlelight dinner, put on a beautiful gown, and have one side totally flat. Whether you like it or not, breasts are very, very important in sex and in the way you present yourself. I'm sure they also affect the way he looks at me. He says it doesn't bother him, and it probably bothers me a lot more than it does him. It is tiresome, looking down there and seeing no cleavage.

You have to realize that I had only been with Scott for 3 months when this occurred. There were still many things I didn't know about him. We became very close, immediately, but I still wasn't completely comfortable. Even now, there are times when I'm shy about the way I look, and I have a hard time dealing with it. I'll tell him, "Kill the lights; I'm coming to bed." I know that is absurd. You would think that your feelings are somehow attached to your eyesight. But, when you are missing a breast, there is definite comfort in darkness.

When I went back to see my surgeon after I had been released from the hospital, I had many questions for him. I wanted to know about the chemotherapy: Who would administer it, and would it be done in his office or in the hospital? He referred me to the university hospital and to a whole new set of specialists. That scared me. I didn't know these people, and I didn't know what to expect from them. He gave me names of the doctors at the hospital and handed me my pathology report in a sealed envelope.

I went home and immediately ripped open the report and read through it. I came to the part that said, "Prognosis: poor," and I went Bing! I had no business reading that report. I didn't know what I was reading, and I didn't know how to interpret it. It scared the hell out of me.

Scott: We both read through the pathology report, but I didn't understand most of it, only words here and there. At the bottom, it read: "Prognosis: Condition poor." That, everyone can read; it was black and white and simple language. It was also very difficult to take. We had both just been through her surgery and were trying to remain positive. Then to have something like that come along is demoralizing. It's like having someone tell you that all of your effort is not worth shit; it doesn't matter what you do, because this is the way it is.

Sheila: Six weeks after my surgery, I went to the hospital to see the doctors about chemotherapy. They told me that the type of cancer I had was poorly differentiated and had a high recurrence rate. That was another blow. I went into a rage. I cursed them and screamed, "Bullshit! You are not telling me that I'm dying! I am only 30 years old. I have a daughter and my own house. For the first time in my life, after a terrible marriage, I have a man that I really love; I have everything to live for: a new job, a new relationship, a child, everything." I really fought it, and I've continued to fight it. I have bad moods, but I'm not going to let it get me.

Scott: I think the chemotherapy was even more of an adjustment for Sheila than the surgery itself. Chemotherapy required a great deal of patience and understanding from me and from everyone around Sheila, especially her daughter. The drugs affected her poorly. She was moody and short-fused. She had a temper and she cried all of the time. She stayed in bed a lot. I could deal with that, and her daughter handled it well. Her daughter showed real understanding and patience for her mother and what she was enduring; I think she knew that Sheila was not always going to act that way and there would be an end to it. We were all relieved when the chemotherapy was over. It really pushed everyone to the maximum. I had to keep telling myself that the drugs were making her react the way she was. She said many dumb things during that time. I think her logic and reasoning were not as clear as they normally were, and she was very emotional.

Sheila: You go through so many emotions with cancer, and chemotherapy does trigger those emotions. You are high at one moment and then lower than a snake the next. My moods were up and down. I don't think I was really rational for many of the things that I did or said. I wasn't altogether there, and I wasn't in control all of the time. Despite my actions and the way life was treating me, Scott moved in with me during my chemotherapy. I really knew he loved me if he could move in at that time.

Chemotherapy was terrible for me. I had very long, luscious blonde hair, and after the first chemotherapy treatment, it started coming out in handfuls. During the second week I had big clumps of hair falling out of my head. I made an appointment to see wigs, and they matched me with several long, blonde wigs. Soon I was practically bald. I looked like Bozo the Clown; I had a strip of hair running along the edges of my scalp. I not only lost the hair on my head, but I also lost the rest of my body hair, every bit, from head to toe. I still had a few eyelashes, but my eyebrows were almost nonexistent. I had to wear a lot of makeup to look normal. I also gained 18 pounds on chemotherapy, which I'm having a hard time losing. So, besides being bald, not getting into my clothes, and losing a breast, I kept saying, "What is next?" It is a tremendous amount to deal with.

Scott: Hair loss was traumatic for Sheila. She seemed to have an enormous amount to cope with, and it was sometimes hard for me to help her.

Sheila: With a breast, you can camouflage your loss, but with hair loss, what can you do? I mean, I couldn't wear wigs to bed. Talk about romance. He had to look at this woman who had one breast and was bald as a billiard ball. I said, "Oh my God, I look like I just stepped out of a circus." We can laugh now, but at the time there were many tears. Finally, all this hair was falling out, and he made the ultimate decision. He said, "Sheila, you're clogging all of the drains. I have to cut off every bit of your hair because it's falling out, and it's getting all over your clothes. Let's just get it over with once and for all." I said, "Okay," and he got the scissors and just snipped off the rest; that was probably the best thing he ever did. He just got rid of it, and I stopped worrying about it falling out.

Scott: There were times when I needed someone to confide in. I have one or two close friends that I can talk to, but they didn't really understand what was happening.

Sheila: We often talked about our relationship. In fact, there were times when we weren't sure that it would last. It had nothing to do with my cancer; it was just his own feelings. He has other commitments; he goes to school, he works, and he loves to travel. It's hard to commit yourself to a woman who has cancer, who is going through chemotherapy, and who has a 13-year-old daughter and a house. That's a lot to ask of anyone. He had to be absolutely sure how he felt about me before he made any kind of commitment to me.

Scott: I needed to work through my own feelings and think about my life. I thought about how I felt about Sheila before surgery and before she had cancer. I had to decide what I was feeling now. I had to confront myself: "Am I staying with this woman because I pity her, or because I love her?" There were times when I really could not answer that question. Finally, I decided that if I left I would never know, and if I stayed, I would have to be very careful about why I stayed. I decided that I wanted to stay. I love her and I wanted to give her 100% of my support and love and see her through this experience. If there were anything that I could do to help her, I would do it. That meant taking care of her, her surroundings, and her daughter. It meant providing moral support and letting her know that she was going to get through this okay. I was determined to keep as optimistic an attitude as I could and to show some strength for her.

Sheila: He was always planning for the future. That was important for me, because when all of this first happened, I didn't take any interest in the house or even in balancing the checkbook. I owned my own house, and we talked about painting it. But I would say things like, "Why should I paint this damn place if I'm going to die? Why should I buy anything?" I didn't want to buy anything: clothes, furniture, paint, anything. Why should I, if I weren't going to be able to enjoy it in 6 months? Toward the end of my chemotherapy, many of these feelings disappeared; we repainted the house, and I started buying clothes again.

Scott: She started living a normal life again. She joined a support group through the American Cancer Society, and she started taking dancing lessons. By remembering that there were other things that she needed to do with her life, she began to get out again and not let this hold her back.

Sheila: You can allow yourself to get depressed and let everyone feel sorry for you. It's easy to have a sad face and then people will say, "Oh, I'm so sorry." I didn't want that crap. I just wanted to be happy and to laugh. Scott and I had funny experiences, and we tried to keep our sense of humor. Our laughter has helped me survive this experience. When I go to my support group, I tell people about the funny things that happen. Like the time I forgot to put the toilet seat down and my wig fell in. I had to shake it out, wash it, and hang it out in the sun to dry. Then I realized that I couldn't go anywhere because I was bald, my other wig was being fixed, and I only had this one. You must laugh at things like that.

Scott: I wanted to take her to a loud dance studio in town, with her dressed like the bald lady in *Star Trek*. She wouldn't have it.

Sheila: He wanted to dress me in silver tights and makeup. He wanted me to be a Trekkie. He told me it would be the chance of a lifetime.

Actually, we did have fun with it. We went to a Kenny Loggins concert in June and I was still pretty bald at the time. I had an eighth of an inch of hair all over my head, so I decided to dress in style. I bought myself a bright lavender headband and put on a black jumpsuit with high heels and makeup. I wore lavender and black jewelry, earrings that were as big as my head, and beads. I didn't wear my wig. We went to the concert and people did double and triple takes. I'm sure they were talking about that bald woman: "A good-looking man like that with a bald woman, yuck!" It was really interesting. The women made derogatory comments about my head, but the men seemed to be complimentary. It was very, very strange. If they had only known why I looked the way I did.

Getting involved with support groups has also helped me to adjust. Women need to know that there are self-help groups available and that we are not alone. The American Cancer Society has a number of these groups going. Reach to Recovery is one, and I am now a volunteer. I'm also in another support group that meets once a month, and we swap stories about our experiences.

It's one of those meetings where you can cry, especially with the women who have just come out of it. We cry, we hold each other, we laugh. You can face a lot of things together.

One of the women in our group just had a recurrence. She had her surgery the same time I did, and she was just getting ready for her yearly checkup when they found an inoperable mass in her chest. She only has 6 months to live. You have to learn that when you are working closely with people, not everyone is going to make it, and that's hard to take. I had to come to grips with that reality this month with her.

We share everything in these meetings. We talk about sex and looks and feelings. Many of these women are single and are dating. They ask, "How do you tell a man that you've had this surgery? Maybe you've only gone out with him two or three times, and it gets to a point where you might end up in bed. What do you do then?" That's a problem that you need to broach, and you need to know what to do. Even with Scott it was difficult for me, because I was still self-conscious.

I learned about breast reconstruction in my support group. One of the women had it done and she told me about her plastic surgeon. I had no idea that there were any alternatives. My surgeon never said anything about reconstruction. After I heard about it though, halfway through my chemotherapy, I started asking doctors at the hospital about breast reconstruction, and they said, "Go for it." They were very supportive. But they also told me that I would have to wait until the chemotherapy was over. Then they said, "Do it. You're young and you want your breast back. It would be a great thing for your mental attitude."

Scott: I really didn't like the idea of her doing it. I'm not comfortable with it. I don't want her going into an operating room again. We've talked about it quite a bit, and I am concerned because I feel that she is doing this entirely for me, and there is no need.

Sheila: Probably he is right to a certain extent. I'm doing this partly for him, but it is also for me. I think that if I have breast reconstruction, I'll feel better about myself and the way I look. After a mastectomy, every time that you look at yourself in the mirror, it's a reminder of cancer. Personally, I don't feel I have cancer anymore; I really don't. It's something I had to deal with at the time, but now it's time to go ahead and get my breast reconstructed and stop worrying about it. I don't want to look down any more and see that there is a breast missing. I miss wearing regular bathing suits and nice lingerie. Actually, the more I think about it, the more I realize that I'm doing it for myself. It is to help me forget this disease.

I like to sleep on my stomach, but with a missing breast this position becomes awkward and off balance. I am also uncomfortable with my prosthesis. I'm an accountant, and just moving my arm to the calculator makes the prosthesis rub; it bothers me. The first thing I do when I get home from work is kick off my shoes and throw out my prosthesis.

In my mind, I made a commitment to investigate breast reconstruction the minute I heard that it was a possibility. I decided that I wanted it if I could have it.

I was really scared when I went to see the plastic surgeon. The first time he saw me, he told me to take off my clothes so he could take some photos. He got out his camera and took about 20 pictures of every angle of my breast. He was also taking pictures of my stomach and my hips. Meanwhile, I'm thinking, "Oh my God, blackmail!" I felt like I was posing for Playboy. But he needed those pictures to decide what to do, and he said that with the weight I had gained during chemotherapy and after having had a child, he felt an abdominal flap was the best operation for me. You see, I don't have an 18-year-old's stomach anymore, and yet my remaining breast has a nice size and shape. If I had this flap surgery, he wouldn't have to touch my opposite breast. He felt he could get the best match for my breast with an abdominal flap reconstruction, and I would be more pleased with it, knowing that I could get rid of my stomach and also get a breast to match my remaining breast.

I had to think a long time about having this operation. Not only am I going in for more surgery, but I am having a major operation; this is one of the most complicated forms of reconstruction. It is a big deal to decide. When you have cancer, you don't have a choice. You go into the hospital, and you get surgery. I'm going into a major operation that is by choice, and that is hard. I'm saying, "Okay, Doc, I'm going to let you rearrange my entire body, and I'm putting it in your hands." If I didn't trust my plastic surgeon, I wouldn't be able to say that. It shows you how much faith I have in him. I am saying, "Do your best. I totally trust you with my life."

Scott: She isn't making this decision based on ignorance, however. Since her mastectomy, we've taken time to learn about reconstruction.

Sheila: Several weeks ago we invited a girl over to our house. She had this same operation by another surgeon, and we wanted to see somebody else's work. She came over 8 weeks after her surgery and she showed Scott and me her breast. She just stripped down and said, "Okay, this is what I look like." It was nice seeing another breast. When you go into this, you have to understand that your body is never going to look exactly the same as it did before. There are going to be some concessions. There are going to be some scars; I will have a scar across my stomach. My main concern is my appearance in clothes; now I'll be able to wear a bra and won't have to wear a prosthesis. I'll be able to fill something out again.

Scott: I'm still having problems with her having more surgery. It's another operation, and it worries me. But if it's going to help her psychologically and improve her self-image, then I want her to have it. It has to be important to her.

Sheila: I'm looking forward to breast reconstruction. I am not interested in having a nipple-areola put on right now; it's not a priority for me. I can always go in later and have it done. I'm not in a hurry. No one would really see the nipple, except Scott. If I feel deprived, I can probably just cut out brown construction paper and stick it on.

I want to be able to wear a normal bathing suit this summer. In fact, the night before my surgery I'm meeting my plastic surgeon at the hospital with my bathing suit. It has a French cut to the legs, and instead of a straight line cut across my abdomen, he is going to give me a "happy face" scar so I can still wear this suit. I'm going to try on my suit for him so he can plan my scars to fall in the right area. Women don't understand that the scar doesn't have to extend straight from hip to hip; it can be curved up. It's nice to know that even these details can be individualized.

Women need to know about breast reconstruction and about the different options for cancer treatment. They need this information before it happens to them. Every woman should be informed about breast cancer. She should know about mastectomies and reconstruction before she has to worry about them. I went into this experience so ignorant. I just said, "Do what you want." I didn't know anything. I didn't know that there were alternatives; I didn't know that there was breast reconstruction. I think if women knew about reconstruction and knew the results, they might not be so hesitant to go in if they felt a lump. I really think that detection is the key, and knowledge about alternatives and treatment will encourage women to report problems as soon as they discover them.

Scott: I agree with Sheila 100%. I think women should be educated. They should know their options, and they should get involved in them. Once you've experienced what we have experienced, you learn to be happy and to make the most of life. You learn that one of the most effective ways of coping with a situation like this is by remaining positive.

FIFTEEN WOMEN
TELL THEIR STORIES

Women are the inspiration behind this book; their voices permeate our writing. Many of these women have been transformed by the specter of breast cancer and have shared their thoughts and feelings to help make this book a reality. Their input has been invaluable, and their sensitivity and generosity are reflected in the stories they have to tell. Following are 15 stories of women who had mastectomies, and in two cases lumpectomies, for breast cancer and sought breast reconstruction. Five of these interviews are new, replacing four of the ones published in the previous edition. As difficult as it was to leave those stories behind, it was a necessity. Procedures for breast reconstruction have changed and improved over the past 10 years, and we wanted our readers to benefit from others' experiences with the latest technical advances. Although some of the narrators of these stories have changed, we have tried to retain the spirit behind the interviews and capture the courage and honesty that typified all of these women. Interestingly, as we compare the original interviews with the more recent ones, many of the same phrases, comments, fears, and emotions are echoed. The operative details may differ, but the concerns remain surprisingly constant. Most striking is the similarity of responses given to questions probing women's reactions to breast cancer, motivations for seeking breast reconstruction, and satisfaction with this operation. We have also been impressed that over the years, women have become better informed about breast cancer and its treatment, and increasingly they have become their own health advocates. As in the previous editions, we have altered names and personal details to protect the privacy of these women.

From the many taped interviews, we have purposely selected women who underwent different reconstructive procedures, some immediately after mastectomy or lumpectomy some delayed-immediate, and others delayed until various times after surgery, to give you some idea of the reconstructive possibilities available and the potential benefits and problems. These women range in age from 28 to 60 years and represent diverse social, cultural, professional, and family backgrounds. We have included single women, widowed and divorced women, women who have a strong family history of breast cancer with a *BRCA1* diagnosis, and married women with and without children. The questions asked of each woman were varied in the interest of providing a wider coverage of topics. Thus one interview focuses on the issue of self-image for the woman seeking breast restoration; another examines the loss of control that is associated with a cancer diagnosis; another discusses the fear and questioning that accompanies a decision for prophylactic mastectomy; and still another discusses the predicaments that a single woman with a mastectomy faces when dating. Patient self-advocacy, coping mechanisms for dealing with complications, the power of positive thinking and spirituality, and the importance of being an informed consumer are also explored. Certain subjects, however, are dealt with in each dialog, including reasons for deciding on breast reconstruction, timing of reconstructive surgery, pain and recuperation after reconstruction, physical and psychological results of reconstructive surgery, and benefits and limitations of reconstructive surgery. An attempt has been made to present an honest, balanced discussion of this option so that women contemplating breast reconstruction will have a realistic understanding of what this surgery offers. Because the female author in this writing team did the firsthand interviewing to facilitate a free and candid discussion, these stories and the questions and observations are presented in the first person.

We begin with Debbie, whose medical background gave her unusual insight into the life-threatening disease that abruptly altered her life and reshaped her perspective.

DEBBIE: CONTROL IS JUST AN ILLUSION

"A lot of positive things have come out of this year, particularly how I view life and treat other people. I think I am more sensitive, but I live with much less illusion that I have control over my life. Loss of control was very difficult for me. I always thought I could manage everything. Breast cancer has a way of bringing you up short and making you face reality."

Control is a big issue for Debbie. Although she expresses a desire to slow down and enjoy life, she is still "going like gangbusters to catch up with many of the things I didn't finish last year." Despite her heavy travel schedule, she has managed to finish her Ph.D. and pass her medical boards all in the same month. Clearly, life is still frenetic, but breast cancer has made her feel vulnerable. It has interrupted her routine and forced her to examine her life. Before, she thought she could handle everything. "I was the total self-contained woman. But breast cancer has changed all that."

Debbie is a pretty, petite 41-year-old. Her short red hair frames her slender face, making her look younger than her years. Her black metal glasses, however, lend an air of seriousness. Debbie was only 39 years old when her breast cancer was discovered. An M.D. with a busy career and hectic schedule, Debbie "just didn't have time for breast cancer." As she relates, "I didn't have time for much routine health care. I have always been extremely busy in my work, and I travel a lot both in the United States and overseas."

Despite her medical background, she knew little about the disease and was shocked when her cancer was diagnosed. As a young single woman, breast loss was a major threat to her. However, her tumor was over 2 cm, and a mastectomy and breast reconstruction seemed the best treatment option, until she heard of neoadjuvant chemotherapy. After further investigation, she opted for this treatment, in which chemotherapy is first given to shrink the tumor and prevent spread. Then she had a lumpectomy, followed by another course of chemotherapy and radiation therapy. Even so, a partial breast reconstruction with an endoscopic latissimus dorsi flap was necessary to correct the defect left after tumor removal. Debbie is delighted with the somewhat unconventional choice she made. She came out of surgery feeling "normal" again.

Our interview traces her story from the time she first heard the shocking diagnosis.

How was your breast cancer discovered? What specialists did you talk to?

I noticed an area in my breast that felt a little different. My doctor said it was fibrocystic disease. So I put it out of my mind. I was doing breast self-exams once a month, but I didn't suspect I had a problem until 9 months later, when I thought I felt a cyst in that area. It was movable and seemed to be filled with fluid. I was too busy to go in to have it checked. Sitting at my desk 3 months later, however, I felt a strong sense of urgency to have the lump checked immediately. This occurred 3 days before I was preparing to present a talk at a major meeting. I saw my physician on Friday and she sent me for a mammogram. After the mammogram the radiologist met with me. He said, "I think that you have a malignancy. I don't see this kind of pattern with anything but cancer." I was stunned.

I decided to see a breast surgeon at the university hospital. I convinced myself that there was nothing to worry about. I would get a biopsy, and everything would be fine. After all, I didn't have a family history of breast cancer, and I was only 39 years old, too young for breast cancer. Lurking in the back of my mind, however, were nagging worries about other risk factors. I was single, had never been pregnant, and was raised on a typical southern diet.

I was referred to a woman surgeon who had a curt, businesslike manner. She was just what I needed. She was a no-nonsense physician who was not prone to mincing words. She said, "Let's do a needle biopsy right now, and if it is negative, we will do an open biopsy."

The needle aspiration was one of the most painful procedures I have experienced. I don't know why. Other women don't find it painful. They didn't get any cells with the first aspiration and had to repeat it. I left for lunch while awaiting the results. When I returned, the nurse, who had been friendly earlier, avoided looking me in the eye. Being a physician, I knew what that meant: the tests must have been positive for breast cancer. So I wasn't totally surprised when the surgeon confirmed the diagnosis.

My breast surgeon called a plastic surgeon in to confer. They determined that they would have to remove most of the breast to get clean margins. At least the whole top part of the breast would have to go, leaving a significant defect. That was devastating to me. I had hoped that I could have breast-conserving surgery; now I would have to face mastectomy. I asked the plastic surgeon about immediate breast reconstruction. I did not want to come out of surgery without a breast. He reviewed my options. I was too slim to have a whole breast constructed out of my latissimus dorsi back muscle. A TRAM flap taken from my abdomen would be a better alternative. He asked me to come by his office later for further discussion and to meet some of his breast reconstruction patients.

How did you react to the news that you had breast cancer? What did you do after you heard the diagnosis and treatment options?

I kept busy. I spent the entire day talking to different specialists. I suddenly remembered that I had a hair appointment at 6 o'clock, and I felt compelled to keep it: "I'll be damned. I'm going to get my hair cut despite all this." While I was at the beauty shop, I called my mother to tell her I had breast cancer. The whole scene was surreal. Why would you get your hair done on the day you find out you have breast cancer? But it seemed a normal thing to do, and I needed that. It was a way of maintaining some semblance of control.

Did you seek a second opinion?

I called a colleague who is a research director for an oncology group in Indiana. She asked me what treatment I had chosen. I told her I was scheduled for a mastectomy and immediate breast reconstruction the next Wednesday. The large size of my tumor and small size of my breast ruled out lumpectomy. She cautioned against making a hasty decision. She said, "Get on a plane. I will schedule appointments for you to talk to the doctors here."

Instead of going to the meeting, I flew to Indiana, where I met with a number of specialists. The diagnosis was the same, but they told me about another option called *neoadjuvant therapy* (also *induction chemotherapy*). With this approach, chemotherapy is given before surgery for women with late-stage or an aggressive form of cancer that is likely to spread (such as inflammatory breast cancer). The chemotherapy is administered early to shrink the tumor and halt possible spread.

I was already scheduled for surgery in 2 days. I thought, why change things now? However, why not get chemotherapy now instead of waiting 4 to 6 weeks after surgery? Nobody can predict when cancer will spread—it could be in 2 days or 2 weeks or even 2 years. So I had some difficult decisions to make.

How did you make your decision?

I went with my instincts. The physicians in Indiana referred me to a local oncologist experienced with neoadjuvant chemotherapy. I went to see him and decided to try this approach. I called off surgery, and on the next Tuesday I started chemotherapy.

Did being a physician make this decision-making process any easier?

It made it harder. Being a physician, I was an integral part of the decision-making process in a way that most patients aren't. Instead of doctors talking to doctors, it was doctors talking to me. I was the person in between. My doctors assumed I knew more than I did. I'm a really good immunologist, but I don't know a thing about breast cancer. I suppose I can understand what I read better than most patients, but still. . . . My doctors gave me enough information, but I am not sure it would have been sufficient for most patients.

When I first talked to my oncologist, he started off with, "I know you've read all about this." I stopped him right there and said, "No, all I have read is some basic material. I haven't read all the medical oncology literature. Yes, I have an M.D. degree, but I don't have any training in that area and can't make critical decisions on whether this or that was a good study. I need you to be my doctor, and I will be the patient. I will ask questions when I don't understand things." Sometimes, however, I do find myself feeling a little intimidated and hesitant to ask questions when I perceive that my doctor is busy. That is a bad attitude; patients need to ask questions, because doctors need to know when a patient is confused.

Was the neoadjuvant (induction) chemotherapy successful? How did this therapy affect your plans for cancer surgery and plastic surgery?

During the first week of chemotherapy, I didn't even touch the lump. I thought, you can't be examining yourself every day to see if the chemotherapy is working. When I finally did touch it, I could barely feel it anymore, and this was a palpable 2.5 to 3 cm lump. That actually frightened me. I don't know why; it was just so amazing to me that it could work so rapidly. I called the oncologist and said you need to tell me what is happening here. I thought I was losing touch with reality. I was sure that I was in denial. But I wasn't. The tumor was shrinking after only the first round of chemotherapy. I had three to four more sessions to go before the surgery.

At this point I decided to visit my breast surgeon to inquire whether I would be a candidate for breast conservation now that the tumor was shrinking.

What was your breast surgeon's reaction to your inquiry about changing your therapy from mastectomy to breast-conserving surgery?

I told her that I was thinking about having breast-conserving surgery instead of a mastectomy because my tumor had shrunk so much that I couldn't feel it anymore. She examined me and couldn't feel it either. We bargained back and forth. She was hesitant to acknowledge that my tumor was smaller. She still wanted to take out a relatively large area of tissue, even though it would be smaller than originally planned. Now she would only remove the area of the tumor, not a wide margin of tissue surrounding it. However, it would still leave me with a big defect, and I would need some type of breast reconstruction. She suggested I talk to the plastic surgeon before I made a final decision.

What did the plastic surgeon recommend?

I went to see the plastic surgeon. Previously he said that I didn't have enough tissue on my back to build a whole breast after mastectomy. Now, however, my tumor was much smaller, and I was considering having a lumpectomy. So I told him how my situation had changed and asked if he thought I had enough back muscle and tissue to fill in the lumpectomy defect. Would I be a candidate for the endoscopic back (latissimus dorsi) flap technique? I learned of this procedure when I visited his office the first time. I had spoken to a woman who had an endoscopic back flap to fill in a lumpectomy defect. She let me see what her reconstruction looked like, and it was amazing. There were only three small scars, and it looked very natural. I thought this might be something that would work for me if I had breast-conserving surgery. He listened carefully, examined my breast, and finally said, "Okay, if you decide to have the lumpectomy, we'll do it."

Did you decide on a mastectomy with immediate TRAM (abdominal) flap reconstruction, or lumpectomy with immediate endoscopic latissimus dorsi (back) flap reconstruction followed by radiation therapy?

Two weeks before I had the surgery, I was still vacillating between lumpectomy and radiation therapy and mastectomy. Although the survival rate is equivalent for both approaches, local recurrence is about 10% higher for lumpectomy and radiation therapy. I had to decide whether I was willing to risk a higher recurrence rate.

My breast surgeon said it depends on what kind of person you are. If you develop a local recurrence after this procedure and can say, "Well, I tried. It seemed like a good option for me at the time," then go for the breast-conserving surgery and the latissimus flap. If you are a person who is going to berate yourself for making a wrong decision, then go with a mastectomy and a TRAM flap. Even then, your recurrence risk doesn't go down to zero.

So I weighed the options. With breast-conserving surgery, my risk for recurrence is 10% higher, but I would have my breast intact and it would match the other side. I also would avoid the major surgery and recovery associated with mastectomy and TRAM flap reconstruction. I tend to be an optimist. I thought this breast-conserving surgery seemed to be a better approach for me. So I went for it. I had a lumpectomy with immediate endoscopic latissimus dorsi flap reconstruction. Then I had a follow-up course of chemotherapy and later 6 weeks of radiation therapy.

Tell me about the operation. What was it like? How long did it take? Were you prepared?

The surgery involved three basic steps. First, I had needle localization to zero in on the exact location of the tumor. Then I had a lumpectomy to remove the tumor, and axillary node dissection to obtain a sampling of lymph nodes in my armpit area to check for tumor spread. Finally, I had breast reconstruction using endoscopic techniques to harvest a portion of my latissimus dorsi back muscle and tunnel it through the axillary incision to restore my breast contour.

The surgery was probably more difficult for me because of the four courses of chemotherapy I had previously. I had taken only 2 or 3 days off work during chemotherapy, and I had traveled when my white blood cell count permitted. I went into surgery quite tired. The night before, I stayed up until 3 AM to get a paper off to a colleague. I thought, "Great, I'm going to have general anesthesia and can catch up on the sleep I lost." What a misconception that was. I wasn't prepared for the needle localization procedure before the lumpectomy.

What does needle localization involve?

The mammogram taken before I had chemotherapy was used to accurately pinpoint the location of the lesion and to guide needle placement. The needles are inserted into the breast, and then they take other mammographic views with the needles inserted. It is quite painful.

Do they give you local anesthesia?

No. Sensation is necessary to ensure the breast can be maneuvered correctly for the mammograms and the needles positioned accurately. Each time they insert a needle they have to do a mammogram. I needed three needles inserted. My breasts are fibrous, and there was a lot of scarring from the chemotherapy, so it was difficult to get the needles in far enough. It was so painful that I passed out. Once the needles were in place, a wire was inserted, and the needles were pulled out over the wire. At this point I was beginning to get the idea that this was not going to be a piece of cake. I was thankful that I was going to be asleep for the rest of it.

What happened after the needle localization?

Before the general anesthesia was administered, the plastic surgeon made preoperative markings. I have scoliosis; the right side of my rib cage bows out a little. He said, "You're probably going to be the only woman I've done this procedure on that I'm going to even out." That made me feel a bit better, although he was partially kidding me. My breast surgeon did the lumpectomy and axillary node dissection and my plastic surgeon performed the breast reconstruction. Afterward my breast still looked and felt like me.

How long did the operation take? Did you experience much pain?

My operation took 3 hours. I was hospitalized for 2 days. They wanted to send me home after the first day, but I wasn't feeling well. I was dizzy and couldn't stand up, so I stayed an extra day. My mother stayed with me the whole time, which helped. I had pain every time I moved my arm and probably should have requested more pain medications.

What was it like being in a teaching hospital? Describe your hospital stay. Did you have any problems?

This was my first experience having surgery at a teaching hospital; before, I was in private hospitals. Even though I had traveled that route myself during training, I forgot what it is like for medical students to come in at 5 o'clock in the morning to look at your wound. At 6 o'clock a resident comes in, at 6:30 the chief resident checks on you, and then the attending comes in. So you have four or five people coming to see you.

I didn't like being on display. I knew that the medical student who came in didn't have a clue as to what she was looking at. Anyway, I was feeling very paranoid. I know that one of the factors that contributes to lymphedema is infection, and I didn't want a lot of people opening up my dressings. There are just so many people all of the time.

I also understand why the plastic surgeon had to take so many pictures of me. But it is difficult. You're standing naked and having pictures taken with this little paper panty on. My distaste for all of this was tempered by knowing why it was necessary. I also knew that some of this routine is not really necessary. There is really no reason for a medical student to wake you up at 5 o'clock in the morning. Why aren't rounds made with at least the resident to cut down on the disruptions? I know that the students need to come in to write the notes in the morning before the resident comes in, but by the end of the first morning, I was ready to slap a few hands and say, "You do not know if this looks good or bad. The only person who can come here and tell me this is okay is my plastic surgeon."

How long did they leave the drains in? Was it painful when they were removed?

I left the hospital with two drains. The first drain came out within a week. If I had to rank the procedure that was the most painful, that is number one; number two is needle localization; and number three is fine-needle aspiration biopsy.

They clip the sutures and say, "Take a deep breath and hold it, because this is going to hurt." Then they just rip the drain out. You have no idea that something that long was inside your back and your scapula. You can't cry, because you have no breath left. It is absolutely excruciating, but it is over quickly, thank goodness. The second drain in your side comes out in 2 weeks; it is not as long as the first one and for some reason is not as painful. Maybe it's because you have more numbness in that area.

Did you have any problems or complications?

After the drains were removed, fluid accumulated all the way up to the scapula. It was like a bag of water. I had to come in every week and have them aspirate it. That wasn't as painful as I would have thought, because I didn't have much sensation there.

Why did you need more chemotherapy after surgery when you had chemotherapy before surgery?

They split the whole course of treatment because they wanted me to have some kind of mop-up chemotherapy after surgery. Then I had the radiation therapy.

How long did you have radiation therapy? What was involved?

Every day, Monday through Friday, for 6 weeks. They place a big target thing around you, like X marks the spot, to focus the therapy. The radiation produces an intense sunburn on your breast that is initially sore and painful to touch. It is red, inflamed, and swollen, and then it tans. They draw marks over your breast area and cover them with plastic to keep them from rubbing off. So you walk around for 6 weeks with lines all over your breast. The redness on my breast has faded now, but the nipple is still somewhat red. For a while the nipple was very sore and inflamed. You couldn't touch it at all.

I actually went to an aesthetician and had her apply superficial peels to this sunburned area on my breast to bleach it. We did six sessions, and I did home bleaching as well, which improved the skin damage from the radiation therapy. The radiation shrank the breast slightly, and I understand that it will continue to shrink a little more over time.

How long was it before you could get back to your normal activities?

I went back to work $2\frac{1}{2}$ weeks after surgery; in another 2 weeks I started physical therapy twice a week. I lifted weights and did exercises to improve my shoulder mobility. The therapists worked with me to try to loosen the adhesions under my arm and improve mobility. My plastic surgeon recommended this. I waited until the radiation therapy and postsurgical chemotherapy were over and my hair grew back before I started playing tennis—it gets hot playing in a wig. Now I'm back to tennis and aerobics. The only reason my schedule is less demanding is because I have chosen to start taking weekends off and not working so late at night. It's a life choice.

My plastic surgeon also recommended massage therapy. Unfortunately, insurance doesn't pay for massage therapy, but I did it anyway.

How often have you had massage therapy? Has it helped?

I have therapy once a week, and I've continued it during my trips to Maine, California, Indiana, and even China. Everywhere I go now, I locate a massage therapist. Before the therapy my scapula was really bound from adhesions. I was stiff and tight—tight to the point where my muscles and ribs hurt. So I have been aggressive with my physical therapy and massage therapy, and it has helped enormously in restoring mobility and flexibility.

Every time I come in for a follow-up, the residents comment on how good my donor site looks. Well, it ought to look good; I've paid thousands of dollars for massage therapy. I recommend it to everybody. It has been one of the best things I have done to keep myself mobile.

Are you pleased with the aesthetic appearance of your breast?

It looks really good. Overall, my breasts are smaller, but they are symmetrical. They have the same droop, and they look very much alike. The scars have faded, and you really have to look to see them. Anybody who didn't know that I had the surgery wouldn't be able to tell.

What do your scars look like?

There is a semicircular incision around the areola. Another incision extends across the axilla or armpit area. It was used for the node dissection and had a drain in it. It was also used at the time of endoscopic surgery to pull the latissimus dorsi flap through to the chest area. You can barely see that scar anymore, because it is in the tissue folds. I also have a 1-inch scar on my side from the drain across my ribs. There was a 1-inch vertical incision on my scapula that I suppose was used to insert the endoscopic instruments. It was sewn up at the time of surgery and did not require drains.

How does your reconstructed breast feel? Is it sensitive?

Most of the sensitivity in my breast has returned. My nipple is not as sensitive as it was. My breast surgeon made an incision around it and dissected under it to do biopsies at the margins of the tumor. During that procedure some of the nerves were cut, especially around the top of the nipple. The nipple still has sensation, but it doesn't always re-act like the other nipple does, for example, when it's cold. It is still sexually responsive. For a while it was very sore. I didn't want to touch it. Part of that soreness was from the radiation therapy.

I didn't realize that the muscle transferred to my chest has its own blood supply, which means that it is still innervated. When I do some-thing that moves the latissimus muscle in my back, my breast moves. When I contract the muscle in back, the muscle in my breast also contracts. The first time I reached up on a shelf to pick something up, this muscle contracted. I thought, "What is that?" Then I remem-bered that a woman in my support group had told me that the muscle continues to function as if it were still on my back. That's been diffi-cult to adjust to; it's a constant reminder that I've had the surgery. I can't do aerobics or cleaning or reach up for something in a cup-board without it contracting. My plastic surgeon tells me this is some-thing that is not going to go away. If I raise my arm in a certain way, it pushes the breast up.

My reconstructed breast is warmer and somewhat firmer than the other one. I guess that's because the muscle is transferred with its blood supply and that healing is going on. The massage therapy helps to soften it a bit.

Do you notice any other physical changes related to your surgery?

My armpit area is flatter and firmer now. It is numb, and yet it feels like something is under my arm. It's a strange sensation, because you can't really feel when you are shaving. I worry about cutting myself. I actually bought a special shaver.

Why did you decide to have immediate breast reconstruction? Did being single influence your decision?

It never crossed my mind not to. Being a single woman, I thought that I would be able to cope better with all the changes if my body image stayed intact. I didn't want to wake up from the surgery without a breast. I also felt immediate reconstruction would produce a better cosmetic result, because the scars would be shorter.

If you had it to do over again, would you have breast reconstruction? Would you choose the same procedure?

Yes, I would do it again, and I would choose the same procedure. The scarring is minimal, and I like the look of my breast. I think that I look close to the way I looked before surgery. I don't have scars that anybody is going to notice. I've been to the beach since then, and you can't tell. Most of the scars are behind the strap of a bathing suit or bra or on my side. Most of the time I don't think that much about having had breast cancer. It only hits me every once in a while. Every day I am reminded that I have had reconstruction, but even that memory is fading. I've been told that it takes a year or so for those tissues to loosen up and become more normal.

How do you tell a man in your life about your breast cancer or breast reconstruction?

I was involved in a relationship when this happened. I told him when I was going in for the biopsy. He knew about it when the lump started nagging at me, even though I was saying it was nothing. I actually had him feel it. I said, "Do you feel that? Doesn't it feel different to you?" He didn't know, but it felt different to me, so he told me to do something about it.

I called him when I was waiting for the results of my biopsy and I called him afterward. He was very supportive the whole time. He said it didn't matter, and I really believed him. I know what your body looks like does matter. And it matters to your partner, but I really got the impression that that wasn't why he cared about me. I really wished at that point that I was either married or that this friend was my partner, but we had both talked about it, and we knew we weren't going to be lifelong partners before this even happened.

I don't know how I'm going to handle this in the future. I don't know if I'm going to tell somebody up front. That's why I wanted to look as much like I did before surgery so it isn't an issue. It's amazing to me how women have complete mastectomies and choose not to have breast reconstruction. They must be truly strong and have an amazing sense of their own self-worth to go through all that and then experience all those body-image changes. I didn't want that. I still worry about it. I know I don't look quite as good as I did. I don't think anybody else would really notice, but I know. Even though I am to the point of thinking I look pretty good now, what would somebody else think about it?

How did your breast cancer therapy affect your desire for intimacy and your sexuality?

During therapy I really did not want any sort of relationship, any sort of intimacy. It just wasn't something that was of interest to me. When you are having radiation therapy, you have marks drawn all over you. If a woman is sensitive or hesitant about pulling her gown off in front of strangers, this would send her through the roof. You go in there every morning and you sometimes see the same technician, sometimes not. I just wish I had a buck for everybody I pulled my clothes off for in the last 18 months. But you become very unemotional about it. It turns the sexual part of it off too. Plus, its very painful during that time. The skin hurts during radiation therapy. You feel like you have a bad sunburn, you're swollen, you have marks all over you, and they put plastic on you so the marks don't come off.

During that time this man and I were still friends, but the relationship just went by the wayside. This is the time you find out if a person is supportive. After this type of experience you know whether you want to spend the rest of your life with a person. My friend and I had already agreed that we did not. So I can't say he left me because I had breast cancer.

What advice would you give to a woman considering breast reconstruction?

For me, the process of dealing with having cancer, facing major surgery, and undergoing chemotherapy and radiation was much easier knowing that I could come out of it perhaps cured and with pretty much the same body. You go into it very frightened. Part of the terror is not knowing exactly what you're going to look like. It was comforting to know that I had this option. To know that reconstruction at the time of the initial surgery would give me a better result was a bonus. I went home with a sense that not much had really changed. I still had my breast; it was just filled in with something different. I would recommend that a woman consider immediate reconstruction. I have never wished that I had waited. I have yet to hear a woman say that she is sorry she had immediate reconstruction, but I have heard some women say they regretted waiting.

It's also important for a woman to know, however, that as good as your doctor is and as many of these procedures as he has done, he has not experienced the surgery himself. There is a tendency for surgeons to minimize the length of recovery and the discomfort that you will feel. Somehow saying, "Oh, you're going to have this discomfort" or "you're going to have this tightness" doesn't cut it. I am always hearing women in the support group say, "I just didn't realize how much pain there would be or how long it would take until I felt better or until I could return to my normal level of activity!" So I would advise women to consider the recovery a yearlong process that you really have to work at to get back to feeling like you did before surgery.

What advice would you like to give to other women?

As a child, when I had something unpleasant to do, I would always say, "I wish it were next week and this was over with." I remember my mother saying, "Deborah, you are wishing your life away." I thought of that when I started therapy, and then I realized that I do not know how much longer I have to live. Nobody does, but once cancer is brought into the equation, it makes life more real. I was so determined during therapy. I thought, "I have no idea what percentage of the remainder of my life this year represents. It could be half of the rest of my life; it could be all of the rest of my life. I am going to try to live it and enjoy it. I am going to try to get something out of every day and give back to people what they have given to me. I have been wishing my life away." I had been putting things off until I was less busy. I think I've learned to treasure the experiences that I have, good or bad, because I learn and grow from them. I've learned to treasure the people that are in my life and to tell them today, because I might not be here tomorrow to say it.

I've also learned to give myself a break. I was hard on myself and afraid of not having control of everything. I wanted perfection, but this experience has taught me that all those things are really an illusion; you never really have control. Things are never really perfect. You might as well go with it and enjoy what you can and try to make it better. Use the resources that you have around you, including the people in your life, and let them help you through this.

I was the epitome of the self-contained woman who didn't really need anybody or anything. I could do everything for myself. I didn't need support. I found out through this that I do need support, and I tell people that I need it now. It has become a very freeing experience. I'm not sure I would say, "Gee, I'm glad I had breast cancer." I have heard women say that. It is a terrible experience, and the fear will stay with you for the rest of your life. But on the whole, many more positive than negative things have come out of it for me. It has helped me to open myself up to life.

LIZZY: WHAT A DIFFERENCE A YEAR MAKES

"One year ago, I was bald and going through chemotherapy. Today, it's a very different story. Time heals. As time passes, you get back to normal. A year makes a huge difference. I'm back to doing everything and feeling good."

Lizzy made these comments to me as she reflected on her recent breast cancer experience. Looking at Lizzy, you would never imagine that she was a breast cancer survivor. She is the picture of health, with rosy cheeks, large, expressive blue eyes, and a full head of curly blond hair framing her slender face. Married with three children, she is thin and fit.

Lizzy had yearly mammograms beginning at age 40, with no problems. That all changed when she was 48, and a routine mammogram identified a suspicious area in her right breast. A subsequent biopsy and MRI revealed cancer in both breasts. She decided to have a double mastectomy to remove the fear of recurrence every time she had a mammogram. For her, breast reconstruction was a logical next step.

Lizzy wanted a simple method of breast reconstruction. Her goal was to return to work and her exercise routine as soon as possible. Therefore she chose immediate bilateral reconstruction (both breasts) with tissue expansion and implant placement. In a second procedure, her nipples were reconstructed and her implants adjusted. Finally, her nipples and areolas were tattooed during an office visit. As she explained, "I am delighted with what I did. When I look in the mirror, I don't see the scars. I think, 'Gosh, they look like breasts!' I'm very pleased with the outcome."

Lizzy's story begins with her initial breast cancer diagnosis.

How was your breast cancer diagnosed?

When I was 48, I went for my annual mammogram and they detected a suspicious area that they wanted to biopsy. The biopsy revealed can-cer in my right breast. An MRI of both breasts detected cancer in my left breast as well. It was too small to be seen on mammogram. When I thought the cancer was confined to one breast, I was trying to choose between lumpectomy and mastectomy. After I found out I had cancer in both breasts, I chose mastectomies to eliminate future worries about cancer recurrence. That was the best approach for me.

Did you require chemotherapy or radiation?

I didn't need radiation therapy, but I did have four sessions of chemo-therapy. Because of my age and premenopausal status, they gave me a blood test to determine whether I should have chemotherapy. My test results came back in a gray area, where they don't definitively recom-mend one course of action; you have to make the decision. That's one of the hardest parts of this whole cancer experience—you have so many decisions to make. There are a lot of options out there, and try-ing to choose the right ones is really tough. I chose to have the chemotherapy, because I was being aggressive in my treatment, first with a double mastectomy and then with chemotherapy to ensure that my body was clear of cancer.

Why did you decide to have breast reconstruction?

My grandma had double mastectomies for breast cancer when she was in her eighties. Because of her age and the times (that was 17 years ago), she didn't have reconstructive surgery and struggled with her prostheses. I saw how my grandmother's chest looked without having anything done. I knew that I wanted some type of reconstructive surgery. I couldn't deal with putting a prosthesis in my bra and feeling bad about my appearance.

How did you investigate your reconstructive options?

When you learn that you have breast cancer, you start talking to other people who have had breast cancer before you. That's very helpful. You think, who do I know who had breast cancer, or who can I call? That's what I did.

Six months before my reconstructive surgery, I visited with a friend who had breast reconstruction with silicone gel–filled implants.

She showed me her breasts and let me feel them. That sounds dumb, but it was helpful to me to see how her breasts looked and felt after implant surgery, nipple reconstruction, and tattooing. Before her mastectomies, she was very busty; she had her breasts rebuilt to the same size they were before, which was bigger than what I wanted. She looked really good. After seeing her, I knew that my breasts would look just fine if I had implants.

My neighbor, who had both of her breasts reconstructed after breast cancer, also visited with me and let me see her breasts. I was amazed at how wonderful they looked. She told me, "You are making these decisions during a stressful time with a lot happening. Once you make your decision, don't look back—just go forward. Whatever decision you make is the right one for you." That was great advice. You can always second-guess yourself and say, "Should I have done something else?" You need to make the best decision and then move on. My decision may not be right for another woman, but it was right for me.

What type of reconstructive technique did you choose? Did cost influence your decision?

I had to decide between reconstruction with implants or with my own tissue. My surgeon gave me a book to read that described the different options. He said that I was a candidate for either approach. I considered the TRAM flap, but I decided against it for several reasons. I talked to other women who had TRAM flap reconstruction. They thought the abdominal surgery was more painful than the breast surgery. Because I was having both breasts reconstructed, they would need to take a substantial amount of abdominal tissue and muscle. I exercise and work out regularly, so I wanted to avoid pain or problems in my abdominal area. I would have loved to have gotten rid of a couple of inches in my stomach and eliminated the roll of fat, but that wasn't sufficient reason to have a TRAM flap.

When a woman is trying to decide what type of reconstructive procedure to select, there are a number of factors to consider, ranging from the length of recovery to the costs of surgery. For me, the TRAM flap was major surgery and cost more than I wanted to spend. You have to check with your insurance company to see what is covered. Even though my insurance company covered my procedures, I still had to pay thousands of dollars before I met my deductible, and there were things my insurance company wouldn't pay for. You have to look at that too when deciding which surgery works best for you.

That's why I decided to have tissue expansion and implants and to have the reconstruction done immediately. I know that implants aren't permanent—in time I may need to have my implants replaced. My plastic surgeon was very upfront about that. I look at that as the same as getting a little tune-up down the road. That's okay with me; I can do that. Or if I have problems with my implants later and decide that I want to have the TRAM flap, I can, although I don't foresee having to do that. By choosing implant surgery, I haven't closed out future options.

How long did the whole reconstructive process take, from insertion of your expanders to final implant placement?

It took approximately 6 months from beginning to end. I had my mastectomies with expanders inserted in October. Then my breasts were expanded over the next few months. My chemotherapy treatments were done in January, February, and March. They recommended that I finish chemotherapy first before my implant surgery. After my chemo was done, about 8 weeks later (at the end of April), I had the expanders removed and the implants put in.

How often were your breasts expanded, and what was involved?

Right after the mastectomies, the expanders were inserted and my plastic surgeon injected a little saline solution in them. Then every time I came to the office he would inject a little more saline to expand them some more, but not too much. I came in every 2 to 3 weeks for a total of four or five expansion sessions. About 50 to 100 cc of saline solution was injected during each visit. I wasn't there very long each time. I would come in, my surgeon would check everything, and then he would put the saline in a syringe, insert the needle into the port under my skin, and just expand my breasts. There is a little area inside the expander where the port is located. My plastic surgeon used a magnetic finder, which was really cool. He would put it on my breast and he could tell exactly where to insert the needle to inject the saline solution.

Did you have input into your final breast size?

Tissue expansion gave me some control in a rather out-of-control situation. I was fairly small-busted to begin with and didn't know exactly how large I wanted to be. I figured I might as well go a little bigger—get something positive out of all this. With tissue expansion, you can make a judgment: "Well, this is a good size for me," or "this isn't." During a very stressful time when you're trying to make so many important decisions, expansion gives you time to figure out what you want to do.

How did the expansion process feel? Was it painful?

My breasts would feel a little tight as the tissues were stretched, but they never hurt. You don't have much feeling with the breast tissue removed, so I couldn't feel the needle and there wasn't any pain. Expanders feel bigger and bulkier than your real breasts, but knowing that they are temporary, you put up with it. I knew that eventually when I got my regular implants, they would be more comfortable.

How did you determine when your breasts had been expanded sufficiently?

My breasts were expanded until they were at a size that was right for my body and my body type—something that I felt comfortable with. Then I didn't come back until I was ready for the implant surgery.

What type of implants did you choose: saline or silicone gel–filled?

I chose the silicone gel. I researched it, and my plastic surgeon and I discussed it. For my body type he really thought that the silicone gel would look and feel softer and more natural.

Describe implant surgery. How long did it take? Were you hospitalized, or was it done on an outpatient basis?

It was done on an outpatient basis, and it didn't take long at all. I was there for 3 or 4 hours, but some of that time was spent in the waiting room before I was taken to the operating room. They put me to sleep and the next thing I knew, I woke up and the procedure was done. It isn't bad at all. They reopen your incisions, remove the expanders, and replace them with implants. I hardly had any pain—just a little discomfort. This was a breeze compared to the original mastectomies. I didn't take any strong pain medication—just Tylenol a couple of times.

Did you have any complications? Was there any swelling or bruising?

No, I didn't have any complications at all. I had a little swelling, but no bruising.

Did you have any drains?

I only had drains when I had the double mastectomy. I had no drains when the expanders were removed or when the implants were put in.

How long did it take you to recover? Were there restrictions on your activities?

I bounced back very quickly. I took it easy for the first week. There were restrictions on weight lifting and exercise. They don't really want you lifting more than 10 pounds—similar to the restrictions I had after the first surgery. I'm a very active person; exercise is a big part of my life. One of the hardest adjustments for me was the restriction on my ability to work out. I could still walk, but I had to forego my weight and step classes, because they would have caused too much pulling through the chest area. I didn't want to exercise and tear out my stitches or damage any part of my body by overdoing it. So I just cut back on my activities. After 6 weeks, I was back to my normal level of activity. Now I can do everything I did before. I feel good.

Did you have your nipples reconstructed? How was it done?

I wanted my breasts to be complete, so nipple reconstruction was a no-brainer. My plastic surgeon used the skin already present on my breast for the reconstruction; he designed flaps of skin, pulled them up, and then twisted them to form a nipple (C-V flap). It's amazing how they do that, because it looks like a nipple when it's done! It really finishes your breast off. Before, I had this noticeable scar across my breasts. After the nipple reconstruction and tattooing (I had that done 1 month later), my breasts were transformed. The tattooing and nipple cover part of the scar, so you only see a little portion of it (not much at all) on each side. When you look in the mirror, you don't notice that big scar anymore and you think, "Gosh, they look normal!" I think the tattooing looks good and the nipples are just right. I'm delighted that I did it all.

Did you have any other revisions or adjustments at the time of your nipple reconstruction?

When I had my nipples reconstructed, I asked to have my implants moved inward, because I felt there was too much space between my breasts. My natural breasts had been oriented to the side with most of the tissue falling near my underarm area. I would wear an underwire bra to move my breast tissue in more centrally—I never really had cleavage. My plastic surgeon told me that he wouldn't be able to create cleavage with the implants if I didn't have cleavage before, but he could move my implants a little closer together and put in some sutures on the side when he reconstructed my nipples. However, I would have to have general anesthesia again. Normally your nipple reconstruction can be done under local anesthesia and you are awake. I decided to go ahead and have the general anesthesia, because I wanted the implants moved and the nipples done at the same time. That worked very well. I had the tattooing 1 month later.

Are you happy with your breast appearance?

I'm very pleased with how everything turned out. My breasts are not like my normal breasts; they are different. But I feel good. I look in the mirror and I'm amazed at what they can do to make you look and feel like a woman. It's just astounding.

Are your breasts warm? Are they sensitive?

Yes, that was one of the other reasons I decided to have the silicone gel implants. I think they feel a little warmer than the saline implants. I don't really have a lot of feeling in my breasts. I know when I'm touching them, but I have lost a lot of the sensitivity, and I haven't really gotten it back.

Have you had genetic testing?

No, I haven't, but I have thought about it for my daughter so she understands our risk status. My oncologist said I could be tested if I wanted to be. In the future, I might. Both my mother-in-law and sister-in-law have had breast cancer. That means my kids have relatives on both sides who have had breast cancer. I'll probably do it at some stage, and maybe my daughter will be tested as well.

I know some people don't want to know if they are at high risk for cancer. They're afraid that they might get a test result that they don't like. Wouldn't you rather know and be able to do something about it ahead of time instead of wait until you already have a diagnosis of cancer or until the cancer has spread? To me, knowledge is power. Once you know where you stand, you can make decisions and explore your options.

Were you satisfied with your choice of a plastic surgeon? What qualities were you looking for?

He has a wonderful bedside manner. When you talk to him in the office, he explains everything—all the different options. He answered all my questions. I knew he had a great reputation, but he has other important qualities. Every time I saw him, he was so kind and compassionate. I could tell he really cares about me as a patient. He wants to make me feel good about myself and to help me feel whole again, like a normal woman. And he succeeded; I feel that way.

Has your husband been supportive? Do you have advice for what a husband should do to be helpful?

My husband was shocked when I told him I had breast cancer. That's a natural reaction, but he was very, very supportive. He came with me to all my visits to the cancer surgeon, and then to the reconstructive surgeon. It helps to have somebody accompany you to your doctor's appointments, because he is hearing everything too, and then you can go home and talk about it.

My husband was great because he didn't tell me what to do. We would talk about my options and he always listened to me, but the final decision had to be mine. He said he would support me in whatever I chose to do, whether I had reconstruction or I didn't; it wouldn't make a difference in how he felt about me. He says I look great. I now have bigger breasts than I did before. That's a bonus from the reconstruction. I thought, if I'm going to have reconstruction, why not make my breasts a little bigger? And I did. They look great, and I feel very good in my clothes.

Was your insurance company difficult to deal with?

My insurance company wasn't difficult at all. I timed my procedures so that they all fell within 1 calendar year, and I had already met all of my deductibles, so I was at the point where everything was going to be paid in full if it was completed before year's end. That's why I hurried to have my nipples reconstructed, my implants moved, and my tattoos done before the end of the year. Insurance coverage is an important factor for women to consider when scheduling the different procedures. It's easy to say, "Oh, I'm not in a big hurry." However, you first need to look at where you are in terms of deductible payments for the year with your insurance. If you wait until the new year, you will start all over with your deductibles for procedures that might have been paid for fully. I didn't have to pay anything for the nipple surgery and tattooing. I'm glad I finished it all in 1 year; that meant considerable savings.

What would you recommend to other women who are considering breast reconstruction?

I would recommend checking out all the different options and talking to your doctor about them. Read books and gather as much information as you can. Then if you want to have breast reconstruction, go for it.

What advice would you like to share with other women?

A year ago, I was bald and going through chemotherapy. At the time, I was overwhelmed, and I wondered, "Am I going to get through this?" But time heals, and as it does, you get back to normal. I look back now and it's hard to believe that a year ago I was going through all this, because I'm back to doing everything and feeling good. It's important to keep your life as normal as possible, even during treatment. That's what I did: I continued to exercise, and that was enormously helpful for me, both mentally and physically. Even on the days when I didn't feel great I'd walk a little; I let my body tell me what to do. When I felt good, I went to the club and exercised. I tried to do as much as I could. I wanted to maintain some normalcy.

When I got breast cancer, I knew there were many things that I couldn't control—but the one thing I had the power over was my attitude. You can be negative and feel sorry for yourself, questioning, "Why me?" or you can be positive and say, "Why not me?" I mean, I am 1 in 8, and I intend to make the best of it. I'm not implying that I didn't have bad days or days when I cried or was upset, because I did. But having a positive attitude and looking to the future helped me get though it.

KATHRYN: IT'S TIME TO FOCUS ON ME

Kathryn is an attractive woman in her mid-forties. Casually dressed in jeans with a gray scarf draped over her shoulders, she is accompanied by her husband, Ted, who has been by her side for the past 2 years. Their mutual affection is obvious. He even went so far as to shave his head when she lost her hair during chemotherapy, a testament to his devotion and support. It seemed only natural that he participate in this discussion as well. Therefore, although this interview focuses primarily on Kathryn, it also includes special insights and comments from Ted. He has been her rock and has played an important role in her recovery. He is teary-eyed as he listens to her recount her breast cancer experience.

Kathryn's story began 2 years ago, when she felt a tender area in her chest. Weeks later, she noticed a nipple discharge and started experiencing radiating pain in her chest. Eventually, after numerous tests and much time had elapsed, a large breast lump was discovered and was diagnosed as invasive ductal carcinoma. Because her lump was large, she had neoadjuvant chemotherapy (administered before her cancer surgery) in an attempt to shrink the breast mass before surgery and reconstruction. Kathryn also decided to have a prophylactic (preventive) mastectomy on her opposite breast, because she did not want to worry about developing another breast cancer. She had bilateral mastectomies, followed by immediate tissue expander reconstruction with her expanders inflated slightly. The final reconstruction was delayed until the radiation was completed and her tissues had time to heal. Then her expanders were removed and she had TRAM flap reconstruction using her own abdominal tissues to restore her breasts. Now, 1 year later, Kathryn is delighted with her reconstructed breasts and laughingly comments that they are larger than before, but she likes the way they look.

How did you discover your breast cancer?

My story started 2 years ago when I felt a tenderness in my chest. I had a mammogram scheduled at my community hospital, and I had some yellow nipple discharge at the time. I was surprised that the technician didn't notice the discharge until I pointed it out. She said that everything looked fine on the x-rays, so I left. A day later, I pulled my seatbelt across my chest and felt a hard, painful lump. I called my gynecologist and she told me to come in so they could see what was going on. She was still able to get some discharge out of my nipple, and she tested it for blood. At that time, my wheels were turning as I tried to understand what was going on. They sent my discharge to the lab, and I returned to work.

When did you begin to realize that something was wrong?

My pain increased, and I started getting streaks of pain that ran through my chest. I have a desk job, and I would be sitting there working when all of a sudden the pain would surge through my breast. I saw my doctor 6 weeks later, and my breast was hard and painful. She did some tests and referred me to a breast cancer surgeon. I remember crying because she had said the dreaded words. I was scheduled to see this surgeon 3 months later. In the meantime, I received my mammogram results from the community hospital; the report said that I had benign calcifications. So I put it out of my mind.

Two months before I was scheduled to see the surgeon, I noticed a bloody discharge in my bra. The next day I went to the Komen Cancer Center and had a needle-guided mammogram, followed by ultrasound. The doctor there examined me, feeling my armpit for my lymph nodes. I suspected what he was looking for. He asked me to come back the next day. But I live an hour and a half away, so I said I'm not coming back just for test results, can you call me? Finally, he told me that he thought I had cancer. He asked me to stick around so they could biopsy my breast right away. I agreed to do that. The next day I came back to find out about the results. My husband and oldest daughter came with me, because I wanted this to be a family thing.

What did they find on biopsy?

I had invasive ductal carcinoma. My breast was enlarged and inflamed, and the lump was huge, over 6 cm; it felt like a golf ball beneath my skin. My primary care doctors never made the connection, and the community hospital did not diagnose it on my mammograms.

What happened once there was a diagnosis?

Things proceeded rapidly. The next day I met with my surgeon, who arranged meetings with the oncologist and the plastic surgeon. I also had more tests. It was impressive how well coordinated these doctors were. By the end of the week I had started chemotherapy.

Why did you have chemotherapy before you had surgery?
How many treatments did you receive?

My tumor was very large. They hoped the preoperative chemotherapy would shrink it so that it was more manageable. I had four treatments, one every 2 weeks. I made it through my first four chemotherapy treatments pretty well. Saturdays I would go back for an injection of a booster to increase my white blood cell count. I was pretty sore on Saturday evenings and into Sunday. By Monday I was ready to go back to work. I tolerated the chemo pretty well.

Did you experience any side effects? Did you lose your hair?

The chemo treatments made my natural hair feel dead and fake; I hated it. My oncologist told me that I would lose my hair within 2 weeks after treatment started. Sure enough, it happened like clockwork 13 days after my first treatment. I got in the shower to get ready for work, and my hair started coming out in my hands. I spent more time cleaning up after my shower than I did actually taking the shower. I called the lady who did my hair; she came to my house that night and we cut it all off. I think my hair stylist thought I was going to cry when she shaved my head, but I was actually relieved not to have that dead weight on my head any more. I had purchased a wig and planned on wearing it.

I wore the wig a few times (mostly at night), but it just didn't feel like hair. I wore my hats to work during the day. At that point I was so tired from the chemo that it was a relief not to have to do my hair. I could just throw on a hat with whatever I was wearing that day and go off to work.

Has your hair grown back?

Yes, and it came back much thicker, with some body. My hair has always been stick straight since I was a child. My mom gave me perms so it would have some life to it. I visited my in-laws in Florida in October, and someone complimented me on my hair. My mother-in-law told them it was a very expensive hairstyle. That was very funny.

What other treatments did you receive? Did these result in any side effects?

My next course of treatment was with Taxol. I was to receive four treatments, one every 3 weeks. I didn't tolerate that very well and had a rash and burning on my hands, legs, and feet. They gave me morphine for the pain. My fingernails developed cracks and bumps, and my nails would actually pull away from my skin. I also had sores in my mouth, my throat, my stomach; they gave me different medicines to help me tolerate all of that.

What impact did the preoperative chemotherapy have on your tumor and on your pain?

That was the amazing part. After my first chemotherapy treatment I realized that my pain had stopped—boom— just like that. My tumor was 6 by 9 cm when I started therapy. When I went back for the second chemotherapy treatment, the tumor had shrunk to 2 by 3 cm. Following two more treatments, they couldn't feel anything.

When did you have your cancer surgery?

When I began taking the Taxol treatments, I noticed more density in my breast, so I went to see the oncologist. He canceled my Taxol treatment for that day, and on the next Wednesday the surgeon performed a double mastectomy. He also removed four lymph nodes from my underarm (axilla). My surgeon came in the next morning after my surgery and told me that there were no signs that my cancer had spread to my lymph nodes. My tumor was a type II B and was estrogen positive, which meant that I would be responsive to hormonal therapy. That's why I'm now on tamoxifen and will be taking it for 5 years.

Did you require any adjunctive therapy after your cancer surgery?

Yes, my doctors recommended radiation therapy. I wasn't happy about this; I didn't want the radiation. I don't smoke, I don't drink much, I exercise, and I live a healthy life. So for them to be telling me I'm going to have all these chemicals pumped into my body and then have radiation on top of it, that was tough to take. I just cried.

Why did you decide to have a prophylactic mastectomy? Did they find something suspicious in your other breast?

No, the other breast was okay. I think it was a mutual family decision. I wanted the best chance for survival, and I didn't want to deal with this again. Frankly, I wanted to be done with it. I have a friend who had cancer in one breast, and she got it again. Now she's got it in her bones. My husband and I have been married so long that we were able to take the double mastectomy in stride, knowing that it would alleviate future cancer worries. After we talked to the plastic surgeon and to the other doctors about the percentages, it was just something that we as a family agreed to. To me, it wasn't a huge issue to do this. I also knew that I could have breast reconstruction and I would be whole again.

Ted: I couldn't imagine being a woman and saying, 'In 2 weeks I have to go back for a mammogram on my other breast.' Who would want the constant worry?

Did you have your breasts reconstructed immediately at the time of the mastectomies?

Yes and no. I had an immediate-delayed reconstruction. My final reconstruction was going to be with the TRAM abdominal flaps, but I needed to have radiation therapy. My plastic surgeon said that radiation damages the tissues for the reconstruction, so I should wait until after I was through with radiation therapy. As an interim measure, he would insert tissue expanders into my breasts and inflate them before the reconstruction. The tissue expanders would keep my skin stretched during the radiation treatments and would provide the semblance of normal breasts. So after my double mastectomy, he immediately inserted the expanders and inflated them slightly.

Did you have any complications after your mastectomies?

Ten days later, they took my drains out. I wasn't feeling well that evening, because I had developed an infection. My surgeon put me on antibiotics, but I ended up being readmitted to the hospital that Monday night and was there through Wednesday. I was given rounds of IV antibiotics. They had to put my drain back in for a few days until there was no more fluid coming out. Once the infection was gone, my plastic surgeon gradually inflated my expanders so that my breasts were expanded before my radiation therapy.

How many radiation treatments did you have? Did you have any side effects?

My radiation started during the first part of June and went through the middle of July. I had 33 treatments. I have a little burn on my collarbone, and my underarm was sore and painful for a few weeks, but I put aloe on it as instructed. I think I came through radiation wonderfully. My plastic surgeon liked what had been done.

How long did you wait after radiation before you could have your reconstructive surgery?

My plastic surgeon said I needed to wait 6 months to heal and allow my tissues to get back to normal before I had reconstruction.

What type of breast reconstruction procedure did you choose and why?

I had a standard pedicle TRAM (abdominal) flap procedure. I didn't want to have to have something foreign in my body. I wanted it to be me—my healthy tissue connected to my body. With the TRAM flap, if I put on weight my breasts will grow with me. I didn't want the maintenance down the road that's associated with implants and the worries that come along with them.

What was done for your reconstruction? How long did it take?

They designed a flap of abdominal muscle and fatty tissue. It was left attached to a strip of muscle in the abdomen and was tunneled up to my chest and used to shape my breasts. It took about 3½ hours to reconstruct both breasts.

How long were you hospitalized?

I was in the hospital for 3 days. I had my surgery on Monday afternoon. My doctor came in the very next day and told me how good I looked; that was all the encouragement I needed. I'm not a very good patient; I wanted to be up and out of bed right away. I had taken some pain medicine that morning, so I was able to start walking up and down the hallway. The next day I woke up and said, "Let's get going." Thursday morning the nurse came back and also commented about how good I looked. I said, "Okay, now I'm ready to go home." My doctor agreed to discharge me, even though I could have stayed another night if I wanted to. That was great news. I had a little sponge bath, got my clothes on, and was checked out by lunchtime.

To feel better, you have to take care of yourself. That's why it was so important in the hospital for me to get up and get moving—not overdoing it, but just getting myself stronger and out of that bed.

Did you have much discomfort on your ride home from the hospital?

I manage pain pretty well with painkillers; I'm not afraid to take them. I knew I would need something for the drive home (we live a distance away), so I took pain medication when I left the hospital and made it home okay. I remember feeling pretty stiff and sore when I climbed out of the truck. My belly was very tender, and my ribcage was even more sensitive. I brought my pillows and blanket to cushion me for the bumpy ride going home.

Ted: Your belly was pretty sore. I would ask, "How does your chest feel?" and you'd say, "Well, it's about a 6." But the belly would be like a 2 or a 3 because of the muscle that the surgeon pulled over.

Did you have a hard time standing up after your reconstruction?

I was pretty tight. Even when I was sitting, I needed to stay hunched over. I wore sweatpants at home, and even now when I put on jeans or my work clothes, it is still a bit of an adjustment, because the waistline doesn't give.

What did you do to help your recovery once you got home?

I tried to slow down a bit and to take care of myself. That's one thing this experience teaches you. The laundry is not going anywhere; it will be there tomorrow. It's like I explained to my mom: I get up and do a few things every day to make myself feel stronger and better. I may not feel up to vacuuming today, but I can do something else and still have a positive attitude and feel like I'm progressing. I also plan ahead and make a stack of stuff that I can do when I sit down. I have a laptop computer and we have wireless in the house, so I could take that and sit on the couch to pay bills, check email, and contact my friends. That is what you have to do for yourself. I would make bargains with myself: "I'll do this one chore, and then as a reward I'm going to sit down and relax for the rest of the day, or just take a nap."

After 6 weeks, how do you feel? Are you back to normal?

I feel fantastic now. I told my plastic surgeon yesterday that I can sit up straight now and put my shoulders back. I'm still a little tender about the ribs, and my stomach muscles are weak. Getting out of my bed at home, I need some help pulling up or an arm for support.

I'm trying to get back into doing a few exercises to work off some of the extra pounds that I put on in my stomach. I gained weight so that my plastic surgeon would have enough tissue to get me back to where I wanted to be. Now my goal is to feel as close to normal as possible.

Have you gone back to work?

I just started back working half-days. I'm still a little limited. It would be hard at this stage to sit in a chair using those muscles all day after being pretty relaxed for 6 weeks. My stomach is still tender, and a full day of work would be too much to handle. Monday was my first day back, and I was sore when I left. Right now the half-days are a god-send. It's nice to be back at work, but it's also reassuring to know that if I'm not feeling well, I can just leave after 12. Yesterday I had a few extra things to get done and I was feeling a little better, so to test the waters a bit, I stayed until 1:30 PM. But in no way would I want to put myself in jeopardy for my healing process, because that will set you back.

Ted: I'm kind of a mother hen. I have focused on making sure that Kathryn doesn't overdo it. She's supposed to be working half-days this week, but yesterday she worked until 1:30 PM. But I know who I'm dealing with, so I have to remind her not to overdo it. If she thinks she's feeling better, the next thing you know, she goes out and does something foolish. Then you're back to ground zero again where she's rehealing. So I tell her, "You just go ahead and do that if you want to. But be aware that if you have a setback, I'm going to take you to our community hospital next time." After our earlier experiences at that hospital, that warning is enough to get her to slow down a little bit. Works every time.

How do your breasts look? Where are your scars?

Right now, my breasts are a tad bigger than they were, which is okay with me. You can still see the circular scars on my breasts, and then there is a curved scar (like a smile) across my abdomen and a belly button scar where it was redone. My friend says it looks like a smiley face, and it does.

How do your breasts feel? Are they soft? Are they sensitive?

They are warm; they feel like my tummy fat. They are very soft. They're not very sensitive right now. I feel pressure. I have some sensitivity on the top part of my breasts, and in through the middle it is a bit more sensitive. That's as far as it goes now; I'm hoping to have more sensitivity, but I really didn't have a whole lot before. It's much better than the expanders. They were nice to have, because they made me look whole on the outside, but they were just not natural. You could feel them, and at first they felt hard. I like this much better.

Have you had your nipples reconstructed?

I'm going later this month to have my nipples reconstructed. My plastic surgeon said he will do the nipples, and then a few weeks later I'll get the tattooing. I've thought about not having my nipples redone. I'm tired of procedures. On the outside, my breasts look normal. But I decided to finish this process. I want to show my daughters that if they ever have cancer or another disease, they can get through it and live a normal life.

If you had to do it all over again, would you have breast reconstruction? Would you choose the same reconstructive technique?

Yes, I would have breast reconstruction, and I'm happy with the TRAM flap technique. It's more natural, and I feel healthier with this approach. I didn't want anything artificial in my body.

Have your family and friends been supportive?

A good support system and a sense of humor, faith, and prayer will help you get through these experiences. My family has always been there for me. If I have a doctor's appointment, they say, "All right, who's driving?" My oldest daughter was still in college at the time I was undergoing chemotherapy, but she could drop me off for my chemo, go to school, and then come back and sit with me. I also had a friend who would come to sit with me. Most of the time I almost needed my own room for chemo because so many people would come to visit me. And my family helped out at home. After my first chemo treatment, Ted shaved his head. It was a sign of solidarity. My daughter joined in also; she donated some of her hair for Locks of Love.

My friends have been outstanding. I got lots of flowers. One of the loan officers at the bank where I work gave me a Christmas ornament for the tree that says "Believe." I set it on my desk as a symbol that you can get through these experiences if you just believe. I'm astounded by the cards and food I have received. At work, they set up a schedule on the calendar after my first surgery so that a different person would bring over food every night of the week. They also offered rides to the doctor, visited me, and called to help. It has been outstanding.

Ted: I have also tried to use humor to lighten things up a bit. Like her hats: I told her that the hats made it easy for me to find her in the grocery store. That pink hat is a standout. When you put on the wig, I can't find you. When we were preparing our Christmas meal, I warned people if they found hair in their food, it wasn't from Kathryn or me. And I ask to borrow her shampoo, even though I don't have any hair. Humor keeps it all in perspective.

What advice would you like to share with other women?

It is important to take care of yourself—first. This is the time to be selfish. It's okay to say no and not feel guilty. I remember feeling horrible when I told my oncologist that I wouldn't participate in a clinical trial. I had been in pain for so long and didn't want to delay my own treatment any longer. My advocate from the Komen Center reassured me that it was okay to take care of myself first. And she was right. This is the time to concentrate on getting better.

When you go through cancer treatment and recovery, you need a goal. For me that goal was healing and getting back to normal. I still have that goal. I'm hoping that after 2 weeks, I'll be working full-time again. In the spring I plan to get out and walk so I can build back up to the miles I did before. If you have those goals, and you are determined that you are going to be okay, then there's really nothing to hold you back.

SANDRA: YOU JUST NEVER THINK IT IS GOING TO BE YOU

"I was standing in the room undressed from the waist up. The technologist came in with my film, and I held it up to the light. I took one look at it, and I saw the breast cancer. I just stood there, and I thought to myself, 'I have breast cancer. I cannot believe this; I never thought it would happen to me. I have breast cancer.' I was almost paralyzed, and I said to her, 'I have breast cancer!' She said, 'You can't know that.' But I knew.

"I got dressed quickly, ran to my office to get my old films, and banged on Jill's door. She is the other radiologist I work with. I banged on her door and said, 'Jill, get over to the breast center. I have breast cancer!' I ran back over to the center, and then I just collapsed and cried while she looked at the films. I kept thinking to myself and saying over and over again, 'You just never think it is going to be you.'"

Interviewing Sandra is an electrifying experience; she is animated and intense, and I sense that she has already anticipated my questions and formulated answers long before I pose them. At 40 Sandra is a slender, energetic brunette whose straight, shiny hair bounces as she talks. She has a busy career, a happy marriage, and three young children. As a radiologist at one of the country's leading medical centers, Sandra spends her working days interpreting breast x-ray films for other women. She is more knowledgeable about breast cancer than most women and has ready access to some of the leading specialists in this field.

As she speaks of that day 2 years ago when she diagnosed her own breast cancer, she is still overwhelmed by a sense of disbelief. A biopsy several days later confirmed her diagnosis. Drawing on her knowledge of breast cancer, she carefully planned her own therapy, choosing to have bilateral mastectomies: a modified radical mastectomy to treat the cancer in her left breast, and a prophylactic mastectomy on her right breast. Although cancer had not yet been detected in her right breast, she knew that her odds of developing a new cancer in her opposite breast were increased, and she preferred to have both breasts removed rather than live with the fear of a more serious cancer. She also knew about breast reconstruction and felt that her chances for breast symmetry would be improved if both breasts were reconstructed simultaneously. Because her cancer was localized, she did not have chemotherapy.

Six months after her cancer surgery, Sandra had bilateral breast reconstruction. Her decisions about breast reconstruction were made with the same care and intelligence that she had applied to her cancer therapy. She interviewed four different plastic surgeons and explored the surgical options for breast restoration. She chose the plastic surgeon and the reconstructive approach that would achieve her personal goals. Although she originally considered a TRAM flap, a major reconstructive procedure, she eventually selected a much simpler technique: intraoperative expansion with implant placement. This approach required less recovery time, promised good results, and allowed her to get back to living a normal life in the shortest period of time. Her story is a compelling one.

Did the fact that you were a physician make it easier for you to deal with your breast cancer and your decisions about treatment?

Most women have to go through a learning phase first. They start out knowing nothing about breast cancer, and suddenly they are diagnosed with it. They struggle with weighing one expert's opinion and recommendation against another; they don't know what to expect next. I knew all that. I was one step ahead of where other women would be. I was trying to guess the pathology, to see whether I had an invasive cancer. I knew exactly what I wanted to know: the good prognostic signs and the bad prognostic signs. I wanted to move as quickly as possible to find out my prognosis. I wanted to know exactly how far along my cancer was, how big it was, and whether there was invasion so I could feel comfortable with what I had to face. This waiting period was not easy for me, perhaps because I knew so much. It was one of the most intense experiences I have ever been through. I was anxious every waking moment; I barely slept until I knew my pathology. At one point I was so tense that I just wanted to cry as loud as I could. But I knew that the kids would hear me and want to know what was wrong. So Bob took them to McDonald's, and then I just cried and cried. I felt much better after that. It is amazing how crying can make you feel better. The unknown, the waiting were very tough for me. Once I knew the pathology I was fine, and it wasn't difficult for me to make a decision about therapy.

How did your family react?

I called my husband right away. I said, "Bob, I just had a mammogram and I have breast cancer, but I don't think I am going to die from it." He was totally speechless, then almost hysterical. We didn't tell the children until after the diagnosis was confirmed.

How did you tell your children?

The biopsy report was back on Monday, and I was in the hospital having my cancer surgery by Thursday. I didn't waste any time, because I knew what I wanted. We told the children on Wednesday night. We sat down in the family room, Bob and I and these three little boys. They knew this was a big deal, because we were having a family conference. Before we said anything, Jonathan, the little one, said, "Okay, who's dying?" Bob and I looked at each other. We thought we had kept a good secret. We tried not to let them know, but they knew anyway; they could sense the tension. We said nobody is dying. Then Bob said that I had a mammogram and Jonathan said, "And you have breast cancer, right?" He knows that mammograms are to find breast cancer. And so we said yes. We told them that there were good kinds of cancer and bad kinds of cancer. Lung cancer, for example, is a bad kind of cancer; breast cancer can be bad or good, but I had a good kind, and we expected that I would be cured of it if we took care of it right. I was going to go into the hospital to have surgery to get rid of the cancer. That would be the end of it. They wanted to know if I was going to get new breasts. I said yes, but at a later time.

They wanted reassurance. They wanted to know if I was going to die. How long was I going to be in the hospital? We told them that I would go into the hospital, and the doctor would take my breasts off and that would take care of the problem. I also told them that they would have to help out after I came home from the hospital, since I wouldn't be feeling well for a while. I would be home for a month and that was good, because I wouldn't be working and they would get to see me a lot. They would have to be very patient and easy on me, and soon I would be strong and feeling well again, and that would be the end of it.

Why did you choose a mastectomy over a lumpectomy with irradiation?

I was diagnosed with intraductal carcinoma of the comedo type. Because this type of cancer tends to have a higher recurrence rate, it doesn't do as well with lumpectomy and radiation therapy as it does with mastectomy, especially if the margins of the resected tumor are positive. Even before I knew that the margins were positive, I elected to have mastectomy because I didn't want to take a chance or worry about the possibility of local recurrence. My decision was also influenced by the fact that this tumor has an excellent prognosis if the whole thing is removed.

Why did you choose a prophylactic mastectomy to remove the tissue from the normal breast before any diagnosis of cancer?

I know, realistically, that people who have had one breast cancer are at higher risk for developing another cancer in the other breast. I wanted to minimize the chance of developing a worse lesion on the other side. This lesion that I had was theoretically curable or highly curable. Why take the risk 5 years from now of developing an invasive cancer in the other breast that might become systemic and threaten my life? That was a compelling reason for me. As it turns out, the prophylactic mastectomy was a smart move. When they removed the opposite breast and biopsied it, it showed atypical hyperplasia, a high-risk lesion. That meant I had quite a significant risk of developing breast cancer on the other side.

The fact that I am a breast imager also factored into my decision. I see women with breast cancer and I see women with second breast cancers all the time. I just couldn't have it on my mind. I wanted to do it and get it over with. I didn't want to wait year after year to see if I was going to get a second breast cancer. I also see many women who have undergone breast reconstruction. I know how difficult it is for a plastic surgeon to make the reconstructed breast and the original breast look symmetrical. To me it wasn't a big deal to have the other breast removed. I wanted my breasts to match, and I wanted to minimize my chance of having a second breast cancer. So I decided to have both breasts removed and then to let a plastic surgeon reconstruct both at the same time to make them symmetrical.

How long did it take you to recover from your mastectomies?

In 4 weeks I was back at work and able to function. I couldn't move my arms very well, but I could drive a car; I certainly could read films. I was glad to be back because I could interact with people. I worked part-time for a few weeks. After 2 months I was back in full swing, although not feeling completely well yet. That took about 3 months.

Did you join any kind of support group?

I didn't really need a support group. I desperately needed people; there's no question about it. I needed the support of people in my daily life. I needed them to visit me, to call me, to be solicitous, to stroke me, and to tell me they were hoping that I recovered. I had lots of support from the people I work with. They relieved me of any clinical responsibility; I wasn't forced into stressful situations. That's the most people can do for you. It helps enormously to have people tell you that they are thinking about you and wishing for the best.

How did your husband help you cope with this experience? Was he supportive?

He helped me by listening, taking me everywhere I needed to go, and not making any demands on me. He totally relieved me of responsibility for the kids and took care of all their needs, because he knew it would be difficult for me and that they would sense my anxiety. As it turns out, they sensed it anyway. He did whatever he could for me. After all, there wasn't anything much he could do.

Why did you decide to have your breasts reconstructed?

I had my breasts reconstructed for convenience, for my own self-esteem, and to look good again in clothes, whether or not I looked perfect in the nude. I wasn't after the perfect cosmetic result. I was annoyed with wearing prostheses. It's difficult to get comfortable prostheses, especially after a bilateral mastectomy. I got the smallest size I could find, so they were as light as possible. Despite my efforts, they were hot and heavy and didn't feel natural. If I wanted to go on a trip, I had to worry about how I was going to pack all this stuff; it wasn't convenient at all. I bought bilateral prostheses that cost over $600 ($300 apiece, plus the price of the bras, a swimsuit, and other items), and I wore them five times in 6 months. A friend of mine said, "Sandra, if you're so uncomfortable in those prostheses, don't wear them.

Everybody who knows you knows that you don't have any breasts, and we don't care. The people who don't know you don't know if you were flat-chested before or what. Just don't wear them." So I didn't.

I walked around flat-chested for 6 months, because I was symmetrical and could get away with it. I didn't wear my prostheses, and I felt perfectly fine and comfortable, except that I looked absolutely dreadful in clothes. There's no way you can get clothes to drape on you; women's clothes are not made for a totally flat-chested look. And we are talking about more than the normal flat-chested appearance of a woman with small breasts. With bilateral mastectomies, there is actually less subcutaneous tissue in front. I decided that I wanted to look more natural and normal and feel good about myself and the way I looked—not necessarily at home, in the nude, but in clothes to walk around every day of my life. I didn't want to wear prostheses to accomplish that purpose.

Was it difficult to face more surgery after you had just had your mastectomies?

Yes, it was. I hurt and I was uncomfortable for so long. You can't sleep very well when you have bilateral mastectomies. I was flat on my back; I couldn't roll over in bed for 6 weeks. I was just trying to get better. I wanted desperately to be able to hug my children again and to cuddle them; they needed me to be able to do that. And I really didn't want to hurt again. I was also very tired for at least 3 months. I'm a fast-moving person who likes to accomplish a lot of things in a day, so it was very annoying to me to spend 3 months dragging around. The prospect of giving up another few months of my life was not appealing. Actually, it was the experience of recuperating from the initial surgery that helped me decide what type of reconstructive method I was going to select. I wanted breast reconstruction, but I also wanted to minimize the time I had to spend recuperating.

Did your husband support your decision to have breast reconstruction?

My husband did not want me to have reconstruction. He said, "You've been uncomfortable enough. Why would you want to have any more surgery?" He made it perfectly clear that if it was for him, not to do it. It didn't matter to him; he didn't care. But I told him that it was really for me. I didn't want to wear prostheses. I wanted to feel comfortable in clothes without having to wear a harness (that's what it feels like). It was entirely for me and not for him. Then he accepted my decision and was supportive.

How did you select the method of breast reconstruction and the plastic surgeon to perform it?

I saw a total of four plastic surgeons, because there was a question as to whether I was a good candidate for all the procedures. I wanted to know about all my options so I could make an informed decision. There are a variety of different methods of reconstruction.

I investigated having the TRAM flap, but I found that it would be very difficult because I didn't have enough abdominal fat. I went to see several plastic surgeons about this. One told me that with as little abdominal fat as I had, he would probably have to put implants under the bilateral TRAM flaps to make my breasts large enough. I decided that if I was going to go through major surgery for the TRAM flap, probably more major than the original mastectomy with a much longer recuperation period, then why put implants under my reconstructed breasts? That would defeat the purpose of natural reconstruction with my own abdominal tissue. In addition to that, I wasn't willing to sacrifice a year of my life: 3 months off work, 3 months feeling lousy, and 6 months of not feeling like myself. That was too much. Time is very precious; I feel a sense of urgency to get on with my life and enjoy what I have. My priorities were totally reestablished after facing a cancer operation.

Tissue expansion was another option I explored. Two plastic surgeons I consulted suggested that I have tissue expanders placed bilaterally, then later in a second procedure, after my tissues had been stretched, have the expanders replaced with implants.

Finally, I went to see a plastic surgeon in another city who reviewed all of the options for me, listened to my expectations, and suggested a different approach. He said that he could use intraoperative expansion and then put the silicone gel–filled implants in to reconstruct my breasts in a single operation, rather than the two-stage reconstruction required for tissue expansion. If I wanted to have nipple-areola reconstruction, I could have that at a later time as a minor outpatient procedure. I elected to have the one-stage intraoperative expansion with implant placement. It was an easier, one-step procedure with a shorter recuperation, and I felt more confident with that particular surgeon.

Was your reconstructive surgery painful, and how long did it take you to recuperate?

After reconstruction I was very nauseated by the narcotics they were giving me. I never pushed the PCA (patient-controlled analgesia) button to get more pain medication; it was already giving me more than I could handle. As soon as I weaned myself from that, I felt much better. Tylenol worked just fine and didn't produce nausea. My level of pain and discomfort, while still significant, was not nearly as bad as with my mastectomies, and I was able to go back to work in 10 days.

How did your breasts look and feel during the first few weeks after surgery?

I have seen so much breast reconstruction that I thought that I would know exactly how I would look and feel when I had it done, but I was wrong. I didn't expect my breasts to be as swollen, tight, and shiny as they became.

The swelling and blueness didn't show up during the 3 days I spent in the hospital. Then my husband and I went to a hotel so I could be watched to make sure everything was okay before I flew back home. In the hospital I was elevated in this nice hospital bed, sitting almost erect, and there wasn't much swelling. At the hotel I just propped myself up on a couple of pillows; I could barely get out of bed because I was sore and bruised. When I woke up the following morning, my reconstructed breasts were so swollen and tight that I was afraid that they were going to just burst open. (This from someone who is informed . . . who knows what happened to her.) I had dreams that if I sneezed or coughed, the seams would open up and the implants would go into orbit. I had this vision of them popping out, so I was afraid to sneeze or cough. Of course, that was totally unfounded. But that's how tight my breasts felt.

They also became totally blue, like two giant, ripe blueberries. That wasn't immediate; the blueness took about a week to develop. They were so swollen and blue. My husband was horrified looking at them. I was blue from my chest above the incisions down to my hips. I spent the weekend looking at those tight, blue, swollen breasts and worrying about them.

Was your plastic surgeon responsive to your concerns?

He was very responsive and reassuring. In fact, the reason we stayed in the hotel was to see the plastic surgeon before we went home. When I told him how I had imagined the implants popping out, he laughed and said, "You know too much to think that's going to happen. This is fine, a normal postoperative course; your breasts will do just great." Then, of course, I was relieved. And he was right. The swelling and bruising resolved, everything softened, and my breasts have turned out fine.

Did you have any late problems or complications?

I had some sutures coming through the skin when I was on vacation. That was a little bit difficult to handle, but it turned out to be relatively minor. I called my plastic surgeon on the phone, and he told me to clip the end of the exposed stitch, and that problem was handled very well. Other than that, I have had no problems. I have healed as expected, and over time my breasts have softened and become more natural looking.

Was your reconstructive surgery covered by insurance?

Yes, it was. We have several policies, but insurance companies are not always happy to pay for breast reconstruction. It makes me very angry. When I first called my insurance company (my husband has coverage with a different company), they gave me the run-around. The first person I spoke to said that they would not cover breast reconstruction because it was cosmetic. I said, "I know better—I am a physician. You are not correct. How dare you say this to anybody on the telephone? Of course it's covered. Let me speak to somebody else." Then they transferred me to somebody else. I said, "I am contemplating having reconstructive breast surgery, and I want to know what you pay. I want to know what my out-of-pocket expenses will be." And this person said, "We can't tell you what we pay. We pay 80% of the usual and customary fee." I said "Okay, what is the usual and customary fee?" They said, "We can't tell you that." I said, "What do you mean you can't tell me? I am contemplating very expensive surgery. When I buy a car, I want to know what it's going to cost before I buy it. I don't expect to get a bill after I buy the car to find out then how much it's going to cost me. I want to know ahead of time." They refused to tell me. So I called the CEO's office, and I told him who I was and described the run-around I had gotten. I asked him how they dared to treat people this way. Didn't they realize there are many people who might forego breast reconstruction because they fear being saddled with enormous bills? It was terrible to do this to people. The CEO said he would call me back, and he did, 48 hours later, to tell me the usual and customary fee they paid for breast reconstruction. It was pitifully poor. Then I called my husband's insurance company to find out what they would pay. They also told me they couldn't tell me, but they did, sooner than my own insurance company. And they provided better reimbursement for the surgeon. So my breast reconstruction was covered by two policies that we had: my major medical policy in addition to my husband's policy. But I was incensed at the way it was handled.

Has reconstruction affected the way you feel about yourself?

In terms of self-esteem and self-image, I can't say that reconstruction has made that big a difference. I value myself enough, with or without my breasts. I did it more for convenience and physical appearance, to feel good about the way I look. I don't feel that my breasts, before or after the surgery, are what makes or breaks me.

Have you had your nipples and areolas reconstructed?

Initially I thought, yes, I'm going to do everything; I'm going to do anything I feel like doing. But I changed my mind. I feel comfortable with my breasts as they are now. It accomplishes what I wanted. I look good in clothes; I don't have to wear prostheses. I don't have to go through any more surgery, and I don't want to. I don't need it; my breasts look very symmetrical. They're soft. They look great in a bathing suit, in a nightgown, and in clothes. That is what I wanted.

Are your reconstructed breasts sensitive? Are they warm?

They're not sensitive. There is pressure sensation, but it's not the same sort of discrimination that you have when you touch the rest of your skin that has normal nerve endings. My breasts are also a little bit cooler than the rest of my body.

Are you satisfied with your breast reconstruction? If you had to do it all over, would you choose to have breast reconstruction again?

Without a doubt, yes. It was worth it for me. It was relatively easy compared to the original surgery, and I am pleased with the results. My breasts are symmetrical, soft, and squeezable. My kids like to snuggle up. I know that when they get cuddly against my chest, they are thinking those are Mom's new breasts, and they feel nice and soft. Nobody can tell. If somebody came up and touched my chest, there is no way to know. My breasts feel very natural and normal.

What advice would you like to give to other women considering breast reconstruction?

Become informed. Investigate all of the options so that you can make a choice that meets your personal needs. Identify your goals. Why are you considering breast reconstruction? What do you expect to get out of it? Do you want to look as natural naked as you possibly can, or just to look good in clothing? How much time do you want to invest? If you are thinking about a more lengthy procedure, you need to assess what it will cost in time and money. How are you going to pay for it? It is crucial to know what your expectations are. Once these questions are answered, you need to know about all of the different reconstructive procedures before choosing a particular method. You can't just go to somebody and have him tell you this is the surgery for you; there is no such answer. You must have input. First, you must be able to state what your goals are. How do you want to look? How much are you willing to go through to achieve that look? Then, when you feel informed, when you know all of your options, and only then, can you make the best decision for you.

RYLIE: YOU NEED TO SPEAK UP

"I'm a tough old broad, and I'm going to be just fine." This gutsy declaration was made to me by Rylie as we talked about her breast cancer experience and the many challenges that she has faced. Her voice is soft and husky, a lingering sign of her years as a smoker, and she spoke in a halting manner, weighing her words and feelings carefully. Rylie is in her mid-fifties, with a loving husband and family. They were a tremendous source of strength to her during her breast cancer treatment and subsequent hair loss, radiation burns, and wound healing problems. But Rylie is a fighter, and she was determined to overcome these problems so she could have her breasts restored and regain her life.

Because of her history of smoking, which was a risk factor for surgery, and because of complications experienced after her radiation therapy, Rylie's choices for breast reconstruction were more limited and more complex. She required a major flap procedure using her own tissues to rebuild her breast but did not want to incur any muscle weakness with one of the standard pedicle flaps. Therefore she chose one of the newer perforator flap techniques: the DIEP (deep inferior epigastric artery perforator) flap, a variation on the TRAM (abdominal wall) flap that spares the abdominal muscles and is performed microsurgically. With this approach she could have the natural full breast she desired without any muscle loss and without the need for implants. Her reconstruction was performed as a delayed procedure, months after her original treatment because of her risk factors and to allow her sufficient time to recover from her chemotherapy, radiation therapy, and wound-healing problems. She later had nipple reconstruction, with an opposite breast reduction and lift for symmetry. She is now scheduled for fat injections to fill the hollow left after lymph node removal and hopefully to improve the quality of the irradiated breast skin. Laser treatments are also planned to improve the rash on her chest wall. Rylie has faced all of these procedures with determination, and in the process she has learned to trust her instincts and to speak up for herself.

Her story begins with her discovery of a lump while showering.

What did you do when you found your breast lump?

I felt it while I was showering. I thought, "This can't be, because I have a mammogram every year." I immediately called my family doctor, who is a wonderful person; she had previously found my biliary cirrhosis. I told her, "I have another crisis to deal with, and I need to see you right away." By that afternoon, I was in the surgeon's office for a biopsy. They called me on my birthday and told me I had cancer.

How did you decide what treatment to have?

I wanted to know what my options were and then to have my cancer taken care of as soon as possible. I was hoping that I could have a lumpectomy, but my cancer was stage IV, too far advanced for conservative surgery. A modified radical mastectomy was the treatment of choice.

Were your doctors helpful as you considered your treatment options?

My cancer surgeon was wonderful. She arranged for me to meet with a plastic surgeon and an oncologist to discuss treatments. They explained my options and the possible outcomes I could expect. This all happened before they even did the biopsy. I found out in mid-November, and by the first week of December I had surgery. They also removed five lymph nodes from my underarm and found that the cancer had spread. It all went very fast.

Was it helpful, having it go so quickly? How did your family react?

It was helpful for me, but it was hard on my family and friends. My friends would call to talk, but I didn't need to keep rehashing things over and over again. To me, it was something private that my husband and I were coping with. My husband is my strength; he was there every step of the way. When it comes time to go, I want him to be the last person I see.

Did you require adjunctive therapy—chemotherapy or radiation?

Yes, because my cancer had spread, I needed both. I had eight treatments with chemotherapy, 28 radiation treatments, and five booster treatments to my incision. It did not go well.

What went wrong? Did you experience side effects from the chemotherapy?

When I was going through chemo, I lost my hair. That worried me, because I didn't know how my grandbabies would react. They were so young; I was afraid they wouldn't know me. My granddaughter was only 2 years old at the time. She came to see me, and I was wearing a baseball cap. It was the first time I had seen her since I lost all my hair. My son handed her to me. She took my hat off, kissed my head, and said, "Memaw, you look just like my daddy now. Let's take a picture." I had to laugh. She didn't have any hair until she was almost 3, so I have a picture of my granddaughter and me and my son—all of us bald. It was no big deal to her. Here I fretted whether she was going to know me, and it didn't even faze her. That has helped me a lot. Kids are so innocent; it's just wonderful how they look at life. I've enjoyed rediscovering life with my grandchildren.

Did you have any problems with the radiation therapy?

The initial treatments went just fine, even though my skin was pretty red afterward. The problems started when they administered the five booster treatments to my scar. They burned badly. I told the doctor that I was being burned, but he didn't listen to me. After investigating this on the computer and reading reports of radiation overdosing in the papers, I feel that I was burned with radiation and that caused other problems. The bottom line is, I understand these doctors are professionals, but over the past 2 years—and it has been 2 very long years—I've learned that you need to make them listen to you. You know your own body.

Shortly after my booster treatments, my mastectomy incision ruptured; that was another major problem to deal with. And it was very ugly; it bothered me. I felt so incomplete. You take a shower and that's the first thing you see. I had hoped that I could have breast reconstruction after my treatment, but my plastic surgeon said I had to wait until the incision healed. That required a whole series of treatments that were very upsetting.

What was done to treat your radiation injury and your open wound? How did you cope?

I needed Wound VAC (vacuum-assisted closure) treatments as well as 54 hyperbaric chamber treatments to promote wound healing. The Wound VAC device was painful, because it had to have an airtight seal over my wound, and it exerted a constant sucking pressure on my wound. I had to have the visiting nurses look at it every day. I couldn't go anywhere, because I had this device hanging on me. I was rock bottom at that point. The doctor I saw at the Wound VAC center referred me to a psychologist. She taught me relaxation techniques that were very helpful in dealing with the Wound VAC and in tolerating my hyperbaric chamber treatments.

What is a hyperbaric chamber?

Basically, it is a large, round, enclosed air pressure chamber. Once you get in this enclosure, you cannot get out unless someone helps you. You have to change into special cotton clothes—like surgical scrubs. You can't have reading material, and you can't even wear your glasses because of the pressure in there. You stay awake while you're in the hyperbaric chamber because of the air pressure on your ears.

Why did you need these treatments?

To promote wound healing. I had radiation injury and a badly rup-tured incision, so I was not in good shape. These treatments were in-tended to help promote wound-healing and improve the quality of my irradiated tissue. But it was not easy.

How many treatments did you receive and how long did they take?

I had 54 treatments. They took 2½ hours each, and I had them 5 days a week. It was grueling. I got to know Roger, the specialist there. When I was in the chamber, I could only communicate with him when he picked up the phone and talked to me. I could see what was going on, and there was a TV on the outside, but I was at their mercy to change the channel or adjust the volume. There's nothing I could do but lie in there. I got to the point where I asked for comfortable pil-lows and blankets; but again, these had to be special pillows and blan-kets to prevent friction. I hated going. So many times driving out there I thought, "Oh, who would know if I didn't go?" Because of my claustrophobia, I took anxiety medicine. It helped me get in the chamber. The worst part was knowing that I was locked in with no way out. Before each session was over, the anxiety medicine had al-ready worn off, and I would start banging on the glass. Roger would hold up his fingers indicating how many minutes remained. There was only one time that I said, "That's it, I've had it—get me out now!" And he did. When he got me out, my blood pressure was sky high, I'd just had enough. The psychologist really helped me deal with this, particularly with the anxiety attacks. She taught me how to close my eyes and go inside myself to calm down.

After enduring these problems, why did you still want reconstructive surgery?

It was just the opposite—I couldn't wait to finish my treatments so I could have reconstruction. Reconstruction was a positive for me. The first thing I did when the treatments were over was call my plas-tic surgeon to say, "It's healed; when can we go?" That's what kept me going. I even lost 25 pounds after my chemotherapy and radiation to help me feel good going into my breast reconstruction. So I was ready. My husband kept telling me, "You don't have to go through this; you don't have to have any more surgery." But I had to; I needed it for me. I wanted to feel normal again.

Was your plastic surgeon supportive? Could he have been more responsive?

He has been wonderful throughout this experience. I met him before I even had the mastectomy. He has been supportive through this whole thing—the open wounds, the Wound VAC, the hyperbaric treatments. He told me, "It's a bump in the road. We're set back a little bit, but we can still do your reconstruction." There was nothing I was afraid to ask him, and he never made me feel stupid. I did what he said because I respected him so much.

What reconstructive procedure did you choose, and why?

Implants were not a good option because of my radiation injury and my smoking history. Anyway, I wanted something natural. First, my plastic surgeon suggested using a flap from my back, but I definitely did not like that idea. My goal was to avoid any muscle weakness. I had read about the different operations and knew that pedicle flaps from the back or abdomen transferred the muscle to the breast. That wouldn't work for me; I didn't want to be left with any muscle weakness. I wanted to be able to lift my grandkids or to garden without worrying about any functional restraints. I just wanted my life to be normal again. So I chose the DIEP flap. This is a variation on the TRAM abdominal flap, but it doesn't use any muscle. It was the perfect choice for me.

What is involved with this procedure?

This is major surgery. The plastic surgeon made an incision that extended from hip bone to hip bone. He then freed up a flap of my abdominal fat and tissue and transferred it microsurgically to my breast area, where he reconnected the vessels and built a breast. When he transferred the flap to my chest area, he removed this horrible, ugly scar that had ruptured on my chest wall; I just didn't want to look at it anymore every time I got in and out of the shower or looked in the mirror. So he cut all that ugliness away.

How long was the operation, and how many days were you in the hospital?

My surgery lasted 5 hours, and I was in the hospital for 5 days. That was probably a little longer than usual, because I developed pneumonia after my surgery. The fact that I was a former smoker made all of these complications more likely. The reconstruction was not painful. I had a pain pump for my discomfort while I was in the hospital. Probably the drains were the most uncomfortable part. They were in my abdomen and in my breast. I hated those drains. I also had to wear compression stockings to prevent the development of blood clots. They monitored my flap regularly to make sure the blood was flowing and that it was healthy. Compared with what I had already been through, my recovery was really not bad at all.

Did you feel pulling in your abdomen after surgery? Was it difficult to stand upright?

I was sore, but there was really no pulling to speak of, because my muscles were still intact. I had no problem standing upright once I felt better.

Did you have any restrictions when you left the hospital?

The main restrictions concerned lifting. I was not to lift any weight over 10 pounds for the first few weeks. I also was not to drive initially, but I believe I was able to drive myself to my first checkup after surgery, so it wasn't too long a time. The recovery after the reconstruction was quicker than after the initial mastectomy. I was fatigued and weak, but that passed quickly and I was just fine. I was frankly just glad that it was over, because I had waited so long.

Did you have any limitations on exercise or physical activity?

As far as exercise is concerned, I was not actively exercising after the mastectomy, but now I get all the exercise I need just running after my grandchildren.

How long did it take before you could resume your normal activities?

Within a month I was feeling okay, and I was ready to have my opposite breast reduced. My plastic surgeon made me wait that long to make sure that everything had healed and that I was ready.

Why did you decide to have your opposite breast reduced?

Because I wanted to. My reconstructed breast was smaller than my opposite one. I asked my plastic surgeon if he could reduce the other one so they would match. He said that he could. I'm delighted that I had this done; I feel so much better. He not only reduced my breast, but he also lifted it. Now my breasts match, and they both have a nice, natural shape.

Have you had your nipple reconstructed? Did you have it tattooed?

Yes, this was done at the time of my opposite breast reduction. He used the skin on my reconstructed breast to form the nipple. In a later office procedure, I had my nipple and areola tattooed. I told my daughter. She got a tattoo when she was in college, and we didn't know about it. So I said, "Now I have one too." She just laughed and said, "Aren't you going to show me your tattoo?" I said, "Sure." I asked my son if he wanted to see it, but he said, "Oh, Mom, please don't share."

Are you finished now, or are there other procedures to be done?

I'm scheduled today to have fat grafting. My chest is sinking in because of the lymph nodes that were removed. The fat injections will be used to fill this defect. My plastic surgeon is also going to resect a wedge of tissue from my right breast for contouring. When that's finished, I'm coming back for a laser treatment to improve the horrible rash from the radiation that I still have on this beautiful reconstructed breast. My doctor says that the fat grafts may also help to improve my skin quality, but it will take time.

Did your insurance pay for these procedures?

They paid for the reconstruction, the nipple, the tattooing, and the opposite breast reduction. However, when it came time for the fat grafting, they denied the claim. I was supposed to have this done in September, once my other procedures were finished. My plastic surgeon said I was in good shape. But the insurance company denied our claim, because they said that fat grafting was cosmetic surgery. We fought them. My plastic surgeon couldn't believe that they said this was cosmetic. I wouldn't have this radiation burn or the indentation in my chest if it weren't for my cancer treatment.

Did the insurance company reconsider and decide to cover the fat grafting procedure?

They did, but they waited until right before Christmas, so it was too late to have the procedure during the same calendar year. I had already met my deductible for the year; that meant I wouldn't have had any out-of-pocket expenses. By delaying until the next year, the insurance company got the final dig: with the new year, I had the expense of meeting my deductible again. Yes, they still had to cover their percentage of the procedures and the doctor bills, but they did stick it to me by making it happen in the new year.

What do your scars look like?

I have a scar around my breast. It actually looks better than it did before, because my plastic surgeon revised the old mastectomy scar to improve its appearance. I also have a scar on my abdomen from one hip to the other.

How does your reconstructed breast feel? Is it warm? Is it soft and sensitive?

It's warm to the touch and soft, but there is limited sensitivity at this stage. If I press on it, I can feel my chest wall muscles underneath.

Is the breast a nice shape? Are you happy with the way it looks?

It's beautiful. The only ugly thing is the rash on my breast. Hopefully, the fat injections and laser treatments will help that.

If you had this diagnosis again and you had to do it over, would you have reconstruction again? Would you have the same operation?

Yes, definitely. I'm very pleased with what I had done. The DIEP procedure was right for me. I didn't want implants, and I didn't want to have any weakness because of muscle transfer. I accomplished my goals. I can now play with my grandchildren and garden without worrying about my movements or thinking about my cancer.

Has reconstructive surgery affected how you feel about yourself? How you dress?

I feel good, very good. This has been great for my self-confidence. Before, I just wanted to hide my body. I would wear my husband's tee shirts, sweatshirts, and baggy sweatpants. I even wore his stocking hat. Then I began losing weight in preparation for my breast reconstruction, and I started thinking, "This is almost over. I'm going to be well again." Now I don't wear my husband's sweatshirts and sweatpants any more—I have my own.

What advice would you like to give to women considering breast reconstruction?

Check out all your options—and learn the positive and negative aspects of each one. Pursue all avenues. This has to be a decision that you are comfortable with. Be happy with your decision. You have to block out everybody else's opinion. You can't pick up a magazine like *Good Housekeeping,* read an article, and make a decision. Get credible, reliable information.

How has breast cancer affected your approach to life?

I feel lucky I'm here. I look forward to every day, and I appreciate my children, my husband, and my grandchildren even more.

Do you have any advice you'd like to share with other women?

Don't be afraid to ask questions. If you feel you're right, pursue it. I felt I was burned during my radiation therapy. I felt I was not listened to by the doctor. During my treatment I would say, "Boy, I sure hurt today." But they would dismiss my comments and tell me, "Oh, it's too soon for you to feel this burned." I feel partially responsible, because I didn't insist on being heard. You know your body. I know you're paying thousands and thousands of dollars to these specialists, but if you're paying all that money, you have the right to be heard. You have the right to tell those doctors how you're feeling and what's going on. Don't let them treat you like a statistic, telling you that this is how it goes, everybody feels this way. I'm not everybody. I don't know how other people feel; I know how I feel. I wish I had insisted, but I learned, and that will never happen again.

TERI: THE FEAR IS GONE

Teri is young and pretty, with shoulder-length blonde hair. She has a natural look that is not enhanced by makeup, making her seem even younger than her 33 years. Slender and of medium height, she was dressed in a purple blouse and gray slacks with big gold hoop earrings and a thin band of gold encircling her neck. She looks like anyone's daughter. Who would imagine that only 2 years ago she chose to have both of her breasts removed prophylactically and then reconstructed?

This decision was not made lightly. Her family was riddled with breast cancer. But it was her grandmother's death from breast cancer that motivated her to have genetic testing, only to discover that she was positive for the breast cancer gene *(BRCA1)*. This genetic finding, along with suspicious mammogram results, prompted her decision to have preventive mastectomies. What a major decision this was for a young divorced mother with a teenage son and a fiancé!

Because Teri was thin and wanted larger breasts, she chose immediate reconstruction with latissimus dorsi (back) flaps and saline implants. Immediate reconstruction was important for her. "I was afraid if I did one breast at a time, the pain from the first operation would keep me from having anything else done. I had to get it over all at once."

Although Teri had spent considerable time researching her options, she had a difficult time coping with the results of her surgery. She hadn't realized that she would hurt in so many places. She had difficulty getting comfortable or sleeping. She cried a lot over the next 2 years and found herself wondering if she had done the right thing. Two years have now passed since her momentous decision to have her breasts removed and reconstructed, and Teri is feeling better about her body with each passing day. Although she cried throughout our interview, she also smiled through the tears. She laughingly told me that she has gained 15 pounds since her surgery, but she said that is a good thing, because now her bottom is in better balance with her enlarged breasts. It has taken her a long time to start laughing again, but she is beginning to feel just fine about her body and her life.

Why did you decide to have your breasts removed prophylactically? Do you have a family history of breast cancer?

My aunt died of breast cancer when I was a teenager, and she was in her thirties. So when my Mom was diagnosed with breast cancer at 37 and had a mastectomy, I assumed she was also going to die; it was a scary time. Then her other sister, who was also in her thirties, got breast cancer and had to have a mastectomy, followed by chemotherapy and radiation therapy. Several years ago, my grandma found a lump and was diagnosed with breast cancer. After her death, I decided that my sister and I needed to be genetically tested. My sister was pregnant at the time and had been diagnosed with thyroid cancer, so it became more urgent that we do this.

We had been getting yearly mammograms ever since my mom had her cancer; they started us early. Every year I went, and it was the same thing—they would see something and I'd have to go back for an ultrasound exam. Then I was told that everything was okay. But on my last mammogram, the surgeon saw a spot on my right breast and wanted me to have another ultrasound. This was after I found out that I was positive for the *BRCA1* gene.

What does it mean to be positive for BRCA1?

It means that I have the same gene that my mom, my grandma, my aunts, and probably everyone else in my family has and that my risk of developing cancer is very high, over 80%. Once I received this information, I did my research; I wanted to know what this meant. The Internet is a wonderful tool; I found lots of information there. I also talked to all of my doctors to get their opinions—not their recommendations. I wanted to know if I were their daughter, what would they think? So I gathered all of the information, and then I made my own decision. From what I learned, it appeared that if I were going to get breast cancer (and my chances were great), it would be when I was in my thirties; I was already 31. My mom and her sister were both 37 when they developed cancer. In my mind, the future held a series of biopsies every time I went for a mammogram. I could do that every year, or I could just have the surgery. Probably if I had not had a son, I wouldn't have been as afraid of getting breast cancer, but I'm not sure. I decided to schedule the surgery for that November.

What type of surgery did you decide to have?

I had bilateral prophylactic (preventive) total mastectomies and immediate breast reconstruction with latissimus dorsi (back) flaps with implants.

Were both breasts operated on during the same operation?

I wanted it over in one operation if possible. Honestly, I was afraid if I only did one side, the pain would prevent me from having the other breast done later. So I was relieved that I was able to have one operation for everything.

What did the operation entail? How long did it take?

It took almost 9 hours to perform. First, my cancer surgeon did the skin-sparing total mastectomies in which she removed all of my breast tissue and my nipples. She also took a sampling of lymph nodes from both underarms. Then my plastic surgeon took over. He transferred latissimus dorsi flaps of skin and muscle from my back and tunneled them to my chest wall to build my breasts. He placed implants under these flaps.

What type of implants were used? Were they saline- or gel-filled?

They were filled with saline. I was nervous about what I had read about silicone gel at the time; I felt more comfortable with saline. Today I might make a different choice, because they have developed a better gel. I think I would like that. I didn't realize that the saline implants ripple as much as they do. I'm not wild about how they feel, either. If you press on the bottom of your breast, you can feel a little pop when the implant moves, kind of like a water balloon. Those are the only problems I've had, though. If I had to make the choice today, I wouldn't be as afraid of silicone, knowing what I do.

What was your reaction when you woke up after surgery?

Going into this, I was fine with what I was doing. People thought I was doing something drastic, but I was determined. I cried a little bit right before the surgery, but generally I was fine.

However, waking up from surgery was very traumatic for me. The pain was so intense that it hurt me to breathe. Both my back and front had been operated on, and I had drain tubes coming out of my sides. I couldn't breathe in or out; I just hurt too much. I could only tolerate very shallow breathing, and I panicked. I wanted my mom. I wanted the implants out. I didn't expect any of that. I never anticipated that I would have that reaction.

What did they do to control your pain?

I had a morphine pump, but I don't do well with pain medications. By the second day, my arm started to burn inside every time I pushed the button on the pain pump, and it kept on getting worse. The last time I pushed it, my arm burned all the way up to my elbow. At that point, I was more afraid of pushing the button than of dealing with the pain. When I told them, they thought my vein had gone bad. Later we discovered that I was having a reaction to the morphine. They stopped the morphine pump and switched me to Tylenol with codeine. I had a reaction to the codeine as well. The only thing that worked at all was a shot of pain medication that they injected after surgery.

What helped you get through it?

My mom and my fiancé helped me through it. My mom had breast cancer, and she has been through the surgery. She kept reassuring me that I could do this. All the while I was thinking, "What did I do to myself?" I had no idea it would affect me that way. That made me cry even more. I didn't go in blind—I knew it would be painful—but it was different when it happened. And then all of the emotions started. I cried more in the first several months after surgery than I had in my entire life.

What was your recovery like? How long were you in the hospital?

I was in the hospital for 4 days. When I got home, I had trouble adjusting. I wasn't sleeping, and I had six drain tubes coming out of me. I barely slept for 13 nights. I couldn't lie on my back because of the drains and the long incisions; I couldn't lie on either side, because the tubes were coming out of my sides, and I couldn't lie on my front where my breast had been reconstructed. So how do you sleep? I sat in a recliner for most of the time. My mom stayed with me for weeks. I would watch everyone get ready for bed, and I knew it would be a long night for me.

I developed a lot of fears after the surgery that I didn't anticipate. The drain tubes were scary. My fiancé, now my husband, and my mom had to measure the fluid accumulation and drain it. I also had home health care, which was very helpful. A nurse came every day to change the dressings. My mom helped with it, but we felt more secure with the nurse checking to make sure nothing was infected.

When were your drains removed? How did that feel?

The week after my surgery, my plastic surgeon removed four of my drains. I was really frightened; I was crying in anticipation of the pain. He clipped the stitches holding the drains in place, and quickly pulled the first ones out. It was so fast, probably no more than 2 seconds. He just ripped them right out. And it surprised me, because it wasn't as bad as I'd thought. Don't get me wrong, the incision area was very sensitive, and the stitches hurt. But when the tubes were pulled out, it just wasn't that bad. He did two of them at the same time, so it was faster for me. The last two had to stay in for another 2 weeks, because I still had drainage. They snaked up through my back and drained a lot, especially on one side. When I came back to have the final drains removed, my cancer surgeon took them out. But what we didn't realize was that these drains were different and more difficult to remove. When she tugged on them, they wouldn't come out. I was screaming at the top of my lungs. Thank goodness for the resident; she held my hand while the surgeon tugged and pulled them out.

Were your breasts swollen or bruised after your operation?

My whole torso was swollen, but I didn't bruise at all. My breasts looked really good as soon as I came out of surgery; at least that's what everyone told me.

How long did you wait before you looked at your breasts?

It was 6 weeks before I looked at them. I waited so long because I was afraid to see my incisions or to deal with the drains. But when I looked, my breasts were awesome. They are better than the breasts I had before, to be perfectly honest. Even my plastic surgeon is proud of the before and after pictures. That makes me feel good.

When were you able to go back to work?

I work as a secretary at the hospital. I was off work for 6 to 8 weeks. When I went back I worked half-days for the first 2 weeks, then I went back full-time. Initially, I thought I could do more with my arms than I could; driving to work was very hard. By the time I would get to the office to park my car, I would be in tears, because my arms hurt from holding them up on the steering wheel. That surprised me. There was no way I could have worked more than half a day at first, because I was worn out. Before that, the only time I was able to get out of the house was to come to my doctor's appointments.

Did you do any exercises to get back your strength?

Not really. My husband and my mom pushed me: "Do this with your arm, do that with your arm." I didn't do any of the exercises; maybe they would have helped more. I just felt like I would do a little bit more each day. One day I would put the dishes in the cupboard and I'd say, "Hey, I can reach the second shelf now." Or in my shower, I would put the shampoo up on the rack. I could see myself improving little by little. I had a son at home, so I had to do the things I normally would; my daily life had to go on. It was a slow healing process.

My plastic surgeon was right on target. He told me that in 18 months I would start to forget what I went through. I would start to feel like myself again, and he was right. Now I have days where I forget what I went through, and I think, "Okay, if I'm forgetting sometimes, that means I'm getting better." There are still things that I can't do that I would like to do. For instance, when I try to lift something, if it's too heavy, it hurts in my back where the muscles were. But it is definitely getting better.

Did you have any complications after your operation?

Yes, I developed capsular contracture in my right breast. It started days after my big surgery—I knew the moment it happened. I was on the couch, and my fiancé went to drain my tube on the right side. I thought he pulled it, but he didn't. He kept telling me that he didn't do anything wrong, but it hurt so bad that it took my breath away. I felt this way the rest of that night, on and off—it was painful. I was afraid to have anyone touch my drains. Right after that, I started noticing that my right breast wasn't jiggling like the left one. When I would move the top of the left one, it was very free, like fluid; the right one wouldn't do that. Each day it got harder and harder.

What did your plastic surgeon do to correct the capsular contracture?

He made an incision in the scar and took the implant out. Then he released and removed the scar tissue that had formed around the implant. When that was done, he put the implant back in and closed my incision again.

Did that fix the problem?

Everything has been perfect since. I mean, it was wonderful. The second I woke up from surgery, I knew he had fixed the problem. The pressure in my breast was gone. It has been much better ever since.

Have there been any surprises with your rebuilt breasts?

I'm adjusting to having larger breasts. When I touch my stomach or raise my hand up to the bottom of my breast, it extends out from my chest like a ledge. I had small breasts before this, so at first I thought, "Whoa, what is that?" They just go straight out, and they're really perky and new. Reaching for things, my arm brushes them. I wasn't used to that either. I never had enough breast tissue to interfere with my movements. So I have a real size difference, but that's what I wanted.

Did you ask him for bigger breasts?

I said, "If you're going to do this, I want something out of it. Do it and do it good!" Previously I wore an A cup bra, and if I gained weight, I would be a B, but most of the time I was an A. We planned on a full C cup, but I have learned since then that I'm a D. So now I've been buying 34D bras, and they fit perfectly. I wasn't expecting to be a D, but I think with the implant and the muscle, that's just what it turned out to be. After 31 years with small boobs, I now have big ones. It's different, but I like it.

Did you have your nipples reconstructed?

After the big surgery, I honestly thought for a long time that I didn't want my nipples reconstructed. I didn't want anything more done to me. It didn't bother me, because I had gotten used to it. I thought, "I can live with this." I was leaning toward not doing it, but I changed my mind.

Why did you change your mind and decide to have nipple reconstruction?

Because of my mom. After her mastectomy she didn't have her nipple reconstructed, so she didn't have one on that side. She said, "I think later down the road, you're going to wish you had done it." So I went ahead and did it, and I'm so glad I did. It was scary, because you are awake during the procedure. It didn't hurt; I was numb anyway. It was just the fear again.

How did he reconstruct your nipples? Where did he get the tissues?

He reconstructed with the skin that was there on my breasts. That was amazing to me. He showed me beforehand what he would do. He designed two triangles of skin that he lifted up, twisted to form a nipple, and then stitched in place (a C-V flap). It took a lot of stitches.

He asked me how big I wanted my nipples to be, and I said that he should decide. I trust him 100%. Whatever he thinks is proportional for me, I'm comfortable with. So he did what he thought best, and they turned out just perfect. At first they were bigger than I wanted, but as they heal, they shrink. Boy, do they! It's absolutely right that they do. I was really happy once they were the right size. I went home with little Dixie cups over my nipples.

Did you have tattooing?

Yes, I waited and then had tattooing done. It was done twice, but it still didn't take very well. I'm not going to do it again; they're fine, and the color is good enough for me.

How are the scars? How do they look?

The scars on my back are long, but my breast scars are nice. After my surgery my plastic surgeon said that he could take the circular scars on my breasts and bring them closer in to my nipples so I wouldn't see them. I asked him about that during my second tattooing session. But by then we were both surprised at how much my scars had faded and lightened up. The pink was gone, and they're white now. They've healed really nicely, so it's not that noticeable. We both agreed that we didn't need to do anything more.

How do your implants feel?

They are heavy, and that was an adjustment—you can definitely tell that I have gone through a healing process. In the beginning, when I would lie in bed, I had to put my arm under my side and kind of bring my breast with me when I turned from one side to the other. It felt as if that part of my body wouldn't come with me, because it was too heavy. I worried that the skin would tear. That's gotten much better; I don't have to do that now. I do sleep in a sports bra for security, and every now and then I'll sleep without it. My breasts don't feel as heavy as they used to, but it's been an adjustment. With your normal breasts, you can lie on your stomach and they just squish to the side. With the saline implants, that doesn't happen. I've gotten to where I can lie on my stomach, but they don't move very much. I feel the hard, circular implants in there—it's definitely noticeable. But I'm getting more comfortable with it, and many days I just feel like me again.

Are your breasts soft? Are they warm?

Yes, they're soft and warm. That surprised me. I had read that sometimes your breasts will feel colder because of the saline implants, but mine have always been warm. Maybe it's because of the muscle cover.

When you touch one part of my body with your hand and then touch my breasts, they feel warm.

Are they numb, or has the sensation come back?

My sensation is beginning to come back. I expected my nipple area to be numb, but I didn't realize that my breasts, chest, and entire back area would also be numb and that the numbness would last this long. My right breast is lagging behind my left breast in the healing process, because the surgeon had to go back in to fix the capsular contracture. It's more numb than the left one. I get so excited every time I notice any sensitivity. I have some feeling now in my upper chest and down between my breasts. I'm beginning to get sensory return in my left breast around the edges. My right one is not there yet, but I'm confident that it will come back. My back around my incisions is still numb, but I now have some feeling under my arms, on my ribcage, and where my drain tubes were. I also have feeling in parts of my back, in a capital I shape. It's getting better each day. My plastic surgeon said that because of my age, I should get a lot of my sensation back. I'm hopeful for that.

Why did you choose this type of breast reconstruction? Are you satisfied with your choice?

I considered just having implants with no back muscle transfer, but my skin is very thin, and my plastic surgeon was afraid that the implants would show through my skin and look like circles. I'm very glad we did the muscle transfer; at the time I didn't have enough fat in my stomach for an abdominal flap, so my back was the best option. Although my recovery was painful, I am happy with the procedure that I chose. I like the look and feel of my breasts. When you look at me, you can't see my implants, my breasts slant down like normal breasts; they're very realistic. Even the nurses in the hospital would comment on how good they look. They just could not believe it.

Are you happy with your decision to have your breasts removed and reconstructed during one operation?

I'm glad I did it in one operation. It was terribly painful, but it's better in the long run. I don't know if I would have gone back for anything else because of the pain.

Has the surgery made you less afraid of getting cancer?

I thought it would take all my fear away; it didn't. Don't get me wrong—it took a lot of it. I don't have the same fears any more. I'll have a little scare now and then. I'll think, "I don't have mammograms now; what if there's still a cell there?" That's in the back of my mind. I think every woman is always going to harbor some worries. That part is going to be there forever, but overall I don't feel like I'm going to get cancer anymore. The fear is gone. When I found out I was *BRCA1* positive, I just knew I would get breast cancer. Now I don't feel that way.

How does your family feel about your decision to have preventive surgery?

My sister (there's two of us girls) had the test, and she was not positive for the gene. That was a big concern for me. If I have it, I can deal with it, but I didn't want her to have it. Both she and my mom were upset that I was positive, but I kept reassuring them, "I'm fine, I can do this." Now I think they're happy I did it. It was hard on my mom, because I cried so much, and she kept trying to reassure me. It was a lot for everyone to handle. I had to be taken care of. I didn't like for my son to see me that way. He was 11 at the time; now he's 13. It scared him seeing me in that condition, but when I came home, he was such a good helper. He did a lot. So now everyone's over it. I'm back to the way I was before. I still have pain sometimes from the severed nerves, but I'm accustomed to it now. It hurts for a moment, and then I'm fine. I can definitely say my pain threshold is much higher now than it was before.

How did your fiancé react to all this?

At the beginning, when I was contemplating surgery, I was nervous. I worried about the effect my surgery would have on our relationship. But he was on board from day one, because he had watched my grandma die and knew what my mom had gone through. He understood what my test results meant. We had been together for almost 10 years; he understood my risk. He was all for it. None of that has changed. We got married shortly after I had the surgery, and he has been wonderful.

How can a man be supportive during this experience?

Every now and then I'll have a feeling that I look ugly. Now I have very good breasts, and I'm very happy with them. You don't see a lot of scar on the front; my back is where the big scars are. So I look at them and it's almost like you can't tell. My plastic surgeon and my husband have both said that if I were on a beach in a bikini, no one would ever know I had this done, unless they looked at my back. So I keep that in my mind. But every now and then I'll wonder deep down, "Does he think, 'Look at those scars,' or 'Those aren't real breasts.' If he touches them now, do they feel normal?" He reassures me as soon as I start to act that way; he puts me in my place right away: "Don't think that, because it's not true." He has definitely been good for me, a source of strength through the whole process.

Has your plastic surgeon been supportive through this process?

He is very proud of me and how everything turned out. That has made me feel better about everything too. When I come in with a worry or call with a question, he instantly reassures me. He has been so supportive for the past 2 years. I know that if I need him, he will always take care of me. That was my fear: I worried that I would go through the whole process, and then he would be done with me, discharge me, and I'd be on my own. I told him that was my concern. He said, "You know what, I'll take care of you for the rest of your life, so don't worry about that."

Do the back muscles that were tunneled to your breasts still move and contract?

Right after the surgery, it was cold outside (I had my surgery in winter), and the muscles in my breasts would contract uncontrollably when I went outside. I had absolutely no control over this. My family would put lots of coats on me; I was really wrapped up so I wouldn't get cold. Regardless, my muscles would contract and squeeze my breasts. When that happened it was hard to breathe, because the muscles are on your chest. Then the pain would sometimes radiate to my back.

Over time, the contractions have lessened. Now I can go outside in the cold, and the muscles might contract for a minute, but it does not hurt like it did, and it takes more for it to happen. It won't happen just walking to my car with my coat on. If I'm out for a long time in the cold, my muscles will start to squeeze a little bit and my breasts will ache.

What advice would you like to share with other women?

I wasn't one to speak up before I did this. Now I want to talk to other women who are thinking about this surgery. I want to say, "This is what happened to me. In case it happens to you, don't be afraid." I want to give them a heads-up. For instance, when I woke up from my surgery and felt like I couldn't breathe, I didn't know that was going to occur. I would have liked for someone to have said, "When you wake up from surgery, your chest is going to hurt, your back is going to hurt, and it might be hard to breathe. But don't worry, we're going to take care of you."

I really didn't expect my emotional reaction. I cried a lot; my dad would sit there and we would be talking about nothing and all of a sudden I would just burst out crying. My doctor would say, "It's going to get a little better every day." He was absolutely right, because I feel nothing like I did then. When you're in that moment after your surgery, you're looking at yourself and you're not sure. You feel like you are going to be in that moment forever; it's hard to imagine a year down the road. You keep thinking, "Am I ever going to be back to normal?" I honestly felt like I would never be normal again, I would never feel like I used to again, and that's not the case—none of that is the case.

Are you happy with the way your breasts look?

I'm very pleased with my breast appearance. I like it when I get compliments. Everyone at home or at work always jokes with me about "the girls," because they're big now. And when someone compliments them, it's amazing to me, because before the surgery I never had that. They were nothing to compliment; they were so little. They were nothing like what they are now. Looking at the before and after pictures that my plastic surgeon took, I think my afters are definitely better. It's a very good outcome and there is no reason for crying anymore.

JEAN: THE FABRIC OF LIFE

Jean arrived at our interview fresh from the health club, still dressed in a black Lycra jumpsuit, an oversized purple tee shirt, and running shoes. She wore no makeup, and her short, light-brown hair curled softly with the perspiration from her recent workout. Her ear buds were draped around her neck, and she turned off her iPod as she lowered herself into the chair. At 48, Jean is the picture of health—youthful, slender, and athletic.

From her demeanor and ready smile, few people would suspect the hardships she has faced. Jean is no stranger to breast cancer and grief. Her mother was diagnosed with the disease when she was still premenopausal, in her forties. She died 10 years later after two bouts with breast cancer, two modified radical mastectomies, and two courses of chemotherapy and radiation therapy. Jean vividly remembers her mother's strength during her 10-year illness and marvels at how truly remarkable she was. Her example has fortified Jean during her own struggles.

Because of her family history of breast cancer, Jean was meticulous about breast monitoring. It was during one of her annual mammograms that her cancer was discovered. She underwent 3 years of treatment—a lumpectomy, bilateral mastectomies, two courses of chemotherapy and radiation therapy, and bilateral breast reconstruction with gluteus maximus free flaps. Throughout this long process, she grew to rely on her own judgment, to research her treatment options, and to express her needs. Her assertiveness was not always welcomed. Her first surgeon made it clear that he was the doctor, and he would make the decisions. They came to a permanent parting of the ways when he refused to perform the bilateral mastectomies she requested to treat her second breast cancer. He suggested that she was crazy to take such action and clearly did not know what she was doing. This was a particularly traumatic time for her. She and her husband had just suffered the unbearable loss of their 16-year-old daughter from cystic fibrosis. But she used her daughter's lifestyle example to move beyond her sorrow.

She refused to lose confidence in her ability to make decisions. She sought a second opinion and found another doctor who was more responsive to her needs. He agreed with her decision for bilateral mastectomies and agreed to perform them. She had the bilateral mastectomies and later, after thoroughly investigating her options, decided to have bilateral gluteus maximus (buttock) free flap breast reconstruction. Jean took control of her health care decisions and gained a new sense of empowerment. As she explained, "For me, the ultimate satisfaction came from being knowledgeable. I participated and made decisions rather than allowing someone to tell me what to do and how to feel. There is a certain amount of power in knowing you are a partner in the decision-making process."

Jean is delighted with the decisions she has made. When I asked about her satisfaction with her results, she slipped off her tee shirt, pulled down her jumpsuit, and proudly let me see for myself. Her story is one of courage and determination.

How old were you when your cancer was diagnosed? How did you react?

I was 42 when I first learned I had breast cancer. It did not come as a total shock to me, because my mother developed premenopausal breast cancer in her mid-forties. She had a modified radical mastectomy with radiation and chemotherapy. In the seventh year, she developed a second cancer in the opposite breast and had the same treatment. She lived 3 years longer. I was 20 when I lost my mother. Breast cancer became part of my life at an early age. She was a wonderful example for me; she joyously marched through life despite the cancer. She was a golfer, and I don't think she ever missed a round of golf because of her illness. With that history, I wouldn't say that I was surprised by my diagnosis.

Considering your family history, what was your routine for monitoring your breasts?

My first mammogram was at age 35, and I got them annually after that. I had small, thin breasts with lots of dense tissue, lumps, and bumps that were hard to read radiographically. When I reached 40, my OB/GYN told me that once a mammogram report becomes a paragraph, you know you're in trouble. He wanted someone besides himself checking me, so he sent me to a breast surgeon. From then on, in addition to my yearly mammograms, I had two physical examinations.

How was your breast cancer diagnosed? What was the proposed treatment? What part did you play in the decision-making process?

The cancer first appeared as a small area of microcalcifications on my yearly mammogram. You begin to learn about those little white spots, and I could see them clearly. Although my surgeon told me that it was highly unlikely that this was breast cancer, I insisted on a biopsy as a precaution. It revealed intraductal infiltrating carcinoma. With my family history, I asked for a mastectomy. Once again, he insisted it was the wrong thing to do. All the research showed that lumpectomy with radiation was as good as mastectomy. I did a literature search and found that to be true. But I still wasn't convinced, so my surgeon sent me to consult with other specialists who supported that treatment approach. They convinced me that I was too young to lose a breast, and the cancer was too small to justify a mastectomy. I had a lumpectomy with follow-up radiation and then started investigating chemotherapy. My oncologist and I reviewed the current research; chemotherapy was not advised for such a small cancer that was node negative. But I had a gem of an oncologist who knew my family history and my feelings. He agreed to support my decision for chemotherapy, even though he wasn't in complete agreement. I felt very good that the decision was being left to me. Since my cancer was microscopic, I decided, "Why not take every precaution, even if I only decrease my risk of recurrence by a small percentage?" So I had the whole ball of wax. I had surgery, radiation, and chemotherapy. I was confident I had made the right decision. Later this decision was confirmed by reports from the breast cancer clinical trial indicating that young women with small, node-negative cancers did well with chemotherapy. I thought, "Yes— I did the right thing."

How was your second cancer discovered?

A year later, a follow-up mammogram revealed the exact same pattern of microcalcifications almost in the identical location, just next to the surgical margin. It was interpreted as normal, with a recommendation for a repeat mammogram in a year. I had heard that story before. Those little spots looked exactly the same as the previous ones. I couldn't believe it! My brother is a radiologist, and I asked him for a second opinion. He reviewed my films and saw the same pattern as before. He recommended follow-up with a biopsy. To confirm that he wasn't being overprotective, he had four other radiologists view the films without telling them whose films they were. They all recommended biopsy. With the force of such unified opinion, my breast care team agreed to do a biopsy. Once again the biopsy revealed in situ cancer. This time I was adamant in my insistence that I wanted mastectomy, not a single mastectomy but bilateral mastectomies—a mastectomy to treat the cancer and a prophylactic mastectomy to remove the other breast as a precaution.

What was your surgeon's response to your request for bilateral mastectomies? Why was your surgeon so resistant?

I had already had several head-to-head confrontations with my surgeon. He said I was still too young, and he would not perform bilateral mastectomies when the cancer was confined to one breast. He didn't think I knew enough to be part of the decision-making process. I would not cooperate. We argued through every decision, starting with the original biopsy and the original surgery. When I read the literature and asked, "Should this test or that test be done? Am I a candidate for this or that?" he literally would get red in the face. One time he stood up and actually screamed at me over the desk, "I understand where you're coming from. I know that women feel like they have to know all there is to know. So when you go through medical school, read every journal, and know how to do surgery, then I'll have this discussion with you. Until that time, you cannot possibly know enough to make such a decision." Clearly, he was the doctor, and he would make the decisions.

How did you handle these confrontations?

I told him that he misunderstood; I only needed to be a specialist in one teeny-tiny subject—my breast cancer. This was linked to one diagnosis, in one area, and I could get all the information I needed, because I knew how to use a library, and I knew how to search the Internet. I didn't need to be a surgeon or an oncologist or know everything there was to know. I only needed to know about my one problem, the clinical trials that were ongoing, and the options for treatment. With this information, I could participate in making decisions about my care. If he didn't want to participate with me, then this relationship was not going to work.

Why did you decide to get a second opinion?

When I chose my first surgeon, I had hoped that he would treat me as a partner in my health care decisions, but here he was telling me that I was incapable of making decisions about my own health care. We had established a tenuous relationship to get through the first surgery. Now, with the second cancer, he was telling me that he'd only do a mastectomy on the side with the double cancer. I couldn't accept that. It kept coming back to me that I had asked him for the mastectomy the first time. Would it have been different if he had done what I requested? I decided I needed to work through this decision with someone who would listen to me and respect my opinions. I felt strongly about the need for bilateral mastectomy after watching my mother die. So I decided to get a second opinion.

What did your second opinion reveal? Why did you decide to switch surgeons?

The surgeon I chose for a second opinion was highly recommended by three or four people whose judgment I respected. I was looking for someone who was thorough, yet conservative. When I went to see this surgeon, I didn't tell him what the other surgeon had said. I told him I wanted a second opinion to see if my request for bilateral mastectomies was wrong or misguided. I gave him my history, mammograms, and biopsy reports. I also told him about my mother. I wanted him to understand all of the factors that influenced my decision for bilateral mastectomies.

After evaluating this information, he recommended bilateral mastectomies. His support for my decision confirmed that I really wasn't as far off the mark as the other surgeon would have me believe. I wasted no time in switching surgeons. My new surgeon agreed to do the bilateral mastectomies, and he welcomed my input in the decision-making process. I now had a surgeon who would listen to me.

Did you consider having immediate breast reconstruction at the time of your mastectomies?

I chose to have the bilateral mastectomies first and take time to investigate whether I wanted breast reconstruction. If I decided to pursue this option, I wanted to locate a surgeon and decide on the best procedure. I have heard of women who cannot bear to come out of surgery without their breasts. I understand that feeling firsthand. I will never forget the shock I experienced when they removed my dressings and I looked at my concave chest. Even so, I don't regret my decision to take things one step at a time.

Why did you decide to have breast reconstruction?

It took some time to adjust to the fact that part of me was gone, but I got used to myself. I joked about my adolescent chest. I felt accepted by my friends and my husband. Having supportive friends helped me feel good about myself. It also freed me to take time to examine my motivation and decide whether I wanted to undergo more surgery.

Ultimately, my reasons for deciding to have breast reconstruction had more to do with my lifestyle than it did with self-image. It was a positive statement about my hope for the future. Exercise and fitness play an important role in my life. Although I had adjusted to my body and had resumed going to the Y to exercise, I came to realize that the world was not ready for a mastectomized woman. It's different when you take off your clothes and there are no breasts there. I felt much like handicapped people must feel. People don't mean to stare, but they do. They don't mean to make this brief, audible sound, but they do. No matter what their motivations, people still stare and ask questions. I like the freedom to exercise without feeling that I am on display. I like being able to exercise in jumpsuits like this one. I enjoy going into the Jacuzzi afterward. I could do that comfortably without breasts, but I increasingly came to realize that people weren't quite ready for that. I couldn't just take off my clothes and walk in the Jacuzzi like everybody else.

Breast reconstruction also represented my proclamation to the world that I had a future and I was getting on with my life. I felt good when I finally decided to have breast reconstruction. I had invested the time to examine my motivation, to find a plastic surgeon, and to select the best technique for me.

How did you select a plastic surgeon and decide on the best breast reconstruction procedure for you?

A number of excellent plastic surgeons with expertise in breast reconstruction practice in my area. I went to see several of them. I had read about the TRAM flap and asked if I would be a candidate. Even though they said I was a candidate for the TRAM flap, I noticed that they sort of wrinkled their noses when they said it. I did not feel particularly reassured. Finally, one plastic surgeon (he had gone through the nose-wrinkling phase also) said that he could do the TRAM operation. However, because my stomach was very flat, there wouldn't be much tissue available for a bilateral reconstruction, and he would only be able to create very small breasts. If that was acceptable to me, then he would do the operation. I needed to be fully aware of the limitations, however. I responded that I wasn't looking for size. It was really to be more natural.

After I left the plastic surgeon's office, I thought about what I had just said. What was I thinking? Why would I go through this major operative procedure to end up with something that's terribly small? Surely there must be some other solution. At that point I hadn't investigated other options, so I started reading books and atlases and learned everything I could about the different reconstructive procedures. I discovered there is excess tissue in many areas of the body that can be used for reconstruction, not just the stomach. When I read about microsurgical breast reconstruction, it seemed the perfect procedure for me. I certainly had other areas to donate from if my stomach was inadequate.

I went back to the plastic surgeon who had been forthright about the TRAM flap and asked if I was a candidate for a microsurgical procedure. He suggested a gluteus maximus free flap (that's a microsurgical procedure using buttock tissue for the breast reconstruction) and called his partner in to examine me and give me his opinion. What followed was very embarrassing.

Why was the examination embarrassing?

I told this plastic surgeon that I probably had plenty of tissue on my buttocks that he could use. He said, "Okay, let's see. Just pull down your underwear and turn around." I did, but it was a horrible feeling. What was worse, however, was his reaction. I had barely turned around when he exclaimed, "Oh yes, no problem." With all I had experienced, his reaction ranks up there as the ultimate embarrassing moment. So I had found the right procedure for me, and the plastic surgeon to perform it. We agreed that I would have gluteus maximus free flaps. Because of the complexity of this procedure, we decided that each breast would be reconstructed in a separate operation.

What did your breast reconstruction involve? How long did it take? Was there much pain or discomfort?

I had been prepared for a long operation, knowing this was considered one of the most complex of reconstructive techniques. They were right; the first operation took more than 8 hours. I do fairly well with pain, and I didn't think the procedure itself or the healing of the wounds was that painful. There was discomfort, however, because you lose the use of one hip and one side at the same time, so it's difficult to get comfortable.

After the operation, you're pretty bundled up; you've lost part of your buttock on one side. The anastomosis where they reattach the vessels restricts what you can do with your arm, how you hold it, and how you move it; you are also restricted as to how you can lie down. It's hard to bear weight and sit on your hip. There is a good deal of discomfort, but it's not actually pain. I coped with these aftereffects just fine, but I was sick from the anesthesia and IV antibiotics.

What was the problem with the anesthesia?

The anesthesia was the only part of my hospital experience that was unacceptable. You come in before the surgery, meet the anesthesiologist, and think you've made a connection. I explained that I did not tolerate drugs or medications well. He listened carefully and took profuse notes. I thought, "Great, he will make sure that everything goes off smoothly." When I got to surgery, I even checked to ensure that they had a record of my concerns about anesthesia. They said sure, but the anesthesiologist that I spoke with the day before was not there, and my special requirements went unheeded. I was put to sleep according to the standard routine. For me it was a disaster. After 8 hours of surgery, it was difficult to wake up from the anesthesia. I was nauseated and felt like I was in a fog. I was violently ill for 5 days; I couldn't eat, and I was throwing up.

What was the timing between the first and second breast reconstruction? Did your reaction to the anesthetic cause a delay?

They usually schedule the second operation after a long delay, but because of my work schedule, I wanted the reconstructions done one after the other. I asked if they could first operate on one breast and I would stay in the hospital for the usual 3 to 7 days. At the end of this time, if I was up to it, I wanted to have the second operation. My plastic surgeon agreed to that schedule, because I was in good physical condition and could handle it.

If the first breast reconstruction had gone like the second one, it would have been a breeze. But the first one went so badly because of the anesthesia that I even considered canceling the other reconstruction. Before I was ready to come back for a second operation, I had to ensure that the method of anesthesia would not have the same after-effects.

I read about anesthesia and interviewed several anesthesiologists to figure what could be done differently. I consulted with another anesthesiologist. He called the hospital to suggest a different approach to avoid the severe reaction that I had suffered during the first operation. They agreed to start me off with a shorter-acting anesthetic that would put me into a light level of anesthesia for as long as it was safe. They would put me into a deeper level of anesthesia for the middle of the procedure, and then they would turn off the anesthetic before I came to. With this approach, I woke up right away, I was out of bed that night, and I asked to go home the next day. It was an amazing difference, because someone had listened and acted accordingly.

Did you take anything for pain after the second operation?

They gave me something when I woke up and after I got back to the room. That was all I needed. It wasn't a painful process, because most areas were numb.

Describe the recovery. What limitations did you have? How long did it take you to get back to your normal level of activity?

I was in the hospital for 7 days with the first operation and for 3 days with the second. Initially, it's almost impossible to get into a car or to sit comfortably anywhere. Your leg hurts a lot, and you compensate by leaning back on couches and chairs because you can't sit up. It's also hard to go up steps. There is a lot of discomfort and tightness, and your movement is restricted. It takes a considerable amount of effort to keep moving and to climb steps. It took a good 3 to 4 weeks at home.

Did you experience any complications?

Fluid accumulated in the hip area after one of the operations. I had to wear a drain for 6 weeks, which I concealed with slacks when I went back to work. That was difficult. It's hard to bandage your buttocks and hips; there really aren't bandages you can put on your hips or strap around them in a comfortable fashion. I had to be really creative with how to wear great big fluffy bandages around my rear end. It was horrible sitting on the drain, moving with it, working with it for so long. I was told to stay home for 4 weeks or longer, but I went back to work both times in 3 weeks. I worked full-time at a busy hospital clinic; there was a lot of activity and I had to move around a lot, but I managed.

How long was it before you felt you were really back to yourself, back to your normal activity level?

That took a very long time. It was great to be able to go back to work in 3 weeks, but it probably took at least 6 months, maybe even 8 months, before I felt like myself physically.

When were you able to resume exercising? Have you returned to your former level of fitness?

It has been important psychologically and physically for me to remain active, but sometimes I got tired of starting over. I'm a runner, and at the time I was also active in lifting weights. The reconstructive surgery greatly restricted those activities. I have never gotten back to the level I was at before. Now I sort of meander a mile or two. I've become a very slow runner. I do more walking outside and on the treadmill. I still lift weights, but not as many or as heavy as I did before. I try to do more cross-training.

Did you choose to have nipple-areola reconstruction?

I almost didn't do that. I actually liked how nice and smooth my breasts felt, and I didn't want to mess that up. Again, it had to do with clothes. I decided that I had gone this far, so why not finish it? I wanted my breasts to look normal under bras and slips and flimsier clothes. I'm glad I did it. The nipple was made from a local flap of excess tissue in the breast area. The areola was created by tattooing, and the nipple was also tattooed.

Are you pleased with the color of the tattoo?

The color needs to be darker, but it's my fault, because they matched my normal areola, which was extremely pale, almost pink. They even commented that it was going to be very light, but they'd told me to select a color that matched my original areola, and this was it. My husband agreed it was the right color, and we decided not to make it darker at the time. It has never turned darker; in fact, it has faded a little over time. At some point I might do it again, but it doesn't matter that much to me.

Are you happy you chose the reconstructive approach that you did? Would you do it again?

Yes, I would do it again. Even though the gluteal free flap was described as a long, difficult procedure with potential complications, I was willing to accept those conditions because I felt it would give me the result I wanted. I wanted my rebuilt breasts to be natural and my own tissue, and that's what I got. The outcome was pretty perfect.

Are you happy with the aesthetic appearance of your breasts?

Absolutely. They're natural, they're well contoured, and they're balanced. I got my wish. Now when I go to the Jacuzzi at the YWCA, nobody stares and I'm no longer self-conscious.

Are you pleased with the size of your breasts?

It seems silly now, particularly since I investigated everything else so carefully, but it never occurred to me to think about my breast size. The subject didn't come up until my preoperative visit, when the nurse said, "What cup size do you think she's going to be?" My first reaction was what a weird, invasive thing to say. I don't care. My plastic surgeon said, "I think it will probably make a B cup." I thought, "Well, I was a B before, so that's pretty good." Later, when I thought about it, I couldn't believe that I never asked. Then I realized how unimportant it was to me. As long as my breasts were somewhat even, I was going to be satisfied. Well, I came out of surgery a size D! My husband to this day keeps saying, "They're just so big!" It's kind of funny that it turned out this way. I tell my husband that I have given him a treat.

Do you have sensation in your breasts? Are they sexually responsive?

If there's anything that I do mourn, it's the loss of my breasts as sexual organs. My husband and I had to talk about that and deal with it. It is a loss to me not to have sensitive breasts. Some feeling on the skin returned right away, and I can feel fine touch in some small areas, but in most areas it's numb. My breasts will never be sexual organs again, and that's a terrible loss.

If your breasts were a sensitive area and were a turn-on to increase your pleasure and stimulate pleasure in other areas, then that feeling cannot be replaced. It's just not there anymore. My husband knows that I have some feeling in some areas, but it's not the same, and he can't stimulate them because there's no feeling. But even knowing that I don't have feeling in my breasts, he thoroughly enjoys them and lovingly handles them, which gives me immense pleasure.

What do your scars look like? Where are they placed?

I ought to show them to you. They are hard to describe. You'd have to be pretty close to see that there are scars around both breasts, and they are getting paler as time goes by. I am not bothered by them. I also have elliptical-shaped scars across my lower buttocks, but they are covered by my underpants.

How do your buttocks feel? Are they numb?

My rear end is numb and uncomfortable. It's a different form of numbness; it's a paresthesia, and it hurts. Since they cut a nerve down the back of the thigh, there's feeling on my skin but numbness underneath. It hurts when skin in the area gets caught or pinched, for example, when I am sitting on a vinyl car seat and my skin tugs or pinches together as I get up. That's enough to make me literally jump out of the car.

I still have residual muscle tightness in my buttocks and thighs as well as my upper body and breast area. This doesn't get any better unless I really stretch, lift weights, and move around to increase flexibility. This is not an operation for someone who isn't fully aware of what they will have to do to get back in shape. If I had only had one side reconstructed, it probably wouldn't seem as much of a challenge, because then you could favor the operated side. We laugh about it, but we now judge restaurants by their chairs. I can't sit on wooden benches or picnic on the ground anymore. I can't sit on something flat. I'm uncomfortable because I've lost the cushioning that reduces the pressure on your buttocks when you are seated.

What advice would you give to women about dealing with breast cancer and breast reconstruction?

Dealing with cancer is no different from dealing with any other life calamity that everyone faces at some point. We all have losses—the loss of a family member, a relationship, a job. I don't believe anyone gets through it alone. I have spent a lot of time soul-searching and questioning why these things happen. What's the use of being a good person who works hard, lives hard, tries hard, and cares about others? What does it stand for? Something must come of it. Yet after all that I experienced, I sometimes feel like it makes no difference. It seems senseless and incomprehensible, and the anxiety is unbearable at times. God cannot make this go away but can give me something back. He can give me the opportunity to experience life—a friend, a thoughtful gesture, an act of kindness, a sunset—all of the pieces that form the fabric of life.

I am now strong enough to totally heal. I have always spent my life developing and investing in meaningful relationships. I didn't think of all those ties as a lifeline, but they were. When I see people who can't deal with trouble, it seems to always come down to the absence of a support system. They don't have a family, they don't have friends, the pieces are missing. You need to have a mutual, caring network to help you deal with life's surprises. That means giving of yourself to other people and knowing and accepting that no one can make it alone.

LYNNE: ARRIVING AT THE OTHER SIDE OF HEALING

The minute you meet Lynne, you are struck by her big laugh and her vivacious, outgoing manner. Lynne is small with short brown hair, an expressive face, and a ready smile. She is a take-charge dynamo who has not let her early breast cancer diagnosis, subsequent operations and complications, and her positive breast cancer gene status deter her from enjoying life to the fullest. Although she is still dealing with the extra weight she gained from taking tamoxifen (hormonal therapy), she is not daunted by a few extra pounds and has taken steps to dance her pounds away. She and her husband, Harvey, are expert ball-room dancers, which has proved a wonderful outlet for them. She has many beautiful ball gowns in her closet and trophies on the mantel as testimony to their dancing skill. They also play racquetball and exercise on a regular basis. As a medical illustrator at a major medical school, she has special access to current medical information and expertise that has been helpful to her in evaluating her options over the years.

Lynne's experience with breast cancer has motivated her to give back to others. She is a long-time volunteer for Reach to Recovery and has developed an inspiring art program for patients at the Cancer Center. Lynne is a virtual whirlwind of activity, but she is also a thoughtful, knowledgeable, and caring individual who worried that she would not live long enough to see her children grow up. Now, 25 years later, both of her children are married, and she has a beautiful grandchild to dote on. Lynne's experience with breast cancer and breast reconstruction involved numerous procedures with a number of bumps in the road that might have deterred other women, but only fortified her in her quest to take control of her situation and get on with her life. Her story is a fascinating one.

How was your breast cancer discovered?

I was only 31 years old when I felt a lump. I had just been to the gynecologist for my checkup a month earlier and had asked him when I should start getting mammograms. He told me 9 years later would be the appropriate time and not to worry until then. I should just do breast self-exams and he would examine me also, which he did and felt nothing.

Four weeks later, as I was getting into the shower, I looked in the mirror and saw a dimple on or slightly behind my nipple. Let me stop here for a moment to mention that I am a medical illustrator, and at that time I was illustrating a breast book and was depicting biopsies, breast lumps, and other potential signs of breast cancer. One of the signs was nipple dimpling, so that alerted me that something was not right. While I was showering and soaping (that's when I usually do a breast self-exam), I felt a lump. My kids at the time were 3 and 6 years old. So I got out of the shower and immediately asked my husband to feel the area and tell me if he felt anything. Sure enough, he did. At first I thought it was a milk gland or I was getting my period or anything else, because I did not have a family history of breast cancer. At that point I didn't have any information. At 7 o'clock the next morning I called the radiology department at the hospital where I work, and they had me come over. Two hours later, they had found the lump on mammography and were 80% sure that it was malignant because of its appearance. I had a biopsy the next day. In 1 week's time I went from feeling a lump, having a mammogram, having a biopsy, and getting a breast cancer diagnosis to having a modified radical mastectomy.

Why did you choose a mastectomy? Did they offer you the possibility of a lumpectomy?

I was fairly small-breasted, and the lump was right in the center of my breast. A lumpectomy would have deformed my breast and would have defeated the purpose of breast conservation. So it was better to do a full mastectomy. It also made me feel more comfortable that they were removing all of my breast tissue. At the time, tissue expanders were becoming popular for breast reconstruction, and not too many people had done them where I live. I contacted a plastic surgeon, and I had one inserted immediately after my mastectomy.

How did you choose your plastic surgeon?

I chose someone at the same hospital where I worked who had performed these procedures before. Back then you made appointments with individual physicians. This was before they developed breast cancer teams where the surgeon, oncologist, and plastic surgeon are all working together.

How did the results of your tissue expansion reconstruction turn out?

Not well at all. The tissue expander was placed too high, toward my clavicle. It was very uncomfortable. The plastic surgeon kept expanding it with saline, saying that gravity would bring it down. But it didn't; it just kept going higher and higher. After a 6-week period, when normally your skin would have been stretched sufficiently to insert an implant, I had the expander deflated. I left the tissue expander in place, because I was told that there was no problem in doing that. I still had the subcutaneous port in place. I decided to just wear a prosthesis for a while and take time to think about what I wanted to do. I was stage II and going through chemotherapy, but I had opted to participate in a clinical trial for stage III treatment, which involved very aggressive chemotherapy. Reconstructive surgery was low on my priority list then, because I had two small children and my focus was on finishing the treatment to cure my cancer.

How long did it take before you thought about breast reconstruction again?

I spent the next 15 years with the deflated expander in place. Over time, scar tissue built up around the port, and I could feel a few little hardened, thickened areas in my breast that I watched. I felt fine. I was comfortable with my body image. With a prosthesis in my bra, I could wear anything; they even offered models that could be velcroed to your body. I was able to get by pretty well for a while. But to be honest, the prosthesis did not complete my body image, even though I didn't admit that to myself. I thought I was doing quite well emotionally and psychologically. Later, when I changed my mind and decided to have reconstructive surgery, I realized that I wished I had not waited so long.

Was there any specific event that made you change your mind and decide to have breast reconstruction?

Time was really the healer. When I was 31, I didn't think I was going to be alive very long; my chances of survival were 40%. Given odds like that, breast reconstruction was pretty low on the list when I was worrying about seeing my children grow up. But over time, after improving my odds with chemo and tamoxifen and surviving for 15 years, my attitude changed. I was ready. My children were now teenagers; they were growing up and life was good. After 15 years, I felt it was time to focus on me.

How did you find a plastic surgeon to perform your reconstructive surgery? What type of reconstruction did you select and why?

I consulted with a few different physicians to determine what approach or operation would work best for me. I started with one plastic surgeon but was quite displeased with the options he recommended. He was very specific about what he wanted to do for me, as opposed to listening to what I wanted done. He was focused on doing one type of procedure that he felt was best for all patients. It was the TRAM flap, but that's a major operation. I had mixed feelings about going through such extensive surgery. This was not a good experience for me, so I consulted with another plastic surgeon several months later.

My consultation with the second plastic surgeon was much more successful. His perspective was more patient oriented. He asked me what I wanted, how I saw my body image, and what my goals were. He explained all of the different options. I decided to have tissue expansion with an implant. I did not want major surgery.

What did you do about the expander that was already in place? Was it removed?

During the examination my plastic surgeon took a syringe filled with saline and said, "Let's just see if we can access the expander port under your skin." I don't even know what kind of expander I had in me. But he could feel the port through my skin, and from knowing when it was inserted, he made an educated guess as to what kind of port it would be. He said that if he could access it, he could then stretch my skin and save me from undergoing one part of the procedure. All I would need was to have the expander removed and an implant inserted, since that was the type of reconstruction that I had decided on. Sure enough, it took about half an hour, and he was able to actually expand this old tissue expander. That meant that rather than inserting a brand new tissue expander, he could use the one that was already in place. So that's what we did.

How often did you have your breast expanded? Was it painful?

I had my existing expander inflated with saline solution during approximately four sessions. My plastic surgeon gradually expanded the skin over a 6-week period. That worked very effectively; the expander was still too high, but he just used it to stretch the skin. He assured me that when he inserted the implant, he would place it in a more natural position. I was very leery during this whole process. After going through surgery and chemotherapy and all of the emotions that are involved, it was somewhat frightening to go back in for surgery again.

There was really no pain involved in the expansion process—just pressure. That part was very easy, and I felt like I was making progress. I felt good that my surgeon was moving forward with me in a positive way, listening to me, and respecting my desire to do the least amount possible to get the best result. That's why he used an old tissue expander to speed the process. That strategy worked very effectively. After the expansion was finished, he presented the different implant options to consider.

What types of implants did you consider? What did you choose?

I could have a saline-filled implant or a silicone gel–filled implant. He had different models in his office, with varying shapes, sizes, and feels. We talked about how my natural breast looked as opposed to the expanded side, where my scar line was, and again, what my expectations were. I felt very secure in the thoroughness of our discussion. I decided to choose a silicone-filled implant. I had to sign papers, because they were still being studied in a clinical trial, which required regular follow-up and testing. I also had to carry a card around with me that identified the type of implant I had. Psychologically, the follow-up process and extra paperwork was somewhat of a burden. It did not allow me to feel free-spirited again.

Did you have your nipple reconstructed?

Initially, I decided not to have nipple reconstruction. I was extremely happy with the implant reconstruction. Ten days later, I went for my first postoperative checkup. I was all wrapped up after having had my drains removed. While I was there, my doctor asked me if I would come next door and talk to another woman. He asked if I would mind being unwrapped so I could show her my reconstructed breast. I said fine, because I was feeling pretty good. She looked at me and said, "Oh my God, you look totally normal." So I walked out thinking, "I look totally normal." I had not heard that in 15 years. I got into my car and was on my way home when I stopped, turned the car around, drove back to the office, and parked. I went back upstairs into the hospital and asked to be scheduled to have the nipple reconstruction. I decided, "Okay, if I'm looking normal, I'm going to finish this entire process." I had an outpatient nipple reconstruction 3 weeks later after my healing was complete.

What was done for the nipple reconstruction?

My surgeon used the tissue right at the site of my reconstruction, so I did not have any grafts taken from other places. I later had tattooing. In planning the nipple reconstruction, we talked about how much projection I wanted so that I would be comfortable in all types of clothing. We also looked at a color palette for the tattooing, and I made the decisions about what I wanted. So once the nipple was reconstructed and I had the tattooing, I felt that I was complete and everything was finished. That put me at about 17 years out.

Were you through with surgery then?

I was for about 3 years, until I ran into a good friend who is a radiologist specializing in breast care. She pulled me aside and said, "You need to get genetically tested; the BRCA1 and BRCA2 test is becoming available for high-risk people." She thought I would qualify, because I was only 31 years old at diagnosis.

Did you have the genetic testing?

Yes, I did. I had to fill out a form about family history, and I had nothing to put down. There was no history of cancer in my family whatsoever that I could recollect. I only had one question in my entire family line, and it was a grandmother who had died very young; nothing else had ever popped up. So I had it done, and I came back positive for BRCA2.

What does it mean to be positive for BRCA2?

Being positive for the BRCA2 gene meant that I had a high risk for breast cancer in the other breast—over 90%. This would pretty much guarantee that I would get breast cancer in the other breast. I was also at high risk for melanoma and pancreatic, lung, and ovarian cancer. I had already had a full hysterectomy, so I didn't have to bother with that one—that was already out of the equation.

What did you do after you received the positive BRCA2 gene results?

Two weeks later, I scheduled a second mastectomy, a prophylactic one, because I wanted to be very proactive and do as much as possible to prevent another cancer. I had the same plastic surgeon who did my last implant reconstruction. He worked with an oncologic surgeon. I had immediate implant reconstruction with the same type of implant that was used in my other breast. Several months later, I had nipple reconstruction. So now I am a perfectly balanced person.

What did they find when they did your preventive mastectomy? Were there any irregularities?

When the pathology report came back, it showed that every single part of the breast tissue was atypical. I asked my oncologist and surgeon what that meant; their feeling was that this was tissue that wanted to become cancerous but had not. I went back to my oncologist and asked if the tamoxifen I had been taking for 20-plus years and still take (longer than the 5 years suggested in the clinical trial) was the reason that the tissue had not turned cancerous. The oncologist said it could be the tamoxifen that was holding everything in check. I will never know, but I have read all the trial studies, and most of the women who participated were postmenopausal women, which I was not. I was too young to fall into the trial study. I had two other doctors read the trial results, and then we made decisions together. That's why I am still taking tamoxifen.

Since your diagnosis with the BRCA2 gene, have your children been tested?

When my test came back positive, I shared that information with my son and daughter. My feeling is that knowledge is powerful, and if you have knowledge, then you know how to make decisions. Given that philosophy and knowing how aggressive I have been in fighting this, both of my kids decided to get tested, because they wanted to know. I was told that there was a 50/50 chance that they would have the gene. My daughter already had a plan if she had tested positive. She said, "I feel that I'm going to be negative." I asked her why she had that feeling. She said, "Because we've already talked this to death, and I have a plan. The plan would be that I would have children early. Then I would have a double mastectomy and a hysterectomy. This would relieve me of future worry, and I could just lead my life in beauty, comfort, and ease." Sure enough, her test results came back negative, so she does not have to be concerned from a genetic standpoint. However, she does have to be concerned as a woman, because 1 in 8 women will get breast cancer in their lifetime.

My son's test, on the other hand, came back positive; he does carry the gene. His first question to me was, if I had known that I carried this, would I have had him? I was absolutely floored by this question, and I said "Absolutely. Absolutely." Just because you carry it does not mean it will exhibit itself in your lifetime. So that alleviated some anxiety for him, but he does worry knowing he's at a higher risk for other cancers as well. But as a boy, as a man, it's a much better statistic than if my daughter had tested positive.

With your prophylactic mastectomy and reconstruction, what was your recovery like? How long did it take you to get back to feeling yourself?

My recovery was very short. I had the tissue expander put in immediately after the mastectomy. I did not have an axillary dissection, so that eliminated a lot of the discomfort that I experienced years earlier with my first mastectomy. Then I went through the expansion process, followed by implant placement and nipple reconstruction. I was back at work and doing everything I wanted to do very, very quickly. So now I feel just great.

How do your breasts look and feel? Are they soft and sensitive?

They feel fabulous. They're soft. They are not sensitive. The sensitivity is on the medial side of my arms; there is no breast sensitivity. I'm perfectly balanced; I don't wear any sort of bra anymore, because I don't need to.

Could anyone tell that you had reconstruction or cancer by looking at you?

The only way that they could tell is if they saw the scar lines on the sides of my breasts. From the front, they cannot tell at all. I go to the gym and take off my clothes in the locker room without feeling self-conscious. Before reconstruction, I would not have done that. That has made a major, major difference.

What would you recommend to women who are thinking about breast reconstruction?

I would recommend breast reconstruction to them. I waited 15 years before doing it, so I really lived every day thinking about my cancer. Every day that I dressed or undressed, I had a visual connection with my cancer. I thought I was doing myself a favor by waiting, and in some ways I was, because I wasn't ready, but it could have been sooner. Reconstruction had an impact on my body image that I was not consciously aware of. Before I had reconstruction, I would be outside gardening and my prosthesis would fall out in the middle of the weeds. So I was limited in my activities and in my clothing. Reconstruction has allowed me to go out there and be myself with my own body image. Now I can exercise, dance, and do whatever I want without being self-conscious. I did not start ballroom dancing until my reconstruction was totally complete. Before that, I felt too restricted. For me, reconstruction helped to complete the process and arrive at the other side of healing.

How has your breast cancer experience affected your attitude about life?

I am a counselor for Reach to Recovery and have visited a lot of women over the years. For me this has proved to be a liberating experience; it made me stronger, it put my values and priorities in perspective, and it let me know what was important in life. As I talk to other women, they validate these feeling about the breast cancer experience. I always tell them that it's very sad for me personally that it took something this tragic, thinking that I was going to die at 31, to set my priorities straight and provide a clear path for how I should live my life. So that's really what it did; it gave me strength, and I can now give hope to others, which I continue to do all the time. Every day is very special. Old clichés such as "live each day to the fullest" suddenly have special meaning for me.

MAGGIE: A WOMAN'S SEXUALITY

"Flamboyant" was the word Maggie proudly used to describe herself, and I had to smile at the accuracy of her self-assessment. An imposing woman of 5 feet 8 inches, she has an air of self-assurance that dominates her conversation. She is also a somewhat flashy dresser, which only serves to complement her personality. The day of our interview, Maggie was dressed in a bright red blouse draped in comfortable folds over her ample bosom. Her waist was cinched by a gold belt, several gold chains encircled her neck, and her long fingers tapered into finely manicured nails, lacquered in bright red to match her lipstick. She wore black slacks and black high heels, and her black hair was carefully coiffured in a short, bouffant style. Her gold bracelets clinked as she talked to me about the importance of breasts and sex appeal to women of all ages and why she, as a widow in her early sixties, felt it was particularly important to have breast reconstruction.

Maggie's striking appearance is consistent with her open and appealingly honest personality. She likes herself and the image she portrays; she was determined not to let breast cancer diminish her body image or make her uncomfortable interacting with others. Her cancer was discovered when she was widowed after 34 years of a happy marriage; one married daughter lived in a nearby town. Although she was involved in a busy career in retail lingerie, she did not want to spend the rest of her life without a partner. She liked socializing and frankly admitted that she liked her breasts just as they were. She had always worn clothing that was "sexy," and she said, "I didn't want to change my image now." Of particular importance was her desire to be able to feel free to engage in an intimate relationship without inhibition. Therefore, when she was diagnosed with breast cancer, she was determined not to delay breast restoration any longer than necessary.

Living in a small town, she did not have an experienced reconstructive surgeon available to consult, so she undertook her own research to find out all she could about the different types of reconstructive operations and the best surgeons to perform them. She decided to have a delayed TRAM flap breast reconstruction. Although this was one of the more complicated procedures, she selected it because she did not want an artificial substance in her body. As Maggie explained, "I'm an original, and I want everything about me to be real." Even though immediate breast reconstruction was not an option for her, she was determined that the delay would be as brief as possible to curtail the period of breast loss. Her deadline was to have her breast reconstruction completed and be totally recovered 1 year after her mastectomy. She set about this goal with style, humor, and determination. Now, 3 years later, this gutsy lady has remarried and is enjoying life more than ever. Sometimes Maggie even forgets that her reconstructed breast is not her original one.

How did you discover your breast cancer?

I found a lump while I was examining my breasts in the shower. I had fibrocystic breasts, so I had lumps before, but this one felt different. It seemed to be attached to the skin; with the others the overlying skin was more movable. I decided to follow up with my gynecologist. He referred me to a surgeon, who sent me for a mammogram and suggested a biopsy. When I came out of the anesthesia after the biopsy, my daughter was there, and she told me they had found a malignancy.

What was your reaction to your cancer diagnosis?

I wanted to know how bad my cancer was and what was going to happen to me. When my doctor told me that I was going to need a mastectomy, I told him that I couldn't have one. I was alone; I was unmarried. My breast was a very important part of my body. I felt that I needed my breast if I was to get on with my life. I just couldn't have a mastectomy, but he said that I must. That's when I started my research. I needed to find out quickly what my options were.

What type of research did you conduct to investigate your options?

I got on the phone and started calling people. I had heard of a lady in my town, a friend of a friend, who had a mastectomy and breast reconstruction; I called her. I contacted everybody I could think of. I even called people in other states. I am the kind of person who wants to know what lies ahead of her and what is the best direction to go. In 3 days I did quite a bit of research, and I learned about cancer treatment and breast reconstruction.

Why was reconstruction so important to you?

My mother's oldest sister had breast cancer. She had her mastectomy many years ago, and she never had reconstruction. To me it was a horrible sight. I felt that I would have to change my image if I lost my breast. I am a flamboyant dresser. I have always liked low, revealing clothes. I am that kind of person, that's just me; I have been that way from the age of 16. I didn't want to lose my breast. I liked me. Even though I was not involved intimately with a man at that time, I did not feel that I could ever be comfortable with the opposite sex if I had only one breast.

How did you learn about reconstruction? What type of reconstructive technique did you select?

I heard about reconstruction through my phone calls to women with cancer. I would call these people and ask them questions: "Did you have reconstruction?" "Where did you have it?" "What was it like?" "Who did your surgery?" "Were you satisfied?" I never spoke to anybody who had anything but implants, but I knew flaps were being done, because I had read about these techniques in some books. I decided early on that I didn't want implants. I am not that kind of person. I've never wanted false teeth. I've never wanted anything artificial if it was possible to have the other. I would settle for implants before I would do without, but I wanted the best, and I felt that my own tissue was best. I also wanted immediate reconstruction so I wouldn't have to go without my breast.

Were you able to have immediate reconstruction?

No. I wanted my doctor in my home town to do my mastectomy, because he had a very good reputation. I also felt that he would take a more personal interest in getting all the cancer. Since there really wasn't anyone in town who could have done the reconstructive surgery, immediate reconstruction was out of the question. So I had my mastectomy, and then I was ready for reconstruction. And despite my cancer surgeon's warning that no plastic surgeon would touch me for 6 months, I was determined to get my breast back sooner.

How long did it take you to recover from your mastectomy? Did you experience much pain? What was your emotional reaction to the surgery?

The pain wasn't too bad. I had my surgery on Tuesday and checked out of the hospital on Friday morning. The mental anguish was much worse than the pain. I didn't let anyone except my mother see me without a breast. I had the surgery at 9 o'clock in the morning, and that afternoon I sent my mother out to get an artificial breast to put in my gown. I still insisted on wearing my low-cut nightgown, and I lay there very straight so that nobody could tell that the prosthesis was pinned in my very sexy nightgown. I wondered if I could go on with my life. After all, I had lost something very important to me, something that made me a whole person. I couldn't concentrate on the pain; breast reconstruction occupied my thoughts. I'm impatient that way. If I have anything facing me, good or bad, I am anxious to get on with it.

How did you find the plastic surgeon to perform your TRAM flap breast reconstruction?

I had heard about him from several women I talked to. He had a good reputation, and he was at a major medical center. I decided to consult with him. If I didn't like him, I could always go to someone else in the city. I live in a small town, and I felt that a major medical center was the best place to go. I went to see the plastic surgeon only 3 weeks after my mastectomy. As it turned out, he suited me just fine, so I didn't need to consult with anyone else.

What was your consultation like? Why did you select this plastic surgeon to perform your breast reconstruction?

I came all dressed up and in my high heels. I was afraid that because of what I had heard about a 6-month delay, he wouldn't operate on me right away. My goal was to have everything complete, behind me, and out of my mind as much as possible within a year. When I was filling out my medical history, I would not write down the month that I had my mastectomy; I just wrote the year. I was determined to stay in control. I wanted to tell him what I wanted and what I could stand; I wanted it my way. If he had not listened to me, I would have gone elsewhere.

At the beginning of our consultation he asked me why I had come to him for reconstruction. I said, "Because I heard you are the best, and I won't have anything but the best. I don't want implants. I want a TRAM flap." I told him exactly what I wanted. Later, when he saw me undressed, he said, "When did you have this done?" I said, "It doesn't matter when I had it done; I want this reconstruction done during your first opening. I want it now." He grinned. He is a quiet, laid-back person, so it was easy for me to stay in control, which I liked. I loved him from day one. A woman in this state of mind doesn't need sympathy, but she needs someone who is calm and gentle. I felt his caring from the time that he started talking to me. He smiled and said, "We'll have to see when I have the next opening." I said, "You're going to do me?" and he said, "Yes, but this type of surgery is not for everybody." He didn't paint a pretty picture.

What did he tell you about the TRAM flap? Did you understand that this was a major operative procedure?

He said that the TRAM flap was painful. You have to be in good health, and it can be time consuming, possibly 4 hours of surgery, with months for full recovery. He also said that several steps or different operations are usually needed to get the breast and abdomen to look just right. He explained that it would probably take close to 9 months to complete it, the nipple and everything. He told me that it was a hard surgery. I would have to be off work for quite a while. He told me about all the possible complications and explained them in great detail so I would understand what I was getting myself into. Of course,

I didn't listen, not really, because I know me, and he didn't. If he would do his job, then I could do mine. My plastic surgeon gave me a book to read when I left his office. Even with all of this information, I did not realize what I was facing; only experience can teach you that. As far as I was concerned, I felt I could tolerate anything for a few days to have peace of mind and to feel whole again.

Did your plastic surgeon take pictures of you during your consultation?

My plastic surgeon took pictures of me from my first visit through my final operation; he took some before and then some each time I had another surgery. It's uncomfortable for any woman to be totally undressed in front of a stranger, no matter if it's your doctor, and have him taking pictures of you. I'd joke about it because I was uncomfortable. I'd say, "Why are you taking all these pictures? Am I going to be in Playboy?"

Was your plastic surgeon reluctant to perform your reconstruction just 3 weeks after your mastectomy?

He said, "You know it's been just 3 weeks since you had this other surgery." I said, "I know, but I'm very healthy despite the breast cancer. I'm also very headstrong and determined to do this." So he agreed to operate on me in 3 weeks; that made 6 weeks to the day since my mastectomy. But he let me know that I was pushing it; I would have to follow his directions to get ready, or else my breast reconstruction would have to be delayed. I was happy with that. I said, "You tell me what to do and I will do it. I will be ready."

Describe your TRAM flap breast reconstruction; what did it involve?

I was cut from one side of my abdomen to the other, all the way in front. The abdominal skin was then grafted from the navel to the pubic hairline to move up to my breast with the accompanying abdominal muscle (the rectus abdominis muscle) and fat to give me enough skin and tissue to build a breast. It is my understanding that this flap of abdominal muscle and tissue was threaded up through a tunnel into the left side; that's where my mastectomy was. Then my plastic surgeon shaped a breast from it. He also had to make a new navel. I have a very pretty navel, almost as good as Mother gave me.

How long did it take you to recuperate from your reconstructive surgery? Did you experience much pain?

The reconstructive surgery lasted 4½ hours. Afterward, when they rolled me to my room, they bumped my bed. I knew then I was in bad shape. I hurt all over, from my breast to my lower abdomen. The pain was concentrated more in my abdomen than it was in my breast, but it was all connected. When they transfer the muscle to the breast, they open a tunnel from the abdominal area to the breast area, so there is a large area that needs to heal.

I had four or five drain tubes coming out of my abdomen and breast, a catheter, a morphine pump for pain, and oxygen. The next morning, when two nurses came to get me up, the pain was almost unbearable. One of the nurses, unfortunately, wasn't well trained in how to get a person back into the bed. She let me fall back, which was the worst thing. I had stitches and it hurt terribly. I know the morphine helped, but by the third day it was making me deathly ill, and I told the nurse to take the pain pump out. I felt I could tolerate the pain better than I could tolerate the nausea. I told them I would ask for a shot if the pain got too bad.

Knowing that they had taken part of a muscle and transferred it, I had this horror of not being able to straighten up, like an old woman. So my next step was to get on my feet to see how far I could straighten up. I was looking forward to that, although I knew it was going to be tough. I surprised myself when I did get up to go to the bathroom on the third day. I was still quite bent over, but I knew if I kept on I would be able to straighten up pretty soon, because I wasn't as bad off as I expected. I am very tall, 5 feet 8 inches. A little person wouldn't have as far to stretch as I did. It was very important to me to be erect again, so I really worked on it. By the fourth day I was in the hall walking, taking tiny steps. I had to hold on to the rail, but I was straight.

I was in the hospital 5 or 6 days. When I left the hospital, I stayed with my mother for a week and a half. During that time I was not always able to dress, because I was so sore that I could hardly stand for anything to touch me. Even so, I exercised. I found a flat place in my mom's yard, and five or six times a day, with just my nightclothes and my tennis shoes on, I would walk one way and then another, and then I would go in and lie down. Then I would walk again. Three weeks after my surgery, my daughter asked me to go to a shopping center with her. I called a hospital equipment store, rented a wheelchair, and went shopping in a wheelchair. I was totally exhausted when I got home. I could hardly stand any bumps, but I did it. I still had on the stretch halter top they had given me in the hospital to wear over the bandage. I wore my clothes and jacket over that.

It took 2 to 3 months before I felt like myself again. As far as the pain was concerned, the first step of the reconstruction was the most painful. The rest was a breeze.

Was your breast what you expected after the first stage of reconstruction?

I had been told what to expect, but it's always a surprise when you see yourself after surgery. It was difficult to face the scars. I didn't expect my stomach to feel so hard; it was also numb, and that lack of sensation was quite disturbing to me. It resembled the numbness you experience after you have Novocain at the dentist; you know you're touching something, but it has no feeling. My breast was also numb, but I was expecting that. Even so, it still felt strange, and it looked funny without a nipple.

I had more swelling than I anticipated. Immediately after my operation, the area under my breast where the flap was tunneled was swollen as big as another breast. I worried if it would ever go down. That was my first question to my plastic surgeon. He assured me that the swelling would go down, and if it didn't, he would take care of it during the next step of surgery. That eased my mind, because I had all the confidence in the world in this doctor. I knew that after a few more operations he could make me look the way I wanted to. I was anxious to get on with it. I kept asking when he planned to do the next step.

What other procedures or steps were required to complete your breast reconstruction?

I had some hardening under the arm; that's where my lymph nodes had been stripped. You could feel stitches. It felt like scar tissue. It was a hard knot, and it pooched out. In the second step he took care of that: he reopened the incision, removed that tissue, and it was fine. It bothered me that he had to make another little scar on my breast to remedy that situation. When I looked at it I thought, "Oh Lord, another scar."

He also suctioned the swollen area under my breast that I was so concerned about. By this time it had shrunk to the size of a lemon, so there wasn't much contouring to do. In the lower abdomen on each side where he started and finished the incision, I had little areas of skin that seemed to hang over. He called them "dog-ears." He told me not to worry about these dog-ears, because he planned to use them to get tissue grafts for my nipple-areola reconstruction. Fortunately, one side leveled out and we didn't disturb it; he got his graft from the other side.

Why did you decide that you wanted nipple-areola reconstruction?

To make the reconstructed breast look like the other breast; it wouldn't have been complete otherwise. I knew I had gone through the worst, and I would never settle for an unfinished job.

Did he tattoo your reconstructed nipple-areola, and if so, was it a good match with your opposite nipple-areola?

Yes, I had a tattoo, and no, the match is not good. I hurried too much for the first tattoo—I was so determined to get it all done. They told me that they felt they were doing the tattoo too soon; it might not take, because the tissue had not healed enough. It didn't. I had to have it done over, but the match still isn't good. My plastic surgeon is not happy with the coloring on the tattoo, and neither am I. It's too dark. I have a lot of yellow tones in my skin, and that's one of the hardest colors to match. My plastic surgeon has said that he can take care of it.

Did you have any complications, any problems?

No. It just took some time to recuperate, but I really didn't have any trouble.

What were your primary goals in having reconstruction?

To be like I was. I never thought that I had the prettiest breasts in the world, but once I had lost one, I wanted a replacement just like the old one. Until you lose something, you never appreciate it; you take it for granted. I didn't really want any miracles. I didn't expect to mess with nature. Nature does a great deal for most people. But once I had lost my breast, then I felt I owed it to myself to find a way to restore what cancer took away.

Are you satisfied with the appearance of your breast? Is it soft, natural? Does it have feeling?

Yes. I cannot tell now that it has not been there forever. I also cannot tell any difference in feeling. I was told by my plastic surgeon that I would probably not have any feeling in this breast, no sensation. However, I do have sensitivity to touch all around the breast and at different places on the breast. The nipple has no sensitivity, and there is no sexual feeling.

Where are your scars located, and how do they look?

The scarring is disturbing. I have a scar completely around the breast on the left side and an inch-long V-shaped scar extending onto my breast from my underarm. I also have a scar that extends across my entire lower abdomen. Now they're fading into hairline scars that are more acceptable.

If you had to do it over again, would you choose to have breast reconstruction? Would you select the same technique?

Yes. I think the direction I took was best for me. I don't know anything that I could have done to make it turn out any better. I have been totally pleased. I feel complete. I feel attractive again. I am comfortable undressing in front of a man. I look good in my clothes again. I can go on with my life.

How does breast cancer and breast reconstruction affect a woman's relationship with a man? Is it difficult when you are single and dating? What are the worries?

Divorced, widowed, or single women have mastectomies and reconstruction just the same as married women who have companions and support. At the time of my mastectomy, I was not involved in a sexual relationship, and it would have been impossible for me to consider one with only one breast. Even though I had reconstruction, I wondered how I could explain what had happened to me. I wondered if a man would feel that I was complete, sensuous. Then I decided that any man who doesn't accept me as I am isn't worth my time. This sounded good, but I still had to give myself a pep talk every time I went out on a date. When I met a guy, I would think about how I would tell him. When you're dating, this is a worry. Most men like to love a woman, and a woman likes to be loved; a breast is an important part of that. Even if you don't have a sexual relationship with a man, the first thing most men do after they get pretty well acquainted with you is fondle your breasts. I didn't tell anybody about my breast, however, unless our relationship developed and I saw that I was going to undress. Then, before I reached that point, I would prepare him for what I had to say. I would begin by telling him that I had breast cancer and had a mastectomy and breast reconstruction. Sometimes I wouldn't go any further. It was surprising how the men related; I don't think it made a difference to anyone I became involved with. And men don't hide their feelings well. Usually they were shocked to hear about it at first, and then they would say, "Well, if it weren't for the scars, you couldn't tell you've had anything done." I said, "That's right, and in time it will be less visible."

When you met your present husband, what was his reaction to your breast reconstruction?

I met him through a friend, and we had several phone conversations before our first face-to-face meeting. Of course, I didn't tell him anything about my surgery at that time. I really didn't even like the guy during our first meeting. He continued to call me, though. Several weeks later, I was coming to the city where he lived, so I called him and told him that I was going to be there. He insisted on taking me to dinner. At dinner we talked and discovered we had mutual interests and that we both liked to travel. When he asked if I wanted to go to Nashville with him that weekend, I surprised myself by saying yes.

I like to dance and sing, and I was looking forward to a good time in Nashville. It didn't worry me that I had this reconstructed breast and would have to tell him about it. That wasn't on my mind until the time came. That's the way I handled it with everybody I met. So I didn't think the breast would make or break my relationship.

That night we checked into a motel and made dinner arrangements at a nice steak place. I thought, "Well, I like this guy, and I'm probably going to wind up in bed with him." Before we went out to dinner, I pointed over to the other bed and told him to sit down, because I had a story to tell him. He sat down and I said, "I had cancer a year ago, and I had to have a breast removed." I was always a little "hyper" about telling someone, even though I never thought I was. As I was telling my story, I looked over and big tears started rolling down his face. He reached over, embraced me, and kissed me. I asked him, "What are you crying for?" Here's this big old 300-pound man crying, and I'm the one who's had the surgery. He said, "You're just the most remarkable person that I have ever met in my life." You know, I had several male friends that I dated after having my breast reconstruction who said the same thing to me. They said, "You're marvelous. I admire you, and there is nothing to be ashamed of." I always told them that I wasn't ashamed of it; I just felt that I should tell them in case they questioned the scars. I think that men accept this better than women accept it themselves.

What advice would you like to give to other women considering breast reconstruction?

A woman at any age owes it to herself to consider breast reconstruction. It does wonders for you mentally. It helps you to bypass self-pity and move on to life.

JUDY: WHY WAIT?

I didn't want to see myself without my breasts, and I didn't see any reason to wait. Why wait and heal, only to be reopened and have to heal a second time? With immediate breast reconstruction, I never felt the terrible devastation of breast loss after bilateral mastectomies. The hard part was over once I had that surgery, and from then on it was an adventure in rebuilding."

It was summer when I interviewed Judy for the first time. Tanned and fit, she was dressed in a white shirt and shorts, with her dark hair pulled back from her face. Married with two daughters, she has an active career as a communications expert at a local high school. Who would ever imagine that breast cancer could strike this beautiful, articulate woman of 47? And yet, true to the statistics, Judy was diagnosed with breast cancer 5 years ago.

Her diagnosis, while shocking, was not totally unexpected, because she had a family history of breast cancer, and had herself been plagued with fibrocystic breasts, a long-standing problem that made breast monitoring difficult. Judy had been under close surveillance by her surgeon for many years and had had numerous biopsies for suspicious lumps.

Just 2 years before her breast cancer diagnosis, after she had three suspicious lumps biopsied at one time, her surgeon suggested that she consider prophylactic mastectomies and reconstruction to reduce the risk of developing breast cancer in the future. She had even seen a plastic surgeon about this option, and he also recommended preventive mastectomies. But Judy was still doubtful; she didn't have cancer, and the thought of having her breast tissue removed was not appealing. Reflecting on this early decision now, Judy admits, "I should have been smarter. My mom has breast cancer, and I have a family history." She went to another surgeon for a second opinion. He told her it would be foolish to let them take her breasts off; she should wait until she had cancer, if indeed she ever did. That was just the news that she wanted to hear, so she decided to wait and see.

Two years later, shortly after her aunt had been diagnosed with a breast malignancy, Judy's breast cancer was discovered during yet another biopsy. This time she took immediate action. She had a modified radical mastectomy on the right side and a prophylactic mastectomy on her left breast, a procedure in which the breast tissue is removed and the nipple cored out. Both breasts were reconstructed immediately with tissue expanders.

Judy's decision to have immediate breast reconstruction was partially explained by her mother's experience with breast loss. "I had seen my mom with her concave figure and staples all across her chest. I watched her battle with a prosthesis. I remember the day that she threw it against the wall. She was so tired of hauling that thing around. She had very big breasts, and after her one breast was removed, she needed a large prosthesis for balance; it weighed 7 or 8 pounds. That's a heavy load to carry. I knew that route was not for me. With immediate reconstruction, I never had to experience breast loss. I never mourned my breasts. My attitude was, "Now that this is out of the way, let's go."

Judy's initial reaction when she woke after her operation was one of relief. "When I woke up, I lifted the sheet immediately, and all I had was two little Steri-Strips on my body. I had expected massive bandages. I had these little mounds, and it was like I didn't lose that much. Even knowing that it really wasn't me under there, it was reassuring to have something there."

How long did it take you to recuperate?

I had my mastectomies and reconstruction on a Thursday, and I went home on a Saturday, but it took a good 4 weeks before I felt like doing much. My mom came and stayed for a week and helped out. I went out in public right away; I attended my daughter's graduation a week later. I went to the grocery store. Raising my arms was a little difficult, however, and I didn't want my scars to stretch. So I was careful about lifting and moving. I didn't vacuum. In fact, I still don't vacuum if I can get out of it.

I was off for the summer, and I didn't go back to work until late August. I was still having my breasts expanded then. The expansion was not hard once I got over the initial part. In October, when I had my expanders replaced with implants, I stayed off work 2 weeks. I really didn't need that full 2 weeks; 1 week would have been fine. But at that point, my priorities were different. I decided that I was going to take all the time I needed to heal. I put myself first probably for the first time in my life.

When I had my nipple reconstruction, it was done the day before Christmas vacation, and I had another 2 weeks to recuperate.

How did you choose your reconstructive technique? What considerations were most important to you in making this decision?

I chose tissue expansion with implant placement because that's what my plastic surgeon recommended. He told me about the other operations and about the tummy flap, but because I was so slender, he didn't think I had enough stomach fat to reconstruct both of my breasts. We also discussed more involved flap procedures for breast reconstruction in which tissue is moved from one part of the body to another and reconnected with microsurgery. I really didn't want to go through the pain of a procedure that involved, and I didn't want all of the scars. So tissue expansion seemed to be the best option for me.

Describe the expansion process. What happened when you had your breasts expanded?

Two weeks after my surgery, I met with my plastic surgeon and his nurse, and we started the expansion process. My plastic surgeon told her how much fluid to inject into my expanders and over what period of time. From then on, his nurse usually took care of me, injecting about 100 ml of fluid into each breast during each session. Expansion proceeded pretty rapidly. It took about 15 minutes each time, and I went every week for the first 7 or 8 weeks and then less frequently. We never cut back on the amount of fluid injected, and we never stopped. But she always gave me the option. She was very responsive to my needs.

Tell me how this nurse helped you. What did she do to make this process easier for you?

She was one of the greatest supports that I had. She allowed me to have control, to make some decisions about my body, and to decide how fast I wanted to have my breasts expanded. Each time she asked if I felt I could handle it. If I told her something didn't feel right, she never brushed me off or dismissed my concerns. Instead, she would say, "Tell me how you feel. Exactly where is the problem?" Not all nurses do that. I had experiences with other nurses during that process, and I never received that kind of compassion. If I was extremely tight, she allowed me to say whether I wanted to be expanded or not. And a lot of nurses don't. They say, "You have to get used to the tightness, because the only way to stretch the skin is to expand it immediately." But that's not necessarily true; sometimes your skin doesn't stretch as fast as they think it should. Sometimes you need the time to allow your skin to relax and work itself loose so that it is more comfortable.

Tissue expansion involves some sense of being violated. This is true especially with the original surgery, but even with the expansion you are not in control of making decisions about what's being done to your body. My nurse gave me control.

How did it feel to have your expanders inflated? Was it painful?

I had more feeling on my right side, where I had the preventive mastectomy. I always felt the pinprick of the needle being inserted into my expander port. Once it was in, I didn't feel a thing. The other side had no feeling. I could feel some pressure. I was not always comfortable, but I was never in pain.

After the first 4 weeks, it felt like I had bricks put in my body. My breasts felt heavier, like I was carrying more weight. That's probably because my expanders were positioned behind my chest muscle and were exerting pressure on it. I just felt my breasts blowing up; I could actually see them as they grew. That was encouraging to me, because I didn't want to be flat-chested. As a teenager I was fairly big-breasted. And I think I would have had a hard time being totally flat-chested. But I could see my breasts as they grew, and each time I would go home and think, "They're getting better."

How long did the expansion process take?

Everything went like clockwork. I wore my expanders for about 5 months. It took me 4 months to have my breasts totally expanded, and then a month to let my breast skin rest so my breasts would become comfortable.

Was it inconvenient?

No, because it was summertime. Had I been in school, it might have been. But my mindset was such that nothing would have seemed an inconvenience. I had tunnel vision with breast reconstruction. Other things went on in my life, but this was a goal; it consumed a large part of my life and my thinking.

Why did you choose to have your nipple-areola reconstructed?

Because I wanted to be complete. I wanted my breasts to look normal and to match. The nipple on my normal breast was preserved after the prophylactic mastectomy, so I wanted one on the mastectomy side also.

How was your nipple-areola reconstructed, and when was it done?

My initial surgery was done in May, my expanders were replaced with permanent saline-filled implants in October, and my nipple was reconstructed in December. The nipple reconstruction was done at a third procedure to allow my breasts to settle. My nipple was reconstructed from the scar tissue extending under my arm. I later had my nipple tattooed as an outpatient procedure.

How do your breasts look? Are you satisfied with the appearance?

My breasts are symmetrical, and I look terrific in my clothes. I asked to be big, and I got bigger than I had planned to be, but I'm very satisfied. Sometimes I have to be careful about buying clothes, because the top doesn't fit the bottom, but that's a minor inconvenience compared to my level of satisfaction.

After the modified radical mastectomy, my armpit was hollowed out, and it looked funny to me in sleeveless clothes. Other people probably wouldn't have noticed if I kept my arm down, but I was self-conscious. To correct this problem, my plastic surgeon removed a piece of muscle from my back (the latissimus dorsi muscle) and swung it under my arm, so I now have a fairly normal-looking armpit.

My nipples still don't match, but that's because I had my nipple skin preserved on my normal side. At the time I didn't want to lose the nipple on my normal side if I didn't have to. That seemed very important then; it isn't now. Sometimes I wish I had gone ahead and had it taken off so there was a little better match. But that side is more comfortable, because I have more skin.

Also, the color of the tattoo on my reconstructed nipple doesn't match the color of my preserved nipple. I have yellow-toned skin, and yellow tones are difficult to replicate. I've heard that they now have tints with more yellow pigment available. After my tattoo fades, I'm going to have my nipple-areola tattooed again to try to get a better match. It is hard to do it again. After all of that surgery, Band-Aids are a real turn-off.

How do your reconstructed breasts feel? Are they sensitive? Are they soft? Are they warm?

I have no feeling in about a 3½-inch diameter. I do have feeling around the outside of my breasts, but only in the skin. All of the good, warm sexual sensations are gone. I miss those most of all. My breasts are cooler than the rest of my body. When it's cold, my breasts get cold. I'm a walker, and I try to counteract that by layering with light-weight clothes. Then my breasts don't get so frigid. On winter nights I use an electric blanket and flannel sheet to keep me warm. The rest of my body isn't cold; I just feel cold when I touch my breasts with my arms, because I have no feeling there.

Is there anything you would change about your reconstruction?

I would like to have the sexual feeling back, and I think someday they probably will know how to do that. If they do it in my lifetime, I'm going to be jealous. But that's the hardest part for me.

Has the mastectomy and reconstruction experience affected your feelings of sexuality and femininity?

Yes. Breasts are important; they are a turn-on. Now that my breasts are no longer sensitive, I don't have that response. As you get older, turn-ons are harder to come by. You are without that, and you have to have a pretty good relationship with the person you have sex with, whether it's a husband or another partner. The woman who goes through this has to know that this is a loss. Your femininity goes with the mastectomy; the reconstruction rebuilds that femininity. I never get in the shower that I don't look at myself and smile. I never feel devastated.

What are your scars like?

I don't scar badly. You would never even notice I had a scar on my right breast. The one on my left breast from the mastectomy is also faded and barely noticeable. It is a very thin line, and the nipple is grafted right over the major part of the scar. I do have a red scar from when the surgeon redid my armpit. It will take several years, but I know it will eventually turn white like the rest of my scars have done.

Did you have any problems or complications after your breast reconstruction?

No, none at all.

What coping mechanisms did you rely on to help you get through this experience?

I went through this experience fairly humorously. When I went in, knowing hospitals the way I do, I wrote "prophylactic" on my right breast and "modified radical" on my left, so that they didn't do the wrong side. When I went in to have my implants put in, I communicated further by writing "big" on my breasts. And when I had my nipple tattooed, I also had a little heart tattoo put on my side. I figured it took a lot of heart to get through it all.

Did you join a support group?

Yes, a breast reconstruction support group, and it was important to me. It has been a vital part of the healing process. You talk about this experience with your family, but they can't really relate. They've never had muscle spasms as the muscle adjusted to having a foreign body behind it. They don't know what it's like to lie on your stomach and feel like you are lying on rubber balls. They don't know when you move from side to side that you feel like you've got to push your breasts back into place, which you really don't. But it's a strange feeling because of the lack of sensation in your breast. I can go to my support group and talk all I want about my breasts and about reconstruction and nobody says, "Here she goes again." It's a group that wraps around you when you have problems. We share more than just our breasts: the good and the bad. With reconstruction, I knew everything that could go wrong. Women in the group share what has gone wrong with them. Doctors will tell you what might possibly happen, but in my support group I could see firsthand what did happen. Some people belong to the group for a short while and then leave, because they don't need it anymore. I still need it, not just as a means to express myself, but because it's payback time. The women in the group were wonderful for me; if I can be there for somebody else, then I want to do it. I am one of the lucky people. My reconstruction was aesthetically successful. It looks fantastic. I've not had any major problems. Not everyone is so lucky. One of my good friends who I brought to the group died 2 weeks ago. That was tough to deal with. But that helps me stay in touch with reality. It scares me, but it helps me.

In retrospect, do you feel that you made the right decision when you had a prophylactic mastectomy on your normal side?

Definitely. If I were allowed more hindsight, I would have done it 2 years earlier, when my breasts were merely high risk. I would recommend that anyone who is diagnosed with precancerous breasts get them taken off. What you gain from early prevention far outweighs the loss of a breast. It is just not worth carrying the time bombs around. And that is literally what I did. As my husband said, "Somebody has to hit you with a 2 by 4 to get your attention."

Was reconstruction worth the time, pain, and money? Would you do it again, and would you choose the same reconstructive approach?

I would do it again in a heartbeat. And if something were to go wrong with my implants tomorrow, I would probably have tissue expanders and implants again. I know that 20 or 30 years down the road I may have different options, but I really don't want any other major surgery unless it's absolutely necessary. Tissue expansion and implant placement are not major surgery. I also know that the flap procedure is available to me if my implants should fail or if something should happen and I cannot have implants anymore.

How did your family react to your mastectomies and reconstruction?

They were with me all the way; they were as involved in it as I was. We engaged in a lot of humor to keep us all going. My youngest daughter is the funny bone in the family, and she kept it light. She called the state motor vehicle department to get me a handicapped parking sticker as a double amputee. They didn't give me one, but that was her type of humor. Even now, she jokes, "Those are the biggest things I have ever seen, Mother; what do you do with them?" My husband chose to stay with me in the hospital and take care of everything, even though my aunt was director of nursing there and offered to stay. But I was more comfortable with him. It was a bonding time for us.

Are your daughters concerned about the threat of breast cancer? How has this experience affected them?

It has brought us much closer together. It has also made us aware of what's in their future. They have to be careful. My oldest daughter is very open and talks freely about her body. She is a tiny person who is very large-breasted. She is aware that her breasts could be time bombs and that cancer could come earlier for her than it did for me. It seems to be hitting younger people all the time. My gynecologist has recommended that she come in every 3 months to have her breasts checked. My younger daughter is 19 and is self-conscious about her body; no one sees her body. We found her a wonderful female gynecologist. Even so, my daughter said it was the most horrifying experience she's ever been through. She has even said things to me in jest, yet not really joking, "Thanks, Mom—look what you have given me to look forward to."

We have a friend who is 25 and was diagnosed with breast cancer in December. That brought it home, but my younger daughter still doesn't talk to me about it. I know that this experience has heightened both of my daughters' awareness of the threat of breast cancer. They talk about it with their friends. Their friends are all aware that I've had it, and when they come over to visit, they never meet my eyes when they are talking to me. Their eyes are right on breast level.

They ask me a hundred questions about how it feels. What does it feel like inside? How does it feel to touch? I'll say, "Why don't you touch my breasts and see?" I don't ever push. They always want to.

Was your plastic surgeon responsive to your needs?

When you are dealing with somebody on a very busy time schedule, you have to come prepared with questions written down or so well implanted in your head that you don't walk out and say, "Oh, I wanted to ask him this." My plastic surgeon hung the moon as far as I am concerned. He is probably the most caring man I've ever been around. He was responsive, but I wish he would slow down a little. He is in and out; he moves like a butterfly. Although all my needs were met, I would like him to sit down in a chair when he comes into my room. I would like him to talk to me after he has examined my breasts. I did learn to express these feelings to him. I would say, "I didn't get my money's worth yet; sit down, I want to talk." I didn't want small talk; I know his time is valuable, but I want to be able to express my concerns, to let him know when my breasts are uncomfortable. Some people are intimidated by doctors. And you can't be. You are paying their bills. You have a right to decide what's going to be done with your body. You have a right to tell your doctors how you are feeling about things and expect them to respond to that.

What advice would you like to give to other women about breast reconstruction?

Most people think reconstruction is just going to be more surgery. But it is different. It is uplifting; it's the healing process. You're back looking like you did. Don't let the threat of cancer stop you from doing it. I think people are so afraid once they have cancer that they worry that reconstruction is just an extension of their illness and it's not; it heals you. Cancer is terrifying, it is horrifying, and I will live with that every day. Wondering what's going to happen next. But reconstruction is nonthreatening; it's a rebuilding process. Although I was a whole person without my breasts, reconstruction restored me physically to the person I was.

JOAN: FROM CATERPILLAR TO BUTTERFLY

"Cancer has taught me to live life to the fullest. I used to be a caterpillar watching life go by, crawling instead of flying. Cancer made me realize that life is to be lived. Now I am a butterfly ready to take flight."

Joan shared these words of wisdom and triumph as she proudly displayed the brightly sequined butterfly that was attached to her equally vivid green sweater. "It's a stick-on," she confided in me, "that goes with anything I wear. It's a sign of hope, and it just makes me feel good. Butterflies are so beautiful. When I see them, I can't be sad." Joan was diagnosed with breast cancer over 5 years ago after a sudden bout of fatigue that literally stopped her in her tracks during her morning walk. A trip to the doctor and a subsequent mammogram resulted in a cancer diagnosis. Joan was stunned but philosophical about the news. Although her doctor originally thought a lumpectomy would suffice, the pathology report showed that the tumor margins were not clear of cancer cells, and she had one positive lymph node. She would require a mastectomy and subsequent chemotherapy. When she learned that she could also have breast reconstruction, Joan decided to have a mastectomy with immediate breast reconstruction with a latissimus dorsi (back) flap of her own natural (autologous) tissue. She chose this form of reconstruction because she did not want an implant and had sufficient back tissue to do the job.

Joan is a soft-spoken, no-nonsense individual. She works in a government office as an administrative assistant and is not a wealthy woman by any means. Now in her fifties, Joan is heavyset, with streaks of gray highlighting her medium-brown hair. Although she is not an animated talker, there is an earnestness about her that makes you lean forward to try to embrace the many layers of her personality. Breast cancer represented a special challenge for Joan. As a single woman, she lacked the support system provided by husband, children, or a significant other to help her cope with recovery or with the grieving process that usually accompanies this type of life-threatening illness. Other life events precipitated by her cancer led to changes that caused substantial stress. She was forced to give up her second job because of doctor's orders to slow down; she found herself strapped economically, unable to meet financial obligations without this supplementary income; and most recently, a job reassignment caused further concern.

Joan's story poignantly illustrates the complex emotions and life changes that breast cancer elicits and the special problems that single women may encounter. Joan prides herself on her optimistic and pragmatic approach to life. However, she also admits that once she let down her guard, fully 1 year after her cancer diagnosis and treatment, she was overcome by a deep, overriding sense of grief and depression unlike any she had ever experienced. Her faith finally pulled her through this particularly dark period. As Joan recalls, "I just gave it to God. I said, now you take it and do what you will." Since that time bouts of depression still overtake her, and she has had counseling to help her cope. She has also gone back to school to recapture her zest for life and her optimism about the future. Her hope is that by helping others she can also help herself.

How did you discover that you had breast cancer?

We have a wellness program at work and are allowed time to exercise. I walked every morning and was up to 2 miles a day. One day, halfway into my walk, I started getting very tired. It just kept getting worse. I finally had to sit down on somebody's wall outside their house. I thought, "Oh, my God, something's wrong with me. I don't know if I am going to be able to get back to work." I sat there for over 20 minutes and then started back real slow. I went to my doctor's office the very next day. I told him, "Something is desperately wrong with me." The fatigue was unbelievable. I had never experienced anything like that. He did some tests, and when he got to the breast exam, I could tell by his face that he had found something. He sent me for a mammogram.

They found a large, fast-growing cancer. I hadn't felt anything myself. Of course, I wasn't very regular about doing breast self-exams then, but I do it regularly now. As soon as they looked at my breast, they could actually see that it was dimpling, sort of pulling in. I thought that I knew all of the signs of cancer, because my mother died of pancreatic cancer. But that was a new one for me. I also never realized that fatigue could be part of it. After examining my breast and looking at my mammogram, the doctors were 99% sure that this was cancer.

How did you cope with your cancer diagnosis? What helped you to deal with this news?

Frankly, it was harder for my doctor to tell me than it was for me to hear it. I was sorry to put him through it, but that's life. I shed a few tears and then drove home. I thought, "Okay Joan, you have two choices. You can go home and cry all night, but then tomorrow you will go to work with red puffy eyes and a migraine. Or you can do something else." So I did something else. It was December 2, and I put up Christmas decorations—the tree, the lights, the candles, the whole deal. I sat there and enjoyed the glow. I said to myself, "You are about to start a long journey. The only way to survive it is to have a positive attitude. Positive energy will heal you, whereas negativity and depression will only make things worse." To me there was no choice; there was only one way to go.

What happened after the diagnosis? How did you find a surgeon?

My internist recommended a surgeon, but I didn't like him. He seemed cold and impersonal. He told me that he was 99% sure I had cancer; whenever he saw dimpling like mine, it was always cancer. I thought to myself, "I deserve better. Cancer is enough to experience; I don't want to be treated like a number." I told this doctor I needed a second opinion.

A friend at work referred me to another surgeon. I went to see him and took a pad of paper and tape recorder to help me remember what he said. I liked him right away. He was willing to talk to me as long as I needed, until all the questions were answered. He was the total opposite of the first surgeon. I said, "This is the one for me."

Did he explain your options?

Yes. He told me that I would probably be a candidate for a lumpectomy or that I could have a mastectomy with breast reconstruction. He was pretty confident that the lumpectomy would take care of it. They would do that in place of a biopsy, in case that was all that I needed.

What did the lumpectomy reveal? Why did you then have a mastectomy?

He did the lumpectomy as an outpatient procedure. When the pathology report came back, one tumor margin was not clear of cancer. My surgeon offered to go back in and clean it up, but I told him to "just take the whole breast. I don't need it. My life is more important." At this point I had entrusted my fate to God. I said "God, I don't know what to do. You guide me. I know you will show me what's best." And God did. Two weeks later I had a mastectomy with immediate breast reconstruction.

How did you learn about breast reconstruction?

The surgeon asked if I were interested in breast reconstruction. I hadn't thought about it. To me, plastic surgery was something that was either done by women who were vain and wanted bigger boobs or smaller butts, or it was for accident victims. You know—either vanity or trauma. After some thought, however, I decided I would like to consult with a plastic surgeon. My surgeon made an appointment for me to see one of the top plastic surgeons in our area.

Why did you decide to have breast reconstruction? What reconstructive procedure did you choose? What did this involve?

I decided that if I could have my breast rebuilt naturally, I would go ahead and do it. It would be something that I would do for myself. When the plastic surgeon explained all of the different types of reconstruction, I was just blown away. I'm going, "Whoa, I didn't know you could do all that, even tattooing and nipples." I thought, "This is neat."

I was determined not to have an implant. I was getting rid of cancer. I didn't want anything else put in, particularly something that might cause further concern. Since I didn't want an implant, a flap of my own tissue was the best option. I was not a good candidate for the TRAM (abdominal) flap because I was too heavy, and it would be a more dangerous operation for me. Fortunately, for once in my life, being overweight was a blessing. I had plenty of fatty tissue on my back. So I chose to have my breast reconstructed with an autologous latissimus dorsi (back) flap. It was a good choice. With this procedure, the plastic surgeon took a back flap of muscle and fatty tissue and tunneled it through my underarm incision to my chest wall to shape my new breast.

Why did you decide to have immediate breast reconstruction?

I was excited that everything could be taken care of in one major operation and I would have a breast when it was over. That meant one less hospital stay. This was my very first experience in a hospital, and I was relieved that I could just get it over with at one time and at less overall expense.

What was your primary goal in seeking breast reconstruction?

I wanted a rebuilt breast that looked like my natural one. I didn't want implants, because they might need to be redone periodically. That didn't make any sense to me. Why not use natural tissue and save yourself a lot of trouble down the road? I joked about it with everyone at the hospital. I said, "Well I went into the hospital with me and came out with me slightly rearranged."

How long were you hospitalized? Did you experience much pain?

I was in the hospital for 3 to 4 days. The pain wasn't bad. With the latissimus dorsi flap, they have to make a midback incision that also cuts the nerves in that area. Therefore I had no pain to deal with, just the strange sensation of dead weight. My new breast didn't hurt; it was just heavy. The nurses had me on the PCA (patient-controlled analgesia) pump so I could give myself doses of pain medicine. I only hit the button twice during the first day. I didn't need it after that.

I was out of bed the next day. From then on, I spent little time in bed. People were surprised to see me roaming around. I don't know what they expected. When someone knows you are a cancer patient, I suppose they expect to see you lying in bed, pale, looking like you're ready to die. I wasn't. I was walking the halls, talking to the nurses, and waving to everyone.

Was hospitalization as frightening as you imagined?

I was pleasantly surprised by the hospital experience; I thought it would be horrible. I had always joked that if I ever had to go to the hospital, someone would have to knock me out and take me there before I had time to think about it. But it wasn't that bad. Anyway, I had so much to do that I really didn't have time to worry about the hospital stay.

Did you go home with drains in place? How long did these stay in?

I had three drains inserted in the hospital. These bother a lot of people, but they weren't a problem for me. They took out two of them in the hospital. I went home with only one drain still in; it was removed after 3 weeks.

Did you have any restrictions on activity after your surgery?

Because my back flap was used to reconstruct my breast, I was not allowed to lift my arm above my shoulder for a while. I was also not allowed to drive for about 7 weeks. What struck me as funny is that I despise driving. I do it out of pure necessity; I really hate it. What I need is a chauffeur, and that's not going to happen any time soon. However, when they said I couldn't drive during recovery, I felt a burning desire to get out there and drive. Boy, did I want to drive a car! I wanted out of that apartment and into my car. I bugged my plastic surgeon every time I came in. Of course, once there was no restriction, I didn't want to do it anymore.

My activity was generally limited for about 3 months. I had to forego exercises until I healed. I got carried away in the hospital with my exercises. I had surgery in the morning and that night they let me walk across the room. The next day I started walking the wall with my fingers as they had instructed. What they hadn't told me was that I had to heal a bit before I began. Every time I did those exercises, I started bleeding. So I had to stop for a short time to make sure I was healed.

Did you have anyone who could help you when you went home? What special accommodations did you have to make for yourself?

Being single, I didn't have somebody to ask, "Honey, do this, Honey, make this appointment, or Honey, help me with this." I had to do it all myself. My father was there for the lumpectomy, but after the mastectomy Dad was getting ready to go into surgery himself, so I had no one I could rely on.

It took me a while to convince my plastic surgeon that I was going home alone and nobody would be there to do for me. He kept assuming that I would have help, and I kept insisting otherwise. After the third time, my message sank in. I said, "Read my lips, I am going home alone; now tell me what to do."

He told me that I should place anything that I normally reach for in my cabinets or above my head on the counter within easy reach. That worked, but the kitchen was a mess for a while. My clothes washer is one that I roll to the sink to hook up, so I had to move it to the middle of the kitchen before surgery so it could be plugged in easily without my having to exert too much effort. It was in the way, but it did the trick until I was able to lift my arm and move more easily.

How long did it take you before you returned to your normal level of activity once you got home? How long before you could return to work?

It was about a year before I was totally back to myself, even though my energy level is still not what it was. However, that never interfered with my work. I am stubborn, so I worked half-days the whole time. I just did what I had to do to save my life. It was important for me to keep working. It gave me a feeling of accomplishing something every day. Even if I only got one stupid letter typed, it was better than sitting at home vegetating.

Were they understanding at work about your illness? Were they supportive?

I work for a government agency and have done so for almost 12 years. They were my support system. They had recently started a program that allowed people to donate personal leave time to others. People at work literally supported me for almost 2 years by donating leave to me. I didn't have to worry about bills or where the money was coming from; all I had to worry about was getting better. So many people offered to help. They came out of the woodwork—people I didn't even know. They gave me a list of people who offered help. If I needed anyone to take me to get groceries, to go to doctors' appointments, or run errands, I could call on these individuals. They bought me a microwave when they learned that I would not be able to raise my arm above my head for a while. They even brought frozen dinners over so I wouldn't have to cook. They were absolutely amazing.

What was your reaction to chemotherapy? Did you experience any problems or side effects?

It wasn't as bad as I thought it was going to be, even though I did have to adjust to feeling queasy all the time. I enjoyed the nurses; we had a good time. I also enjoyed going to the treatments. I know that sounds crazy, but for me it represented one step closer to getting better.

At the first chemotherapy treatment they had trouble finding good veins. It took a very long time. To avoid having this problem each time, they decided to put a port in. It's a type of tube that is inserted in your chest and goes into your veins or one of your main arteries. It stays in for the whole course of treatment. The part that you can feel in your chest is about the size of a quarter, and it's slightly raised. They were able to insert the needle directly into the port rather than into my veins. The port stayed in for 1 year.

I was pleasantly surprised at how far chemo has come since I witnessed my mother's treatment for pancreatic cancer. She was deathly ill and hospitalized for an entire week, throwing up the whole time. I thought, "Oh God, I guess this is what I have to look forward to." But it wasn't that bad. I had a treatment every few weeks for a couple of hours each time. Then I knew that I had about 2 hours before I was going to be sick. So I would get something I enjoyed eating on the way home, and I would totally indulge myself until I started vomiting. I only became really ill and vomited once during treatment; after that, I was just queasy and tired. The fatigue has stayed with me even today. Most of the people I know who've had chemo never fully regain their energy. I thought I would. I thought that once the chemicals were out of my system, everything would go back to the way it was—plenty of energy. But it isn't the same.

I also lost all of my hair except for a few strands. I wore turbans until my wig was ready. I had three different turbans and decorated them with various pins and brooches. People started saying, "What's she got on today?" and they would check my turban to see what I had pinned to it that day. That was fun.

Did you have your nipple-areola reconstructed? Did you require any additional adjustments or secondary procedures?

Yes, I had my nipple and areola redone. That was part of the package. My nipple was rebuilt with the same tissue that they used for the reconstruction—the local tissue on my breast. The areola was created later by tattooing.

Some other adjustments were made during the same outpatient surgery. I had swelling under my arm after the first surgery that felt like a ball of extra tissue. It was really annoying. My plastic surgeon kept assuring me that the swelling would go down, but it didn't. It bothered me a lot. Finally I said, "This swelling needs to go." My plastic surgeon said he could remove it with liposuction when he did the nipple reconstruction. I said, "While you are in there suctioning, could you just slide the suction down and get some of the fat out of my stomach and hip area?" He said that a lot of women make that request, and he could do it all at the same time. So at the time I was having my nipple reconstructed, they also removed the swelling under my arm and suctioned my stomach area.

When I healed, my areola was tattooed in the office. That was fun. The nurse who was doing the tattooing used the good breast as a palette to match the different colors. We mixed the colors to get as close a match as possible. I chose the final color.

Did your breast reconstruction meet your expectations? Would you choose to have reconstructive surgery again?

Yes, I would do it again in a heartbeat. Reconstructive surgery exceeded my expectations; it was much better than I thought it would be. I would also choose the same operation. It was the right one for me.

Are you satisfied with your breast appearance? Are your breasts symmetrical?

I'm very satisfied. I thought the reconstructed breast would look different from the other one, but it really doesn't. I was just amazed at how careful he was to make sure they are exactly the same. They even droop the same; I couldn't believe it. I really expected some sort of a difference because one is natural. The other one is natural tissue, but it is back tissue. My results are amazing; you can't even tell I had it done. The scars are barely noticeable. My new breast looks just like the other one.

How does your reconstructed breast feel? Does it have sensation?

That's the only thing that's different. It's warm like the other one, but there is no feeling in it. It doesn't get hard when I get cold like the natural one does. I can feel pressure, but if I scratch it, I can't feel that.

What do your scars look like? Where are they located?

I have one back scar, two breast scars, and one underarm scar. The first time I saw the scars I said, "Whoa!" But now they have faded. There are just little tiny marks. They are not a big deal.

Did you have any surprises from your breast reconstruction?

Because they used my back muscle and fatty tissue to make a breast, it still functioned as if it were a back muscle moving my arm. In other words, when I move that arm, my breast moves automatically, because it is all connected. It is strange. The first time it happened I thought, "Hey, what was that?" It just looks funny, and I told myself, "Well maybe it's a good thing I'm not married. I guess I'd better get used to it, because it always happens." No one told me this would happen. I just reached for something one day and all of a sudden that breast went boing! I figured it out, once I stopped laughing. It was really funny; it took me by total surprise. I was thinking, "Okay, why is my breast doing that?" and then I sat and thought about it and figured it out. It's back tissue; it's still connected, so it seems only natural that when I move my arm, the muscle still works.

Were your doctors helpful to you through this process?

Yes, I got the information that I needed, but sometimes I had to practically stand in the doorway to get my plastic surgeon to stay put. He is very busy, I know, but sometimes I just needed to get his attention. I had to say, "Wait a minute, I have some questions." Then he was fine. He would stop and answer whatever questions I had. The oncologist learned early on that I was somebody who wanted to know absolutely everything; I didn't want anything hidden from me at all. Once he realized that, our relationship was 100% better. He was not accustomed to people wanting to know everything. He said most of his patients don't really desire that much information; they just want enough to get by, just a little bit. But I said, "I don't want you to hide anything. This is my body, it's my life, and I want to know everything." I went in with questions every time, and after the first two or three visits, he realized that this was the pattern. This was who I was, and this was how I worked. Then it was okay. He would do the examination and say, "Okay, hit me with the questions. I'm ready." Then we would go through my list, and he would answer every question.

How could your doctors have been more helpful?

They talked to me, explained my options, but didn't direct me to any outside resources. I have always felt that every doctor needs to be prepared to hand a patient diagnosed with cancer a booklet with questions and answers and available resources. I didn't have a clue. You've heard this terrible thing, and you say, "I have cancer? What do I do about it?" Somebody needs to be there immediately to tell you. Someone said, "Make sure you ask the right questions." But I didn't know what the right questions were, and that's where most people are. Doctors should be a resource for patients.

Do you think there are special challenges for a single woman coping with something like this?

Most of my friends who have gone through this experience are married with children. They have family right there—that's both good and bad. It is hard for the family, but at the same time you have people there to help you do things. You have shoulders to cry on, somebody to hug you and tell you it's going to be okay. When you're single and alone, you don't have that; you have to find it elsewhere. I was lucky, because I received a lot of that support at work. Also, I wasn't as needy, because I just didn't go through the emotional thing at the beginning. I never do anything like anybody else. It was not until I hit my 1-year anniversary that I fell apart.

How did you fall apart? Why do you think it happened?

I just fell apart. I was caught completely unaware. At first, after I was diagnosed and then after the surgery, I kept waiting for the stages of grief that everyone told me to expect. They said that you have to go through all the steps, just like a death. So I waited and I waited, but it never happened. And I really didn't see the point anyway, because I never asked, "Why me?" For me, the question was always, "Why not me?" I mean really, there is no point in denying cancer. It's just something that happens.

Then one day I was sitting in front of my computer at work, and one minute I was talking and the next minute I was sobbing for no apparent reason. I was fine; I knew that. I knew I would be cured. I just lost it. I went to one of the ladies I work with and she hugged me and said, "Just let it out. It's all right. You took care of all the technical stuff, and now your body is making you listen to it, because you have ignored it so far." She was right; she was absolutely right. I needed somebody to tell me it was okay to give in to my emotions. I had been thinking, "This is stupid. I'm fine. What am I doing this for? This is unnecessary; I don't need this." But I was wrong. I had to go through it.

Was there someone you could talk to about your feelings?

That has proved to be a problem for me. I am an excellent listener, and I can help other people, but it is really difficult for me to reach out to somebody when I need help. One of the biggest challenges was confronting this whole disease process by myself. I've lived alone for a long time, and I'm accustomed to being the one doing everything for myself and being totally self-sufficient. All of a sudden, however, I wasn't self-sufficient anymore. Cancer has a way of making you dependent. I didn't want to admit that, and it took a couple of friends sitting me down and saying, "Joan, you have to realize you do need help now. We all need help sometimes. We have all these people who want to help you, and when you tell them no, you are not allowing them that chance to feel good because they helped you. It makes them feel good if they can do something." It is such a helpless feeling when you see someone you care about going through something and there is nothing you really can do. I try to help others now whenever I can to make this coping process a little easier for them.

Have you had any further problems with depression?

Although I am feeling positive now, you would have seen another side of me if you had been here 3 weeks ago. Then I was in total depression, crying all the time. I had been that way for about 3 months. I don't really know why I get depressed. The first depression started with the cancer recovery process. I expected to go through a grieving process, which is part of the loss and the cancer experience; however, I never expected that the depression would come back. Since that time, I have found out that this depression recurs for some people. Evidently that's the way it is for me, because this is the third or fourth time I've had this, and it got worse. I have seen a therapist, and that didn't help. I had to let God help me get through it. After all, he got me through this whole thing in the first place. So I let him handle it, and the depression went away. It comes out of the blue; I can't point to anything in particular that triggers it. Now I realize that this is something I am going to have to deal with. Recently I talked to a few ladies, and they said they have also experienced these bouts of depression. That's kind of hard to deal with; you don't function like you should. You aren't happy, but you aren't really sad, either. I am fine one minute and the next minute, bam! Kind of like a little gray cloud that follows you around and once in a while drops a little rain on you.

What contributes to these depressive feelings?

There are so many pressures and stresses to deal with that coping is not always easy. It's difficult when you're single. You only have one income to depend on. My doctors won't let me work a second job anymore. I used to do that, but now, because of the stress I am prone to, they have said no. I don't earn much, and with the additional expense of my illness, I can't pay the bills, and creditors are calling. I leave the answering machine on all the time, but I just can't live that way. I also have more pressure at work. They assigned me to a new job 6 months ago; it was either that or no job at all. They have given me a year to learn it. I like it better than I did at first, but it's not what I want to be doing. So there have been a number of pressures that have probably contributed to my depression.

What do you do to help yourself stay positive and to keep your spirits up?

I try to be good to myself. Sometimes I treat myself to movies or buy something pretty that I might not have purchased before. It is just an extravagance, something that captures my fancy, like a lovely scarf. It's all about enjoying life. I like to get out and walk, to take pleasure in nature, to sit and meditate, to talk to the birds, to read good books, to listen to nice music, to dance, to indulge myself in activities that bring joy. I have joined a singing group: it relaxes me and helps to relieve stress. I have also gotten back into childhood pursuits, such as coloring books. Some people say, "At your age, with a coloring book?" But why not? I've found the little child in me again. I had lost that child for a while. But she's back now. So I color sometimes. When I get a chance, I go to a special camp for adult cancer patients; it is just wonderful. It's on a lake in a gorgeous setting. They pamper you there. It is a safe haven. No explanations are ever needed, because we are all coming from the same place.

Going back to school has been a big step for me; it is a symbol of my effort to improve my life. It is probably the most significant, positive action I've taken to reverse the pressures that cause my depression. It's both frightening and exciting, but I'm committed to it.

Why are you going back to school? Has the adjustment been difficult?

People ask me, "Why is someone your age going back to college?" My response is, "Why not?" If you are happy with your life, terrific, but I am not, and I intend to do something to change it. I'm trying to reclaim my opportunities; cancer has given me the second chance that I needed.

I am just starting and there are challenges. I had 2 years of college 30 years ago. I was a sophomore, and believe it or not, after 30 years I'm still a sophomore. They accepted almost all of my former credits. It's easier going back now, because schools are gearing themselves toward older students. Increasingly, they offer special programs to help us and they seem to have respect for older students, so that's good. The problem I'm having now is that I have 30 years of catch-up to do. It's also tough finding the money to go to school; I rob Peter to pay Paul. I can't pay the creditors, but I know I have to go to school if I want to have a better life. It's an investment in my future.

What impact has cancer had on your life?

Cancer has totally turned my life around. I used to consider myself a caterpillar; now I'm a butterfly, experiencing the beautiful flowers, the world, and life itself. I used to just inch my way along and watch the world go by. I'd say, "I'd like to try that someday. Oh, well, I'll get to it later." Now I know that there are no guarantees. I seize the opportunity of the moment. If there is something I want to do now, I do it if at all possible. Life is so much better now. I've gone back to school, I've spread my wings, and I'm intent on finding a new direction in life.

Cancer made me realize that I was on the wrong path. God wanted me doing something else. I used to sit and wait and wonder why people did not do for me. Now I reach out to others, and I do for them. You heal yourself when you help others to heal. It is a process that grows and blossoms. Now I have a goal: I am going to use my education to counsel cancer patients. At this time I'm doing it as a volunteer until I have the training to do it as a professional. I get so much joy out of it, much more than I give. It is a gift to be able to help someone in need.

People think of cancer as a negative, but it can become a positive. It has for me. Cancer was a wake-up call. It refocused me and redirected me to the right path, the one I am on now. I don't know where it is going to lead me, but I am going to enjoy the journey.

MARCY: YOU CAN'T TELL THE DIFFERENCE

"It's amazing! If you didn't know that I had breast cancer and reconstruction, you could never tell. Just look at these pictures; aren't they great? My husband is so proud; he shows them to everyone."

Slim and pretty, Marcy's face is framed by bobbed dark hair. This former teacher is married with two small children. She blushes as she pulls several photographs out of her purse and hands them to me. Her delight in her restored appearance is infectious. "These were taken of me wearing the same bathing suit before my mastectomy and after my tissue expansion reconstruction, and you just can't tell the difference. If anything, I look better now."

Marcy's breast cancer was discovered on her first mammogram, right before her fortieth birthday. Fortunately, it was in its earliest stages, making her prognosis excellent. Nevertheless, decisions about which treatment approach was best for her were not always easy, even though her husband, a cancer specialist, helped her to sort through her options and find the best care possible. She is well informed and the type of woman who wants to know all the facts. Because of her husband's profession, she looks to physicians for expertise and sound advice and does not come to the doctor-patient relationship with the trepidation that many others exhibit. Even so, Marcy frequently found herself puzzled and needing more information and direction in selecting the best treatment for her breast cancer and the right reconstructive technique.

How did you decide between lumpectomy and mastectomy?

That was frustrating. I kept asking my cancer surgeon what he would recommend. I said, "If I were your wife, what would you do?" All he could say was, "I can't tell you what to do."

I realize it's hard, especially for male doctors, because they feel that breast cancer is a uniquely female problem and they don't know what to make of it. But patients come to doctors for their expertise. I hope that doctors haven't become afraid to recommend a course of action for their patients or to say that mastectomy can cure. I wanted some direction, and I persisted in asking him what he would do. He said, "I can't tell you what to do." I protested, "I want you to tell me what is the best thing to do. That's why I'm here; you're the expert—you should know." We kept going around in circles; it was frustrating. He said, "You have to do what you feel is right. You have to make that decision." But I was coming to him for an answer, and he wasn't willing to give me one. He said, "You can have a mastectomy or a lumpectomy, or at this point you can choose to do nothing. We can watch it; it is so early."

I said, "Does a mastectomy guarantee me better results than a lumpectomy?" He replied noncommittally, "Lumpectomy is an option many people have chosen, and they have done well after 5-year and 10-year follow-up." I saw another cancer surgeon for another opinion, and he said the same thing.

It was frustrating not to be able to have my doctor tell me what the best course of action was. There is so much controversy surrounding breast cancer, so many different options. I wanted him to say, "This is the way to go." But I guess maybe they really don't know.

Why did you choose mastectomy over lumpectomy? Are you happy with your choice?

I knew in my heart that a mastectomy was the best choice for me. I didn't want to worry about a possible recurrence. I couldn't put more value on saving a breast than on saving my life. Long-term survival is important; I want to watch my children grow.

I'm very happy with my decision; I would do the same thing tomorrow. Knowing that I could have the reconstruction made my decision for mastectomy that much easier. It took away the anxiety. The only anxiety I experienced throughout the whole ordeal was when I had to wait those 2 days in the hospital before I got the final pathologist's report back. My cancer was so early that it would have been 4 to 5 years before I would have felt it on self-exam.

I would recommend what I did to anyone. After the mastectomy they were able to study the whole breast, and they discovered that the cancer was multifocal. Had I had the lumpectomy, they would not have gotten every little area of cancer. For me, the procedure I had was the right one. Of course, I didn't know that 100% until after it had been done, but in hindsight, it was.

Why did you seek breast reconstruction?

It is comparable to someone losing a limb and wearing an artificial leg, losing an eye and wanting a glass eye. Your breast is a part of you. It doesn't define who you are sexually, but you want it back. You want to be whole.

Sexual feelings between my husband and me were fine following the mastectomy and before reconstruction. I didn't have reconstruction to feel sexy, just to feel complete—to be normal, not necessarily bigger or better than before. I wanted to dress normally, to not be concerned with what I could wear and what I couldn't. I felt I was young, just 40, and I wanted to look normal for me, for my husband, and for my children.

How did you learn about breast reconstruction?

One of my husband's scrub nurses gave him your book to give to me. It turns out she had a double mastectomy and reconstruction. My husband was astounded. He said, "I operate with you every day. I never noticed anything different, and you never mentioned it." She said, "Well, I don't talk about it, but this book was a tremendous help to me. I thought it would be a big help to your wife."

I came home that weekend and read the book from cover to cover and said, "Thank goodness, everything is going to be fine." That next week I went in to have my mastectomy and never once gave it a second thought or felt that I was making a mistake.

How did you select your plastic surgeon?

He was recommended by my husband's surgical colleagues. When I was diagnosed with breast cancer, my husband called everyone he knew and asked, "Where should we go? Who is the best?" They said we had the best right here. It made it easy. My surgeon also recommended the same plastic surgeon. We kept hearing his name so often that it gave us a feeling of confidence and security. We never thought to look elsewhere.

Have you been happy with your plastic surgeon? Was he responsive to your needs?

He was just wonderful. He went over the different reconstructive options with me, talked about immediate versus delayed reconstruction, answered my questions, and was very reassuring. He was confident in his ability to reconstruct my breast, and he took away any fear or doubt that I had. His staff was also wonderful, especially the nurses. When I have problems, I call. It has been a terrific experience.

Why did you decide not to have immediate reconstruction?

My surgeon and plastic surgeon were at two different hospitals, and I felt comfortable with the surgeon at the local hospital; it was where my husband practiced. We were well known there. I wasn't sure what operation I would choose for reconstruction, but I knew I wanted to go ahead with the mastectomy. I decided to get that out of the way and then take time to read the book, talk to other people, and decide what type of reconstruction I wanted. The plastic surgeon also gave me names of former patients and suggested that I call them and talk to them.

Did your plastic surgeon and cancer surgeon coordinate your care, even though they were at different hospitals?

Yes. They spoke before my cancer surgery, and my plastic surgeon told my cancer surgeon what type of incision would be best for the reconstruction and how much skin to leave.

What type of reconstructive operation did you choose?

I considered all of the options and decided on tissue expansion with simple reconstruction with an expander implant. During my recovery from the mastectomy, I met a woman who had the abdominal flap. She was unhappy with it. She had her reconstructive surgery a number of years ago, and I'm sure it was not the state-of-the art operation it is today. Even so, she said that she still can't sit up straight in bed; she can't bend over and pick up a basket of laundry. She has never felt right; she has a very uncomfortable feeling in her midchest area, where she thinks the flap was turned. She said that if she had it to do over, she would not have such an elaborate operation. It was a huge surgery with a long recovery period. I didn't want anything that dramatic. Also, I wasn't rebuilding a huge breast. I didn't need a lot of tissue. I am not that large physically, so I didn't feel they would have a whole lot to work with anyway. So I eliminated the possibility of an abdominal flap.

We talked about the latissimus dorsi back flap. Implants are often used along with that flap. I rejected that option, because I figured why subject myself to a major flap procedure with additional scars on my back. I decided I might as well just go with the simple implant.

My husband and I came back to see the plastic surgeon with our decision and said, "What do you think of this; would tissue expansion with an implant be good?" He said he thought it would work in my situation. This was really a good solution for me, because it gave me control over my breast size with minimal discomfort.

Why did you decide that implant reconstruction was the right choice for you?

I wanted reconstruction; I wanted the breast back, but I didn't want to go through a horrendous process to get it. I wanted the simplest, easiest operation. I wanted a nice cosmetic effect with the least amount of trauma and disruption in my life. My children are young, 7 and 11; I wanted as little time away from them as possible.

Did you have any surgery on your opposite breast?

Yes, I had an augmentation. We decided to do a small saline implant on the other side to give that breast the same type of lift and look; plus, since I was going to have implants, I thought it would be a nice bonus if I could go a little bit bigger than I was. My plastic surgeon thought he could do that without any trouble. Augmentation was not what I initially requested, however. Originally I wanted to have a prophylactic mastectomy with an implant on the other side.

Why did your surgeon dissuade you from having a prophylactic mastectomy? Why did you want a preventive mastectomy?

My surgeon said that my type of cancer is not normally bilateral, and he discouraged it. Even so, I knew by just having breast cancer in one breast you have a higher risk of getting it in the other breast, and why would I want that? Why not just do both? But all the doctors said that I was being a little too reactionary, because of my type of cancer and the fact that I had no family history. I was not in a high-risk group.

I thought, "Well, if it happened once, why wouldn't it happen again?" They told me yearly mammograms would be able to catch it soon enough. They said that the pocket for the implant would be already made, and it would be a very easy procedure. So I didn't have a prophylactic mastectomy and implant. Instead, I just had an augmentation with an implant. I still think that the prophylactic mastectomy would have given me more peace of mind.

Describe your hospitalization.

I went into the hospital at 6:00 AM and had the procedure done at 8:00 AM; I went home at 9:00 the next morning.

Did you have much pain after reconstruction? How did it compare with the pain you experienced after your mastectomy?

The mastectomy was a breeze. I was in the hospital for 3 nights, and when I went home I felt almost no pain. I was back doing almost everything I wanted to do within 10 days. I had no complications. It went great. I wanted to start reconstruction as soon as possible. We waited 3 months, because my plastic surgeon felt that would allow enough time for my tissues to heal.

I had a lot of pain after reconstruction. That was surprising; none of the other women I spoke with mentioned that reconstruction was painful. When I came for the preoperative workup, I was asked if I generally have a lot of pain. I said no; generally I have a very high tolerance for pain. With the mastectomy, I was pain free after the first day, and then I took Tylenol. So they didn't order any special pain medicine for me, and I agreed with that decision. But I was wrong. I can remember waking up in recovery and not being able to move, not being able to take a breath. I think I was hyperventilating. The nurse kept telling me to calm down. If anyone touched me, I just gasped. I felt a tremendous burning sensation in my chest. I would try to take a breath and it would hurt. Both sides hurt. When the nurse asked if I would like something for pain. I said, "Yes!" She said, "They have nothing ordered for you. They didn't think you would need it." That was my fault. It was very painful, and I don't know why. I talked to people who didn't think it was that painful. When I spoke with people later, they admitted that it might have hurt at first, but they really didn't remember anymore, and since I didn't seem to think it would hurt, they hadn't wanted to tell me any different. I thought, oh, thanks!

They gave me pain medication when I went home and that took care of the pain, but it would wear off. It took about 4 days before I felt better. I could move around, but trying to sit up or turn over in bed was painful.

Did you have much bruising after your reconstruction?

The breasts themselves were not black and blue. But on my side and across the front of my chest there was a little bruising; it healed fairly quickly.

Did you experience much swelling with the reconstruction and augmentation?

Yes, after my surgery, my breasts were huge and swollen. At first I was petrified. I said, "Oh, my God, I've gone overboard. What am I going to do? This is terrible." My husband said, "This is great." I thought, "This is too much." But then the swelling started going down and my reaction was, "No, stop—it's going too low—they're not going to be big enough!" I went from one extreme to another, but then things leveled out and everything was fine.

How long before you could return to normal activity?

After 7 days I started feeling better and I wanted to drive; they said I could try it if I felt up to it. We have a Ford Explorer with no power steering, and the steering wheel was hard to turn, but I wanted to drive. I wanted to get back on the road, pick up my children. I knew as soon as I left my driveway it was a mistake. We have a curve in the driveway, and I could barely make the turn. I couldn't turn the wheel. As long as I was going straight, I was fine; a turn really hurt. I continued on and then got back home; I didn't drive for another week. I think I set myself back a few days. After the second week I could do just about anything. I don't do aerobics or jog; I'm not big into physical activity right now, so I wasn't anxious to get back to something strenuous. For me, normal activity was just regular housework, driving, walking, and riding my bicycle.

Describe the expansion process. When did it begin, and how often was your expander inflated? How long did it take?

I started about 2 weeks after my reconstructive surgery. My skin was expanded about every 3 weeks. I went to the office and it took about 20 minutes. It was very easy. They have a device inside of you, and they plug the syringe into this device that hooks up like an IV line. Saline is injected to expand it. You just lie on the exam table, and they infuse whatever quantity they have determined is needed to expand your breast that day. You can feel it gradually dripping in. One time they were going to put a little more in, but it was feeling tight and a little sore, so I asked to stop for the day. I had a busy weekend coming up. It was nice to have that control.

I had three sessions, then further expansion was delayed because the incision opened up. I started in January, and the expansion process was completed by May, so the total process took approximately 4 months. Then during an outpatient procedure my tissue expander was exchanged for a permanent saline implant.

Was tissue expansion painful?

It is a full feeling—not painful, just tight every time it's expanded. Then after a few days it gives and feels normal until the next expansion. I guess the tissues stretch so they will be ready for the permanent implant and so the breast will appear more normal. Sometimes I took Tylenol right after it was done, but that is all I ever needed.

Have you had any problems?

No problems on the right side with the augmentation. The only problem I had was on the left side with the expander. My incision opened a little bit; it wasn't a serious problem, but we had to delay the tissue expansion for several weeks.

Did your surgeon know why that happened?

After the first expansion session I still had Steri-Strips covering the incision; we didn't take them off and reapply them. When the breast tissue stretched, my plastic surgeon thinks the expansion process might have caused a tape burn, causing my incision to open. After a few weeks it healed, and then we left all the Steri-Strips off. I've never had another problem.

Do you have any restrictions now?

No. We went to Florida after my surgery, and I tried to swim; that was difficult because it was hard to stretch. But everything else I can do fine.

Are you going to have nipple-areola reconstruction?

Yes; I want my breast to be complete. When we were in Florida, I wore a regular bathing suit. The only time there was a noticeable difference between my breasts was when I came out of the water and was cold, and you could see that I had a nipple on one side and not on the other. I have seen reconstructed nipples on other women, and they looked beautiful. Someone described it as "the icing on the cake." If you're going to go this far, why stop? Why not take it through to completion? People who see the pictures think my breast reconstruction is marvelous. I tell them I am a work in progress; I am not finished yet. They are very impressed. A lot of women I've talked to who have seen the bathing suit pictures say now we know that if it happens to us, we won't be so afraid, because we can see what can happen afterward.

Aesthetically, are you pleased with your breast appearance?

Yes. Here are some pictures of me wearing the same bathing suit before the mastectomy and after the reconstruction. My husband took these to the hospital and showed them to the nurses on the floor who had taken care of me. I was so embarrassed. The results are marvelous.

Does the reconstructed breast have any feeling or sensation? How does it compare to the opposite breast that was augmented?

Sensation is normal in the right breast that had no mastectomy and a simple implant. There is feeling in the left reconstructed breast, but it's blunted. When I push on my left breast, I can feel the pressure, but not much sensation.

Is there any sexual feeling or sensitivity?

To be perfectly honest, I have avoided sexual contact on the left side; I don't feel right yet. My husband has no problems with it. But I don't feel finished yet. The shape of the breast still needs some adjustment; it is fuller on the top and below. There is no nipple. I still feel we are working on it.

If you had to do it over, would you have reconstruction again? Would you have the same kind of reconstructive approach?

I would do exactly the same thing. It was the right approach for me, and I'm very happy with what I did.

Was your husband supportive? How did he react to the idea of your having breast reconstruction?

He was wonderful. Being a cancer surgeon himself, he understood what we had to face. My husband deals with cancer every day, and he has to tell patients they have cancer. The idea of disfigurement never entered into it; the total focus was on the cure. The minute we found the cancer it was, "We can take care of it," and "If you want, you can have reconstruction," and "This isn't the end of the world." He was finding out as much information as he could and as quickly as he could so we could make the decisions we needed to make.

He supported me all the way and went through the whole learning process with me. I remember one funny incident when my husband and I were looking over the pictures of some patients that the plastic surgeon's nurse was showing us. My husband asked, "Where are the photos of women who've had their mastectomies and were reconstructed?" It turned out that was just what we were looking at, but you couldn't tell. It was very reassuring.

It was a learning experience for both of us. Right before I was to have reconstructive surgery, one of my plastic surgeon's patients who also had a simple implant reconstruction came to see my husband for a medical problem. As he was taking her history, he asked her what other surgeries she had had. When she said that she had a mastectomy and reconstruction, he asked her who her plastic surgeon was and if she was happy with him. She said that she had gone to my plastic surgeon and thought he was wonderful. My husband told her that I had just had a mastectomy and was about to have breast reconstruction and she just said, "Well, let me show you!" She was so proud and thrilled with her result. He immediately had her call me on the phone, and she talked to me from his office for 20 minutes, telling me how wonderful everything was, what a positive experience she had, and how terrific my plastic surgeon was. She offered to meet with me and show me how she looked. My husband came home and said, "She looked incredible. She looked wonderful, and you would never have known." He said, "I'm a doctor looking, and I would never have known. She looked that good."

What about this experience would you like to share with other women?

I would like to tell women not to risk their lives to save a breast. I was never very big-breasted. That was never the focus of my feelings of self-worth or femininity. Maybe if it had been, I would have felt differently. Not all women feel that way. In fact, I talked to a woman doctor who had breast cancer; her husband also was a doctor, and he said mastectomy was the way to go for her type of cancer. She said she couldn't or wouldn't have a mastectomy. She couldn't do it; it would be very difficult. I said, "But Susan, when you are faced with the statistics?" She said, "I know, but I don't think I could deal with it emotionally." Even her husband admitted that her breasts had always been very important to her, and that is why she couldn't face breast loss. I never had that feeling. Anyway, with what can be accomplished with reconstruction today, I wouldn't take the risk of keeping my breast; I wouldn't want to live day in and day out worrying if the cancer is still there. Is it coming back? I wouldn't want to make cancer an everyday part of my life. I'd want to take the form of treatment that would be the most definitive and proceed with my life.

Did knowledge about reconstruction make it easier to cope with your cancer surgery?

Knowing that it could be fixed made all the difference. Knowing that, my attitude was let's get on with it—take care of it, get rid of it, and move ahead, as opposed to, "Oh no, this is terrible." I went to my mastectomy almost jubilant; I wanted to get this breast off and rebuilt again. So I coped pretty well, because I knew I could have reconstruction. I could do something.

It's the feeling of powerlessness that gets you. Around Christmas we were having company, and a string of Christmas lights went off on the tree. When that happened, I just lost it. I decompensated; I panicked. My sister was astounded. She laughed at me and said, "You had cancer, had a mastectomy, and you never said anything. Now you are getting upset about your Christmas tree?" Well, this was important, because I couldn't fix it. I had people coming, and I couldn't get the lights on. But my breast I could fix. I could take care of it. That made all the difference. I was in control.

How have your friends reacted to your breast reconstruction?

They didn't realize how easily breast reconstruction could be accomplished. They never expected me to continue to look so normal throughout the whole procedure, even with the expansion. My friends have just been amazed. They think breast reconstruction is marvelous. Knowing about my experience and about the possibility of breast reconstruction has done wonders for their peace of mind. Now they know that should it happen to them, it is not the end of the world.

FAITH: I COULDN'T FACE BREAST LOSS

"Please be sure to tell your readers that not only people with beautiful bodies are vain. We with the run-of-the-mill-type bodies also want to have the best image of ourselves that we can."

Thus began the letter that I received from Faith several weeks after our interview at her plastic surgeon's office. Faith is a pretty young woman with short, dark hair and glasses. She was only 28 when her breast cancer was discovered. She courageously investigated her treatment options. As a young, single woman, Faith was unwilling to face breast loss. Unfortunately, living in a small town, she had few people to consult about reconstructive options. There was only one general surgeon in town, and no plastic surgeons. The only women she knew who had had mastectomies were considerably older than she was. Therefore she took it upon herself to contact a Cancer Helpline in a neighboring state and request information on breast cancer and breast reconstruction. The information she received proved a godsend, and she studied everything she could until she found the procedure that she felt was right for her. She used the same research methods to locate a medical center, surgeon, and plastic surgeon to do an immediate breast reconstruction. Faith braved this trauma alone, traveling to the hospital by herself.

She cried through most of our discussion, taking off her glasses to wipe her eyes periodically. This experience was still very fresh and her emotions overwhelming. As she explained, "Doctors and nurses really need to stress that a person is going to be very emotional after any surgery, especially this one. I'd like to see a person assigned to the breast cancer team whose function is to provide emotional support.

Because you already have a permanent breast shape in place, people tend to believe you're 'all well.' You are not. You still have to cope with surgery, with having a mastectomy, and with having cancer."

Faith chose one of the most complex and extensive methods of breast reconstruction: an immediate TRAM free flap, a microsurgical operation in which her abdominal tissue and muscle were transferred to her breast and the nerves and blood vessels were reconnected under an operating microscope. She was in surgery for approximately 10 hours, and although she would have liked to have had better information about her operation, she is delighted with the technique that she selected.

How did you discover your breast cancer?

I found a lump on January 1. Three days later, I went to see my family doctor. He felt two lumps and I had a mammogram, but nothing showed up. My doctor said, "It's just fibrocystic disease. It's common in big-busted women. Nothing to worry about." He referred me to a surgeon who also thought they were just cysts. But I wasn't satisfied. My gut told me something was wrong, and I wanted the lumps out. The surgeon tried to discourage me. He said, "You're 28. You'll have a scar." I told him, "I don't care; let's get these lumps out and see what they are." So he removed them, and he was right: what we had felt were cysts. But when he lifted the cysts, he found extensive intraductal carcinoma.

How did you get your information about breast cancer and breast reconstruction?

I saw a breast cancer documentary on TV. It was presented by a hospital in North Carolina. They had an 800 number; I called it and they sent me a packet of literature on breast cancer and breast reconstruction. This information was wonderful, because it gave me something to read to base my decisions on. I also searched the Internet. There is a wealth of information there—almost too much. I'm a research person. I have to know all the options before I make the decision. By the time I got my second opinion, I knew what I wanted done.

Why did you decide to have a mastectomy to treat your cancer?

The doctor in my town suggested a lumpectomy and irradiation, but I went to a neighboring city for a second opinion. That doctor said I needed a mastectomy for the type of cancer I had. I took the pathology slides to this second surgeon, and he had a complete pathology report done on them. I was devious, however; I took the old report out and said, "Here are the slides; tell me what this is." They had another pathologist look at them, and his diagnosis came back word for word the same as my other pathology report. The surgeon told me to have a mastectomy and get it over with. He said, "If you were my wife, there would be no way I would let you have a lumpectomy. This type of cancer cannot be felt, because it is so deep within the tissue." So I said, "Okay, but I want a TRAM flap breast reconstruction done at the same time."

How did you select the TRAM free flap breast reconstruction? Why did you choose to have microsurgery?

I knew that's what I wanted done because I had read about it in the material I received from the American Cancer Society; it contained a pamphlet on reconstruction with about a 3-inch paragraph, no pictures or anything, describing the TRAM flap reconstruction technique. I wasn't really sure about the difference between the regular TRAM flap and the free TRAM flap, but I knew that I liked the idea of using my stomach tissue. I have severe allergies, and I was afraid of the implant technique. With my luck, I'd be allergic to them. Anyway, I have plenty of extra abdominal tissue, and this seemed to be the right approach for me.

Why did you want immediate breast reconstruction? What did you do when your surgeon was unwilling to perform an immediate TRAM flap reconstruction?

I could not face leaving the hospital without a breast. This surgeon I went to for the second opinion told me to have the mastectomy done and to come back in 3 to 6 months and have the TRAM flap. I said, "No, I want to go home with something. I cannot handle just having a skin flap with an expander underneath to stretch the skin. I want to have a breast when I leave the hospital." He told me that he had never done an immediate TRAM breast reconstruction.

I said, "It's being done somewhere, and I'm going to find out where." I called the American Cancer Society and got the name of a good plastic surgeon and cancer surgeon in a nearby city at a major medical center. Then I called my doctor back and said, "I want a referral." This was about 4:00 PM on a Friday afternoon. He called me back at 4:15 and said, "Be in there Monday morning at 9:00." So I went in and on March 5, 2 months after I found my lump, I had an 8-hour operation.

Did your plastic surgeon explain the different reconstructive options to you? Did you know that you were having a free TRAM flap and not a pedicle TRAM flap?

I came in with my mind made up. This procedure was my choice. They saw how hardheaded I was. I came in and told them I wanted a TRAM flap. I even had a booklet with me with information about TRAM reconstruction. I think they assumed I knew everything about it; they just agreed to do it. I qualified with my weight; I had a stomach for them to use. I heard them refer to it as a free flap, but I didn't understand that it was a more complicated form of TRAM flap operation. Nobody explained the difference to me, but I think I fooled them; they thought I was much better informed than I really was.

Did you require blood transfusions?

Yes. Before the surgery I had to have 3 units of blood donated. At first I couldn't think of someone we could trust to give blood, so I had to give my own. They kept telling me, "We'll never get the 3 units out of you in this short period of time." So I called my pastor, and within 3 hours there were 10 people from my church volunteering to give blood for me; it was great! And so many people called and came to see me; I saved the cards and counted them. I think I have 900 cards. People just pulled together.

How long did the operation take?

It took about 8 hours total. The only thing I remember in recovery is the nurse leaning over me and asking, "Can you tell me what they did?" I got so indignant with her, because I thought she should have known what they did to me. Then she said, "Send her to her room; she's okay." So I'm sure I had to talk to them before I got to my room.

Describe your hospital stay. Did you experience much pain?

I was in the hospital 6 days. My surgery was on a Tuesday, and I was much better and functioning on my own by Sunday. I came out of surgery with three drain tubes and a catheter; at one time I had nine items going into three needles for IVs. I also had a morphine pump.

The incisions themselves did not hurt, because they were so deep and the nerves had been cut. Most of the pain was through the stomach, where they had done the "tummy tuck" to take the tissue. My stomach was very tight. I would try to sit up and I couldn't. I guess my pain resembled the pain of childbirth. A person never realizes how the simplest movements use the stomach muscles. A sneeze will just about kill you. Reaching is impossible. You don't even want to think about lying down flat. I also had trouble from my back. I had hurt it years ago, and it really ached from having to sit and lie in the same position. I had difficulty finding a comfortable position, and I had to sleep on my back, propped up with pillows. I'd never have made it without my aunt staying with me during the days and my mother staying at night. After all, the nurses can't be by your side at all times.

I think the main contributor to my pain was the length of surgery. Eight hours is a very long time. I had two major surgeries in one. I remember feeling as if I had been beaten. Every muscle hurt. To help get rid of the aches I did what the doctor advised: I exercised. That meant I shuffled back and forth down the hospital corridor.

I also had trouble with my veins and the IVs. Because I had so many needles in, my veins started rupturing. I was taken back to surgery and had a jugular vein IV line inserted. Believe it or not, this made me feel much better. It gave me back the use of my one good arm. Until this was done, I couldn't even reach to get my own water or get into bed by myself.

I decided that the next time I have major surgery, I will have the jugular IV installed during surgery. The larger needle and blood supply in my jugular vein let them draw blood samples directly out of the IV instead of being stuck again when they needed to see if I needed another transfusion. Also, all other medications could be placed directly into the IV.

Did you require any special monitoring because you had microsurgery?

When you have microsurgery, they need to see if the blood vessels have been connected and that there is blood flow through the tissue. They check this by implanting a little Doppler probe. This is a device that monitors the blood flow. Before you leave the hospital, they pull it out. They also touch the reconstructed breast to check its temperature. If there's a cold spot, they'll know that the blood is not flowing through that area correctly.

Did you have to adjust to any surprises during your hospital stay?

In a medical center you have to get used to these young doctors always coming to see you in groups of five or six. I think that's one thing people need to be prepared for. Even though you have one doctor, he comes attached with five behind him. They're not all students; these are people who are already doctors, but they are studying that particular field and training specifically with someone. It was intimidating at first, but eventually you lose all inhibitions. They just come in and give orders: "Unsnap the top of your gown." You're just sitting there, and you're thinking, "Excuse me—who are you?"

How long did you recuperate before returning to work?

After my 6 days in the hospital, I was at home for 4 weeks before I returned to work. My job requires a lot of lifting. I'm on my feet, and it is hot where I work. So I stayed home for 4 weeks to make sure everything was fine.

Did you have any problems or complications?

I had an infection; it was the kind you get when you cut yourself and the surrounding area swells. It occurred because the knots from some of the stitches weren't dissolving; the stitches dissolved, but the knots didn't. The infection spread. Because I live some distance from the medical center, I went to my family doctor and he gave me an antibiotic for it. The next week, when I saw my plastic surgeon for a checkup, the incisions were already looking better. My plastic surgeon told me to continue on that medicine because the infection was healing just fine. It was just a skin infection. There was never any chance of losing the flap, even though that's the first thing that went through my mind: "I can't lose this. I don't have anything else to replace it with, so let's get this infection out of here!"

How long did it take until you were standing straight again and feeling like yourself?

Everybody kept saying that I was going to walk bent over at first, and they were right. But I thought I would be bent over by choice, not because I couldn't stand up. You should be told that. The muscle is gone. You have to stretch it out in order to stand upright again.

At first I was miserable every time I stood up, but I made myself do it. Each time I would try to stand up just a little bit straighter. I noticed by the end of the day that as I got tired, I also got more slumped over. It was very hard to stand erect. We live on a farm, so I would go out and take walks to try to get my energy back. Within 3 weeks I was standing up straight. It has taken about 5 months to really feel like myself again.

Did you have nipple-areola reconstruction? Did you have any other adjustments made during that operation?

I came back for the nipple reconstruction 3 months after my initial surgery. My plastic surgeon reconstructed the nipple and areola from the little patches of skin (dog-ears) that he left where he made my initial abdominal incision. I felt better before we did the nipple reconstruction than after. The scars were healing. I had some bad scar tissue from the infection. During the nipple reconstruction, he cut the skin all over again and took out tissue; so now I have new scars. The nipple looked gross when I first had to start changing the bandages. I thought, "Yuck, I shouldn't have had this done. We should have left it the way it was." But now that some time has passed, the nipple reconstruction looks better, and the more I see myself in the mirror, the more I like it.

He also did liposuction to smooth my stomach and hip area. That hurt worse than any of the other surgery. I never knew liposuction could hurt so much. My whole hip area was black and blue where they had just rounded it and trimmed it off.

Are you satisfied with your breast appearance? Is it what you expected?

Now that my breast has been shaped and trimmed and my nipple has been reconstructed, it looks pretty normal. As time passes, my breast appears more natural. It's not perfect, but I am pleased. My breasts still don't match; they aren't exactly the same shape. My new breast is too full in some aspects. My plastic surgeon is not happy with the shape, but I don't want to be put back to sleep again unless it's absolutely necessary to reduce the fullness. When I have a bra on, you can't tell. When I put on a swimsuit for the first time, I was like, "Yuck, I can tell it." I could notice that the shapes were not the same.

But I'm not in a swimsuit that much, so I don't mind. The cancer surgeon had to cut so low to get part of the breast tissue out that even when I have my bra on, you can see the lower part of the scar. I keep thinking I need to pull my bra down.

What do your scars look like? Where are they placed?

I have a circular scar all the way around the right breast area and underneath the arm. I'm also cut from behind one hip all the way across the abdomen to behind the other one. When you see this scar in the mirror, it's like somebody railroad-tracked you; it looks just like a pair of braces, only it's scar tissue. But my scars are doing better. Every week they seem to fade a little bit more. I'm sure that in a couple years, they will be fine. I have seen pictures of women who had this technique, and I could barely see any scarring. You could tell that their breasts didn't look exactly the same, but who could tell which was the reconstructed breast? I'd have to look on the back of the photographs to see which one was the reconstructed one and which one was the natural breast. Hopefully, one day people will look at mine and comment, "I can't tell which one it was. They don't look exactly the same, but. . ."

How does your reconstructed breast feel? Is it sensitive?

The new breast is more solid feeling and looks a little different from my other breast. It also has some sensitivity, and as time goes by it's getting more sensitive.

If you had it to do over again, would you have reconstruction? Was it worth the pain and trouble?

Yes. The results are so important and lasting that the memory of the pain fades. I look natural in my clothes. My breast feels natural; it jiggles when I walk. When I had the surgery, it didn't move at all at first, and my plastic surgeon kept telling me that when it was healed, it would start jiggling like the other one does. The first time it jiggled, I was so excited! I was like, "It's attached, it works!" My mother said, "What's wrong with you?" and I said, "Watch it, watch it. It jiggles!"

It's been worth it, most definitely. I feel more confident, because I feel like it is natural. I'm not going to be allergic to it; I'm not going to reject it. I'm not going to have to go back in 2 years to have an implant taken out and another one put in because the first one sprang a leak. It's done.

Are you pleased with the technique that you chose?

Wonderfully. I am very happy. I'm very pleased because now I consider mine finished, whereas some women are still having to go through the process of having the skin stretched and the implant inserted and they're just not finished. Mine's finished.

Do you think your age had some impact on your desire for immediate reconstruction?

Most definitely. Most people my age are healthy and vibrant. If you've got something wrong or you've got a prosthesis, it makes you a lot more self-conscious. Psychologically I couldn't have handled going home from the hospital with nothing there. I probably would have gone bananas if I had gone home with the scar and a hole.

Do you feel you were fully informed about the details of your breast reconstruction? Was there more information you could have had? Are there questions you think a woman should ask?

Personally I wish I had been supplied with all the gory details, not just simple before and after pictures. I would like to see the information written out in simplified medical terms so you can understand what is going on, so you can anticipate what will happen, and so you will know how your appearance will change. They should tell you that it is going to take three or four surgeries to get your breasts to look right. I was told there would be more than one operation, but it seems like every time I come here, there is going to be another one. You should know that you are going to have a year of bad scarring, so when you wake up you'll know what to expect. I was able to handle it, but I know some women who would be horrified to wake up and see all the stitches and scars. Their response would be, "What did they do to me!" A lot of times, unless you know what you want or are good at asking questions, the doctors won't tell you everything. It simplifies things for them; they just go ahead and do their little procedure and you wake up and that's it. I would like to see the information written out, so if you knew you were going to have the TRAM flap, they would explain in detail what they would do. I didn't really understand fully until after I had the surgery what it meant to have the TRAM done with microscopes and to have the blood vessels sewn together. I wish I had known beforehand, but I still would have had the procedure done. It was the perfect operation for me. Still . . . I needed more information. After all, these are life-changing decisions.

LOUELLA: MAKE THE BEST OF IT

"My philosophy has always been that as long as you feel sorry for yourself, things are not going to get a whole lot better. You will just sink deeper and deeper into those moods, and it will be harder and harder to pull yourself out. You need to break the pattern. Reach out to someone else, get involved, draw on your inner spiritual resources. Do anything to get your mind off yourself. As long as I am on this earth, I will do the best I can to take one day at a time, because that is all we are promised. None of us knows what tomorrow is going to bring. It is time to enjoy life."

Louella expressed these sentiments as she related her breast cancer experience and the series of complications that she weathered during her recovery. Louella is a licensed practical nurse with a big smile and a hearty laugh. She is a striking African American woman with short, cropped hair, large, expressive eyes, and a full, well-proportioned figure. She came to our interview clad in a bright red sweater and dangling pearl earrings that contrasted beautifully with her dark complexion.

Louella's cancer was discovered during a long-overdue checkup. A routine mammogram was the harbinger of shocking news. Her cancer was advanced and she had one positive node. Treatment involved lumpectomy with immediate latissimus dorsi breast reconstruction and then chemotherapy and radiation therapy. She was devastated and angry with herself for having neglected her health care so long that it had led to this. "If I hadn't been so negligent and had checked myself and gotten yearly mammograms, perhaps this could have been caught sooner." As a health care professional, Louella is well aware of the advantages of early detection for breast cancer, and she admonishes herself for being foolish. She knows that breast cancer survival statistics for African American women are far worse than for the general population, possibly because less attention is paid to routine screening and checkups. She admits she should have known better.

Considering all that Louella has suffered in the past few years, it is truly astounding that she can be so positive about life. She has faced a series of complications, including edema, hematoma, radiation burns, and lymphedema. Most of these were transient problems that have now resolved except for the lymphedema she developed after axillary dissection. The lymphedema is an ongoing reminder of her bout with breast cancer. It is a chronic problem that requires constant care to prevent debilitating fluid buildup. She accepts the problems she encountered philosophically as a small price to pay for the gift of life. As she explains, "I'm grateful to God that I'm here."

How did you discover your breast cancer?

Realizing I had been negligent about my own health while taking care of others, I resolved to take care of myself. Three months later, I made an appointment with an internist for a full checkup. During that process I had a mammogram that revealed some suspicious areas. That was followed by an ultrasound and an ultrasound-guided biopsy. These three tests confirmed that I had cancer, and I was referred to a cancer surgeon, who broke the news to me. It was mind-boggling; you just fall apart. You really don't know what to do, what to say, or how to react. My first reaction was, "Let's get it out as soon as possible." I was in a state of shock. Since I thought this was just a routine mammogram, I had no one with me. I pulled myself together long enough to call my husband, and he joined me. We then went to see the support nurse. I cried and wept for quite awhile; it was a very emotional time. It was hard pulling myself together, but I had to, because I had another doctor to see.

Did your doctors present you with various treatment options? Which ones did you select, and why?

I saw a total of three doctors that day: a cancer surgeon, a radiologist, and a plastic surgeon. The cancer surgeon explained my options to me. I wanted to preserve my breast and requested lumpectomy with radiation therapy if my cancer could be treated with this procedure. Initially they thought that a mastectomy would have to be done because of the type of cancer I had. As it turned out, I was able to have the lumpectomy and radiation that I desired. However, the resulting defect would be large, because I had a clump of three tumors. I would need a filler breast reconstruction with a latissimus dorsi back flap if I wanted a normal breast appearance. I also would have to have an axillary dissection so that my lymph nodes could be checked for cancer. With those procedures, my breast was preserved. Once I recovered from surgery, I would have radiation therapy, and if there were positive nodes, I would have chemotherapy. The axillary dissection revealed one positive lymph node, so I had the full course of chemotherapy. Radiation therapy was given next after my body recovered.

When I first found out that I had cancer, I just wanted to get it out. If I had allowed myself more time to think, I might have explored the alternative of holistic medicine or having chemotherapy first to see if the tumor size could be decreased before I decided on surgery.

Why did you decide to have a partial breast reconstruction?

I knew I didn't want to wake up with no breast or a partial breast and have to deal with the trauma of a scar. I wanted my body to look as much as possible as it did before surgery.

Did your doctor inform you of the different options for breast reconstruction? Why did you choose the latissimus dorsi (back) flap?

I was given several options. I could have implants or tissue expanders, or I could have flap surgery with tissue taken from other donor sites. Because I am a heavy, full-figured person, I had abundant tissue in all the right areas. I chose the back as my donor site. If I'm going to hurt, I prefer it to all be in one location—just the chest and back area as opposed to the chest and stomach area or the chest and buttock area, which are other areas where donor tissue can be obtained.

Describe your operation. How long did it take? How long were you hospitalized? Did you experience much pain?

The surgery took 4 hours. That included the lumpectomy, axillary dissection, and reconstruction. I was in the hospital for 2 days, which wasn't long enough, but that's the way it is with insurance coverage today. I was sore and stiff, and my right arm was swollen and tender. I had two drains, one in my underarm incision and one in my side incision; those drains remained in until I was discharged.

Did you experience any complications after surgery?

I had a number of small problems after surgery. Fluid accumulated in my armpit. My drains were removed too soon. They should have remained in 3 to 4 days after I was discharged; I paid a price for that. The surgery was done on Wednesday, I was discharged on Friday, and by Sunday fluid had built up in my armpit. It was just jiggling and sloshing around like water in a balloon. I was not physically hurting anymore, but just experiencing a lot of discomfort. I could not lie on that side; my right arm was already swollen, and the surgical sites were still painful. I called my plastic surgeon and he told me to come in. For the next 5 weeks, I had to have fluid withdrawn every other day. There was no discomfort when the fluid was being withdrawn, because I was still numb. However, I did experience a pulling sensation and pressure in that area. During this time I also felt dizzy and flushed. On two of the trips I was able to walk in but left in a wheelchair because I was so weak. I had to drink liquids each time before I left to ensure adequate fluid replacement. Then I would immediately go home to take pain medication, settle down, and let my body adjust to the stress of it all.

I also developed blood clots (hematomas) under one of the incisions; those had to be aspirated under local anesthesia. The actual aspiration of those blood clots was deep enough that the local anesthesia didn't numb the area very well. It was painful. I also had an adverse reaction to the antibiotics, which resulted in my losing my sense of taste. Fortunately, it came back after the antibiotics were discontinued. Those complications lasted about 6 to 8 weeks.

The most serious complication, which developed a few months later, was lymphedema, a swelling of my arm that remains an ongoing concern.

What caused the lymphedema? What are the symptoms? How is it managed?

Once the lymph nodes were removed (they took 15) and the nerve endings were cut, the lymphatic system in my arm shut down, causing ongoing fluid buildup as well as swelling and tenderness in my arm and hand. Unlike the initial fluid buildup caused by early drain removal, this will not go away. As a result, I must wear a Jobst elastic compression sleeve and do exercises. I also use a sequential compression sleeve and pump. I put my arm into the sleeve and turn on the machine. It slowly squeezes the arm in segments all the way up to the armpit. It forces the fluid up and out.

When arm fluid starts accumulating, my right arm gets stiff, and the hand and arm swell. It's very uncomfortable. You know it's time for another treatment, so you just do it and get it over with. The fluid is usually excreted through the kidneys, and you feel fine for another 24 or 36 hours before the process starts again. For the most part, it's a minor payment for one's life. Some of the ladies in my support group have a much harder time adjusting to lymphedema. They say it is a terrible inconvenience to have to get into that machine all the time. But you have to make time despite your busy lifestyle. This is a problem that stays with you, and you can't neglect it.

How long did it take before you were performing normal activities? When could you return to work?

I was physically unable to work for some time. I took a hiatus of about 9 months. I had not planned to take that long, but complications and problems kept coming up. Once I recovered from the initial surgery and the complications, I started chemotherapy.

What was your reaction to the chemotherapy? Did you experience any side effects? How did your family react?

I started chemotherapy in early December. After the first treatment my hair started coming out in large clumps. That really surprised me. I didn't expect it to happen so quickly. By Christmas I was completely bald, clean as an onion. I was wearing turbans, berets, scarves, you name it.

Most of us don't appreciate our hair until it's gone. You feel breezes stirring around the ears and the nape of the neck that you didn't know existed. I even had to resort to a sleeping cap. I bought a lacy one; I wanted something fancy. I figured, "If I have to sleep in this thing, why not wear a pretty one?" It would get too hot and I would take it off. Then in the middle of the night I would get chilly again and I would grope for it under my pillow and slip it back on. I don't think any of us ever realizes how much heat is lost through the head until your hair is gone. Then you really can appreciate the hair that you have and realize it has a real purpose other than just looks.

During the chemo I also had mood swings, insomnia, upper gastric problems, and minor lesions. My appetite was not good, but the nausea and vomiting were kept to a minimum by medications.

Why did you need to have radiation therapy?

Radiation is the treatment of choice after lumpectomy. It is just one more treatment to help kill any remaining cancerous cells in the breast area after the tumor has been removed during the lumpectomy. Radiation therapy consists of daily treatments 5 days a week for 5 weeks. I tolerated the first 20 treatments pretty well, except that my breast and underarm area became red (like a bad sunburn) and tender. The next treatments did not go as well; I developed problems and painful complications.

What complications did the radiation therapy cause?

From the twenty-first treatment on, the skin rolled off my breast like a peel coming off an onion. It just blistered and burned. There were burned areas across my breast, under it, and in the armpit area. They were treated as if they were thermal burns. My dressings were changed three to five times a day and Silvadene cream was applied. My plastic surgeon has pictures documenting all of this. He immediately put me on medication and antibiotics to prevent infection. One of the problems with lymphedema is that you really have to guard against skin irritations and infections, because the lymphatic system cannot drain lymph as efficiently as before surgery, so bacteria can take hold. If you develop an infection, you're susceptible to much more serious problems.

It took about 6 to 8 weeks for my burns to heal, and during that time I was still undergoing radiation treatments. I would see the doctor before the treatment, get the treatment, see the doctor afterward so he could change the dressing, and then I'd go home. Then I would repeat the process the next day. That pain was excruciating. If you've ever had a burn, you know how it feels, especially when it affects tender areas such as the breast and armpit. They hurt constantly. I had to shower every day, because I didn't want to get it infected. I would take off those slimy dressings, shower, swab on big clumps of Silvadene cream, and put more dressings on. My husband and I dealt with that. I was not a good patient. I cried, screamed, and pulled on his clothes. He'd just hold on to me and we'd do it. Nothing that I took really helped the pain, because once you took off the dressing, it started to hurt all over again. It was the same thing if water touched my skin. The pain was terrible.

How did you cope with the pain from the radiation burns?

I stopped trying to think about anybody else during that time. It was just me, me, and me! I tried to be a good sport about it. I listened to a lot of music and did a lot of praying, because at some point it just seemed like the medicine wasn't working. It seemed like the more medication I put on, the more it hurt and the bigger the area got. I was going through dressings right and left. I started buying them in bulk. I recall the day I came in to see my plastic surgeon for a follow-up visit. When he saw what the radiation had done, he closed his eyes, kind of shuddered, and said, "My goodness!" He took pictures and immediately ordered medication. He told me to come back in 2 weeks so he could see how I was healing. He was very pleased once it started to heal.

Are you on hormonal therapy? Are there any side effects?

I started taking tamoxifen in September. This is one more tool to help fight the cancer. I will take it for 5 years. It increases your hot flashes, but I have developed a solution for that problem. I have a little foldup fan that I pull out and just fan away. No matter what the weather, I can cool down. I keep fans around wherever I am, even at work. I get a big glass of water and fill it with ice. It usually chills me down quickly. I've noticed, however, that sometimes it cools me down so fast I get chills and have to drink some hot tea. Since I work nights, nobody is really aware of what I go through to get comfortable. If I were around a lot of folks in the daytime, fanning one minute, chilling the next, they would really have second thoughts about me.

Were you satisfied with the results of your breast reconstruction?

My plastic surgeon has done a beautiful job. I'm heavy-breasted, and from the beginning he said to me, "Louella, we're not gods, but we will do the best we can to match them up." He did an excellent job. My reconstructed breast is a little larger on the right side, but I can accept that.

Did you have nipple-areola reconstruction?

No, I didn't need nipple reconstruction because my nipple was preserved. Everything was done from the side: the muscle was brought from the back through the incision that was in the front, and everything was connected. So I never had to have nipple reconstruction, tattooing, or anything of that sort.

Describe your scars. What do they look like?

The scars are minimal. I wasn't sure they were going to be, since I tend to have keloids. I was very concerned about this and told both the cancer surgeon and the plastic surgeon about it. But nothing developed, and the scars are fine. Even the places where the drains were inserted have healed beautifully, leaving only hairline incisions.

My reconstructive scar is about 6 inches long. The scar for the axillary area where the lymph nodes were removed and the latissimus flap tunneled through is approximately 12 to 14 inches long, extending the full width of the armpit. I also have a tiny, 2- to 2½-inch scar over the top of the nipple. This is where they initially went in to remove the tumors. So I have three scars, all of which are aesthetic. The one in the underarm can't really be seen unless I raise my arms when I have on a swimsuit or a low-cut dress. The one in the latissimus area is in such a spot that it's hidden with a bra, and of course, the one over the nipple is also hidden.

Do you have any sensitivity in your breast and nipple on that side?

I wouldn't say I have full sensitivity or sexual responsiveness, but it's nearly normal. It's been over a year, and the way it's going, I hope to have full sensitivity within the next few months.

Do you have any other side effects?

Because my back muscle was transferred to the front of my chest, there is actually a certain little area on my breast I can press and it will push out. I told my plastic surgeon, "I can do things nobody else can do. I think I have a marketing tool here."

I still have a certain degree of numbness in the axillary area where all the lymph nodes were removed and in my arm. The arm numbness used to extend from the elbow to the shoulder, but slowly it's getting better. The numbness in the armpit is still there. I don't perspire in that area anymore.

Was lumpectomy and breast reconstruction the right choice for you?

I think that was my best choice. I didn't feel that I could deal with the scar or the flat chest after surgery. Psychologically it made a difference to me to have a breast, at least something there, and not have to worry about wearing a prosthesis in my bra.

Was your husband supportive and helpful during this experience?

My husband did his best to empathize, but he really couldn't understand. That's why I joined a support group. I needed to talk to somebody who could relate to my experience. He kept saying, "Why do you keep crying? Why don't you just cry and get it over with?" I would say, "You don't understand, because it's not your breast. It's not your body." He has found strength in talking to the other husbands and boyfriends and loved ones who share their feelings and experiences in dealing with the women they care about.

Initially after the surgery my husband seemed to need to hug and squeeze me all the time. I had a certain way I turned to block him if he squeezed too tight. He would say, "You know I want to hug you, but I always hurt you." Finally, he said, "I'll tell you what, you hug me. You know how tight you can hold me without hurting yourself. Show me how tight to squeeze, and I'll take your lead." That was what worked. I can remember many days after that when I would look at him and say, "I need my hug, I really do." Then I would squeeze him so he would know how tight to hold me. That solved our problem. We were able to have our little "hug sessions" after all.

Communication is particularly important at a time like this. You need to talk things out, because you don't know how he feels, and he doesn't understand how you feel. You can yell at each other and have your little temper tantrums, but when that's over, you need to talk to each other, to open up, to share, to say, "Hey, this is how I feel, how do you feel? What do you think about this? What should I do here? I need you to help me. I need you to talk to me. Let's talk this thing through so we can get it resolved and go on." We all have busy schedules and sometimes feel like there just is not enough time in a day, but 30 minutes, even 15 minutes sharing a cup of tea sprinkled with a little conversation goes a long way. That's basically how I've dealt with having cancer and being a cancer patient.

My husband has been a terrific help with my physical recovery. He has never been helpless. He knows how to cook and clean and wash and iron. He was raised by a mom who taught him to do for himself. So that was never a problem for us. He was there every day to fix breakfast, lunch, and dinner. Finally, I said it was too much. "You have to have time away. Why don't you just do breakfast and dinner and I will manage lunch."

What can people do to help you recover?

One of the most important things people can do is just to listen and be empathetic. I don't say sympathetic, because you don't want their sympathy. You just want them to listen and not shy away or be afraid of you. I don't hear from some of my friends anymore; I am not sure why. I think they feel my cancer is contagious. Most people, however, have been caring. Once they found out about my breast cancer, they called, offered suggestions, offered help, and compared experiences. They consoled me when I was hurting and laughed with me when I felt better. It was a wonderful outpouring of love.

How did your faith help you cope with this experience?

I keep my radio tuned to the gospel station. There is something about music that soothes your soul. If nothing else reaches you, the music does. I meditate to some songs. I also believe in prayer and fasting.

I am a member of the First Christian Fellowship Church, which I joined 2 years ago while visiting my daughter in another town. It's a small church where everybody knows everybody, and everybody shares feelings and emotions. They do not yet have a branch church in my city, so I have a long-distance spiritual relationship.

When I learned I had cancer, I called my pastor and he immediately prayed for me and asked to be kept apprised of my progress. Ever since I joined the church and was baptized, I had received frequent letters, sometimes six a week, from all of the sisters there. When my cancer was diagnosed, I was flooded with correspondence. They found time to pour out their emotions and offer their prayers. I also got letters from the pastor and I was on the prayer list, on altar call, and in the tape ministry. They send me CDs of the weekly service, and I listen to those since I am not physically able to attend church. I feel united with the other church members when I put on the CDs on Sunday, which is the hardest time, because that's when everyone goes to church. I have gotten all my strength from these sources of faith and spirituality.

How has your breast cancer experience affected your relations with others?

It has made me want to reach out to other people and to share my experiences. I have phoned all my relatives and urged them to take care of themselves, to get their daughters to do breast self-examination, and to go for mammograms. I even extended myself to friends, co-workers, and church members. Surprisingly, some of these women were also breast cancer patients who needed to talk about their experiences and to share.

What advice would you like to share with other women?

We all live in a bubble of sorts. We think that nothing will invade our bodies, and we will always be fine and live forever. We tend to neglect ourselves, and it can be harmful. Several people have told me that they don't know how I talk about my experiences and about breast cancer. I find it easy. Keeping things bottled up is a real killer; it just destroys you. I don't say run to every street corner and say, "Guess what I have," but sharing, quiet sharing will heal you.

BETH ANN: MIND OVER MATTER

"My husband and I have many good memories from our breast cancer experience. I know that sounds crazy, but it's true. Even though breast cancer was a terrible blow, it was not all bad. We managed to enjoy ourselves throughout the whole process and were unwilling to become victims. We took the offensive and attacked the problem. We surrounded ourselves with positive energy, controlled our environment as much as possible, and refused to give in to negativity."

These comments were made to me by Beth Ann as she recounted her experience with breast cancer and the strategies that she and her husband, Dean,* used to cope with her diagnosis and therapy. A striking woman with a peaches-and-cream complexion and a halo of red hair, Beth Ann's voice is soft and compelling. She is stylishly dressed in a periwinkle suit that shows off a trim figure. One would be hard pressed to believe that she is a breast cancer survivor who at 48 years of age has faced some serious challenges. A loving, participating partner has made her journey easier. It is clear from her story that a positive attitude and a supportive relationship can make all the difference.

Beth Ann and her husband have been together for almost 28 years now, first as friends, then as lovers, and during the last 12 years as married partners. Life seemed complete until 4 years ago, when a routine physical examination led to a mammogram, a biopsy, and a diagnosis of DCIS (ductal carcinoma in situ) in her left breast. Two separate surgeons recommended a mastectomy.

Beth Ann opted to have a skin-sparing mastectomy combined with immediate breast reconstruction with a TRAM (abdominal) flap to avoid permanent breast loss. Following surgery, she had a 6-month course of chemotherapy.

Beth Ann and her husband have a particularly close and sharing relationship. It was only natural that her breast cancer diagnosis should be viewed as their problem, their challenge, their disease. So intent was Dean on becoming actively involved that he initially pushed too hard and assumed too much control. Beth Ann had to tell him to back off and to allow her to do the talking and make the decisions. Despite these initial missteps, Dean's ongoing support served as a lifeline for Beth. As she recalls, "He kept me comfortable and

*An interview with Dean is included in Chapter 17.

confident. I knew that he loved me, not my breast. He did all of those romantic things that make a difference. He also took care of me when I needed it and provided a shoulder to cry on when my spirits were flagging."

As a former military professional, Dean's instinct was to aggressively attack the problem, and that is what he and Beth Ann did. They did extensive research, developed decision trees outlining available options, and laid out "battle plans" to wage their own personal war against breast cancer. Dean was intent on helping Beth Ann maintain a positive attitude. Cheers to rally her spirits, exotic nature posters to help counteract the hospital environment, and motivational CDs to focus energies on recuperation were some of the strategies they adopted to cope with surgery and recovery. They used the same methods during chemotherapy to keep their positive energies flowing and to mitigate the side effects of nausea and hair loss. They refused to let their fears overshadow their zest for life.

As Beth Ann recalls, "I was diagnosed with breast cancer right before the Christmas holidays. My husband gave me the news while I was lying in the recovery room." Maybe I was dopey, but I said, "Well, we'll face it and we'll take care of it." At this point he was more devastated than I was. Then I started to cry. Overall, I took it pretty well. I knew that I had no choice. You just have to take care of these things. I'm not the type of person who goes into denial; I face what life holds and move on. I had delayed going to the doctor for a routine Pap smear, so I was probably lucky I went when I did, because my cancer was discovered in its earliest stages.

Why did you choose to have a mastectomy and breast reconstruction rather than a lumpectomy?

When they removed the tumor, they did not get clean margins. I had a ductal carcinoma in situ (DCIS), and the surgeon recommended a mastectomy. Of course, I wanted a second opinion. A friend sent me to another surgeon for a consultation. He took another mammogram and confirmed my diagnosis and treatment recommendation. You could actually see a golf ball–sized area on the mammogram. If they tried to remove wedges of breast tissue or do a lumpectomy, they would have to remove so much of my breast to get clean margins that I would be deformed and would likely be very unhappy with the aesthetic appearance. Mastectomy seemed the best choice.

Why did you want to have breast reconstruction?

I didn't want to lose my breast, and I let the surgeon know that keeping my breast was important to me. I knew that I would be unhappy without any breast at all. I was too young and enjoyed my sexuality too much to be satisfied with that kind of result. My surgeon recommended a skin-sparing mastectomy and immediate breast reconstruction.

What is a skin-sparing mastectomy? What are its advantages when combined with immediate breast reconstruction?

With a skin-sparing mastectomy, they leave most of the breast skin intact and only remove the nipple and areola skin and all of the breast tissue underneath. Then they fill the skin in immediately for the breast reconstruction.

Why did you choose to have immediate breast reconstruction at the time of your mastectomy?

I didn't want to wait. I could see from the pictures the plastic surgeon showed me that the scarring was different when you delayed the breast reconstruction. If I had a standard modified radical mastectomy and delayed the breast reconstruction, they would have to remove a lot more skin, and my breast scars would have been longer and more noticeable. With a skin-sparing mastectomy and immediate breast reconstruction, I could minimize my scars and still have a breast. Anyway, I just didn't see any point in having another operation. If my surgeon and plastic surgeon did not see a problem with doing the mastectomy and breast reconstruction at the same time, then that was my preference.

How did you find a plastic surgeon and decide on the right reconstructive approach for you? Why did you select the TRAM (abdominal) flap?

The surgeon referred me to a plastic surgeon who is part of his breast management team. He called this plastic surgeon, who came over for a consult. After he looked at the mammograms and examined me, the plastic surgeon concurred that mastectomy was the right choice for me. Then he reviewed the various options for reconstructive surgery. When he told me about the possibility of using my own tissue to build a new breast without having to use implants, I was delighted. I have allergies and am prone to developing rashes; even Band-Aids tend to irritate my skin. Therefore I did not want anything foreign in me like an implant. When he described the TRAM flap, I knew instantly that it was the approach for me. It was just perfect. I have plenty of fat on my stomach, and I could have a totally natural breast. Even though it was a major surgery, I was eager to do it.

How many hours did your surgery take? How long were you hospitalized?

It's tough surgery. Recovery is slow, but I really didn't have a bad time with it. The operation took about 5 to 6 hours. I was hospitalized a little less than 6 days. I went in on Wednesday and went home the next Monday, with drains hanging out of me, because I still had fluid buildup. These stayed in for the next week or two.

Describe your hospital stay. Did you experience much pain after surgery?

Recovery wasn't bad. I had a private room with a great view. As I woke up on the first day, my husband was putting posters on my wall so people could sign them when they came to visit. I was hot, and he placed cold compresses on my forehead to cool me off. I had compression stockings around my legs that were expanding and contracting to keep the blood moving and to prevent blood clots. I also was told to press a pillow against my breast to keep it warm and to maintain good circulation.

I started my period when I was in the hospital. That caught me off guard, because it was early. They tell me it happens all the time and is probably caused by stress. Women need to know that this is likely to happen. I wish I had known ahead of time so I could have planned for it.

I was up sitting in a chair the very next day after surgery. I had tubes hanging out of me, but I didn't really have any breast pain; that area was numb, because nerve endings are cut when the breast tissue is removed. The pain came from the abdomen. You are very sore in your abdominal area, and you are not able to stand up straight, which is very difficult. Everything you do expands and contracts your abdomen. A sneeze or a cough produces a violent pressure. It just hurts. I had an automatic IV drip for pain medicine (PCA), but I didn't need it very often. They'd tell me that I had to "keep ahead of the pain," so I needed to keep using it. I'd say okay, and I'd do it. I didn't take many of the pain pills after they took out the PCA line.

The pain was more tolerable than I thought it would be. Some of that was probably a result of the positive reinforcement that I got from the motivational messages I was listening to on my iPod and from the positive reinforcement that surrounded me. We made a special effort to control the environment, and I think that helped me to control my pain and to come through this experience with an upbeat attitude.

How did you take control of your environment? What types of motivational messages did you listen to? Did they help to make your recovery easier?

Dean brought in posters to decorate the hospital room. One of the posters had an absolutely gorgeous scene showing a stream rushing through a forest. We used to go backpacking, so I could put myself in this scene. When I went to chemotherapy, we took this poster to hang in front of me. I listened to my iPod, and I just tried to chill out and put myself there instead of here. I'd talk to my body and tell it to accept the medicine and kill the cells. I don't know if it works, but I feel I did okay with it, so maybe it does.

During surgery, chemotherapy, and throughout this whole process, we took control of our environment and made it as comfortable as possible. We planned the chemotherapy treatments so we could spend the whole afternoon together before I started to feel queasy and had to go home. It really wasn't that bad.

I also listened to Dr. Bernie Siegal's motivational messages on my iPod to help me remain positive and hopeful. They give you a message that you're going to get well, that you're content with your progress, and that this is for your own good. That positive reinforcement helped me in my recovery. (Beth Ann stops for a minute to wipe her eyes, apologizing for her tears.) I still get emotional thinking about it. I listened to these messages before I went to surgery and during the operation itself. The whole time I was in surgery I had my iPod with me. I also listened to them all during my hospital stay. When people weren't around to talk to me, I listened, and Dean and I kept that stuff going. I think that makes a difference.

I later gave some motivational CDs to my sister, who had a hysterectomy, and everyone was surprised at how fast she recovered. Who knows, maybe we just have good bodies. All I know is that you use what works; these motivational messages seemed to do the trick for me. The power of suggestion is important when you are feeling so fragile and afraid.

How soon were you able to move around, to wash your hair, and to shower? Did you need any assistance?

Before my surgery I had talked to a friend who had abdominal surgery, and she told me that it really wasn't so bad. What I needed to do was to get up and walk as soon as the doctors would let me and that would speed my recovery. That kind of mental preparation helped. I did very well with her advice. At first you can't do much. You can't even stand up straight until your stomach muscles stretch. However, as soon as they told me I could get up and walk, I made an effort to walk as much as I could. I walked around the hospital. I walked to my windows to just watch the birds outside. I did that a lot, and it made me feel better.

Dean and I also figured out a way to clean me up a bit and to wash my hair. That was a tremendous help psychologically. I had to pull my knees up and lean my head back so he could wash my hair in the sink. One of the worst parts of recovery is that you feel so sweaty and grungy after surgery. I felt great when I was able to put some makeup on, and I toddled over to visit a woman down the hall who was feeling depressed. I mean, at that point I was already thinking that I needed to pass this on to people as much as I could to help people out.

I had a catheter in for the first day or two, which didn't bother me in the slightest, even when they took it out. My first shower turned out to be really funny. Dean helped me wash myself, but he didn't want to get wet, so he took off his long pants and put on a hospital gown and got in with me. In the middle of the shower someone from the pain therapy department came looking for me. You can imagine how shocked he was to see Dean answer the door in a nightgown when he was expecting to see a woman recovering from breast surgery. We had a good laugh about that one.

Did you need to make any special preparations when you were ready to leave the hospital?

When I tried to get dressed to go home from the hospital, I discovered that I didn't have the right clothes. My waist was swollen from the abdominal surgery, and my pants wouldn't fit because they didn't have an elastic waist. I had to leave the hospital in my nightgown. I didn't know to buy anything ahead of time to wear after surgery. That's important information for a woman to have. You need something that buttons up the front, because you can't lift your hands above your head for a while. It also hurts to try to pull something over your head. I went home on Monday, and on Thursday my sister took me clothes shopping. I picked two or three things from the rack and then I sat down in the dressing room while my sister brought clothes in for me to try on. I just sat for most of the time, because I really didn't have the energy to walk around and shop. I bought clothing that I could get in and out of easily: three pairs of elastic-waist pants and three shirts that buttoned up the front. That's what I wore for the next few weeks and months until the swelling in my waist subsided.

What limitations did you have? Did you need help initially with household chores? How did you cope with them?

During the first few weeks my mother or my sister was there to help me. It's important to have somebody there to assist you when you get home, because you really can't do much for yourself. After a while, when I was able to go out to the grocery store, I still could not push my cart to the car, particularly since the lot is situated on a hill. I had to have one of the kids from the store put the stuff in the car. I couldn't carry the bags into the house either. I had to shop when my husband was at home so he could bring them in. I had to pick up the groceries I wanted one item at a time, because you can't lift very much weight. I know you're not supposed to do laundry and things like that, but I just made do. I didn't lift, but I did kick the laundry basket across the room with my foot, and then I picked up one piece of clothing at a time for folding. I could still cook, but I had to be careful not to lift anything heavy. You just have to pay attention to what the doctor says you should do. It gets better as time passes.

Because of the pulling in your abdomen, you can't lie flat in bed. We had a big floor pillow (about 2 feet square) that we covered with a sheet, and I propped it behind me and slept in a sitting or partially reclined position. At first you can't even get out of bed, so it helps to have somebody there for the first few days. Then after a little while you start to develop strategies for getting yourself out of bed. I managed by using my leg as a fulcrum. I would pick my knee up and then pull it down; that way I would be able to sit myself up as long as I was holding on to something. Then I could turn my body around and get out of bed. My fulcrum technique is really helpful to know when you are recovering from this operation, because you can't pull from your abdomen.

I took a nap every day. You're tired from being bent down, and you just have to relax periodically. I would sit on the couch, and before long I'd be asleep. For diversion, I went out to lunch with my girlfriends, who would pick me up.

When were you allowed to start exercising?

Within a few weeks, when I had healed, they let me start doing the hand/arm exercises; I also started walking the parking lot at my apartment complex. I tried to walk as much as I could. One time I walked too far and I had to call a cab to get me back to the apartment for a $2.00 fare. I was so embarrassed, but I was just too worn out to get back on my own. You have to learn your endurance; you can't walk for very long at a time since you get worn out easily, partly because you are not standing up straight. After the tummy tuck your stomach is pulled really tight, and you lean over to counteract the pulling. It hurts to straighten up. It takes a while for your skin and muscles to stretch back out so you can stand upright.

How long was it before you could drive? When were you able to go back to work?

It took about 6 or 7 weeks before I could drive. I have a stick shift, so it might have been even more difficult for me. You can't drive at first, because you need to be more flexible and to be able to turn your abdomen a bit along with your head to see better. Things like that slow you down. I went back to work after 7 weeks, which I think is probably an average time. I worked only part-time for the first 2 weeks, because it was very tiring for me.

Did you have any problems or complications after your breast reconstruction?

Several weeks after I was home, I felt a hardness in my breast. The weight of my husband's body hurt me when we were close to one another. The doctor said that a part of the flap had died and my body had formed a capsule around it. It was a little hardened area, the size of a marble, but it hurt, so I decided to have it removed. This was done at the same time I had my nipple reconstructed.

Why did you decide to have your nipple-areola reconstructed? What was done? Were any other adjustments made at the same time?

Before I had the nipple done, my reconstructed breast was just a round shape formed with abdominal skin. I just didn't feel done. A lot of women decide not to go any further, but I wanted to do it. The plastic surgeon created a nipple from the available skin on my breast. I know that some women worry that a reconstructed nipple will look funny because it sticks out prominently, but the projection goes down and it looks quite natural after a time.

My plastic surgeon also used liposuction to smooth out the hip area where it was still a little puffy around the ends of the abdominal incision. That hurt. You are bruised after the liposuction, and it hurts to even scrape against things for the first few days. It takes about 10 days for the bruising to go down. Once I had the nipple tattooed, I felt like I was done.

Are you happy with the aesthetic appearance of your reconstructed breast? Is the contour good? Is it symmetrical with your natural breast?

Aesthetically, my new breast looks very good now. It has a wonderful shape. It's not perfect, but it's very similar to the other one, and it hangs symmetrically. If I gain weight it sort of swells and is tender, so it's important for me to keep my weight down as much as I can. That's harder to do now, because I am not as good about exercising as I once was.

The nipple-areola tattooing did not produce a very good color match. The colors are just not the same as those on my natural breast; they keep fading. I had the color put on twice. During the second time there was a lot of scar tissue, and it was difficult to get the color to take. It's not the same beige-brown tone as my normal breast. In my eyes, however, it's perfectly fine, and I don't think it makes a difference to my husband. So I don't consider it a problem.

How many scars do you have? Where are they located? What do they look like?

I have a scar under my arm that comes up across the breast in the middle and then goes around the nipple. That has faded to such a fine white line that it's barely noticeable. (I also applied cocoa butter and vitamin E oil to help the healing process.) There's a small pucker under the arm where things were put together again, but it's not much of anything. I have a bigger scar on my abdomen. It extends from hip to hip and looks like a big smile. It's redder, but I'm sure that's because it's still healing. As soon as the doctors said it was okay, I massaged my abdominal scar to improve the blood flow to that area and to help me recuperate faster.

Do you have any sensation in the breast? Is your nipple sensitive to touch? Is it responsive to sexual stimulation?

Oh, I have regained a lot of the sensitivity. I even have sensitivity in the nipple. The nerves have grown back. It's never going to be the same as the other side; it certainly isn't going to have the sexual responsiveness. I can still tell that someone's touching it. I can tell I have clothes on. But it still does not have complete sensory return, and I doubt that it ever will. Even so, it is definitely getting better as the nerves grow back. The same is true for my abdomen. I lost a lot of feeling in that area, but it is coming back.

What impact did the loss of sexual sensitivity in your breast and nipple have on your sex life? Did you have to make any special accommodations?

Actually, this didn't change my sex life at all, other than having to be careful of positioning to avoid undue weight or pressure in the beginning.

How long did you have to wait before you could resume sexual relations? Was it awkward? Were you worried about your husband's reaction?

You don't have to wait a particular length of time; it's a comfort issue more than a privacy issue. My husband was careful not to pressure me about sex. In fact, I pushed him into having sexual relations again. He would say, "Do you want to right now?" and I would say, "Sure." He was very funny about it at first, because he didn't want to hurt me. I also had to shift around a bit until I found a comfortable position; it was a little awkward that way. I didn't feel less of a sexual woman because of it, however.

My husband's a special man. He had told me long before any of this came up that he really liked my breasts, but it wasn't my breasts he wanted or that he was married to. He wanted me, not just them. So I was not totally fearful of that. You always have some doubt, because you don't know how people will really react. But I felt his background would make him understanding. My breast also looks good. It looks so real, so much like the other one, and it's got the same feel. From that perspective, and because I did go the distance and do the nipple reconstruction, I look pretty much the way I did. It's not perfect, but it's very nice for both of us.

Have you had to change your clothing because of the reconstruction? Can you still wear the same things?

I really haven't had to make major changes. I wasn't supposed to wear an underwire bra, and I thought that would be an inconvenience in the beginning, because I have been wearing underwire bras for years now. However, I was starting to feel a little pinch around the side, and I thought I should do what they recommended if it would be more comfortable. So I bought one that doesn't have an underwire, and I do believe that I'll be happy with that. Other than that, all my other clothes are about the same. I've always kept in shape and done my arm exercises, so I haven't had problems with arm swelling

Was breast reconstruction worth the pain, time away from work, and recovery? Did it meet your expectations?

I tell women who ask me about breast reconstruction that it is a personal decision. It made a difference to me; it made me feel like I was complete. You know your reconstructed breast is different when you look in the mirror, but that's okay, because I love the way it turned out. I'm very happy, very content with the result, and it makes a difference in my attitude and in all of the things that I do.

If you had this decision to make again, would you choose the same type of reconstruction? What would you advise other women about this approach?

I would do it in a minute with the same techniques. The younger you are, the more likely you are to choose this approach. It is a difficult surgery, and there's a lot of recovery time; some people might not be up to it. I know I have talked to women on the phone whose husbands and boyfriends say, "Why would you want to do anything that takes so long to recover from?" I know it's not right for everybody. However, I can honestly say it was right for me. If I develop another breast cancer, I couldn't use my abdomen again, but I would use my back (the latissimus dorsi flap) or another donor area. I would do it again, because I like the effect; I like the way it looks and I like getting it over at the same time as the cancer surgery. I also knew that I didn't want to cope with looking at myself in the mirror without a breast or to deal with putting a prosthesis in every day to feel matched. For some women that wouldn't be a problem, but I was young, in my forties, and to me the thought of it was shocking.

Were your doctors responsive to your needs? Did they communicate well? What could they have done better?

Every doctor is in a hurry; that is why we must take responsibility for our own health care. If a doctor is talking while starting to walk out and I'm not done, I say, "Please, I have more questions," and I make him come back in. Some of them can't help it because they're just in a hurry, and they look at you and tell you that you are doing just fine. My advice is always to make them sit back down. And they will, they always do. I now have a great relationship with my surgeons and my oncologist. I feel secure in their knowledge and their abilities. It made a difference to me knowing that these doctors are respected in the medical community and that they have wonderful reputations. I knew that I was getting the best of everything. I felt in good hands. Plus, with my husband's medical background, he was always looking at my charts and trying to keep track of what was happening. A lot of people aren't going to be able to do that, but I would suggest that you take the time to go to the medical library and get some information so that you feel like you know the topic and you're not totally befuddled by what the doctor is telling you. I realize that may be a younger person's attitude. My mother doesn't do that; she just listens to what the doctor has to say. She doesn't want to know any more. But you miss things that way; you need to educate yourself. There is a lot of information out there to help you feel that you can gain control of your situation and make an informed decision. This is your life, and you need to make the best of it.

What kind of advice would you give other women about breast cancer and breast reconstruction?

First, I'd tell them to get periodic checkups. It's important not only to do breast self-exams, but also to have your doctors examine your breasts and to get routine mammograms. Do not be an ostrich with your head in the sand, afraid of finding things. The sooner you find something, the earlier you can take care of it.

The second thing I would say is that a cancer diagnosis is not a death sentence. You can recover from this. You need to go into this experience with a mindset that says that you can do this; you can take care of it. Then you'll come through it. Breast cancer is not the end of anything. I do as much as I have ever done before. I've done a lot of things in my life, and now I am able to continue to do them. I flew home 2 days after my biopsy; I did that as soon as I could go. Within a year, while I was still wearing my wig, I took trips to Florida and took a vacation inner-tubing down a river. I realize that's no big deal, but it has a symbolic meaning. It shows that you can do a lot; cancer is no reason to stop living and to stop enjoying yourself.

How can a man be supportive of a woman during this experience? What works and what doesn't?

The first thing a man is going to have to realize is that he can't make all the decisions for you. Men tend to want to be problem-solvers and, like my husband, they want to gather all the information, make a decision, and then provide the direction: "Let's do it this way." But you can't do that. The woman has to take the lead. This is a woman's body we are talking about and a woman's prerogative. She has to be the one to say this is what I want to do or not do. And in the end the man needs to be able to go along with what she decides.

I was very happy that my husband could actually be with me in the hospital the whole time. He cheered me up and helped me keep a positive attitude. We actually had fun, and I don't think many people could say that. He spent the night there every night, and he did a lot of things for me. He was just there and took care of things; he brought me flowers, and he was always showing my breast to everybody. It was great just having him there when I needed him to put cold compresses on my head or to help me shower or wash my hair or just get out of bed. The nursing staff can't run to you the second you want a glass of water and you can't reach it. They are busy. Having someone in the room with you, a husband, a relative, a friend, makes a big difference and is very helpful. You need someone you are comfortable with who will be there with you to let you talk and cry if you need to—someone who will also give you the freedom to choose your own options.

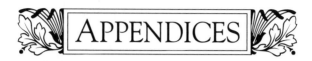

APPENDICES

A   *Quick Guide to Key Online Resources*

B   *Breast Cancer Information and Support Services*

C   *The Patient's Rights*

D   *National Cancer Institute Cancer Centers Program*

E   *The Histopathologic TNM Classification of Breast Carcinoma*

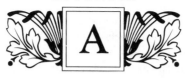

QUICK GUIDE TO KEY ONLINE RESOURCES

*T*here is an enormous amount of information on breast cancer available online. It can be overwhelming to sort through the various websites to try to find credible information and helpful support services. The following quick guide is meant to simplify this process. It contains a select group of websites that we have found to be enormously helpful to breast cancer patients and their families. A more comprehensive list of credible resources is included in Appendix B.

Comprehensive Resources

American Cancer Society: www.cancer.org
Contains a wealth of excellent resources and educational materials on a wide range of topics from basic cancer statistics to cancer support groups. Many of these materials are also available in print (see bibliography).

National Cancer Institute (NCI):
www.cancer.gov/cancertopics/types/breast
Provides an enormous amount of timely and valuable information for patients and their families on topics ranging from breast cancer facts to current treatment options, risk factors, clinical trials, and much, much more. Many of these materials are also available in print (see bibliography).

Physician Data Query (PDQ): www.cancer.gov/cancertopics/pdq
NCI's comprehensive online cancer database. It contains information on a wide range of cancer topics, a registry of 8000-plus open and 19,000-plus closed cancer clinical trials from around the world, and a directory of professionals who provide genetics services.

Breast Cancer Organization: www.breastcancer.org
Provides information on treatment options.

My Cancer Advisor: www.mycanceradvisor.com
Provides electronic versions of timely and informative booklets written for cancer patients, their families and caregivers, as well as links to "trusted sources" that are accurate and balanced. (See Appendix B for a list of My Cancer Advisor's free booklets on breast cancer.)

Patient Resource: www.patientresource.net
A blog site that contains professionally prepared informative video materials for cancer patients, as well as commentary from cancer experts.

Support Services

The Susan G. Komen Breast Cancer Foundation: www.komen.org
Offers support, patient advocacy, information, and a wide range of resources for breast cancer patients and their families.

Breast Cancer Network of Strength (formerly Y-Me):
www.networkofstrength.org
Provides information and emotional and peer support to anyone affected by breast cancer.

FORCE: www.facingourrisk.org
Provides support and information to BRCA-positive women.

Young Survival Coalition: www.youngsurvival.org
Provides support, education, and resources to young women with breast cancer.

Sister's Network for African-American Women:
www.sistersnetworkinc.org
Provides information and support to African-American women facing breast cancer.

Sharsheret: www.sharsheret.org
Provides information and support to Jewish women facing breast cancer.

Nueva Vida, Inc.: www.nueva-vida.org
Provides support, education, and resources to Latina women with breast cancer.

National Asian Women's Health Organization (NAWHO):
www.nawho.org
Provides information about a range of health issues, including breast cancer, for Asian-American women.

Living Beyond Breast Cancer: www.lbbc.org
Provides services and educational information to women of all ages and ethnic backgrounds.

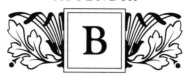

BREAST CANCER INFORMATION AND SUPPORT SERVICES

The following organizations and resources offer a wealth of information and support to cancer patients and their families. Information is easily accessed online and through the contact information provided. This is a comprehensive list, but unfortunately it is not all inclusive, because there are just too many worthwhile organizations providing breast cancer services. Therefore we have highlighted some of the best ones available that serve a variety of different needs. We have also included a section on some of the international organizations providing care throughout the world.

NATIONAL CANCER SUPPORT SERVICES

Adjuvant!
Website: *www.adjuvantonline.com*
Adjuvant! helps health professionals and patients who have early cancer discuss the risks and benefits of receiving additional therapy after surgery (adjuvant therapy: usually chemotherapy, hormonal therapy, or both).

African American Breast Cancer Alliance, Inc. (AABCA)
P.O. Box 8981
Minneapolis, MN 55408
Phone: 612-825-3675
Fax: 612-827-2977
Website: *www.aabcainc.org*
Email: aabca@aabcainc.org
Founded by African American women who had experienced breast cancer, the AABCA is a nonprofit organization dedicated to providing education and emotional and social support to breast cancer survivors, their family members, and the community.

American Cancer Society (ACS)
National Office
250 Williams Street
Atlanta, GA 30303
Phone: 404-315-1123
Toll free: 800-ACS-2345 (227-2345)
Website: *www.cancer.org*
The ACS is a nationwide, community-based, volunteer health organization dedicated to eliminating cancer as a major health problem by preventing cancer, saving lives from cancer, and diminishing suffering from cancer through research, education, and service. Services include:

1. Public and professional information on a broad range of topics
2. Service and rehabilitation
   - **Reach to Recovery:** Support program for breast cancer patients. For more information or to locate a Reach to Recovery program in your area, visit the "In My Community" section at *www.cancer.org,* or call 800-227-2345.
   - **Road to Recovery:** Provides transportation to and from treatment for people who have cancer and do not have a ride or are unable to drive themselves. Call 800-227-2345 to find out whether Road to Recovery is available in your community.
   - **Hope Lodge:** Lodging
   - **TLC:** Hair loss and mastectomy products
   - **Look Good . . . Feel Better:** Help with appearance-related side effects of treatment
   - **I Can Cope:** Cancer education classes

American College of Radiology (ACR)
1891 Preston White Drive
Reston, VA 20191
Phone: 703-648-8900
Toll free: 800-227-5463
Website: *www.acr.org*
Email: info@acr.org
The ACR provides patients with information on important questions to ask about treatment, safety, and locating an accredited facility.

American Hospital Association (AHA)
155 North Wacker Drive
Chicago, IL 60606
Phone: 312-422-3000
Website: *www.aha.org*
The AHA represents and serves hospitals, health systems, and other organizations committed to health improvement. Their goal is to advance the health of individuals and communities.

American Institute for Cancer Research (AICR)
1759 R Street, NW
Washington, DC 20009
Phone: 202-328-7744
Toll free: 800-843-8114
Fax: 202-328-7226
Website: *www.aicr.org*
Email: aicrweb@aicr.org
AICR focuses exclusively on the link between diet and cancer. In addition to supporting research in this field nationwide, AICR provides a wide range of educational publications.

American Society of Breast Surgeons
5950 Symphony Woods Road, Suite 212
Columbia, MD 21044
Phone: 410-992-5470
Toll free: 877-992-5470
Fax: 410-992-5472
Website: *www.breastsurgeons.org*
The American Society of Breast Surgeons is the primary leadership organization for general surgeons who treat patients who have breast disease.

American Society of Clinical Oncology (ASCO)
2318 Mill Road, Suite 800
Alexandria, VA 22314
Phone: 571-483-1300
Toll free: 888-282-2552
Website: *www.asco.org*
Email: membermail@asco.org
ASCO is a nonprofit organization with the goals of improving cancer care and prevention. Members include physicians and health care professionals in all levels of the practice of oncology.

American Society of Plastic Surgeons (ASPS)
444 East Algonquin Road
Arlington Heights, IL 60005
Phone: 847-228-9900
Website: *www.plasticsurgery.org*
The ASPS is the largest plastic surgery specialty organization in the world. ASPS publishes numerous informational brochures and maintains a website to provide public education about plastic surgery.

State Laws on Breast Reconstruction
Search for "state laws on breast reconstruction" from the ASPS home page to access information for specific states regarding insurance coverage for postmastectomy breast reconstruction. Insurance coverage is required for postmastectomy reconstruction if the mastectomy is covered. Additional information is available by following state government links provided.

Association of Oncology Social Work (AOSW)
100 North 20th Street, Suite 400
Philadelphia, PA 19103
Phone: 215-599-6093
Fax: 215-564-2175
Website: *www.aosw.org*
Email: info@aosw.org
The AOSW is a nonprofit, international organization whose mission is to provide psychosocial services to cancer patients and their families.

Breastcancer.org
Website: *www.breastcancer.org*
Breastcancer.org is a nonprofit organization dedicated to providing reliable, complete, and up-to-date information about breast cancer. Their online message boards can be accessed at *community.breastcancer.org*.

Breast Cancer Network of Strength
135 South LaSalle Street, Suite 2000
Chicago, IL 60603
Phone: 312-986-8338
YourShoes English hotline: 800-221-2141 (interpreters available in 150 languages)
YourShoes Spanish hotline: 800-986-9505
Fax: 312-294-8597
Website: *www.networkofstrength.org*
The Breast Cancer Network of Strength (formerly known as Y-ME National Breast Cancer Organization) provides immediate emotional relief to anyone affected by breast cancer. Their mission is to ensure, through information, empowerment, and peer support, that no one faces breast cancer alone.

YourShoes is a 24/7 breast cancer support center staffed by trained breast cancer survivors providing peer support through a toll-free hotline, email, and support groups. Online information is provided through interactive brochures and newsletters. The *Breast Cancer Survivor Match* program, available through the YourShoes Support Center, pairs women with peer counselors who had the same diagnosis and are the same age, or have experienced similar challenges; YourShoes also provides a *Partner Match* program for those who are supporting a woman through breast cancer. These confidential, free-of-charge services are available to anyone who calls the hotline at the numbers given above.

Breast Cancer Research Foundation (BCRF)
60 East 56th Street, 8th floor
New York, NY 10022
Phone: 646-497-2600
Toll free: 866-FIND-A-CURE (346-3228)
Fax: 646-497-0890
Website: *www.bcrfcure.org*
Email: bcrf@bcrfcure.org
The BCRF provides critical funding for innovative clinical and translational research to advance the effort to prevent and eventually cure breast cancer.

Breast Cancer Support
P.O. Box 1521
Montague, NJ 07827
Website: *www.bcsupport.org*
Email: bcsurvivors@gmail.com
An online breast cancer support group for survivors. The website has message boards and chat rooms.

CancerCare
275 Seventh Avenue, Floor 22
New York, NY 10001
Toll free: 800-813-HOPE (4673)
Fax: 212-712-8495
Website: *www.cancercare.org*
Email: info@cancercare.org
This organization provides free professional counseling, support groups, education, information, and referrals to cancer patients and their families. All services are provided by professional oncology social workers and are free of charge.

Cancer Information (formerly Yes, I Can)

Website: *www.cancerinformation.com*

Cancer Information (formerly Yes, I Can) is designed especially for people with concerns and questions about cancer, including information about treatment options. Their website provides information on managing the side effects of chemotherapy; it also offers a customized doctor discussion guide, and financial assistance information.

Cancer.Net

American Society of Clinical Oncology
Attn: Communications and Patient Information Department
2318 Mill Road, Suite 800
Alexandria, VA 22314
Phone: 571-483-1780
Toll free: 888-651-3038
Fax: 571-366-9537
Website: *www.cancer.net*
Email: contactus@cancer.net

Cancer.Net (formerly People Living With Cancer) provides oncologist-approved information from the American Society of Clinical Oncology. The website offers timely information to help patients and families make informed healthcare decisions.

Cancer Research Institute

One Exchange Plaza
55 Broadway, Suite 1802
New York, NY 10006
Phone: 212-688-7515
Toll free: 800-99-CANCER (992-2623)
Fax: 212-832-9376
Website: *www.cancerresearch.org*

This independent organization supports the most significant advances in cancer immunology research for preventing, treating, and curing cancer. It is a good resource for answering medical and research questions.

Cancer Support Community (CSC)

1050 17th Street, NW
Washington, DC 20036
Phone: 202-659-9709
Toll free: 888-793-9355
Fax: 202-659-9301
Website: *www.cancersupportcommunity.org* or *www.thewellnesscommunity.org*
Email: help@cancersupportcommunity.org

The CSC is an international nonprofit organization dedicated to providing support, education, and hope to people affected by cancer. As the world's largest employer of psychosocial oncology mental health professionals, based in the United States, the organization offers a network of personalized services and education for all people affected by cancer.

CenterWatch
100 North Washington Street, Suite 301
Boston, MA 02114
Phone: 617-948-5100
Toll free: 866-219-3440
Fax: 617-948-5101
Website: *www.centerwatch.com*
Email: sales@centerwatch.com
CenterWatch is a source for accessing news, directories, analysis, and proprietary market research for clinical research professionals and patients. This organization also provides patients with information on clinical trials, drugs, and other essential health and educational resources.

Centers for Disease Control and Prevention National Breast and Cervical Cancer Early Detection Program (NBCCEDP)
Centers for Disease Control and Prevention
Division of Cancer Prevention and Control
4770 Buford Highway, NE MS K-64
Atlanta, GA 30341
Toll free: 800-CDC-INFO (232-4636)
Fax: 770-488-4760
Website: *www.cdc.gov/cancer/NBCCEDP*
Email: cdcinfo@cdc.gov
The NBCCEDP provides access to breast and cervical cancer screening services for underserved women in all 50 states, the District of Columbia, five U.S. territories, and 12 Native American tribes.

Coalition of Cancer Cooperative Groups
1818 Market Street, Suite 1100
Philadelphia, PA 19103
Toll free: 877-520-4457
Fax: 215-789-3655
Website: *www.cancertrialshelp.org*
Email: Info@CancerTrialsHelp.org
The Coalition of Cancer Cooperative Groups is a nonprofit organization whose mission is to increase patient awareness of cancer clinical trials, facilitate access, and promote participation.

Coping With Cancer
P.O. Box 682268
Franklin, TN 37068-2268
Phone: 615-790-2400
Fax: 615-794-0179
Website: *www.copingmag.com/cwc*
Email: info@copingmag.com
Coping is a source of knowledge, hope, and inspiration to people with cancer worldwide. The *Coping With Cancer* website provides information by specific cancer type and focuses on living with cancer, wellness, and inspirational topics. *Coping With Cancer* magazine includes news, FDA updates, resource lists, and stories from patients, caregivers, and survivors about their coping strategies.

Corporate Angel Network
Westchester County Airport
One Loop Road
White Plains, NY 10604-1215
Phone: 914-328-1313
Toll free: 866-328-1313
Fax: 914-328-3938
Website: *www.corpangelnetwork.org*
Email: info@corpangelnetwork.org
This nationwide volunteer program provides free long-distance air transportation for cancer patients (and one accompanying family member) who need to travel for their treatment by using available space on corporate and private jets. Eligibility is not based on financial need, and patients may travel as often as necessary. To obtain free air transportation, call the CAN Patient Line at the toll-free number given above within 3 weeks of a specific appointment at a recognized cancer treatment center, or send them an email with a phone number where you can be reached.

ENCOREplus
YWCA of the USA
Office of Women's Health Initiative
2025 M Street NW, Suite 550
Washington, DC 20036
Phone: 202-467-0801
Fax: 202-467-0802
Website: *www.ywca.org*
Email: info@ywca.org
The YWCA offers a national program called ENCORE*plus*, a breast cancer program that provides outreach, education, and screening mammograms to women who lack access to needed breast health services. The program is run by women for women. To find an ENCORE*plus* program, call the YWCA headquarters, or search online at *www.ywca.org* to find a location near you.

Facing Our Risk of Cancer Empowered (FORCE)

16057 Tampa Palms Boulevard West, PMB #373
Tampa, FL 33647
Toll free: 866-288-RISK (7475)
Help line: 866-824-RISK (7475)
Fax: 954-827-2200
Website: *www.facingourrisk.org*
Email: info@facingourrisk.org
FORCE is a national nonprofit organization devoted to providing support, education, and advocacy and promoting awareness and research specific to hereditary breast and ovarian cancer.

FertileHOPE

Toll free: 866-965-7205
Website: *www.fertilehope.org*
FertileHOPE is a national LIVESTRONG initiative dedicated to providing reproductive information, support, and hope to cancer patients and survivors whose medical treatments present the risk of infertility.

The Hereditary Cancer Center

Department of Preventive Medicine
2500 California Plaza
Omaha, NE 68178
Toll free: 800-648-8133
Fax: 402-280-1734
Website: *medschool.creighton.edu/medicine/centers/hcc*
The Hereditary Cancer Institute at Creighton University is a nonprofit institution dedicated to research on hereditary cancers. It also disseminates information on cancer genetics and research and evaluates families to identify hereditary cancer and to predict cancer risk to family members and their offspring. This group maintains a registry of families with a pattern of familial cancer.

Living Beyond Breast Cancer (LBBC)

354 West Lancaster Avenue, Suite 224
Haverford, PA 19041
Phone: 484-708-1550 or 610-645-4567
Toll free: 888-753-5222
Fax: 610-645-4573
Website: *www.lbbc.org*
Email: mail@lbbc.org
The LBBC is a national education and support organization whose mission is to empower all women affected by breast cancer to live as long as possible with the best quality of life. They offer specialized programs and services for the newly diagnosed, young women, women with advanced breast cancer, women at high risk for developing breast cancer, and African American and Latina women.

MedlinePlus

U.S. National Library of Medicine
8600 Rockville Pike
Bethesda, MD 20894
Website: *www.medlineplus.gov*
Email: custserv@nlm.nih.gov
MedlinePlus brings together information from the National Library of Medicine, the National Institutes of Health, and other government agencies and health-related organizations. Preformulated MEDLINE searches are included in MedlinePlus, providing easy access to medical journal articles. MedlinePlus also has drug information, an illustrated medical encyclopedia, interactive patient tutorials, and current health news.

My Cancer Advisor and Patient Resource

Websites: *www.mycanceradvisor.com* and *www.patientresource.net*
My Cancer Advisor and Patient Resource are patient-empowering websites with the mission of informing and educating cancer patients and their caregivers to better navigate their treatment. Patient Resource focuses on patient advocacy and empowerment through education. It produces a number of comprehensive publications (in print and on their website) that are of interest to cancer patients and their families. These include *Patient Resource Cancer Guide*, a comprehensive 160-page guide for patients that describes all aspects of cancer diagnosis and treatment as well as a listing of more than 2000 websites that are trusted and reliable, cancer treatment facilities, and cancer specific advocacy groups. It also publishes three companion publications, the *Patient Resource Breast Cancer Guides*, with more than 100 pages specific for breast cancer patients.

These free booklets are available from the above websites, or call 816-333-3595, ext 26:

- *Patient Resource Cancer Guide: A Treatment and Facilities Guide for Patients and Their Families*
- *Patient Resource Cancer Guide: Metastatic Breast Cancer*
- *Patient Resource Breast Cancer Guide: Her2+ & ER/PR+ Personalized Therapy Options*
- *Patient Resource Breast Cancer Guide: A Treatment and Facilities Guide for Patients and Their Families*

National Breast Cancer Coalition
1101 17th Street, NW, Suite 1300
Washington, DC 20036
Phone: 202-296-7477
Toll free: 800-622-2838
Fax: 202-265-6854
Website: *www.stopbreastcancer.org*
Email: info@stopbreastcancer.org
This grassroots advocacy movement is working toward increased federal funding
for breast cancer research and finding a cure.

National Breast Cancer Foundation, Inc. (NBCF)
2600 Network Boulevard, Suite 300
Frisco, TX 75034
Website: *www.nationalbreastcancer.org*
NBCF is committed to spreading knowledge and fostering hope in the fight
against breast cancer. Their mission includes increasing awareness through education, providing diagnostic breast care services for those in need, and providing support services. They fund free mammograms for women who are unable to
afford them and support research programs in leading facilities throughout the
country.

National Cancer Institute (NCI)
NCI Office of Communications and Education
Public Inquiries Office
6116 Executive Boulevard, Suite 300
Bethesda, MD 20892-8322
800-4-CANCER (422-6237)
Website: *www.cancer.gov*
Email: cancergovstaff@mail.nih.gov
The NCI is a division of the National Institutes of Health and is the federal government's principal agency devoted to researching cancer prevention, diagnosis,
treatment, and rehabilitation and to dissemination of information on prevention, detection, and treatment. The NCI provides free information on cancer detection, treatment, rehabilitation, NCI-supported clinical trials, and research
programs, all available online or by phone. The NCI supports treatment centers throughout the country and conducts breast cancer research. In addition to
its Cancer Information Service, the NCI also conducts clinical studies. The
online booklet, *What You Need To Know About Breast Cancer,* is available for review and at-home printing and includes information about breast cancer symptoms, diagnosis, treatment, and questions to ask the doctor.

Knowledgeable cancer information specialists can answer your questions about cancer and can help you use the website, as well as tell you about the NCI's printed and electronic materials. The specialists are available by phone, live online chat, email, or mail. (See the contact information above.)

National Cancer Institute Clinical Trials
An online resource from the NCI for obtaining information about cancer clinical trials designed to help users find and select a treatment trial. It also posts information about clinical trial results and other educational material. For more information, visit *www.cancer.gov/clinicaltrials*.

LiveHelp
Cancer information specialists from the NCI's cancer information service offer online assistance on the NCI website. Visitors participate in a confidential online text chat. This service is available Monday through Friday from 8:00 AM to 11:00 PM Eastern time.

Cancer Information Service
The NCI's Cancer Information Service provides scientifically based, balanced information about all aspects of cancer to patients, their families and friends, health professionals, and the general public. They educate people about clinical trials and facilitate their participation by identifying clinical trials for all aspects of cancer care from prevention through treatment and rehabilitation. NCI-supported trials are available at institutions across the country. Information specialists are trained to answer cancer-related questions by phone, live online chat, and email. These services are free.

NCI Cancer Bulletin
The *NCI Cancer Bulletin* is a biweekly online newsletter designed to provide useful, timely information about cancer research to the cancer community. The newsletter is published approximately 24 times per year by the NCI. Subscribe online at *www.cancer.gov/ncicancerbulletin*.

Physician Data Query (PDQ)
PDQ is the NCI's comprehensive cancer database. It contains summaries of a wide range of cancer topics, a registry of 8000-plus open and 19,000-plus closed cancer clinical trials from around the world, and a directory of professionals who provide genetics services. PDQ also contains the NCI Dictionary of Cancer Terms, with definitions for more than 6000 cancer and medical terms, and the NCI Drug Dictionary, which has information on 1200-plus agents used in the treatment of cancer or cancer-related conditions. The NCI's PDQ database is available online at *www.cancer.gov/cancertopics/pdq*.

National Center for Complementary and Alternative Medicine (NCCAM)

P.O. Box 7923
Gaithersburg, MD 20898
Toll Free: 888-644-6226
Fax: 866-464-3616
Website: *www.nccam.nih.gov*
Email: info@nccam.nih.gov
The NCCAM is the federal government's leading agency for scientific research on complementary and alternative medicine (CAM).

National Coalition for Cancer Survivorship (NCCS)

1010 Wayne Avenue, Suite 770
Silver Spring, MD 20910
Phone: 301-650-9127
Toll free: 888-650-9127
Fax: 301-565-9670
Website: *www.canceradvocacy.org*
Email: info@canceradvocacy.org
The NCCS is a network of independent groups and individuals offering support to cancer survivors and their loved ones. It provides information and resources for people diagnosed with cancer and publishes a quarterly newsletter, *The Networker*, for its members.

Online NCCS Resources

Provides information that cancer survivors need to know about health insurance.

National Comprehensive Cancer Network (NCCN)

275 Commerce Drive, Suite 300
Fort Washington, PA 19034
Phone: 215-690-0300
Fax: 215-690-0280
Website: *www.nccn.com*
The National Comprehensive Cancer Network is a not-for-profit alliance of 21 of the world's leading cancer centers. The goal of their website is to educate cancer patients to engage in more informed conversations with health care providers so they can live longer and better quality lives. The website provides information to help patients, families, friends, and cancer survivors make treatment decisions, locate financial assistance for cancer care, learn how to find the best types of insurance plans, make decisions about palliative care, and track and maintain medical records. They also give tips for managing fatigue, eating a healthy diet, and exercising during and after treatment.

National Consortium of Breast Centers (NCBC)
P.O. Box 1334
Warsaw, IN 46581-1334
Phone: 574-267-8058
Fax: 547-267-8268
Website: *www.breastcare.org* or *www.ncbcinc.org*
Email: NCBC@breastcare.org
The NCBC is a professional membership organization of comprehensive breast centers throughout the nation. One of their goals is to serve as an informational resource and provide support services to those rendering care to people with breast diseases through educational programs, newsletters, a national directory, and patient forums.

National Hospice and Palliative Care Organization (NHPCO)
1731 King Street, Suite 100
Alexandria, VA 22314
Phone: 703-837-1500
Fax: 703-837-1233
Website: *www.nhpco.org*
Email: nhpco_info@nhpco.org
This organization's hospice help line assists callers in locating a hospice in their area. To search for a provider, visit their website.

National Lymphedema Network, Inc. (NLN)
116 New Montgomery Street, Suite 235
San Francisco, CA 94105
Phone: 415-908-3681
Toll free: 800-541-3259
Fax: 415- 908-3813
Website: *www.lymphnet.org*
Email: nln@lymphnet.org
The NLN provides a quarterly newsletter, *LymphLink,* with cutting edge articles and information about medical and scientific developments, support groups, pen pals/net pals, an updated resource guide, and more. Their website provides referrals to lymphedema treatment centers, health care professionals, training programs, and support groups, as well as educational materials for health care professionals and patients.

National Patient Travel Center
4620 Haygood Road, Suite 1
Virginia Beach, VA 23455
Phone: 757-512-5287
Toll free: 800-296-1217
Fax: 800-550-1767
Website: *www.patienttravel.org*
Email: info@nationalpatienttravelcenter.org
The National Patient Travel Center's mission is to ensure that no financially needy patient is denied access to distant specialized medical evaluation, diagnosis, or treatment for lack of a means of transportation. This group provides information about all forms of charitable, long-distance, medical air transport services and provides referrals to all appropriate sources of help available in the national charitable medical air transportation network.

National Society of Genetic Counselors, Inc. (NSGC)
401 North Michigan Avenue
Chicago, IL 60611
Phone: 312-321-6834
Fax: 312-673-6972
Website: *www.nsgc.org*
Email: nsgc@nsgc.org
The NSGC's mission is to promote the availability of quality genetic services. They provide referrals to health centers with genetic counselors on staff and can also provide information about BRCA1 and BRCA2 and genetic testing.

The National Women's Health Network
1413 K Street, NW, 4th Floor
Washington, DC 20005
Phone: 202-682-2640 or 202-682-2646
Fax: 202-682-2648
Website: *www.nwhn.org*
Email: healthquestions@nwhn.org or nwhn@nwhn.org
This organization is a national consumer group devoted to women and their health needs and to protecting the rights of women in areas of health care. The group acts as a strong advocate for legislative and medical issues, including breast cancer. They also produce the newsletter *Women's Health Activist*, which provides current information on a variety of women's health issues.

Patient Advocate Foundation
421 Butler Farm Road
Hampton, VA 23666
Toll free: 800-532-5274
Fax: 757-873-8999
Website: *www.patientadvocate.org*
Email: help@patientadvocate.org
This foundation provides effective mediation and arbitration services for patients to remove obstacles to health care, including medical debt crises, insurance access issues, and employment issues for patients with chronic, debilitating, and life-threatening illnesses.

Co-Pay Relief (CPR)
421 Butler Farm Road
Hampton, VA 23666
Phone: 757-952-0118
Toll Free: 866-512-3861
Fax: 757-952-0119
Website: *www.copays.org*
The CPR program is provided through the Patient Advocate Foundation. It provides direct financial support to insured patients, including Medicare Part D beneficiaries, who must financially and medically qualify to access pharmaceutical copayment assistance. The program offers personal service to all patients through call counselors, who personally guide patients through the enrollment process.

Patient Resource Publishing
440 West 62nd Street
Kansas City, MO 64113
Phone: 816-333-3595
Fax: 816-386-2909
Website: *www.patientresource.net*
Email: prp@patientresource.net
The goal of Patient Resource Publishing is to empower cancer patients and their families by giving them access to comprehensive information and resources (see p. 634 and the Bibliography for more information.)

R.A. Bloch Cancer Foundation, Inc.
Bloch Cancer Hotline
One H&R Block Way
Kansas City, MO 64105
Phone: 816-854-5050
Toll free: 800-433-0464 (Hotline)
Fax: 816-854-8024
Website: *www.blochcancer.org*
Email: hotline@blochcancer.org
This foundation provides a hotline that matches newly diagnosed cancer patients with someone who has survived the same kind of cancer. It offers free information, resources, and support groups and supplies three books at no charge: *Fighting Cancer*, *Cancer . . . There's Hope*, and *Guide for Cancer Supporters*.

SHARE
1501 Broadway, Suite 704A
New York, NY 10036
Phone: 212-719-0364
Toll free: 866-891-2392
Website: *www.sharecancersupport.org*
Email: info@sharecancersupport.org
SHARE's mission is to create and sustain a supportive network and community of women affected by breast or ovarian cancer. SHARE brings these women and their families and friends together with others who have experienced breast or ovarian cancer and provides participants with the opportunity to receive and exchange information, support, strength, and hope.

Sisters Network, Inc.
2922 Rosedale Street
Houston, TX 77004
Phone: 713-781-0255
Toll free: 866-781-1808
Fax: 713-780-8998
Website: *www.sistersnetworkinc.org*
Email: infonet@sistersnetworkinc.org
Sisters Network, Inc., is a national African American breast cancer survivorship organization that is committed to increasing local and national attention to how breast cancer affects the African American community.

Susan G. Komen for the Cure
5005 LBJ Freeway, Suite 250
Dallas, TX 75244
877-GO-KOMEN (465-6636)
Website: *www.komen.org*
The Komen Foundation is the world's largest grassroots network of breast cancer survivors and activists. They offer a comprehensive program for the research and treatment of breast disease. Information on screening, breast self examination, treatment, and support is available by telephone. They are fighting to eradicate breast cancer as a life-threatening disease through chapters and Race for the Cure events, and by funding national breast cancer research, project grants, and local education, screening, and treatment projects in communities nationwide.

KomenLink
This is an online newsletter that provides timely information about breast health, breast cancer, and Komen's programs and initiatives. Their website also includes an informative section on Understanding Breast Cancer, which includes topics on risk, prevention, and more. The Komen breast care help line provides free, professional support services to anyone with breast health or breast cancer questions or concerns.

Linking ARMS (Assistance & Resources Made Simple)
The Linking ARMS program is dedicated to helping underserved women with breast cancer. A partnership between CancerCare and Susan G. Komen for the Cure, Linking ARMS provides financial assistance, education, and support services to low-income, underinsured or uninsured women across the country. Patients can access the Linking ARMS program by calling the CancerCare toll-free line at 800-813-HOPE (4673).

U.S. Food and Drug Administration (FDA)
10903 New Hampshire Avenue
Silver Spring, MD 20993
Toll free: 888-INFO-FDA (463-6332)
Website: *www.fda.gov*
The FDA provides safety information on drugs and other FDA-approved products and devices, such as breast implants.

Young Survival Coalition (YSC)
61 Broadway, Suite 2235
New York, NY 10006
Phone: 646-257-3000
Toll free: 877-YSC-1011 (972-1011)
Fax: 646-257-3030
Website: *www.youngsurvival.org*
Email: info@youngsurvival.org
YSC is an international organization dedicated to the critical issues that are unique to young women and to breast cancer. YSC works with survivors, caregivers, and the medical, research, advocacy, and legislative communities to increase the quality and quantity of life for women younger than 40 who have been diagnosed with breast cancer.

SECOND OPINION CENTERS

A number of major hospitals throughout the country offer second opinion consultation services at varying costs. A multidisciplinary team of specialists meets with the patient and the family to review the diagnosis and tests to provide the patient with a recommended second opinion for the course of treatment. Call the Cancer Information Service at 800-4-CANCER, or visit their website at *www.cancer.gov/aboutnci/cis*, to locate the center nearest you.

INFORMATION ON HEALTH INSURANCE

America's Health Insurance Plans (AHIP)
601 Pennsylvania Avenue, NW, South Building, Suite 500
Washington, DC 20004
Phone: 202-778-3200
Fax: 202-331-7487
Website: *www.ahip.org*
Email: ahip@ahip.org
AHIP is a national association representing nearly 1300 member companies providing health insurance coverage to more than 200 million Americans. The organization provides a unified voice for the community of health insurance plans.

The Center for Medicare Advocacy, Inc.
P.O. Box 350
Willimantic, CT 06226
Phone: 860-456-7790
Fax: 860-456-2614
Website: *www.medicareadvocacy.org*
The Center for Medicare Advocacy, Inc. is a national, nonprofit, nonpartisan organization that provides education, advocacy, and legal assistance to help elders and people with disabilities obtain Medicare and necessary health care.

Centers for Medicare and Medicaid Services
7500 Security Boulevard
Baltimore, MD 21244
Phone: 877-267-2323
Website: *www.cms.gov*
The goal of the CMS is to ensure effective, up-to-date health care coverage and to promote quality care for beneficiaries. They provide information on Medicare and Medicaid and their benefits, how they work together, and what is covered. Patients can also read and print Medicare publications and find regional offices for more information.

Insurance Information Institute (I.I.I.)
110 William Street
New York, NY 10038
Phone: 212-346-5500
Website: *www.iii.org/individuals/healthinsurance*
Email: members@iii.org
The mission of the I.I.I. is to improve public understanding of insurance—what it does and how it works. The I.I.I. publishes a number of helpful pamphlets and books and provides information on health insurance basics, buying insurance, and a glossary of insurance topics.

INTERNATIONAL RESOURCES

Australian New Zealand Breast Cancer Trials Group
Clinical Trials Group
Department of Surgical Oncology
Calvary Mater Newcastle
Locked Bag 7
HRMC NSW 2310, Australia
Phone: 61 2 4985 0136
Fax: 61 2 4985 0140
Website: *www.anzbctg.org*
Email: enquiries@anzbctg.newcastle.edu.au
This group's mission is to promote breast cancer research in Australia and New
Zealand. They provide information on the latest clinical trials being conducted.

Breast Cancer Care
5–13 Great Suffolk Street
London SE1 0NS, United Kingdom
Phone: 0845 092 0800
Helpline: 0808 800 6000
Website: *www.breastcancercare.org.uk*
Email: info@breastcancercare.org.uk
This United Kingdom organization provides information and support to cancer
patients and their families. They offer a national help line, volunteer service,
and a wide range of information and audio tapes.

Canadian Breast Cancer Foundation
375 University Avenue, 6th Floor
Toronto, Ontario M5G 2J5, Canada
Phone: 416-596-6773
Toll free: 800-387-9816
Website: *www.cbcf.org*
Email: NationalHealthPromotion@cbcf.org
This organization provides financial support for breast cancer research and treat-
ment as well as comprehensive breast cancer information for patients, their fam-
ilies, and the public at large.

Canadian Breast Cancer Network
331 Cooper Street, Suite 300
Ottawa, Ontario K2P 0G5, Canada
Phone: 613-230-3044
Toll free: 800-685-8820
Fax: 613-230-4424
Website: *www.cbcn.ca*
Email: cbcn@cbcn.ca
CBCN is a national network of organizations providing support, education and awareness to breast cancer survivors.

Canadian Cancer Society
National Office
Suite 200, 10 Alcom Avenue
Toronto, Ontario M4V 3B1, Canada
Phone: 416-961-7223
Fax: 416-961-4189
Website: *www.cancer.ca*
Email: info@cis.cancer.ca
A national community-based organization that provides a wide range of cancer information, peer support, and financial information to cancer patients and their families to promote an enhanced quality of life.

Cancer Council Australia
GPO Box 4708, Sydney NSW 2001
Level 1, 120 Chalmers Street
Surry Hills, NSW 2010, Australia
Phone: 61 2 8063 4100
Fax: 61 2 8063 4101
Website: *www.cancer.org.au*
Email: info@cancer.org.au
This organization is the Australian counterpart to the American Cancer Society, providing valuable information and support to cancer patients and their families.

Macmillan Cancer Support
89 Albert Embankment
London SE1 7UQ, United Kingdom
Phone: 020 7840 7840
Hotline: 0808 808 00 00
Fax: 020 7840 7841
Website: *www.macmillan.org.uk*
This is a leading United Kingdom organization that provides support, counseling and information for cancer patients and their families and friends. It also publishes booklets on specific cancers and their diagnosis and treatment.

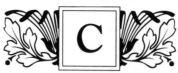

THE PATIENT'S RIGHTS

The two documents that follow confirm the rights and standard of care that women should expect from their doctors and from the medical personnel who treat them.

A Breast Cancer Patient's Options and Rights*

- To receive a simple and clear diagnosis of her condition
- To receive all available diagnostic procedures and a complete workup before surgery
- To have the consent form clearly explained to her before she signs it
- To have the biopsy performed first (under local anesthesia), including the right to see the pathologist's report and have it explained to her; surgery may be performed at a later date
- To be aware that, for certain patients, the future option of reconstructive plastic surgery exists and to have the surgeon take that option into consideration
- To receive consideration from the surgeon and other medical personnel for the physical and emotional trauma she is undergoing
- To receive an explanation of any viable alternative treatments—including biopsy with radiation therapy as primary treatment, chemotherapy, mastectomy, etc.—and the risks, disadvantages, and advantages of each treatment
- To receive a satisfying explanation for why the surgeon has decided on a particular surgical procedure rather than a less mutilating one
- To be referred to a therapist for physical or psychiatric therapy following surgery
- To receive competent follow-up care after surgery and to know who is going to be responsible for that care
- To be referred to a support group for information and assistance with her personal concerns
- To be always treated as an adult

*Prepared by Women for Women, a nonprofit West Coast organization.

The Patient Care Partnership*

The Patient Care Partnership was developed by the American Hospital Association (AHA) to inform patients about what to expect during their hospital stay with regard to their rights and responsibilities. It offers the following guidelines:

1. The patient has the right to high-quality hospital care. She has the right to know the identity of doctors, nurses, and others involved in her care, and to know when they are students, residents, or other trainees.

2. The patient has the right to a clean and safe environment.

3. The patient has the right to be involved in her care. When decision making takes place, it should include:

   - A discussion of her medical condition and information about medically appropriate choices. To make informed decisions, she needs to understand the benefits and risks of each treatment, whether a treatment is experimental or part of a research study, what to reasonably expect from treatment with any long-term effects on the quality of life, what the patient and her family need to do after leaving the hospital, and the financial consequences of using uncovered services or out-of-network providers.

   - A discussion of the treatment plan. When the patient enters the hospital, she signs a general consent to treatment. In some cases, such as for surgery or an experimental treatment, the patient may be asked to confirm in writing that she understands what is planned and agrees to it. This process protects the patient's right to consent to or refuse a treatment. The doctor will explain the medical consequences of refusing the recommended treatment. It also protects the patient's right to decide if she wants to participate in a research study.

   - Getting information from the patient. The patient's caregivers need complete and correct information about her health and coverage so that they can make good decisions about care. This includes: past illnesses, surgeries, or hospital stays; past allergic reactions; any medicines or dietary supplements (such as vitamins and herbs); and any network or admission requirements under the patient's health plan.

   - Understanding the patient's health care goals and values. The patient's health care goals and values or spiritual beliefs will be taken into account as much as possible throughout her hospital stay. The patient's doctor, family, and care team should know her wishes.

*Prepared by the American Hospital Association.

- Understanding who should make decisions when the patient cannot. If the patient has signed a health care power of attorney stating who should speak for her if she becomes unable to make health care decisions for herself, or a "living will" or "advance directive" that states her wishes about end-of-life care, copies should be given to her doctor, family, and care team. If help is needed making difficult decisions, counselors, chaplains, and others are available to help.

4. The patient has the right to have her privacy protected. The hospital must respect the confidentiality of her relationship with her doctor and other caregivers, and the sensitive health and health care information that are part of that relationship. State and federal laws and hospital operating policies protect the privacy of the patient's medical information. The patient should receive a Notice of Privacy Practices that describes the ways that hospitals use, disclose, and safeguard patient information and that explains how to obtain a copy of information from the hospital's records about patient care.

5. The patient and her family have the right to plan for the care she will receive after leaving the hospital. A patient can expect the hospital to help her identify sources of follow-up care and to let her know if the hospital has a financial interest in any referrals. As long as the patient agrees that the hospital can share information about her care with them, the hospital will coordinate their activities with the patient's caregivers outside the hospital. The patient can also expect to receive information and, where possible, training about self-care that will be needed when she goes home.

6. The patient has the right to expect help with her bill and with filing insurance claims. Hospital staff members file claims for patients with health care insurers or other programs such as Medicare and Medicaid. They also help the doctor with needed documentation. Hospital bills and insurance coverage are often confusing. If the patient has questions about a bill, she can contact the hospital's business office. If help is needed understanding insurance coverage or the health plan, the patient can start by contacting her insurance company or health benefits manager. If the patient does not have health coverage, hospitals should try to help patients and their families find financial help or make other arrangements. Hospitals will request the patient's help with collecting needed information and other requirements for obtaining coverage or assistance.

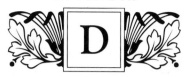

NATIONAL CANCER INSTITUTE CANCER CENTERS PROGRAM

The National Cancer Institute (NCI) Cancer Centers Program* comprises more than 65 NCI-designated cancer centers engaged in multidisciplinary research to reduce cancer incidence, morbidity, and mortality. This program supports three types of centers through Cancer Center Support Grants:

- Comprehensive Cancer Centers that conduct programs in all three areas of research: basic research, clinical research, and prevention and control research. They also have community outreach and education programs.
- Clinical Cancer Centers that conduct programs in clinical research and may also have programs in other research areas.
- Cancer Centers (formerly called Basic Science Cancer Centers) that focus on basic research or cancer control research, but do not have clinical oncology programs.

Each type of cancer center has special characteristics and capabilities for organizing new programs of research that can exploit important new findings and address timely research questions. All NCI-designated cancer centers are reevaluated each time their cancer center support grant comes up for renewal (generally every 3 to 5 years).

To attain recognition from NCI as a Comprehensive Cancer Center, an institution must pass rigorous peer review. Under guidelines revised in 2008, a Comprehensive Cancer Center must perform research in three major areas: basic research; clinical research; and can-

*Information on the NCI Cancer Centers Program is being reprinted with permission from the National Cancer Institute.

cer prevention, control, and population-based research. It must also have a strong body of interactive research that bridges these research areas. In addition, a Comprehensive Cancer Center must conduct activities in outreach, education, and information provision, which are directed toward and accessible to both health care professionals and the lay community.

Clinical Cancer Centers have active programs in clinical research and may also have programs in another area (such as basic research or prevention, control, and population-based research). Clinical Cancer Centers focus on both laboratory research and clinical research within a single institutional framework. This interaction of research and clinical activities is a distinguishing characteristic of many Clinical Cancer Centers.

The general term *Cancer Center* refers to an organization with scientific disciplines outside the specific qualifications for a comprehensive or clinical center. Such centers may, for example, concentrate on basic research, epidemiology and cancer control research, or other areas of research.

Since the passage of the National Cancer Act of 1971, the Cancer Centers Program has continued to expand. Today, NCI-designated Cancer Centers continue to work toward creating new and innovative approaches to cancer research. Through interdisciplinary efforts, Cancer Centers can effectively move this research from the laboratory to clinical trials and into clinical practice.

Patients seeking clinical oncology services (screening, diagnosis, or treatment) can obtain those services at Clinical Cancer Centers or Comprehensive Cancer Centers. They can also participate in research studies (clinical trials) at these centers. Most Cancer Centers engage almost entirely in basic research and do not provide patient care.

A list of the NCI-designated Cancer Centers follows. Information about referral procedures, treatment costs, and services available to patients can be obtained from individual cancer centers. Additional information about the Cancer Centers Program can be found online at *http://cancercenters.cancer.gov.*

Comprehensive(*) and Clinical(†) Cancer Centers Supported by NCI

Alabama

UAB Comprehensive Cancer
  Center*
University of Alabama at
  Birmingham
1802 Sixth Avenue South, NP 2555
Birmingham, AL 35294-3300
205-934-5077

Arizona

University of Arizona Cancer
  Center*
1515 North Campbell Avenue
P.O. Box 245024
Tucson, AZ 85724-5024
520-626-7685

California

Chao Family Comprehensive
  Cancer Center*
University of California–Irvine
101 The City Drive
Building 56, Route 81,
  Room 216L
Orange, CA 92868
714-456- 6310

Beckman Research Institute
City of Hope National Medical
  Center*
1500 East Duarte Road
Duarte, CA 91010-3000
626-256-HOPE (4673)

Jonsson Comprehensive Cancer
  Center*
University of California–Los Angeles
Factor Building, Room 8-684
10833 Le Conte Avenue
Los Angeles, CA 90095-1781
310-825-5268

Salk Institute Cancer Center†
10010 North Torrey Pines Road
La Jolla, CA, 92037
858-453-4100, Ext. 1385

Sanford-Burnham Medical Research
  Institute†
10901 North Torrey Pines Road
La Jolla, CA 92037
858-646-3100

Stanford Cancer Center†
Stanford University
800 Welch Road, Room 284
Stanford, CA 94305-5796
650-736-1808

UC Davis Cancer Center†
Universtiy of California–Davis
4501 X Street, Suite 3003
Sacramento, CA 95817
916-734-5800

UCSF Helen Diller Family Compre-
  hensive Cancer Center*
University of California–San
  Francisco
1450 3rd Street
Room HD-371, UCSF Box 0128
San Francisco, CA 94158-9001
415-502-1710

Moores Cancer Center
University of California–San Diego*
3855 Health Sciences Drive,
  Room 2247
La Jolla, CA 92093-0658
858-822-1222

USC Norris Comprehensive Cancer
    Center*
University of Southern California
1441 Eastlake Avenue, NOR 8302L
Los Angeles, CA 90089-9181
323-865-0816

Colorado

University of Colorado Cancer
    Center*
University of Colorado at Denver
    and Health Sciences Center
P.O. Box 6508, Mail Stop F434
13001 East 17th Place
Aurora, CO 80045
303-724-3155

Connecticut

Yale Cancer Center*
Yale University School of Medicine
333 Cedar Street, Box 208028
New Haven, CT 06520-8028
203-785-4371

District of Columbia

Lombardi Cancer Research Center*
Georgetown University Medical
    Center
3970 Reservoir Road, NW
Research Building, Suite E501
Washington, DC 20057
202-687-2110

Florida

H. Lee Moffitt Cancer Center and
    Research Institute*
University of South Florida
12902 Magnolia Drive, MCC-CEO
Tampa, FL 33612-9497
813-615-4261

Georgia

Winship Cancer Institute†
Emory University
1365C Clifton Road
Atlanta, GA 30322
888-WINSHIP (946-7447)
404-778-5669

Hawaii

Cancer Research Center of Hawaii†
University of Hawaii at Manoa
651 Ilalo Street, BSB 231-H
Honolulu, HI 96813
808-440-4596

Illinois

Robert H. Lurie Comprehensive
    Cancer Center*
Northwestern University
303 East Superior Street, Suite 3-125
Chicago, IL 60611
312-908-5250

University of Chicago Comprehen-
    sive Cancer Center*
5841 South Maryland Avenue,
    MC 2115
Chicago, IL 60637-1470
773-702-6180

Indiana

Indiana University Melvin and Bren
    Simon Cancer Center†
Indiana Cancer Pavilion
535 Barnhill Drive, Room 455
Indianapolis, IN 46202-5289
317-278-0070

Purdue University Center for Cancer
   Research†
Hansen Life Sciences Research
   Building
South University Street
West Lafayette, IN 47907-1524
765-494-9129

Iowa
Holden Comprehensive Cancer
   Center*
University of Iowa
5970 "Z" JPP
200 Hawkins Drive
Iowa City, IA 52242
319-353-8620

Maine
The Jackson Laboratory Cancer
   Center†
600 Main Street
Bar Harbor, ME 04609-0800
207-288-6041

Maryland
Greenebaum Cancer Center†
University of Maryland
22 South Greene Street
Baltimore, MD 21201
410-328-7904

Sidney Kimmel Comprehensive
   Cancer Center*
Johns Hopkins University
401 North Broadway
The Weinberg Building, Suite 1100
Baltimore, MD 21231
410-955-8822

Massachusetts
Dana-Faber/Harvard Cancer Center*
Dana-Farber Cancer Institute
44 Binney Street, Room 1628
Boston, MA 02115
877-420-3951
617-632-2100

David H. Koch Institute for Integra-
   tive Cancer Research at MIT†
Massachusetts Institute of Technology
77 Massachusetts Avenue, Room
   E17-110
Cambridge, MA 02139-4307
617-253-8511

Michigan
The Barbara Ann Karmanos Cancer
   Institute*
Wayne State University School of
   Medicine
4100 John R
Detroit, MI 48201
800-KARMANOS (527-6266)

University of Michigan Comprehensive Cancer Center*
6302 Cancer Center
1500 East Medical Center Drive
Ann Arbor, MI 48109-0942
800-865-1125
734-936-1831

Minnesota
Masonic Cancer Center*
University of Minnesota
MMC 806, 420 Delaware Street, SE
Minneapolis, MN 55455
888-226-2376
612-624-8484

Mayo Clinic Cancer Center*
Mayo Clinic Rochester
200 First Street, SW
Rochester, MN 55905
507-266-4997

Missouri

Siteman Cancer Center*
Washington University School of
    Medicine
660 South Euclid Avenue
Campus Box 8109
St. Louis, MO 63110
314-362-8020

Nebraska

University of Nebraska Medical
    Center/Eppley Cancer Center†
600 South 42nd Street
Omaha, NE 68198-6805
402-559-4238

New Hampshire

Norris Cotton Cancer Center*
Dartmouth-Hitchcock Medical
    Center
One Medical Center Drive, Hinman
    Box 1920
Lebanon, NH 03756-0001
603-653-9000

New Jersey

The Cancer Institute of New Jersey*
Robert Wood Johnson Medical
    School
195 Little Albany Street
New Brunswick, NJ 08903-2681
732-235-8064

New Mexico

University of New Mexico Cancer
    Research and Treatment Center*
1201 Camino de Salud NE
MSC 07-4025, Room 4642
Albuquerque, NM 87131
505-272-5622

New York

Albert Einstein Cancer Research
    Center†
Albert Einstein College of Medicine
Chanin Building, Room 209
1300 Morris Park Avenue
Bronx, NY 10461
718-430-2302

Cold Spring Harbor Laboratory†
P.O. Box 100
Cold Spring Harbor, NY 11724
516-367-8383

Herbert Irving Comprehensive
    Cancer Center*
College of Physicians and Surgeons
Columbia University
1130 St. Nicholas Avenue
Room 508
New York, NY 10032
212-851-5273

Memorial Sloan-Kettering Cancer
    Center*
1275 York Avenue
New York, NY 10021
800-525-2225
212-639-2000

NYU Cancer Institute†
New York University Medical Center
550 First Avenue
New York, NY 10016
212-263-6485

Roswell Park Cancer Institute*
Elm and Carlton Streets
Buffalo, NY 14263-0001
716-845-5772

North Carolina
Duke Comprehensive Cancer
   Center*
Duke University Medical Center
Box 2714
Durham, NC 27710
919-684-5613

UNC Lineberger Comprehensive
   Cancer Center*
University of North Carolina at
   Chapel Hill
102 Mason Farm Road, CB 7295
Chapel Hill, NC 27599-7295
919-966-3036

Wake Forest Comprehensive Cancer
   Center*
Wake Forest University
Medical Center Boulevard
Winston-Salem, NC 27157-1082
336-716-7971

Ohio
Case Comprehensive Cancer Center*
Case Western Reserve University
11100 Euclid Avenue, Wearn 151
Cleveland, OH 44106-5065
216-844-8562

Comprehensive Cancer Center*
The Ohio State University
OSU James Cancer Hospital
300 West 10th Avenue, Suite 519
Columbus, OH 43210
614-293-7521

Oregon
OHSU Knight Cancer Institute†
Oregon Health and Science
   University
3181 Southwest Sam Jackson Park
   Road, CR145
Portland, OR 97239-3098
503-494-1617

Pennsylvania
Abramson Cancer Center*
University of Pennsylvania
16th Floor Penn Tower
3400 Spruce Street
Philadelphia, PA 19104-4283
215-662-6065

Fox Chase Cancer Center*
333 Cottman Avenue
Philadelphia, PA 19111
215-728-3636

Kimmel Cancer Center†
Thomas Jefferson University
233 South 10th Street
Bluemle Life Science Building,
   Room 1050
Philadelphia, PA 19107-5799
215-503-5692

University of Pittsburgh Cancer
    Institute*
UPMC Cancer Pavilion
5150 Centre Avenue, Suite 500
Pittsburgh, PA 15232
412-623-3205

The Wistar Institute †
3601 Spruce Street
Philadelphia, PA 19104-4268
215-898-3926

South Carolina
Hollings Cancer Center†
Medical University of South
    Carolina
86 Jonathan Lucas Street
Charleston, SC 29425
843-792-8284

Tennessee
St. Jude Children's Research
    Hospital*
262 Danny Thomas Place
Memphis, TN 38105-3678
901-595-3982

Vanderbilt-Ingram Cancer Center*
Vanderbilt University
691 Preston Research Building
Nashville, TN 37232-6838
615-936-1782

Texas
Cancer Therapy and Research
    Center†
University of Texas Health Science
    Center at San Antonio
7979 Wurzbach Road, Mail Code
    8026
Urschel Tower, Room U627
San Antonio, TX 78229
210-450-1000

Dan L. Duncan Cancer Center†
Baylor College of Medicine
One Baylor Plaza
Mail Stop BCM305
Houston, TX 77030
713-798-1354

Harold C. Simmons Cancer Center
UT Southwestern Medical Center
2201 Inwood Road
Dallas, TX 75390
800-460-HOPE (4673)
214-645-HOPE (4673)

M. D. Anderson Cancer Center*
University of Texas
1515 Holcombe Boulevard, Box 91
Houston, TX 77030
713-792-2121

Utah
Huntsman Cancer Institute†
University of Utah
2000 Circle of Hope
Salt Lake City, UT 84112-5550
801-585-0303

Virginia

Massey Cancer Center†
Virginia Commonwealth University
P.O. Box 980037
Richmond, VA 23298-0037
804-828-0450

UVA Cancer Center†
University of Virginia, Health
   Sciences Center
MSB West Complex
Jefferson Park Avenue, Room 6171E
Charlottesville, VA 22908
434-243-6784

Washington

Fred Hutchinson/University of
   Washington Cancer Consortium*
Fred Hutchinson Cancer Research
   Center
P.O. Box 19024, D1-060
Seattle, WA 98109-1024
206-667-4305

Wisconsin

UW Paul P. Carbone Comprehensive Cancer Center*
University of Wisconsin
600 Highland Avenue, Room K4/610
Madison, WI 53792-0001
608-263-8610

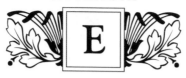

THE HISTOPATHOLOGIC TNM CLASSIFICATION OF BREAST CARCINOMA

The following classification was prepared by the American Joint Committee on Cancer (AJCC) and the International Union Against Cancer (UICC). It describes the tumor, the condition of the lymph nodes, and the presence of metastasis individually and then combines that information to classify breast cancer into four stages.

PRIMARY TUMOR (T)

TX   Primary tumor cannot be assessed
T0   No evidence of primary tumor
Tis   Carcinoma in situ

Tis (DCIS)	Ductal carcinoma in situ
Tis (LCIS)	Lobular carcinoma in situ
Tis (Paget's)	Paget's disease of the nipple *not* associated with invasive carcinoma and/or carcinoma in situ (DCIS and/or LCIS) in the underlying breast parenchyma; carcinomas in the breast parenchyma associated with Paget's disease are categorized based on the size and characteristics of the parenchymal disease, although the presence of Paget's disease should still be noted

T1   Tumor ≤20 mm in greatest dimension

T1mi	Tumor ≤1 mm in greatest dimension
T1a	Tumor >1 mm but ≤5 mm in greatest dimension
T1b	Tumor >5 mm but ≤10 mm in greatest dimension
T1c	Tumor >10 mm but ≤20 mm in greatest dimension

T2   Tumor >20 mm but ≤50 mm in greatest dimension
T3   Tumor >50 mm in greatest dimension

T4   Tumor of any size with direct extension to the chest wall and/or to the skin (ulceration or skin nodules)

NOTE: *Invasion of the dermis alone does not qualify as T4*

T4a   Extension to the chest wall, not including only pectoralis muscle adherence/invasion

T4b   Ulceration and/or ipsilateral satellite nodules and/or edema (including peau d'orange) of the skin, which do not meet the criteria for inflammatory carcinoma

T4c   Both T4a and T4b

T4d   Inflammatory carcinoma

REGIONAL LYMPH NODES (N)

NX   Regional lymph nodes cannot be assessed (e.g., previously removed)

N0   No regional lymph node metastasis

N1   Metastasis to movable ipsilateral level I, II axillary lymph node(s)

N2   Metastasis to ipsilateral level I, II axillary lymph node(s) that are clinically fixed or matted, or in clinically detected* ipsilateral internal mammary nodes in the *absence* of clinically evident axillary lymph node metastasis

N2a   Metastasis in ipsilateral level I, II axillary lymph nodes fixed to one another (matted) or to other structures

N2b   Metastasis only in clinically detected* ipsilateral internal mammary nodes and in the *absence* of clinically evident level I, II axillary lymph node metastasis

N3   Metastasis in ipsilateral infraclavicular (level III axillary) lymph node(s) with or without level I, II axillary lymph node involvement, or in clinically detected* ipsilateral internal mammary lymph node(s) with clinically evident level I, II axillary lymph node metastasis; or metastasis in ip-

*NOTE: *Clinically detected* is defined as detected by imaging studies (excluding lymphoscintigraphy) or by clinical examination and having characteristics highly suspicious for malignancy or a presumed pathologic macrometastasis based on fine needle aspiration biopsy with cytologic examination. Confirmation of clinically detected metastatic disease by fine needle aspiration without excision biopsy is designated with an (f) suffix, such as: cN3a(f). Excisional biopsy of a lymph node or biopsy of a sentinel node, in the absence of pathologic T assignment, is classified as clinical N, such as: cN1. Information regarding the confirmation of the nodal status is designated in site-specific factors as clinical, fine needle aspiration, core biopsy, or sentinel lymph node biopsy. Pathologic classification (pN) is used for excision or sentinel lymph node biopsy only in conjunction with a pathologic T assignment.

silateral supraclavicular lymph node(s) with or without axillary or internal mammary lymph node involvement

N3a   Metastasis in ipsilateral infraclavicular lymph node(s)

N3b   Metastasis in ipsilateral internal mammary lymph node(s) and axillary lymph node(s)

N3c   Metastasis in ipsilateral supraclavicular lymph node(s)

PATHOLOGIC CLASSIFICATION (PN)*

pNX   Regional lymph nodes cannot be assessed (e.g., previously removed or not removed for pathologic study)

pN0   No regional lymph node metastasis identified histologically

    pN0(i−)   No regional lymph node metastasis histologically, negative immunohistochemical stain [IHC]

    pN0(i+)   Malignant cells in regional lymph node(s) no greater than 0.2 mm (detected by hematoxylin and eosin stain [H&E] or IHC including isolated tumor cell clusters [ITCs])†

    pN0(mol−)   No regional lymph node metastasis histologically, and negative molecular findings (RT-PCR)‡

    pN0(mol+)   Positive molecular findings (RT-PCR),‡ but no regional lymph node metastasis detected by histology or IHC.

pN1   Micrometastasis; or metastasis in one to three axillary lymph nodes, and/or in internal mammary nodes with metastasis detected by sentinel lymph node biopsy but not clinically detected§

    pN1mi   Micrometastasis (greater than 0.2 mm and/or more than 200 cells, but not greater than 2.0 mm)

    pN1a   Metastasis in one to three axillary lymph nodes, at least one metastasis greater than 2.0 mm

    pN1b   Metastasis in internal mammary nodes with micrometastases or macrometastases detected by sentinel lymph node biopsy but not clinically detected§

---

*Classification is based on axillary lymph node dissection with or without sentinel lymph node biopsy. Classification based solely on sentinel lymph node biosy without subsequent axillary lymph node dissection is designated (sn) for *sentinel node*, such as pN0(sn).

†*Isolated tumor cell clusters* are defined as small clusters of cells not greater than 0.2 mm, or single tumor cells, or a cluster of fewer than 200 cells in a single histologic cross-section. ITCs may be detected by routine histology or by IHC methods. Nodes containing only ITCs are excluded from the total positive node count for purposes of N classification but should be included in the total number of nodes evaluated.

‡*RT-PCR*: reverse transcriptase/polymerase chain reaction.

§*Not clinically detected* is defined as not detected by imaging studies (excluding lymphoscintigraphy) or not detected by clinical examination.

pN1c   Metastasis in one to three axillary lymph nodes and in internal mammary lymph nodes with micrometastases or macrometastases detected by sentinel lymph node biopsy but not clinically detected*

pN2   Metastasis in four to nine axillary lymph nodes, or in clinically detected† internal mammary lymph nodes in the *absence* of axillary lymph node metastasis

pN2a   Metastasis in four to nine axillary lymph nodes (at least one tumor deposit larger than 2.0 mm)

pN2b   Metastasis in clinically detected† internal mammary lymph nodes in the *absence* of axillary lymph node metastasis

pN3   Metastasis in ten or more axillary lymph nodes; or in infraclavicular (level III axillary) lymph nodes; or in clinically detected† ipsilateral internal mammary lymph node(s) in the *presence* of one or more positive level I, II axillary lymph node(s); or in more than three axillary lymph nodes and in internal mammary lymph nodes with micrometastases or macrometastases detected by sentinel lymph node biopsy but not clinically detected*; or in ipsilateral supraclavicular lymph nodes

pN3a   Metastasis in ten or more axillary lymph nodes (at least one tumor deposit greater than 2.0 mm); or, metastasis to the infraclavicular (level III axillary) lymph nodes

pN3b   Metastasis in clinically detected† ipsilateral internal mammary lymph nodes in the *presence* of one or more positive axillary lymph node(s); or in more than three axillary lymph nodes and in internal mammary lymph nodes with micrometastases or macrometastases detected by sentinel lymph node biopsy but not clinically detected*

pN3c   Metastasis in ipsilateral supraclavicular lymph nodes

---

*Not clinically detected is defined as not detected by imaging studies (excluding lymphoscintigraphy) or not detected by clinical examination.

†Clinically detected is defined as detected by imaging studies (excluding lymphoscintigraphy) or by clinical examination and having characteristics highly suspicious for malignancy or a presumed pathologic macrometastasis based on fine needle aspiration biopsy with cytologic examination.

DISTANT METASTASIS (M)

MO   No clinical or radiographic evidence of distant metastasis

cM0(i+)   No clinical or radiographic evidence of distant metastasis, but deposits of molecularly or microscopically detected tumor cells in circulating blood, bone marrow, or other nonregional nodal tissue that are no larger than 0.2 mm in a patient without symptoms or signs of metastases

M1   Distant detectable metastasis as determined by classical clinical and radiographic means and/or histologically proven larger than 0.2 mm

NOTE: The MX designation has been eliminated from the AJCC/UICC TNM system.

R CLASSIFICATION

The absence or presence of residual tumor at the primary tumor site after treatment is indicated by the symbol R. The R categories for the primary tumor site are as follows:

R0   No residual tumor
R1   Microscopic residual tumor
R2   Macroscopic residual tumor
RX   Presence of residual tumor cannot be assessed

The margin status may be recorded using the following categories:
- Negative margins (tumor not present at the surgical margin)
- Microscopic positive margin (tumor not identified grossly at the margin, but present microscopically at the margin)
- Macroscopic positive margin (tumor identified grossly at the margin)
- Margin not assessed

AJCC/UICC STAGE GROUPING OF PRIMARY TUMOR, REGIONAL LYMPH NODES, AND DISTANT METASTASIS

The descriptions are combined to define four stages:

Stage 0	Tis	N0	M0
Stage IA	T1*	N0	M0
Stage IB	T0	N1mi	M0
	T1*	N1mi	M0
Stage IIA	T0	N1†	M0
	T1*	N1†	M0
	T2	N0	M0
Stage IIB	T2	N1	M0
	T3	N0	M0
Stage IIIA	T0	N2	M0
	T1*	N2	M0
	T2	N2	M0
	T3	N1	M0
	T3	N2	M0
Stage IIIB	T4	N0	M0
	T4	N1	M0
	T4	N2	M0
Stage IIIC	Any T	N3	M0
Stage IV	Any T	Any N	M1

*T1 includes T1mi.
†T0 and T1 tumors with nodal micrometastases only are excluded from Stage IIA and are classified Stage IB.

Notes

- M0 includes M0(i+).
- The designation pM0 is not valid; any M0 should be clinical.
- If a patient presents with M1 before neoadjuvant systemic therapy, the stage is considered Stage IV and remains Stage IV regardless of response to neoadjuvant therapy.
- Stage designation may be changed if postsurgical imaging studies reveal the presence of distant metastases, provided that the studies are carried out within 4 months of diagnosis in the absence of disease progression and provided that the patient has not received neoadjuvant therapy.

- Postneoadjuvant therapy is designated with a *yc* or *yp* prefix. Of note, no stage group is assigned if there is a complete pathologic response (CR) to neoadjuvant therapy; for example: ypT0ypN0cM0.

HISTOPATHOLOGIC GRADE (G)

GX   Grade cannot be assessed
G1   Low combined histologic grade (favorable)
G2   Intermediate combined histologic grade (moderately favorable)
G3   High combined histologic grade (unfavorable)

HISTOPATHOLOGIC TYPE

The histopathologic types are as follows:

In Situ Carcinomas
    NOS (not otherwise specified)
    Intraductal
    Paget's disease and intraductal

Invasive Carcinomas
    NOS
    Ductal
    Inflammatory
    Medullary, NOS
    Medullary with lymphoid stroma
    Mucinous
    Papillary (predominantly micropapillary pattern)
    Tubular
    Lobular
    Paget's disease and infiltrating
    Undifferentiated
    Squamous cell
    Adenoid cystic
    Secretory
    Cribriform

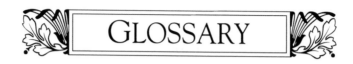

GLOSSARY

AC   Chemotherapy combination of two different drugs: Adriamycin and Cytoxan.

adenocarcinoma   Cancer arising in gland-forming tissue. Breast cancer is a type of adenocarcinoma.

adjuvant chemotherapy   Anticancer drugs used in combination with surgery and/or radiation as an initial treatment before there is detectable spread, to prevent or delay recurrence.

adjunctive (adjuvant) therapy   A secondary treatment in addition to the primary therapy. For example, chemotherapy is often an adjunctive therapy to mastectomy.

Adriamycin (doxorubicin)   A commonly used chemotherapy drug administered to kill cancer cells.

Adrucil (5-fluorouracil)   A commonly used chemotherapy drug, administered to kill cancer cells.

advanced breast cancer   Stage of cancer in which the disease has spread from the breast to other body systems by traveling through the bloodstream or the lymphatic system.

alopecia   Hair loss, a common side effect of chemotherapy.

Aloxi (palonosetron)   A long-acting antinausea medication in the class called $_5HT_3$ agonists; it is given intravenously before chemotherapy treatments.

amenorrhea   Absence or stoppage of a menstrual period.

androgen   Hormone that produces male characteristics.

anemia   The condition of having a low red blood cell count that results in fatigue.

anesthesia   Procedure used to make surgery painless, either by local numbing or by rendering the patient unconscious. It is usually performed by an anesthesiologist or nurse anesthetist.

angiogenesis   The process of growing new blood vessels.

antibiotics   Medications that fight bacterial infections.

antiemetic   An antinausea medication.

antioxidants   Compounds that slow the deterioration (or oxidation) of cells in the body. Vitamins C and E and beta-carotene are antioxidants.

Anzimet (dolasetron)   An antinausea medication in the class of $_5HT_3$ antagonists that can be taken by mouth or given intravenously.

apoptosis   Cell suicide.

Aranesp (darbepoetin alfa)   A medication given by subcutaneous injection every 2 to 3 weeks, used to correct chemotherapy-caused anemia.

areola   The circle of pigmented skin on the breast that surrounds the nipple.

Arimidex (anastrozole)   A drug for treatment of advanced breast cancer in postmenopausal women.

aspiration   Withdrawal of fluid or tissue from a cyst or lump in the breast, performed by inserting a needle and drawing (aspirating) fluid into a syringe.

assay   Test.

asymmetrical   Not having the same shape and size on both sides.

asymptomatic   Without obvious signs or symptoms of disease.

atypical cells   Not usual; abnormal.

atypical ductal hyperplasia (ADH)   A condition of abnormal breast ducts that can only be diagnosed by biopsy and leads to a higher risk of breast cancer in the breast containing the abnormality.

atypical hyperplasia   Excessive growth of cells, some of which are abnormal.

augmentation mammaplasty (breast augmentation)   An operation to enlarge a woman's breast, usually by placing a silicone breast implant behind the breast.

autologous   From the same person. An autologous blood transfusion is blood removed and then transfused back into the same person at a later date.

autologous flap breast reconstruction   Breast reconstruction with a woman's own natural tissues. Common donor sites for flaps are the abdomen, back, buttocks, and thigh.

axilla   The underarm or armpit area behind the anterior axillary fold. It contains the axillary lymph nodes.

axillary lymph node dissection   Surgical removal of lymph nodes from the armpit. This tissue is then sent to a pathologist to determine whether the breast cancer has spread.

baseline mammogram   A woman's first mammogram to use as a standard reference for evaluating changes in future mammograms.

benign   Opposite of cancerous or malignant. A benign tumor is a non-cancerous growth. It is self-limiting and does not spread to other areas of the body.

bilateral   Involving both sides, such as both breasts.

bilateral mastectomy   Surgical removal of both breasts.

biomarker   Characteristics of tumor cells that provide information on tumor behavior. These are used to predict a patient's prognosis and, in some cases, predict the outcome after specific therapy.

bone marrow   The soft inner part of large bones in which blood cells develop.

bone marrow analysis   A test in which bone marrow is removed from the back of the pelvic bone to look for involvement by cancer or to assess how blood is being made.

bone scan   A test to determine whether there is any sign of cancer in the bones.

brachial plexus   A bundle of nerves in the underarm area; these nerves supply sensation to the arm.

brachytherapy   A form of radiation therapy in which the source of the radiation is placed close to, or implanted in, the body.

BRCA1 and BRCA2   Breast cancer genes that have been linked to familial breast cancer.

breast-conserving surgery and irradiation   Treatment option for breast cancer whereby the tumor, a small margin of surrounding tissue, and the sentinel lymph nodes are surgically removed. Most of the breast is preserved, and the remaining tissue is then treated using a course of radiation therapy.

breast implant   A soft, silicone form that can be placed in the body to simulate a breast.

breast reconstruction   An operation to create or rebuild a natural-looking breast shape after mastectomy.

breast self-examination (BSE)   Monthly, methodical self-inspection of the breasts in which a woman becomes familiar with the normal look and feel of her breasts.

CAF   Chemotherapy combination of three different drugs: Cytoxan, Adriamycin, and 5-fluorouracil.

calcifications   Small calcium deposits in the breast tissue that can only be seen by mammography.

cancer   A general term for more than 100 diseases characterized by abnormal and uncontrolled growth of cells.

cancerphobia   An exaggerated fear of cancer.

capsular contracture   A capsule or shell of scar tissue that may form around a woman's breast implant, giving it a feeling of firmness, as her body reacts to the implant.

carcinoembryonic antigen (CEA)   Blood test used to follow women with metastatic breast cancer to help determine whether the treatments are working.

carcinogen   A substance that can cause cancer.

carcinoma   Most cancers are carcinomas. These are cancers arising in the epithelial tissue, including the skin, glands, and linings of the internal organs.

carcinoma in situ   A carcinoma that has not spread outside the area where it began.

cathepsin-D   An enzyme present in breast tissue and in other cells that helps break down tissue. Large quantities of this enzyme in breast tissue may indicate a high degree of invasion into surrounding healthy tissue.

catheter   A tube implanted or inserted into the body to inject or withdraw fluid.

cells   Individual living units of which all organisms are composed. Cells are organized into tissues and organs.

cell cycle   The steps a cell goes through in the process of reproducing itself.

cellulitis   Infection of the soft tissues.

centigray   Unit of measure of radiation dose.

chemotherapy   Treatment of cancer with powerful anticancer drugs capable of destroying cancer cells. The term usually refers to *cytotoxic* drugs given for cancer treatment.

circulatory system   The system consisting of the heart and blood vessels that provides blood to all parts of the body.

clavicle   Collarbone.

clinical trials   Studies designed to evaluate new cancer treatments.

CMF   Chemotherapy combination of three different drugs: Cytoxan, methotrexate, and 5-fluorouracil.

cohesivity   Thickness or rigidity.

cohort study   Scientific study of a group of people who have something in common when they are first assembled and who are then observed for a period of time to see what happens to them.

combination chemotherapy   Use of two or more chemicals to achieve maximum damage to tumor cells.

comedo   Type of DCIS in which the cells filling the duct are aggressive looking.

Compazine (prochlorperazine)   A commonly used antinausea medication.

complete blood cell count (CBC) Test to measure the number of red blood cells, white blood cells, and platelets in a blood sample. This test helps evaluate the effect of chemotherapy on the bone marrow where the blood cells are produced.

computed tomography (CT) scan A computer-generated x-ray study that permits visualization of internal body structures. Typically, contrast material is given by mouth and intravenously to highlight internal organs.

concordance The pathologist's findings agree with the imaging appearance.

core biopsy Type of needle biopsy in which a small core of tissue is removed from a lump without surgery.

cyclical In a cycle, like the menstrual period, which is every 28 days, or chemotherapy treatment, which is periodic.

cyst A saclike structure within the body that is filled with liquid or semisolid material.

cystosarcoma phyllodes Unusual type of breast tumor.

cytology Study of cells under a microscope.

Cytoxan (cyclophosphamide) A drug used to kill cancer cells.

cytotoxic Causing the death of cells. The term usually refers to drugs used in chemotherapy.

designer estrogens A class of drugs, such as raloxifene, developed to replace traditional estrogen therapy without some of the associated risks.

DIEP flap A type of perforator flap breast reconstruction using skin and fat from the abdomen, but sparing the muscle. The tissue is freed from the abdomen, transferred to the patient's chest, reconnected using microsurgery, and shaped to create the new breast.

differentiated Clearly defined. Differentiated tumor cells are similar in appearance to normal cells.

donor site A part of the body from which tissue is taken and transferred to another part of the body for reconstruction.

dose-dense chemotherapy A technique of giving chemotherapy in which the treatments are compressed and given more frequently.

double-blind A research study method in which neither the participants nor the researchers know which subjects are in the control group and which subjects are in the test group.

drain Tubes or suction devices inserted after surgery to drain the fluids that accumulate postoperatively. Drains may be left in place for several days, as needed.

duct   In the female breast, milk travels through a system of tubelike ducts from milk glands to milk reservoirs in the nipple area. The duct is the site of most breast cancers.

ductal carcinoma in situ (DCIS)   Cancer cells present in the breast ducts that have not grown beyond their site of origin; sometimes referred to as precancer.

early-stage breast cancer   When cancer is limited to the breast and has not spread to the lymph nodes or other parts of the body. Also called in situ, or localized breast cancer.

edema   Swelling caused by a collection of excess fluid in the soft tissues.

electrocautery   Instrument used in surgery to cut, coagulate, or destroy tissue by heating it with an electric current.

Emend (aprepitant)   An antinausea medication given in pill form and started before chemotherapy is administered.

endoscopic surgery (or minimally invasive surgery)   Operation performed through short incisions using special, long instruments. The operative cavity is visualized through small video cameras attached to the endoscope; these cameras project a video image of the tissues beneath the skin via fiberoptic light. This technique is commonly used in many general surgery operations and can also be used for plastic surgery to obtain distant tissue for breast reconstruction.

engorgement   An area of the body that is filled and stretched with fluid or distended with blood.

epidermal growth factor receptors   Indirect measurements of the rate of tumor growth. Along with hormone receptor tests, these can be used to predict how a patient will respond to hormone therapy.

estrogen   A female hormone produced mainly by the ovaries.

estrogen receptor (ER)   Protein found on some cells to which estrogen molecules will attach. If a tumor is positive for estrogen receptors, it is sensitive to hormones and therefore can be affected by changes in hormone levels.

Evista (raloxifene)   A hormonal drug in pill form from the class of drugs called SERMs. Evista blocks estrogen and progesterone receptors.

excisional biopsy   Procedure in which the whole lump is taken out.

familial cancer   Cancer that occurs in families more frequently than would be expected by chance.

Fareston (toremifene)   A hormonal drug in pill form with tamoxifen-like activity, a *SERM*. Fareston blocks estrogen and progesterone receptors.

fascia A sheet or broad band of fibrous or connective tissue that covers muscles and various organs of the body and attaches the breasts and other body structures to underlying muscles.

fat necrosis Area of dead fat, usually following some form of trauma or surgery. May appear as lumps or thickened areas.

Femara (letrozole) A hormonal drug in pill form in the class of aromatase inhibitors; used for receptor-positive postmenopausal patients only.

fibroadenoma A benign, firm, identifiable breast tumor commonly found in the breasts of young women.

fibrocystic breasts A recurring benign condition characterized by breast tenderness, pain, swelling, and the appearance of cysts or lumps.

fibrous Gristlelike; often applied to strands of tough tissue that can grow in the body. In breast reconstruction, this usually refers to the scar tissue formation sometimes found around implants.

5-fluorouracil (5-FU) A drug used to kill cancer cells. Also available in pill form under the name Xeloda.

flap A portion of tissue with its blood supply moved from one part of the body to another. Flaps of muscle, fat, and skin are frequently used to provide additional tissue for reconstructing a woman's breasts. Common donor sites for flap reconstruction are the abdomen, back, buttocks, and thigh.

flow cytometry Test that measures DNA content in tumors.

follicle stimulating hormone (FSH) Hormone from the pituitary gland that stimulates the ovaries.

Food and Drug Administration (FDA) The U.S. government agency that enforces laws on the manufacturing, testing, and use of drugs and medical devices. The FDA must approve a drug for marketing before it is made commercially available to the public.

frozen section Tissue that is sliced and frozen to make a slide for immediate diagnosis by a pathologist.

G-CSF (granulocyte colony-stimulating factor) Abbreviation for Neupogen, a drug given subcutaneously on a daily basis to raise white blood cell counts.

gene A unit of DNA that determines the manufacture in the body of a particular protein.

general anesthesia A state of unconsciousness produced by anesthetic agents, resulting in absence of pain sensation over the entire body and a greater or lesser degree of muscular relaxation; the drugs producing this state are typically administered by inhalation, intravenously, or intramuscularly.

genetic Relating to genes or inherited characteristics.

genetic code A code contained in genes that determines the manufacture of proteins.

genetic material Genes and the DNA from which they are made.

genome All of the chromosomes that together form the genetic map.

gluteus maximus musculocutaneous flap Breast reconstruction operation that uses a distant flap of the patient's own tissue (autologous) from the buttock area to build a new breast.

gracilis flap breast reconstruction (also known as TUG or TMG flap) Microsurgical (free) flap breast reconstruction operation that uses the fat that sometimes accumulates in the upper inner thigh. The flap also includes the gracilis muscle through which the blood supply reaches the skin. The tissue is freed from the abdomen, transferred to the patient's chest, reconnected using microsurgery, and shaped to create the new breast.

grading Classification of cancers according to the appearance of cancer cells under the microscope. Low-grade cancers often grow more slowly than high-grade cancers.

growth rate factors Markers used to predict the growth rate of cancerous cells and the likelihood that the cancer will spread.

gynecomastia Swollen breast tissue in a boy or man.

harvest To obtain distant tissue for use in reconstructive surgery, such as breast reconstruction.

hematoma A collection of blood that can form in a wound after an injury or operation.

hemorrhage A rapid, uncontrolled outflow of blood.

***Her-2/neu* gene** An oncogene that, when overexpressed, leads to more cell growth. This oncogene is often associated with a poor breast cancer prognosis and is known to have a high growth rate.

Herceptin (trastuzumab) An antitumor agent that targets the *Her-2* tyrosine kinase receptor and is most effective in patients in whom this protein is overexpressed.

heterogeneous Composed of many different elements. For breast cancer, heterogeneous indicates numerous different types of breast cancer cells within one tumor.

hormone A chemical substance produced by the body that can turn organs on and off, thus regulating many body functions, such as growth and sexual functions. Synthetic forms of many hormones are administered to treat hormone deficiencies, such as those caused by menopause.

hormone-receptor assay   Diagnostic test to determine whether a breast cancer's growth is influenced by hormones.

hormone therapy   Treatment of cancer by removing or adding hormones to alter the hormonal balance; some breast cancer cells will only grow in the presence of certain hormones.

hot flashes   Sensation of heat and flushing that occurs suddenly. May be associated with menopause or as a side effect of some medications.

HRT   Abbreviation for hormone replacement therapy.

hyperplasia   Excessive growth of cells.

hysterectomy   Removal of the uterus (not necessarily the ovaries).

IGAP flap   An inferior gluteal artery perforator flap. An autologous tissue flap procedure that uses fat and skin from the lower buttock to reconstruct a new breast mound after a mastectomy.

immune system   System by which the body is able to protect itself from foreign invaders.

immunotherapy   Therapy that works by enhancing the body's own defense system.

incisional biopsy   Biopsy procedure in which a piece of the lump is removed.

infiltrating cancer   Cancer that can grow beyond its site of origin into neighboring tissue. Infiltrating does not imply that the cancer has already spread outside of the breast. Infiltrating has the same meaning as invasive.

infiltrating ductal carcinoma   Also known as invasive ductal carcinoma. This is the most common type of invasive breast cancer.

inflammatory breast cancer   An aggressive form of invasive breast cancer that causes redness and swelling of the breast.

informed consent   Legal standard that states how much knowledge a patient must have about the potential risks and benefits of a therapy before being able to undergo the treatment. Many states have informed consent laws regarding breast cancer that require physicians to provide treatment options to patients before any medical treatment is given.

infraclavicular nodes   Lymph nodes lying beneath the collarbone.

inframammary crease or fold   The crease where the lower portion of the breast and chest wall meet.

in situ   In the site of. In regard to cancer, in situ refers to tumors that have not grown beyond their site of origin and invaded neighboring tissue.

intraductal   Within the duct. Intraductal can describe a benign or malignant process.

intraductal carcinoma in situ (DCIS)   A preinvasive cancer located in the milk ducts of the breast.

intravenous (IV) line   A needle inserted into a vein to administer blood products, nutrients, and medications directly into the bloodstream through a tube.

invasive cancer   Cancer that has spread outside its site of origin to infiltrate and grow in surrounding tissue.

inverted nipple   The turning inward of the nipple. Usually a congenital condition, but if the nipple was previously projecting and suddenly becomes inverted, this can be a sign of breast cancer.

irradiation   A form of ionizing energy that can destroy or damage cells. Cancer cells tend to be more easily destroyed than the normal cells in the surrounding tissue. For breast cancer treatment, this therapy can be used as an adjunct to breast-conserving surgery to reduce the chance of cancer recurrence.

Ki-67   A test performed on biopsied breast cancer cells that measures the potential growth rate of a cancer. A higher number indicates a faster growing cancer.

Kytril (granisetron)   An antinausea medication in the class of $_5HT_3$ antagonists that can be given in pill or intravenous form.

lactation   Production of milk from the breast.

latissimus dorsi flap   Flap of skin and muscle taken from the back used for breast reconstruction after mastectomy or partial mastectomy.

latissimus dorsi muscle   Triangular back muscle that is transferred with some overlying skin as donor flap tissue for reconstructing a breast after mastectomy.

lobular carcinoma in situ (LCIS)   Abnormal cells within the lobule that do not form lumps but can serve as a marker of future cancer risk.

lobules   Parts of the breast capable of making milk.

local treatment of cancer   Treatment only of the tumor.

localized cancer   Cancer confined to its site of origin.

lump   Mass of tissue found in the breast or other parts of the body; 80% of all breast lumps are benign.

lumpectomy   Surgical removal of a cancerous tumor along with a small margin of surrounding tissue.

lymph Fluid that flows through the body, much like the blood, but in a separate system of vessels called the lymphatic system. Lymph fluid contains some waste products that are filtered through the lymph nodes, then this tissue fluid is returned to the blood.

lymphedema A condition characterized by the collection of excess fluid in the hands and arms after lymph nodes are removed or blocked from breast surgery.

lymph nodes Structures in the lymphatic system that act as filters, catching bacteria and cancer cells, and contributing to the body's immune system, which fights infection and disease. Lymph nodes can be a location of cancer spread.

magnetic resonance imaging (MRI) A computerized image created using electromagnetic fields rather than x-rays.

malignant Cancerous.

mammaplasty Breast operation to alter breast size.

mammogram Breast x-ray film detailing the structure of breast tissue; requires only low doses of radiation.

mammography Process of taking breast x-ray films to detect breast cancer.

mammosite A technique of limited or partial radiation therapy of the breast.

margins The area of tissue surrounding a tumor when it is removed by surgery. Positive margins indicate that this area of tissue is not clear of tumor.

mastectomy Surgical removal of the breast, usually for treatment of cancer.

mastitis Infection of the breast.

mastodynia Pain in the breast.

mastopexy Breast lift procedure that tightens the breast by removing sagging skin caused by the forces of gravity and the effects of aging.

Mediport A temporary device that is surgically implanted in the chest or arm to accept an IV line during chemotherapy.

menopause The cessation of menstruation, usually as a result of aging. The level of female sex hormones is reduced in menopausal women.

metastasis Spread of cancer from one part of the body to another. It can spread through the lymphatic system, the bloodstream, or across body cavities.

metastatic cancer Cancer that has spread beyond the breast to other parts of the body.

metastasizing   Spreading to a distant site.

microcalcification   Tiny calcifications in the breast tissue, usually seen only on a mammogram. The presence of these clusters may be a sign of ductal carcinoma in situ.

micrometastasis   Microscopic and as yet undetectable but presumed spread of tumor cells to other organs.

micropapillary   Type of DCIS in which the cells filling the duct take the form of fingerlike projections into the center.

microsurgical breast reconstruction   Method of breast reconstruction whereby a flap of a woman's own tissue is moved from a distant area of the body such as the abdomen, back, thigh, or buttocks to the chest wall to build a breast. Once this tissue is transferred, the blood vessels are sutured and reattached under the magnification of the operating microscope.

microsurgery   Sewing together hair-thin blood vessels with the aid of a microscope.

mitosis   Cell division.

modified radical mastectomy   Surgical removal of the breast, some fat, and the sentinel lymph nodes in the armpit, leaving the chest wall muscles largely intact.

Montgomery's glands   Sebaceous glands in the areola of the nipple. Also known as areolar glands.

multicentric   Having more than one origin. Cancer cells may grow in several locations within the breasts and not be related to each other.

muscle flap   A muscle or portion of muscle that can be transferred with its blood supply to another part of the body for reconstructive purposes.

muscle-sparing free TRAM flap   A hybrid of the DIEP (abdominal perforator) flap and the free TRAM flap that is known as a muscle-sparing free TRAM flap.

mutation   An alteration to the structure of a gene.

myocutaneous flap   Flap of skin and muscle and fat transferred from one part of the body to another for reconstruction.

nausea   The sensation of needing to vomit.

necrosis   Death of a tissue.

needle aspiration   Diagnostic method of removing fluid or tissue from a breast tumor or cyst with a fine needle for microscopic examination.

needle biopsy   Removal of a small sample of tissue with a wide-bore needle and suction.

needle localization   Procedure for pinpointing a lump before biopsy.

negative nodes   Lymph nodes that are free of cancer cells.

neoadjuvant chemotherapy   The use of chemotherapy before surgery, usually to shrink the tumor.

nipple   The pigmented, central projection on the breast containing the outer opening of the breast ducts.

nodular   Forming little nodules.

Nolvadex (tamoxifen)   An antiestrogen drug that may be given to women with estrogen-receptor–positive tumors.

nonsurgical biopsy   A biopsy in which samples of a lump or tumor are removed with a needle under local anesthesia.

nuclear magnetic resonance (NMR or MRI)   Imaging technique using a magnet and electrical coil to transmit radio waves through the body.

nulliparous   Never having given birth to a child.

oncogenes   Growth-regulating genes that can cause tumors when activated. (*Onco* comes from the Latin root meaning "tumor.")

oncologist   A physician who specializes in treating cancer. There are medical, surgical, and radiation oncologists.

oncology   The study and treatment of cancer.

oncoplastic surgery   Use of plastic surgery techniques to achieve both cancer control and improvement in the aesthetic appearance of the breast.

oncotype DX   A test of gene function used to try to predict breast cancer behavior and relapse risk. The test is performed on material collected by biopsy.

one-step procedure   Breast biopsy and mastectomy performed in a single operation.

oophorectomy   Surgical removal of the ovaries; sometimes performed as part of hormone therapy or as a possible preventive procedure for patients at high risk for breast and ovarian cancer.

oral chemotherapy   Chemotherapy administered in pill form instead of by intravenous injection.

orange peel skin   Skin that has the appearance of an orange peeling. This pitting and coloration is caused from inflammation and edema and may be a sign of cancer.

osteoporosis   Softening of bones that occurs with age, calcium loss, and hormone depletion. After menopause, women are particularly susceptible to this condition unless they receive some form of hormone supplement.

p53   A tumor suppressor gene.

Paget's disease   DCIS within the nipple.

palliative   Affording relief of symptoms such as pain, but not a cure.

palpable   Distinguishable by touch.

palpate   To feel with the fingertips.

palpation   Examining with the hand.

partial breast irradiation   Radiation just to the bed of the tumor rather than the whole breast.

partial or segmental mastectomy   Breast surgery that removes only a portion of the breast, including the cancer and a surrounding margin of breast tissue.

pathologist   A physician who specializes in the diagnosis of disease via the study of cells and tissue.

pathology   The study of disease through the microscopic examination of body cells and tissues. Any tumor suspected of being malignant must be diagnosed by pathologic examination.

pathology report   The pathologist's written record of the analysis of the tissue.

patient-controlled analgesia (PCA)   Pain control method that allows the patient to be in charge of her own pain relief. When pain relief is needed, the patient pushes a button on the PCA machine that delivers a predetermined dose of pain medication.

PDQ   Information published by the National Cancer Institute listing all clinical trials currently underway.

pectoralis muscles   Muscles located under the breast and attached to the chest wall.

pedicle   A connection of nourishing blood vessels from the body to a flap of tissue.

perforator   Small veins that connect the deep veins to the superficial veins, allowing blood to drain from the skin into the deep veins.

perforator flap   A flap composed of skin and fatty tissue that is based on a single set of blood vessels (the perforator vessels) that pass through the underlying muscle. For breast reconstruction, these flaps are taken from the patient's abdomen (DIEP and SIEA flaps) or buttocks (IGAP or SGAP flaps). Perforator flap techniques preserve the patient's underlying musculature. The tissue is then transferred to the patient's chest, reconnected using microsurgery and shaped to create the new breast.

permanent section   A tissue sample removed in a biopsy and embedded in wax or paraffin before thin slicing and staining for microscopic examination (compare *frozen section*).

phlebitis   Inflammation of a vein.

platelets   A blood component that prevents bleeding.

ploidy   Measurement of the amount of DNA in a tumor cell that helps to predict tumor behavior.

polygenic   Relating to more than one gene.

port   A device surgically inserted under the skin and connected to a large vein to obtain intravenous access for injection of chemotherapeutic drugs and other medications.

positive nodes   Lymph nodes that have been invaded by cancer cells.

positron emission tomography (PET) scan   A nuclear medicine test used to determine cancer location within the body based on different rates of blood sugar (glucose) use by cancer versus normal tissue.

postmenopausal   After menopause.

precancerous (premalignant)   Abnormal cellular changes that are potentially capable of becoming cancer.

predisposition   A latent susceptibility to disease that may be activated under certain conditions.

primary   The first.

progesterone   Female hormone produced by the ovaries during the menstrual cycle.

progesterone receptor (PR)   The binding site of progesterone on breast cancer cells, which indicates the ability of the cancer to be affected by changes in hormone levels.

prognosis   Forecast as to the expected outcome of disease.

prophylactic mastectomy   Removal of high-risk breast tissue to prevent the development of cancer. This procedure is usually combined with breast reconstruction. Also called preventive mastectomy and risk-reducing mastectomy and increasingly recommended for high-risk patients as a possible means of preventing breast cancer.

prosthesis   Any artificial body part. A breast-shaped form may be worn outside the body after a breast has been removed because of cancer. It fits into the woman's brassiere in a specially designed pocket. Prostheses are made of different materials.

protein   A substance found in all cells. Different proteins are used to drive different types of events in cells. The manufacture of each protein is specified by a different gene.

ptosis   Sagging or drooping. Breast ptosis is usually the result of normal aging and the pull of gravity, or changes caused by pregnancy or weight loss.

quadrantectomy   Removal of one fourth of the breast.

radiation oncologist   A physician who specializes in treating cancer patients with radiation therapy.

radiation oncology (radiation therapy)   Treatment of disease by x-rays or other ionizing energy forms.

radical mastectomy   Removal of the breast, underlying muscles, and underarm (axillary) lymph nodes. This procedure is rarely performed today.

radiologist   A physician with special training in diagnosis of disease by studying x-ray films and other images and using these procedures to facilitate treatment.

radiolucent   A characteristic allowing x-rays to pass through.

radiopaque   A characteristic that blocks x-rays; appears white on an x-ray film.

randomized   Chosen at random. In a randomized research study, subjects are chosen to receive a particular treatment by means of a computer programmed to randomly select names.

reconstructive mammaplasty (breast reconstruction)   Rebuilding of the breast by plastic surgery techniques.

rectus abdominis muscles   The vertical, paired muscles on either side of the midline of the abdomen. These muscles can be used as donor tissue for breast reconstruction (see *TRAM flap breast reconstruction*).

recurrence   Return of a tumor after the initial treatment of the primary tumor.

reduction mammaplasty   Operation for reducing the size of the breasts by removing glandular and fatty tissue.

remission   Complete or partial disappearance of the signs and symptoms of disease in response to treatment. The period during which a disease is under control.

retraction   Often referred to as skin dimpling; describes the process of skin pulling in toward breast tissue.

risk counselor (genetic counselor)   A trained health care professional who can advise a woman on her risk of developing breast cancer and other cancers.

risk factors   Anything that increases an individual's chance of getting a disease.

risk reduction   Techniques used to reduce chances of getting a certain cancer.

saline solution   Saltwater; used in some types of breast implants.

segmental mastectomy   A lumpectomy in which only the portion of the breast containing cancer is removed.

sentinel node(s)   The first lymph node (or nodes) to receive drainage from a tumor, identified by means of dyes or radioactive tracers. Used to determine whether there is lymphatic metastasis in certain types of cancer. If this node is negative for malignancy, others "upstream" from it are usually also negative.

sentinel node biopsy   A procedure in which only the first draining node or nodes are removed through a small incision instead of an entire axillary node dissection.

SGAP flap   Superior gluteal artery perforator flap. A tissue flap breast reconstruction procedure that uses fat and skin from the upper buttock to create a new breast mound after a mastectomy.

SERM   An abbreviation for selective estrogen receptor modulators, a class of hormonal therapy that includes tamoxifen, Fareston, and Evista.

seroma   A fluid collection caused by the localized accumulation of lymph fluid within a body part or area. This condition sometimes occurs after an operation. In breast surgery, it may occur after an axillary dissection.

side effects   Reactions to drugs or treatments that are usually temporary and reversible.

SIEA flap   Superficial inferior epigastric artery flap. A breast reconstruction perforator flap procedure that uses fat and skin from the abdomen to create a new breast mound after a mastectomy.

silicone   A chemical polymer that is used to replace numerous body parts. Breast implant envelopes are made of silicone.

silicone gel   Silicone produced in a semisolid state, used as a filling in breast implants; similar in consistency to a normal breast.

simple or total mastectomy   Removal of the breast only; the lymph nodes and pectoralis muscles are preserved.

skin-sparing mastectomy   Removal of the breast with less skin removed and shorter incisions; only the nipple and areola are excised as well as the overlying skin in those areas. Appropriate only for individuals who have no tumor involvement of the skin area to be spared. Usually combined with immediate breast reconstruction.

sloughing   The process by which the body rids itself of dead tissue. Frequently this happens when the tissue being used does not have an adequate blood supply.

S-phase fraction   Measurement of how fast a tumor is growing.

spiculated   Appearing on mammography as small projections into surrounding tissues from a mass.

sporadic cancer   Cancer occurring in individuals without a family history of cancer.

staging   System for classifying cancer according to the size of the tumor, its stage of development, and the extent of its spread.

stereotactic core needle biopsy   A biopsy performed using two mammographic views to pinpoint the site of the tumor.

subcutaneous tissue   The tissue under the skin.

suppressor gene   A gene that can reverse the effect of a specific type of mutation in other genes.

supraclavicular nodes   The lymph nodes located above the collarbone.

suture   A surgeon's stitch.

symmetrical   Balanced. When one side matches the other. One of the chief goals of the patient and plastic surgeon for breast reconstruction.

systemic   Involving the entire body.

systemic treatment   Treatment involving the whole body, usually with drugs.

targeted therapy   An antibody directed to a specific molecular target, such as Herceptin.

Taxol (paclitaxel)   A chemotherapy drug in the class called taxanes.

Taxotere (docetaxel)   A taxane, drug used for treatment of breast cancer.

thoracic   Concerning the chest (thorax).

tissue expander   An adjustable implant that can be inflated with saltwater to stretch the tissues at the mastectomy site.

TNM   The staging system for cancers including breast cancer (stands for tumor, node, metastasis). The system takes into account the size of the cancer, lymph node involvement, and whether metastases are present.

total mastectomy with axillary dissection   A mastectomy in which the breast tissue and the sentinel lymph nodes are removed. Another name for modified radical mastectomy.

TRAM flap breast reconstruction   Breast reconstruction operation that uses a flap of the patient's own lower abdominal tissue (transverse rectus abdominis musculocutaneous flap) to build a breast. The TRAM flap can be a pedicle flap in which the tissue is moved while still attached to its blood supply, or it can be a free flap, in which the flap is totally separated from its donor site and moved to its new location and the vessels reattached microsurgically. The DIEP flap also uses a flap of abdominal tissue but does not remove any muscle.

Tru-Cut biopsy Type of core needle biopsy in which a small core of tissue is removed from a lump without performing surgery.

tumor An abnormal growth of tissue that can be benign or malignant.

tumor markers Substances released by the tumor or in response to the presence of a tumor. They are studied as potential diagnostic and prognostic tools.

tumor suppressor gene A gene that prevents cells from growing if they have a mutation.

two-step procedure Breast biopsy and breast cancer treatment performed as two steps, allowing diagnosis of cancer and treatment to be separated by hours, days, or even longer periods.

ultrasound High-frequency sound waves used to locate a tumor inside the body. This technology is helpful in determining whether a breast lump is solid or filled with fluid.

ultrasound-guided biopsy The use of ultrasound to guide a biopsy needle to remove a sample of tissue from a suspicious area (seen on mammography but not palpable) for pathologic analysis.

unilateral Involving one side, such as one breast.

vascular epidermal growth factor (VEGF) A protein that stimulates new blood vessels to grow.

x-ray High-energy radiation used in high doses to treat cancer or in low doses to diagnose the disease.

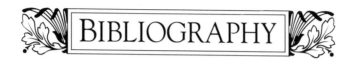

BIBLIOGRAPHY

This bibliography includes consumer books and articles and professional articles that we thought would be helpful to you.

Breast Cancer Information: Diagnosis, Treatment, and Rehabilitation

American Cancer Society. Breast Cancer Clear & Simple: All Your Questions Answered. Atlanta: American Cancer Society, 2007. *(See Appendix B for comprehensive information available online.)*

Bonner D. The 10 Best Questions for Surviving Breast Cancer: The Script You Need to Take Control of Your Health. New York: Fireside, a division of Simon & Schuster, 2008.

Breast Cancer Overview. New York: The New York Times, 2009.

Brody JE. A Breast Cancer With a Built-In Quandary. New York: The New York Times, Feb 22, 2005.

Brown ZK, Boatman KK. 100 Questions & Answers About Breast Cancer, 3rd ed. Sudbury, MA: Jones & Bartlett Publishers, 2009.

Chan D. Breast Cancer: Real Questions, Real Answers. New York: Marlow & Company, 2006.

Grobstein RH. The Breast Cancer Book: What You Need to Know to Make Informed Decisions. New Haven: Yale University Press, 2005.

Health Guide: Breast Cancer. New York: The New York Times, 2008.

Hirshaut Y, Pressman P. Breast Cancer: The Complete Guide, 5th ed. New York: Bantam Books, 2008.

Kolata G. Sharp Drop in Rates of Breast Cancer Holds. New York: The New York Times, Apr 19, 2007.

Ozols RF, Herbst RS, Colson YL, et al. Clinical cancer advances 2006: major research advances in cancer treatment, prevention, and screening—a report from the American Society of Clinical Oncology. J Clin Oncol 25:146-162, 2007.

Ravdin PM, Cronin KA, Howlader N, et al. The decrease in breast-cancer incidence in 2003 in the United States. N Engl J Med 356:1670-1674, 2007.

Shockney LD, Shapiro GR. Johns Hopkins Patients' Guide to Breast Cancer. Sudbury, MA: Jones & Bartlett Publishers, 2010.

Sokolowski N, Rossi V. The Breast Cancer Companion: A Guide for the Newly Diagnosed. New York: Demos Medical Publishing, 2010.

Detection and Diagnosis: Breast Examination, Breast Imaging, and Biopsy

Albertini JJ, Lyman OH, Cox C, et al. Lymphatic mapping and sentinel node biopsy in breast cancer. JAMA 277:791-792, 1997.

Bakalar N. Second Opinion May Aid Breast Cancer Treatment. New York: The New York Times, Dec 5, 2006.

Black ST. Specter of breast cancer: don't sit home and be afraid. McCall's, Feb, 1973.

Boyd NF, Guo H, Martin LJ, et al. Mammographic density and the risk and detection of breast cancer. N Engl J Med 356:227-236, 2007.

Burns RB, McCarthy EP, Freund KM, et al. Black women receive less mammography even with similar use of primary care. Ann Intern Med 125:173-182, 1996.

Burns RP. Image-guided breast biopsy. Am J Surg 173:9-11, 1997.

Castleman M. Early detection: the best defense. Family Circle 105:107, Oct 13, 1992.

Castleman M. What's normal, what's not. Family Circle 105:101, Oct 13, 1992.

Ellerbee L. Our 50s: yes! Mammography saved my life; it can save yours, too! New Choices Magazine, Oct, 1996.

Feig SA. Mammographic screening of elderly women. JAMA 276:446, 1996.

Ferraro S. Self-Exams Are Passé? Believers Beg to Differ. New York: The New York Times, Dec 26, 2006.

Foster RS Jr, Costanza M. Breast self-examination practices and breast cancer survival. Cancer 53:999-1005, 1984.

Godbey F, George SC. Sooner screening: why women under 50 need mammograms. Prevention 49:32, Apr, 1997.

Hatada T, Aoki L, Okada K, et al. Usefulness of ultrasound-guided fine-needle aspiration biopsy for palpable breast tumors. Arch Surg 131:1095-1098, 1996.

Kolata G. Confronting Cancer; Breast Cancer: Mammography Finds More Tumors. Then the Debate Begins. New York: The New York Times, Apr 9, 2002.

Kuhl CK, Schrading S, Leutner CC, et al. Mammography, breast ultrasound, and magnetic resonance imaging for surveillance of women at high familial risk for breast cancer. J Clin Oncol 23:8469-8476, 2005.

McGuinn KA. The Informed Woman's Guide to Breast Health. Palo Alto, CA: Bull Publishing, 2001.

Partridge AH, Winer EP. On mammography—more agreement than disagreement. N Engl J Med 361:2499-2501, 2009.

Pettine S, Place R, Babu S. Stereotactic breast biopsy is accurate, minimally invasive, and cost effective. Am J Surg 171:474-476, 1996.

Pollack A. Findings May Alter Care for Early Breast Cancer. New York: The New York Times, June 7, 2010.

Sack K, Kolata G. Breast Cancer Screening Policy Won't Change, U.S. Officials Say. New York: The New York Times, Nov 19, 2009.

Smith RA. The evolving role of MRI in the detection and evaluation of breast cancer. N Engl J Med 356:1362-1634, 2007.

Genetics, Risk, and Prevention

Altman LK. High Level of Insulin Linked to Breast Cancer's Advance. New York: The New York Times, May 24, 2000.

Altman LK. New Study Links Hormones to Breast Cancer Risk. New York: The New York Times, Aug 8, 2003.

The Associated Press. Study Tracks a Little-Explored Genetic Path of Breast Cancer. New York: The New York Times, June 20, 2007.

Bakalar N. Breast Cancer Not Linked to Abortion, Study Says. New York: The New York Times, Apr 24, 2007.

Bakalar N. Gene Study Helps Explain Link to Breast Cancer. New York: The New York Times, Dec 11, 2007.

Bakalar N. Isolating the Factors Involved in Breast Cancer. New York: The New York Times, Aug 21, 2007.

Bakalar N. Vitamin D and Calcium Intake Found to Affect Breast Cancer. New York: The New York Times, June 5, 2007.

Brody JE. Red Flags for Hereditary Cancers. New York: The New York Times, May 27, 2008.

Collaborative Group on Hormonal Factors in Breast Cancer. Alcohol, tobacco and breast cancer—collaborative reanalysis of individual data from 53 epidemiological studies, including 58,515 women with breast cancer and 95,067 without the disease. Br J Cancer 87:1234-1245, 2002.

Devilee P, Rookus MA. A tiny step closer to personalized risk prediction for breast cancer. N Engl J Med 362:1043-1045, 2010.

Domchek SM, Friebel TM, Singer CF, et al. Association of risk-reducing surgery in BRCA1 or BRCA2 mutation carriers with cancer risk and mortality. JAMA 304:967-975, 2010.

Drug Cuts Recurrence Risk in Breast Cancer Patients. New York: The New York Times, Mar 11, 2008.

FitzGerald MG, MacDonald DJ, Krainer M, et al. Germ-line BRCA1 mutations in Jewish and non-Jewish women with early-onset breast cancer. N Engl J Med 334:143-149, 1996.

Grady D. Breast Cancer Drug Is Approved for Early Cases. New York: The New York Times, Nov 17, 2006.

Grady D. Breast Cancer Study Points to Differences in Recurrence. New York: The New York Times, Jan 15, 2000.

Grady D. Drug Found to Help Lower Breast Cancer Risk. New York: The New York Times, Apr 18, 2006.

Grady D. Racial Component Is Found in a Lethal Breast Cancer. New York: The New York Times, June 7, 2006.

Grady D. Sorting Out Pills to Reduce Breast Cancer Risk. New York: The New York Times, May 9, 2006.

Grady D. Tests for Breast Cancer Gene Raise Hard Choices. New York: The New York Times, Mar 5, 2002.

Grady D. Women With Genetic Mutation at High Risk for Breast Cancer, Study Confirms. New York: The New York Times, Oct 24, 2003.

Harmon A. Fear of Insurance Trouble Leads Many to Shun or Hide DNA Tests. New York: The New York Times, Feb 24, 2008.

Jetter A. Breast Cancer in Blacks Spurs Hunt for Answers. New York: The New York Times, Feb 22, 2000.

Key J, Hodgson S, Omar RZ, et al. Meta-analysis of alcohol and breast cancer with consideration of the methodological issues. Cancer Causes Control 17:759-770, 2006.

Kolata G. Bone Drugs May Help Fight Breast Cancer, Study Shows. New York: The New York Times, Feb 12, 2009.

Kolata G. Hormones and Cancer: Assessing the Risks. New York: The New York Times, Dec 26, 2006.

Kolata G. In War on Cancer, Old Ideas Can Lead to Fresh Directions. New York: The New York Times, Dec 29, 2009.

Kolata G. New Drug Regimen Greatly Cuts Risk of Recurring Breast Cancer. New York: The New York Times, Oct 10, 2003.

Kolata G, Marshall C. Breast Cancer News Brings a Range of Reactions. New York: The New York Times, Dec 18, 2006.

Li C, Chlebowski RT, Freiberg M, et al. Alcohol consumption and risk of postmenopausal breast cancer by subtype: the Women's Health Initiative Observational Study. J Natl Canc Inst. Early online publication Aug 23, 2010.

Nagourney E. Breast Cancer History Is a Two-Sided Family Tree. New York: The New York Times, July 25, 2006.

National Briefing—Science: Drug Effective Against Breast Cancer. New York: The New York Times, Oct 20, 2005.

National Briefing—Science and Health: Breast Density a Cancer Risk. New York: The New York Times, Jan 18, 2007.

National Briefing—Science and Health: Gene Sheds Light on Breast Cancer. New York: The New York Times, Apr 23, 2003.

O'Neil J. Prognosis: A Breast Cancer Reassurance. New York: The New York Times, Aug 12, 2003.

Park A. Halting Hormone Therapy Reduces Breast Cancer Risk Quickly. New York: Time, Feb 4, 2009.

Pollack A. New Drug Holds Promise for Type of Breast Cancer. New York: The New York Times, June 4, 2006.

Pollack A. Promising Results in Stomach and Breast Cancer Drugs. New York: The New York Times, June 1, 2009.

Pollack A. Quality of Life Found Equal With 2 Breast Cancer Drugs. New York: The New York Times, June 6, 2006.

Pollack A. Study Suggests Switching Drugs Could Aid Breast Cancer Patients. New York: The New York Times, Dec 4, 2003.

Pollack A. Test to Predict Breast Cancer Relapse Risk Is Approved. New York: The New York Times, Feb 7, 2007.

Rabin RC. Reducing Your Risk for Breast Cancer. New York: The New York Times, May 13, 2008.

Rabin RC. Smoking May Have Role in Breast Cancer After All, a Science Panel Says. New York: The New York Times, Apr 24, 2009.

Rennert G, Bisland-Naggan S, Barnett-Griness O, et al. Clinical outcome of breast cancer in carriers of BRCA1 and BRCA2 mutations. N Engl J Med 357:175-176, 2007.

Robson M, Offit K. Management of an inherited predisposition to breast cancer. N Engl J Med 357:154-162, 2007.

Rubin Erdely S. When to do BRCA testing. New York: Self Magazine, Mar, 2007.

Saxena T, Lee E, Henderson K, et al. Menopausal hormone therapy and subsequent risk of specific invasive breast cancer subtypes in the California Teachers Study. Cancer Epidemiol Biomarkers Prev. Early online publication Aug 10, 2010.

Schwartz MD, Lerman C, Brogan B, et al. Impact of BRCA1/BRCA2 counseling and testing on newly diagnosed breast cancer patients. J Clin Oncol 22:1823-1829, 2004.

Trichopoulou A, Bamia C, Lagiou P, et al. Conformity to traditional Mediterranean diet and breast cancer risk in the Greek EPIC (European Investigation into Cancer and nutrition) cohort. Am J Clin Nutr 92:620-625, 2010.

Triple-negative breast cancer rate is triply high in black women. Harv Womens Health Watch 16:7, 2009.

Wade N. Genome Researchers Find New Indicators of Breast Cancer Risk. New York: The New York Times, May 29, 2007.

Preventive (Prophylactic) Mastectomy for the Woman at Risk

Goin MK, Goin JM. Psychological reactions to prophylactic mastectomy synchronous with contralateral breast reconstruction. Plast Reconstr Surg 70:355-359, 1982.

Hoogerbrugge N, Bult P, de Widt-Levert LM, et al. High prevalence of premalignant lesions in prophylactically removed breasts from women at hereditary risk for breast cancer. J Clin Oncol 21:41-45, 2003.

Lerner M. Some Women Removing Healthy Breasts to Prevent Recurrence of Cancer. Minneapolis: Star Tribune, 2009.

Metcalfe KA, Semple JL, Narod SA. Satisfaction with breast reconstruction in women with bilateral prophylactic mastectomy: a descriptive study. Plast Reconstr Surg 114:360-366, 2004.

Parker-Pope T. After Cancer, Women Remove Healthy Breast. New York: The New York Times, Mar 9, 2010.

Rabin RC. More Women With Breast Cancer Choosing Double Mastectomies, Study Finds. New York: The New York Times, Oct 13, 2009.

Rebbeck TR, Lynch HT, Neuhausen SL, et al. Prophylactic oophorectomy in carriers of BRCA1 or BRCA2 mutations. N Engl J Med 346:1616-1622, 2002.

Tercyak KP, Peshkin BN, Brogan BM, et al. Quality of life after contralateral prophylactic mastectomy in newly diagnosed high-risk breast cancer patients who underwent BRCA1/2 gene testing. J Clin Oncol 25:285-291, 2007.

Lymphedema

Carter BJ. Women's experiences of lymphedema. Oncol Nurs Forum 24:875-882, 1997.

Swirsky J, Nannery DS. Coping With Lymphedema. New York: Avery Publishing Group, 1998.

Personal Accounts of Breast Cancer and Breast Reconstruction

Akande D. Personal breast cancer journal: a record for life and health. CreateSpace, 2009.

Alboher M. Experience-Based Ventures Help Fight the Frustrations of Fighting Breast Cancer. New York: The New York Times, Oct 25, 2007.

Baruchin A. In Breast Cancer, There Is a Single Agenda: Stay Alive. New York: The New York Times, Oct 31, 2006.

Brinker NG. Winning the Race: Taking Charge of Breast Cancer: My Personal Story and Every Woman's Guide to Wellness. Wyomissing, PA: Tapestry Press, 2001.

Brinker NG, Rodgers J. Promise Me: How a Sister's Love Launched the Global Movement to End Breast Cancer. New York: Random House, 2010.

Delinsky B. Uplift: Secrets From the Sisterhood of Breast Cancer Survivors. New York: Washington Square Press, 2003.

Dunnavant S. Celebrating Life: African American Women Speak Out About Breast Cancer. Dallas: USFI, 1995.

Ellerbee L, Veselka V. Hello dear; I have cancer. Good Housekeeping 225:74, Oct 1997.

Ford B. The Times of My Life. New York: Harper & Row, 1978.

The Healing Project. Voices of Breast Cancer: The Healing Companion: Stories for Courage, Comfort and Strength. New York: LaChance Publishing, 2007.

Hodara S. A Breast Cancer Survivor's Story, Told in E-Mail Messages. New York: The New York Times, Jan 14, 2001.

Kushner R. My side. Working Woman 8:160, May, 1983.

Orenstein P. Twenty-five and mortal: a breast cancer diary. The New York Times Magazine, June 29, 1997.

Peltason R. I Am Not My Breast Cancer: Women Talk Openly about Love and Sex, Hair Loss and Weight Gain, Mothers and Daughters, and Being a Woman With Breast Cancer. New York: HarperCollins, 2008.

Rollin B. First You Cry. Philadelphia: JB Lippincott, 1976.

Shockney L. Stealing Second Base: A Breast Cancer Survivor's Experience and Breast Cancer Expert's Story. Boston: Jones & Bartlett Publishers, 2007.

Silver JK. What Helped Get Me Through: Cancer Survivors Share Wisdom and Hope. Atlanta, GA: American Cancer Society, 2008.

Verna B. Single With Breast Cancer: My Journey. Bloomington, IN: Author-House, 2008.

Zalon J. I Am Whole Again: The Case for Breast Reconstruction After Mastectomy. New York: Random House, 1978.

Treatment Options (*see also* Breast Cancer Information)
General

Breast Cancer and Choices. New York: The New York Times, Jan 1, 2008.

Doheny K. Breast Cancer Vaccines Look Promising. New York: Living.Health.com, June 26, 2008.

Grady D. Therapies Cut Death Risk, Breast-Cancer Study Finds. New York: The New York Times, May 13, 2005.

Khatcheressian JL, Wolff AC, Smith TJ, et al. American Society of Clinical Oncology 2006 update of the breast cancer follow-up and management guidelines in the adjuvant setting. J Clin Oncol 24:5091-5097, 2006.

Kolata G. Bone Drugs May Help Fight Breast Cancer. New York: The New York Times, Feb 12, 2009.

Kolata G. Shift in Treating Breast Cancer Is Under Debate. New York: The New York Times, May 12, 2006.

Miller KD. Choices in Breast Cancer Treatment: Medical Specialists and Cancer Survivors Tell You What You Need to Know. Baltimore: The Johns Hopkins University Press, 2008.

Surgery: Lumpectomy, Mastectomy, and Axillary Lymph Node Dissection

Bakalar N. Talking Out the Choices for Breast Cancer Surgery. New York: The New York Times, Dec 26, 2007.

Carlson GW, Bostwick J III, Styblo TM, et al. Skin-sparing mastectomy: oncologic and reconstructive considerations. Ann Surg 225:570-575, 1997.

Fisher B. Five-year results of a randomized clinical trial comparing total mastectomy and segmental mastectomy with or without radiation in the treatment of breast cancer. N Engl J Med 312:665-673, 1985.

Krag DN, Anderson SJ, Julian TB, et al. Primary outcome results of NSABP B-32, a randomized phase III clinical trial to compare sentinel node resection (SNR) to conventional axillary dissection (AD) in clinically node-negative breast cancer patients. Presented at the 2010 Annual Meeting of the American Society of Clinical Oncology (ASCO), Chicago, June, 2010.

Land SR, Kopec JA, Julian TB, et al. Patient-reported outcomes in sentinel-negative adjuvant breast cancer patients receiving sentinel-node biopsy or axillary dissection: National Surgical Adjuvant Breast and Bowel Project Phase III Protocol B-32. J Clin Oncol. Early online publication Aug 2, 2010.

More or less? Lumpectomy and radiotherapy found as effective as mastectomy on breast cancer. Sci Am 253:59, 1985.

Nagourney E. Choosing Breast Cancer Surgery. New York: The New York Times, June 15, 2004.

Punglia RS, Morrow M, Winer EP, et al. Current concepts: local therapy and survival in breast cancer. N Engl J Med 356:2399-2405, 2007.

Veronesi U, Paganelli G, Galinberti V, et al. Sentinel-node biopsy to avoid axillary dissection in breast cancer with clinically negative lymph-nodes. Lancet 349:1864-1867, 1997.

Chemotherapy and Hormonal Therapy

McKay J, Schacher T. The Chemotherapy Survival Guide: Everything You Need to Get Through Treatment, 3rd ed. Oakland, CA: New Harbinger Publications, 2009.

Muss HB, Berry DA, Cirrincione CT, et al. Adjuvant chemotherapy in older women with early-stage breast cancer. N Engl J Med 360:2055-2065, 2009.

O'Shaughnessy JA. Chemoprevention of breast cancer. JAMA 275:1349-1353, 1996.

Piccart-Gebhart MJ, Procter M, Leyland-Jones B, et al. Trastuzumab after adjuvant chemotherapy in HER2-positive breast cancer. N Engl J Med 353:1659-1672, 2005.

Pollack A. Breast-Cancer Study Finds Benefit in Chemotherapy Every Two Weeks Instead of Three. New York: The New York Times, Dec 13, 2002.

Wilkes GM, Ades TB, Krakoff I. Consumer's Guide to Cancer Drugs. Jones & Bartlett Publishers, 2003.

Yen TW, Kuerer HM, Ottesen RA, et al. Impact of randomized clinical trial results in the National Comprehensive Cancer Network on the use of tamoxifen after breast surgery for ductal carcinoma in situ. J Clin Oncol 25:3251-3258, 2007.

Radiation Therapy

Bartelink H, Horiot JC, Poortmans PM, et al. Impact of a higher radiation dose on local control and survival in breast-conserving therapy of early breast cancer: 10-year results of the randomized boost versus no boost EORTC 2281-10882 trial. J Clin Oncol 25:3259-3265, 2007.

Briefer Regimen May Fight Breast Cancer. New York: The New York Times, Nov 27, 2001.

Buchholz TA. Radiation therapy for early-stage breast cancer after breast-conserving surgery. N Engl J Med 360:63-70, 2009.

Grady D. Shorter Radiation for Cancer of the Breast. New York: The New York Times, Sept 23, 2008.

Breast Reconstruction (*see also* Breast Cancer Information; Treatment Options)

Boehmler JH IV, Butler CE, Ensor J, et al. Outcomes of various techniques of abdominal TRAM flap breast reconstruction. Plast Reconstr Surg 123:773-781, 2009.

Cordeiro PG. Breast reconstruction after surgery for breast cancer. N Engl J Med 359:1590-1601, 2008.

Djohan R, Gage E, Bernard S. Breast reconstruction options following mastectomy. Cleve Clin J Med 75(Suppl 1):S17-S23, 2008.

Elliott LF, Seify H, Bergey P. The 3-hour muscle-sparing free TRAM flap: safe and effective treatment review of 111 consecutive free TRAM flaps in a private practice setting. Plast Reconstr Surg 120:27-34, 2007.

Eskenazi LB. New options for immediate reconstruction: achieving optimal results with adjustable implants in a single stage. Plast Reconstr Surg 119:28-37, 2007.

Goin MK. Discussion of Stevens LA, McGrath MH, Druss RG, et al. The psychological impact of immediate breast reconstruction for women with early breast cancer. Plast Reconstr Surg 73:619-626; discussion 627-628, 1984.

Granzow JW, Levine JL, Chiu ES, et al. Breast reconstruction with perforator flaps. Plast Reconstr Surg 120:1-12, 2007.

Hamdi M, Blondeel P, Van Landuyt K, et al. Bilateral autogenous breast reconstruction using perforator free flaps: a single center's experience. Plast Reconstr Surg 114:83-89, 2004.

Jones GE. Bostwick's Plastic & Reconstructive Breast Surgery, 3rd ed. St Louis: Quality Medical Publishing, 2010.

Levinson J. Breast reconstruction: a patient's view. Plast Reconstr Surg 73:703, 1984.

Schain WS, Edwards BK, Gorrell CR, et al. The sooner the better: a study of psychological factors of women undergoing immediate versus delayed breast reconstruction. Am J Psychiatry 142:40-46, 1985.

Stevens LA, McGrath MH, Druss RG, et al. The psychological impact of immediate breast reconstruction for women with early breast cancer. Plast Reconstr Surg 73:619-628, 1984.

To be whole again: mastectomy treated Peggy McCann's cancer, but breast reconstruction made her well. Life 10:78, May 1987.

Zalon J. I Am Whole Again: The Case for Breast Reconstruction After Mastectomy. New York: Random House, 1978.

Breast Implants

American College of Rheumatology Statement on Silicone Breast Implants. Oct 1995.

American Society of Clinical Oncology. American Society of Clinical Oncology and Cancer Patients Seek to Ease FDA Restrictions on Silicone Breast Implants [press release]. Sept 19, 1996.

Angell M. Science on Trial: The Clash of Medical Evidence and the Law in the Breast Implant Case. New York: WW Norton & Co, 1996.

Angell M. Shattuck lecture: evaluating the health risks of breast implants—the interplay of medical science, the law, and public opinion. N Engl J Med 334:1513-1518, 1996.

Birdsell DC, Jenkins H, Berket H. Breast cancer diagnosis and survival in women with and without breast implants. Plast Reconstr Surg 92:795-800, 1993.

Brody GS, Conway DP, Deapen DM, et al. Consensus statement on the relationship of breast implants to connective-tissue disorders. Plast Reconstr Surg 90:1102-1105, 1992.

Brown MH, Shenker R, Silver SA. Cohesive silicone gel breast implants in aesthetic and reconstructive breast surgery. Plast Reconstr Surg 116:768-779, 2005.

Burton TMA. Harvard Study Finds No Major Link Between Implants and Immune Illnesses. New York: The Wall Street Journal, June 22, 1995.

Council on Scientific Affairs, American Medical Association. Silicone gel breast implants. JAMA 270:2602-2606, 1993.

Elkund GW, Busby RC, Miller SH, et al. Improved imaging of the augmented breast. Am J Roentgenol 151:469-473, 1988.

Fee-Fulkerson K, Conway MR, Winer EP, et al. Factors contributing to patient satisfaction with breast reconstruction using silicone gel implants. Plast Reconstr Surg 97:1420-1426, 1996.

Fisher JC. The silicone controversy—when will science prevail? N Engl J Med 326:1696-1698, 1992.

Fisher JC, Brody GD. Breast implants under siege: an historical commentary. J Long Term Eff Med Implants 1:243-253, 1992.

Gabriel SE, O'Fallon WM, Kurland LT, et al. Risk of connective-tissue diseases and other disorders after breast implantation. N Engl J Med 330:1697-1702, 1994.

Green S. A Woman's Right to Choose Breast Implants. New York: The Wall Street Journal, Jan 20, 1993.

Karns ME, Cullison CA, Romano TJ, et al. Breast implants and connective-tissue disease. JAMA 276:101-102, 1996.

Psychological and Sexual Considerations After Breast Cancer

Brody JE. Travel Companion on the Breast Cancer Journey. New York: The New York Times, Nov 9, 2004.

Dackman L. Up Front: Sex and the Post-Mastectomy Woman. New York: Viking Press, 1990.

Greenberg M. Invisible Scars: A Guide to Coping With the Emotional Impact of Breast Cancer. New York: Walker & Co, 1988.

Kahane DH. No Less a Woman: Femininity, Sexuality & Breast Cancer, 2nd ed. Alameda, CA: Hunter House, 1995.

Lee K. Facing breast cancer before 50. Essence 28:36, Oct 1997.

Peltason R. I Am Not My Breast Cancer: Women Talk Openly About Love and Sex, Hair Loss and Weight Gain, Mothers and Daughters, and Being a Woman With Breast Cancer. New York: HarperCollins, 2008.

Family and Friends and Breast Cancer

Braddock S, Edney JJ. Straight Talk About Breast Cancer From Diagnosis to Recovery: A Guide for the Entire Family, 3rd ed. San Diego: Addicus Press, 2006.

Fincannon JL, Bruss KV. Couples Confronting Cancer: Keeping Your Relationship Strong. Atlanta: American Cancer Society, 2003.

Harpham WS. When a Parent Has Cancer: A Guide to Caring for Your Children. New York: HarperCollins, 1997.

Loscalzo MJ, Heyison M. For the Women We Love: A Breast Cancer Action Plan and Caregiver's Guide for Men. Savage, MD: Bartleby Press, 2007.

Silver M. Breast Cancer Husband: How to Help Your Wife (and Yourself) Through Diagnosis, Treatment and Beyond. New York: Rodale Press, 2004.

Virag I, Berger E. We're All in This Together: Families Facing Breast Cancer. Kansas City: Andrews McMeel, 1995.

Recovery, Rehabilitation, and Survival

Bonner D. The 10 Best Questions for Surviving Breast Cancer: The Script You Need to Take Control of Your Health. New York: Random House, 2008.

Domar AD, Dreher H. Healing Mind, Healthy Woman: Using the Mind-Body Connection to Manage Stress and Take Control of Your Life. New York: Holt Rinehart & Winston, 1996.

Grady D. Another Way to Fight Breast Cancer Relapse. New York: The New York Times, Nov 16, 2004.

Gray R, Fitch M, Davis C, et al. A qualitative study of breast cancer self-help groups. Psychooncology 6:279-289, 1997.

Mickley J, Soeken K. Religiousness and hope in Hispanic and Anglo-American women with breast cancer. Oncol Nurs Forum 20:1171-1177, 1993.

Rosenfeld R. Dr. Rosenfeld's Guide to Alternative Medicine: What Works, What Doesn't—And What's Right for You. New York: Random House, 1996.

Schnipper HH. After Breast Cancer: A Common-Sense Guide to Life After Treatment. New York: Bantam Books, 2006.

Weiss MC, Weiss E. Living Well Beyond Breast Cancer: A Survivor's Guide for When Treatment Ends and the Rest of Your Life Begins, 2nd ed. New York: Three Rivers Press, 2010.

Nutrition and Exercise

Daniels E, Tuthill K. You Can Do This! Surviving Breast Cancer Without Losing Your Sanity or Your Style. Kansas City: Andrews McMeel, 2009.

Demark-Wahnefried W. A Weighty Matter—Lifting After Breast Cancer. N Engl J Med 361:710-711, 2009.

Diet as a Treatment for Breast Cancer. New York: The New York Times, May 18, 2005.

Exercise and Breast Cancer Risk. New York: The New York Times, May 14, 2008.

Irwin ML, Aiello EJ, McTiernan A, et al. Physical activity, body mass index, and mammographic density in postmenopausal breast cancer survivors. J Clin Oncol 25:1061-1066, 2007.

Kaelin C, Coltrera F, Gardiner J, et al. The Breast Cancer Survivor's Fitness Plan: Reclaim Health, Regain Strength, Live Longer. New York: McGraw Hill, 2007.

Kolata G, Altman LK. Study of Breast Cancer Patients Finds Benefit in Low-Fat Diets. New York: The New York Times, May 17, 2005.

Kollak I, Utz-Billings I. Yoga and Breast Cancer: A Journey to Health and Healing. New York: Demos Medical Publishing, 2010.

Obesity Linked to Breast Cancer Risk. New York: The New York Times, Aug 20, 2003.

Olivier S. Breast Cancer Prevention and Recovery Diet: Practical, Accurate Advice From a Breast Cancer Survivor. Pleasant Grove, UT: Woodland Publishing, 2002.

Pierce JP, Natarajan J, Caan BJ, et al. Influence of diet very high in vegetables, fruit, and fiber and low in fat on prognosis following treatment for breast cancer: the Women's Healthy Eating and Living (WHEL) randomized trial. JAMA 298:289-298, 2007.

Pierce JP, Stefanick ML, Flatt SW, et al. Greater survival after breast cancer in physically active women with high vegetable-fruit intake regardless of obesity. J Clin Oncol 25:2335-2337, 2007.

Clinical Trials

(*See Appendix A for NCI and ACS information.*)

Finn R. Cancer Clinical Trials: Experimental Treatments and How They Can Help You. Sebastopol, CA: O'Reilly & Associates, 1999.

References for Locating Articles in the Popular Literature

Articles appearing in the popular literature can also be found through the *Readers' Guide Full Text Mega Edition* (formerly *Readers' Guide to Periodical Literature*) and the Public Affairs Information Service (PAIS) International database, available in most public libraries.

References for Locating Articles in Health Science Journals

For articles appearing in the scientific literature, check the Index Medicus, which is found in medical libraries, most university and college libraries, and some public libraries. This book lists articles appearing in over 2500 science journals. The National Library of Medicine has a series of medical databases called MEDLARS, which are also helpful. These include the following:

MEDLINE. A database with over 4 million citations and abstracts taken from approximately 3200 medical journals published in the United States and throughout the world.
www.nlm.nih.gov/medlineplus

Physician Data Query (PDQ). A database providing current cancer information. PDQ is discussed in Appendix A.
www.cancer.gov/cancertopics/pdq

CANCERLIT. A database containing approximately 550,000 citations and abstracts of articles published since 1978 on all aspects of cancer.
www.cancer.gov/search/cancer_literature

INDEX